FROM THE EXPERTS IN ENDOCRINOLOGY

ENDO 2022
MEET THE PROFESSOR

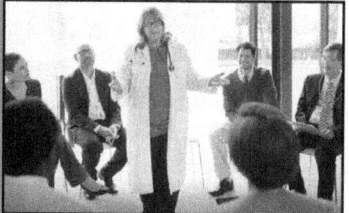

REFERENCE EDITION

ENDOCRINE
CASE MANAGEMENT

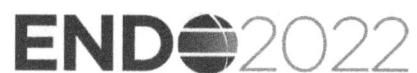

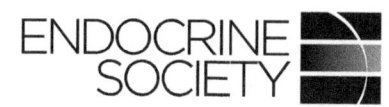

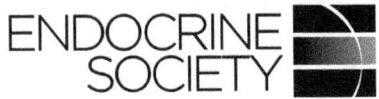

2055 L Street, NW, Suite 600
Washington, DC 20036
www.endocrine.org

Other Publications:
endocrine.org/publications

The Endocrine Society is the world's largest, oldest, and most active organization working to advance the clinical practice of endocrinology and hormone research. Founded in 1916, the Society now has more than 18,000 global members across a range of disciplines.

The Society has earned an international reputation for excellence in the quality of its peer-reviewed journals, educational resources, meetings, and programs that improve public health through the practice and science of endocrinology.

Clinical Practice Chair, ENDO 2022
Bulent O. Yildiz, MD, PhD

ISBN: 978-1-943550-13-5
eISBN: 978-1-943550-15-9
Library of Congress Control Number: 2022942203

On the Cover: © Shutterstock. Doctor Meeting Teamwork Diagnosis Healthcare Concept. (By Rawpixel.com).

ENDO 2022
CONTENTS

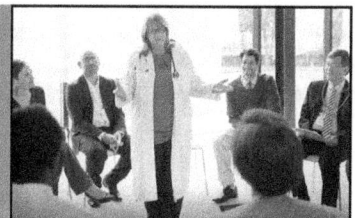

ADIPOSE TISSUE, APPETITE, AND OBESITY

ADRENAL

BONE AND MINERAL METABOLISM

CARDIOVASCULAR ENDOCRINOLOGY

DIABETES MELLITUS AND GLUCOSE METABOLISM

NEUROENDOCRINOLOGY AND PITUITARY

PEDIATRIC ENDOCRINOLOGY

REPRODUCTIVE ENDOCRINOLOGY

THYROID

MISCELLANEOUS

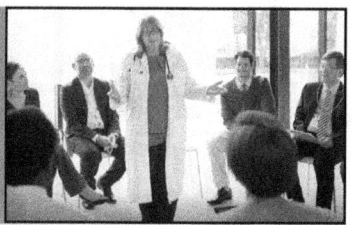

2022 Endocrine Case Management: Meet the Professor Faculty

Bradley Anawalt, MD
University of Washington

Wiebke Arlt, MD, DSc, FRCP, FMedSci
University of Birmingham

Ambika Ashraf, MD
Children's Hospital/University of Alabama at Birmingham

Annika M. A. Berends, MD
University Medical Center Groningen

Nienke Biermasz, MD
Leiden University Medical Center

Maria Brandi, MD, PhD
FIRMO Foundation

Sue Brown, MD
University of Virginia

Jonathan Campbell, PhD
Duke University

Uriel Clemente-Gutierrez, MD
University of Texas
MD Anderson Cancer Center

Marc-Andre Cornier, MD
Medical University of South Carolina

Ricardo Correa, MD, EdD
University of Arizona College of Medicine Phoenix

Melanie Cree-Green, MD, PhD
University of Colorado and Children's Hospital Colorado

David D'Alessio, MD
Duke University School of Medicine

Caroline Davidge-Pitts, MD, MBBCH
Mayo Clinic

Diva Del Carmen De Leon-Crutchlow, MD, MSCE
Children's Hospital of Philadelphia

Ilene Fennoy, MD, MPH
Columbia University

Maria Fleseriu, MD
Oregon Health & Science University

Rachel Gafni, MD
NIH

Benjamin Gigliotti, MD
University of Rochester
School of Medicine & Dentistry

Mark Gurnell, MD, PhD
University of Cambridge, Wellcome Trust-MRC Institute of Metabolic Science & School of Clinical Medicine

Bryan Haugen, MD
University of Colorado
Denver Medical Campus

Kathleen Hoeger, MD, MPH
University of Rochester

Bernice L. Huang, MD
University of Texas
MD Anderson Cancer Center

Sean Iwamoto, MD
University of Colorado
School of Medicine & Rocky Mountain Regional VA Medical Center

Channa Jayasena, MD
Imperial College London

Michiel Kerstens, MD, PhD
University Medical Center Groningen

Julia Kharlip, MD
University of Pennsylvania

Bente Langdahl, MD, PhD, DMSc
Aarhus University Hospital

Lawrence Clarke Layman, BS, MD
Medical College of Georgia at Augusta University

Mike Lewiecki, MD
New Mexico Clinical Research & Osteoporosis Center

Sarah Mayson, MD
University of Colorado
School of Medicine

Elizabeth McAninch, MD
Stanford University
School of Medicine

Manpreet Mundi, MD
Mayo Clinic

Connie Baum Newman, MD, MACP
New York University
School of Medicine

Rocio Pereira, MD
Denver Health Medical Center

Nancy Perrier, MD
University of Texas
MD Anderson Cancer Center

Alessandro Prete, MD
University of Birmingham

Martin Reincke, MD
Medizinische Klinik und Poliklinik IV

Jane Reusch, MD
Rocky Mountain Regional
VA Medical Center

Micol Rothman, MD
University of Colorado
School of Medicine

David Saxon, MD
University of Colorado &
Rocky Mountain Regional
VA Medical Center

Ismat Shafiq, MD
University of Rochester

Ashley Shoemaker, MD
Vanderbilt University Medical Center

Jennifer Sipos, MD
Ohio State University

Savitha Subramanian, MD
University of Washington

Adina Turcu, MD, MS
University of Michigan

Varsha Vimalananda, MD, MPH
Center for Healthcare Organization
and Implementation Research

Danica M. Vodopivec, MD
University of Texas
MD Anderson Cancer Center

Maria Vogiatzi, MD
Children's Hospital of Philadelphia

Philip Zeitler, MD, PhD
Children's Hospital Colorado/
University of Colorado

Annual Meeting Steering Committee (AMSC)

**Stephen Hammes, PhD,
MD – AMSC Chair**
University of Rochester

**Bulent O. Yildiz, MD, PhD –
Clinical Practice Chair**
Hacettepe University
School of Medicine

**Lauren Fishbein, MD, PhD
– Clinical Science Chair**
University of Colorado
School of Medicine

Annual Meeting Steering Committee Clinical Peer Reviewers

Andrew Bauer, MD

Ernesto Bernal-Mizrachi, MD

Antonio Bianco, MD, PhD

Kristien Boelaert, MD, PhD

Massimiliano Caprio, MD, PhD

Bart Clarke, MD

Dawn Davis, MD, PhD

Daniel Dumesic, MD

Stephanie Fish, MD

Lauren Fishbein, MD, PhD

Matthew Freeby, MD

Adda Grimberg, MD

Niki Karavitaki, FRCP, PhD

Marta Korbonits, MD, PhD

Maria Veronica Mericq, MD

Gabrielle Page-Wilson, MD

Robin Peeters, MD, PhD

Margareta Pisarska, MD

Philipp Scherer, PhD

Jennifer Sherr, MD, PhD

Robert Wermers, MD

Selma Witchel, MD

Bulent O. Yildiz, MD

Maria-Christina Zennaro, MD, PhD

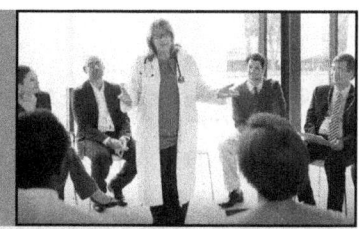

OVERVIEW

The *Endocrine Case Management: Meet the Professor* reference book is intended primarily for consultation relating to endocrinology. As a reference book, educational credits are not available. For information on educational products that include educational credit, please visit endocrine.org/store.

LEARNING OBJECTIVES

Endocrine Case Management: Meet the Professor will allow learners to assess their knowledge of all aspects of endocrinology, diabetes, and metabolism.

Completion of this educational activity enables learners to accomplish key objectives:

- Recognize clinical manifestations of endocrine and metabolic disorders and select among current options for diagnosis, management, and therapy.

- Identify risk factors for endocrine and metabolic disorders and develop strategies for prevention.

- Evaluate endocrine and metabolic manifestations of systemic disorders.

- Use existing resources pertaining to clinical guidelines and treatment recommendations for endocrine and related metabolic disorders to guide diagnosis and treatment.

TARGET AUDIENCE

Endocrine Case Management: Meet the Professor provides case-based education to clinicians interested in improving patient care.

STATEMENT OF INDEPENDENCE

The Endocrine Society has a policy of ensuring that the content and quality of this educational activity are balanced, independent, objective, and scientifically rigorous. The scientific content of this activity was developed under the supervision of the Endocrine Society's Annual Meeting Steering Committee.

DISCLOSURE POLICY

The faculty, committee members, and staff who are in position to control the content of this activity are required to disclose to the Endocrine Society and to learners any relevant financial relationship(s) of the individual or spouse/partner that have occurred within the last 12 months with any commercial interest(s) whose products or services are related to the content. Financial relationships are defined by remuneration in any amount from the commercial interest(s) in the form of grants; research support; consulting fees; salary; ownership interest (e.g., stocks, stock options, or ownership interest excluding diversified mutual funds); honoraria or other payments for participation in speakers' bureaus, advisory boards, or boards of directors; or other financial benefits. The intent of this disclosure is not to prevent planners with relevant financial relationships from planning or delivery of content, but rather to provide learners with information that allows them to make their own judgments of whether these financial relationships may have influenced the educational activity with regard to exposition or conclusion. The Endocrine Society has reviewed all disclosures and resolved or managed all identified conflicts of interest, as applicable.

The Endocrine Society has reviewed these relationships to determine which are relevant to the content of this activity and resolved any identified conflicts of interest for these individuals.

The faculty reported the following relevant financial relationship(s) during the content development process for this activity: **Sue Brown, MD,** Grant Recipient: Dexcom, Tandem Diabetes Care, Insulet Corporation. **Jonathan Campbell, PhD,** Advisory Board Member: ShouTi; Grant Recipient: Eli Lilly & Company, Novo Nordisk, Proteostasis; Speaker: Eli Lilly & Company. **Marc-Andre Cornier, MD,** Advisory Board Member: Regeneron Pharmaceuticals; Grant Recipient: Novartis Pharmaceuticals. **David D'Alessio, MD,** Advisory Board Member: Eli Lilly & Company; Grant Recipient: Merck & Co., Applied Therapeutics, Inc., Boehringer Ingelheim, Eli Lilly & Company, Genentech, Inc., Hanmi, Janssen Research & Development Company,

Metacrine, Novartis Pharmaceuticals, Novo Nordisk, Oramed, Pfizer, Inc., REMD Biotherapeutics Inc., Sanofi, VTV Therapeutics. Research Investigator. **Diva Del Carmen De Leon-Crutchlow, MD, MSCE**, Consulting Fee: Ultragenyx, Zealand Pharma, Hanmi Pharmaceuticals, Heptares Therapeutics, Eiger Pharma, Crinetics Pharmaceuticals; Grant Recipient: Twist Pharma, Crinetics Pharmaceuticals; Stock Owner: Merck & Co. **Maria Fleseriu, MD**, Consulting Fee: Ionis Pharmaceuticals Inc., Ipsen, Pfizer Global R&D, Crinetics, Amryt, Recordati; Grant Recipient: Ionis Pharmaceuticals Inc., Crinetics, Recordati. **Channa Jayasena, MD**, Grant Recipient: Logixx Pharma Ltd. **Bente Langdahl, MD, PhD, DMSc**, Advisory Board Member: Amgen, UCB, Gedeon-Richter; Grant Recipient: Novo Nordisk, Amgen; Speaker: Amgen, UCB, Gedeon-Richter, Astra-Zenica, Astellas. **Mike Lewiecki, MD**, Consulting Fee: Amgen Inc; Speaker: Amgen Inc. **Elizabeth McAninch, MD**, Owner/Co-Owner: Equilibrate Therapeutics. **Ashley Shoemaker, MD**, Advisory Board Member: Radius Health Inc, Saniona, Rhythm Pharmaceuticals. **Savitha Subramanian, MD**, Advisory Board Member: Abbott Laboratories, Akcea Therapeutics, Amarin. **Adina Turcu, MD, MS**, Advisory Board Member: Novartis; Consulting Fee: CinCor, PhaseBio. **Philip Zeitler, MD, PhD**, Consulting Fee: Boehringer Ingelheim, Daiichi Sankyo, Eli Lilly & Company, Janssen Research & Development Company, Merck.

The following faculty reported no relevant financial relationships: **Bradley Anawalt, MD; Wiebke Arlt, MD, DSc, FRCP, FMedSci; Ambika Ashraf, MD; Annika M. A. Berends, MD; Nienke Biermasz, MD; Maria Brandi, MD, PhD; Uriel Clemente-Gutierrez, MD; Ricardo Correa, MD, EdD; Melanie Cree-Green, MD, PhD; Caroline Davidge-Pitts, MD, MBBCH; Ilene Fennoy, MD, MPH; Rachel Gafni, MD; Benjamin Gigliotti, MD; Mark Gurnell, MD, PhD; Bryan Haugen, MD; Kathleen Hoeger, MD, MPH; Bernice L. Huang, MD; Sean Iwamoto, MD; Michiel Kerstens, MD, PhD; Julia Kharlip, MD; Lawrence Clarke Layman, BS, MD; Sarah Mayson, MD; Manpreet Mundi, MD; Connie Baum Newman, MD, MACP; Rocio Pereira, MD; Nancy Perrier, MD; Alessandro Prete, MD; Martin Reincke, MD; Jane Reusch, MD; Micol Rothman, MD; David Saxon, MD; Ismat Shafiq, MD; Jennifer Sipos, MD; Varsha Vimalananda, MD, MPH; Danica M. Vodopivec, MD;** and **Maria Vogiatzi, MD**

The following AMSC peer reviewers reported relevant financial relationships: **Andrew Bauer, MD**, Speaker: Hexal, AG. **Antonio Bianco, MD, PhD**, Consulting Fee: Allergan, BLA Technology, IBSA Foundation, Synthonics. **Kristien Boelaert, MD, PhD**, Advisory Board: Pfizer, EISAI. **Massimiliano Caprio, MD, PhD**, Grant Recipient: Bayer AG. **Bart Clarke, MD**, Advisory Board: Bristol-Myers Squibb; Consulting Fee: Shire/Takeda, Inc., Calcilytix, Inc., Amolyt, Inc. **Dawn Davis, MD, PhD**, Employee: Department of Veterans Affairs; Grant Recipient: Department of Veterans Affairs, NIH. **Daniel Dumesic, MD**, Advisory Board: Spruce BioSciences Inc.; Grant Recipient: NIH. **Lauren Fishbein, MD, PhD**, Advisory Board: PheoPara Alliance; Consulting Fee: Lantheus/Azedra. **Matthew Freeby, MD**, Grant Recipient: Novo Nordisk, Abbott Diabetes. **Adda Grimberg, MD**, Advisory Board: Pfizer; Consulting Fee: Sandoz; Grant Recipient: Eunice Kennedy Shriver National Institute of Child Health and Human Development. **Niki Karavitaki, FRCP, PhD**, Advisory Board: Recordati Rare Diseases, Pfizer, Ipsen; Speaker: HRA Pharma, Pfizer, Ipsen. **Marta Korbonits, MD, PhD**, Consultant Fee: ONO, Novo Nordisk, Corcept; Speaker: Pfizer, Ipsen. **Maria Veronica Mericq, MD**, Advisory Board: Pfizer, Sandoz, Merck, Novo Nordisk; Consultant Fee: Novartis/Sandoz; Grant Recipient: Merck. **Gabrielle Page-Wilson, MD**, Advisory Board: Strongbridge Biopharma, Recordati Rare Diseases, Inc. **Robin Peeters, MD, PhD**, Advisory Board: Sanofi Genzyme, Bayer; Speaker: Berlin-Chemie, Goodlife Fertility BV, Institut Biochimique SA (IBSA), Sanofi Genzyme, Bayer, EISAI. **Jennifer Sherr, MD, PhD**, Advisory Board: Bigfoot Biomedical, Lilly, Insulet, Cecelia Health; Consultant Fee: Medtronic Diabetes, Sanofi; Grant Recipient: JDRF

The following AMSC peer reviewers reported no relevant financial relationships: **Ernesto Bernal-Mizrachi, MD; Stephanie Fish, MD; Margareta Pisarska, MD; Philipp Scherer, PhD; Robert Wermers, MD; Selma Witchel, MD; Bulent O. Yildiz, MD, PhD;** and **Maria-Christina Zennaro, MD, PhD**

The Endocrine Society staff associated with the development of content for this activity reported no relevant financial relationships.

DISCLAIMERS
The information presented in this activity represents the opinion of the faculty and is not necessarily the official position of the Endocrine Society.

USE OF PROFESSIONAL JUDGMENT:

The educational content in this enduring activity relates to basic principles of diagnosis and therapy and does not substitute for individual patient assessment based on the health care provider's examination of the patient and consideration of laboratory data and other factors unique to the patient. Standards in medicine change as new data become available.

DRUGS AND DOSAGES:

When prescribing medications, the physician is advised to check the product information sheet accompanying each drug to verify conditions of use and to identify any changes in drug dosage schedule or contraindications.

POLICY ON UNLABELED/OFF-LABEL USE

The Endocrine Society has determined that disclosure of unlabeled/off-label or investigational use of commercial product(s) is informative for audiences and therefore requires this information to be disclosed to the learners at the beginning of the presentation. Uses of specific therapeutic agents, devices, and other products discussed in this educational activity may not be the same as those indicated in product labeling approved by the Food and Drug Administration (FDA). The Endocrine Society requires that any discussions of such "off-label" use be based on scientific research that conforms to generally accepted standards of experimental design, data collection, and data analysis. Before recommending or prescribing any therapeutic agent or device, learners should review the complete prescribing information, including indications, contraindications, warnings, precautions, and adverse events.

ACKNOWLEDGMENT OF COMMERCIAL SUPPORT

This activity is not supported by educational grant(s) or other funds from any commercial supporter.

PUBLICATION DATE: June 2022

COMMON ABBREVIATIONS

ACTH = corticotropin

ACE inhibitor = angiotensin-converting enzyme inhibitor

ALT = alanine aminotransferase

AST = aspartate aminotransferase

BMI = body mass index

CNS = central nervous system

CT = computed tomography

DHEA = dehydroepiandrosterone

DHEA-S = dehydroepiandrosterone sulfate

DNA = deoxyribonucleic acid

DPP-4 inhibitor = dipeptidyl-peptidase 4 inhibitor

DXA = dual-energy x-ray absorptiometry

FDA = Food and Drug Administration

FGF-23 = fibroblast growth factor 23

FNA = fine-needle aspiration

FSH = follicle-stimulating hormone

GH = growth hormone

GHRH = growth hormone–releasing hormone

GLP-1 receptor agonist = glucagonlike peptide 1 receptor agonist

GnRH = gonadotropin-releasing hormone

hCG = human chorionic gonadotropin

HDL = high-density lipoprotein

HIV = human immunodeficiency virus

HMG-CoA reductase inhibitor = 3-hydroxy-3-methylglutaryl coenzyme A reductase inhibitor

IGF-1 = insulinlike growth factor 1

LDL = low-density lipoprotein

LH = luteinizing hormone

MCV = mean corpuscular volume

MIBG = *meta*-iodobenzylguanidine

MRI = magnetic resonance imaging

NPH insulin = neutral protamine Hagedorn insulin

PCSK9 inhibitor = proprotein convertase subtilisin/kexin 9 inhibitor

PET = positron emission tomography

PSA = prostate-specific antigen

PTH = parathyroid hormone

PTHrP = parathyroid hormone–related protein

SGLT-2 inhibitor = sodium-glucose cotransporter 2 inhibitor

SHBG = sex hormone–binding globulin

T_3 = triiodothyronine

T_4 = thyroxine

TPO antibodies = thyroperoxidase antibodies

TRH = thyrotropin-releasing hormone

TRAb = thyrotropin-receptor antibodies

TSH = thyrotropin

VLDL = very low-density lipoprotein

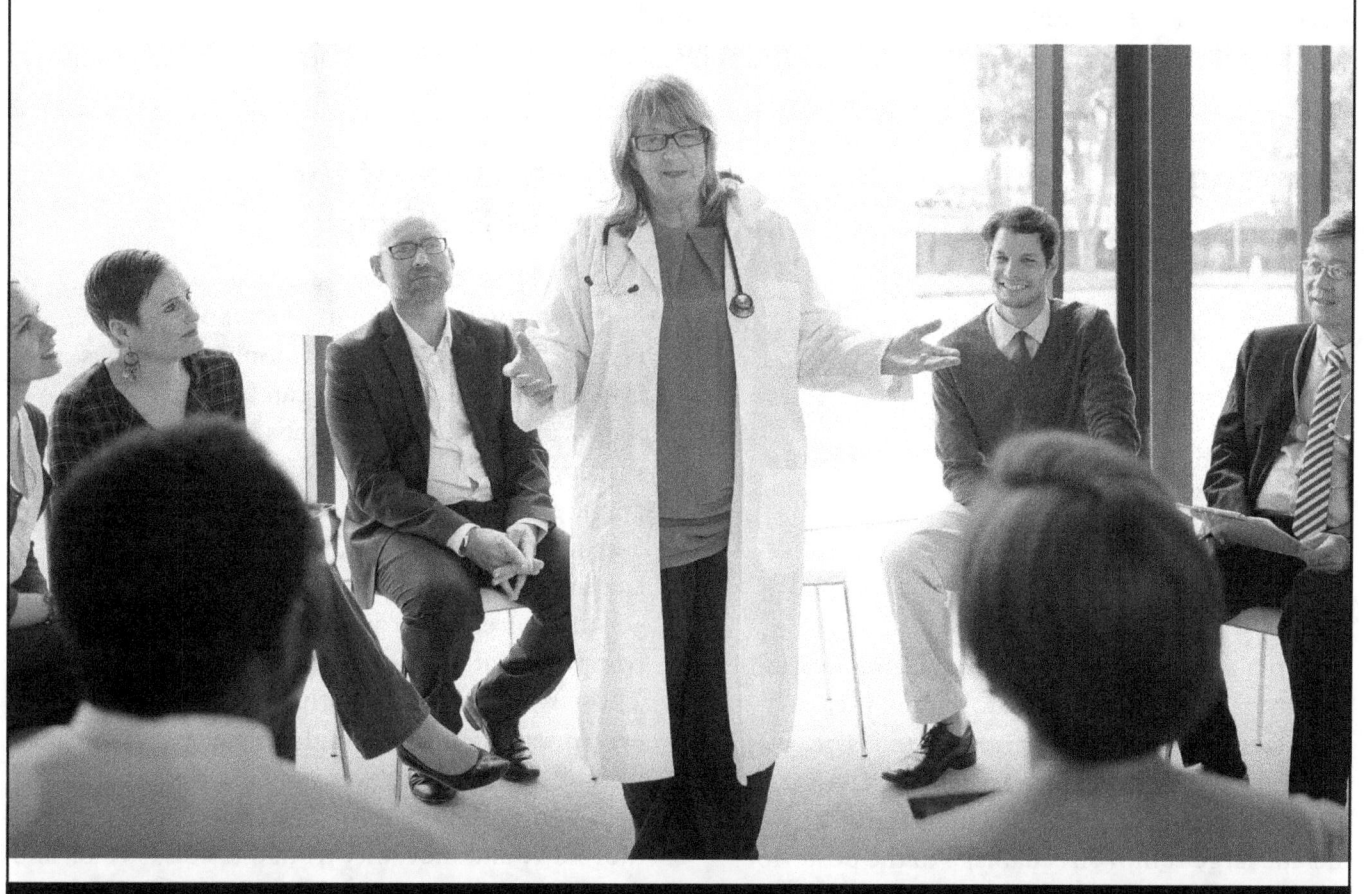

ADIPOSE TISSUE, APPETITE, AND OBESITY

Hypothalamic Obesity

Ashley H. Shoemaker, MD, MSCI. Department of Pediatrics, Endocrinology, and Diabetes, Vanderbilt University Medical Center, Nashville, TN; E-mail: ashley.h.shoemaker@vumc.org

Learning Objectives

As a result of participating in this session, learners should be able to:

- Identify signs and symptoms of hypothalamic obesity.
- Explain the risks and benefits of available treatment options for hypothalamic obesity.

Main Conclusions

Hypothalamic obesity is a common complication of tumors in the hypothalamic region. It is characterized by rapid weight gain and is often accompanied by hypopituitarism. Risk factors for development of hypothalamic obesity include large tumor size, damage to the posterior hypothalamus, hypopituitarism, pretreatment obesity, and younger age. Hypothalamic obesity is refractory to treatment and is highlighted by variable hyperphagia, reduced energy expenditure, and hyperinsulinemia. Lifestyle modifications including a reduced calorie, low-carbohydrate diet, and regular physical activity are recommended but are unlikely to lead to significant weight loss. Medications such as GLP-1 receptor agonists have shown potential to mitigate weight gain in patients with hypothalamic obesity, although weight loss is still difficult. Bariatric surgery can be a safe and effective option for long-term weight loss and weight-loss maintenance.

Significance of the Clinical Problem

Hypothalamic obesity occurs in up to 60% of patients with tumors in the hypothalamic region, most commonly craniopharyngiomas. Hypothalamic dysfunction can be due to tumor infiltration or be a consequence of surgery or radiation therapy. Survival rates for craniopharyngiomas are excellent with an overall 5-year survival rate of 80%, but survivors still face a 5-times greater overall mortality rate and a 3-times greater cardiovascular mortality rate compared with rates in the general population.[1] Those who develop hypothalamic obesity have even greater morbidity and mortality than normal-weight survivors.[2] Prevention and treatment of obesity in this population is vital to decrease the morbidity and mortality from diabetes, stroke, and myocardial infarction.

Barriers to Optimal Practice

Multiple abnormalities in energy balance lead to hypothalamic obesity. Patients with craniopharyngioma who have obesity may have decreased resting energy expenditure compared with control patients who have obesity, most likely due to decreased sympathetic tone,[3] although this has not been a consistent finding. Resting energy expenditure represents approximately two-thirds of daily energy expenditure, with physical activity and other nonexercise activities accounting for the remaining one-third. Patients with hypothalamic obesity typically have a decreased daily activity level. Patients with craniopharyngioma have decreased movement counts as measured by accelerometry and rate their physical capabilities lower than those of healthy control participants.[2]

We used accelerometry to measure physical activity over a 1-year period in 31 children and young adults with hypothalamic obesity enrolled in a clinical trial.[4] Overall, patients spent the most of the time in sedentary activity and low-intensity activity with an average of only 24 minutes per day of moderate or vigorous activity—well below the recommendation of 60 minutes per day. Other studies have also shown decreased quality of life scores in the areas of physical mobility, fatigue, and energy.

Along with the reduction in daily energy expenditure, there is a failure to reduce food intake. While some patients with hypothalamic obesity have significant hyperphagia, most patients do not report extreme hunger or food-seeking behaviors.[3,5] Hyperphagia questionnaire scores are similar to those of patients with common obesity.[5] Patients with hypothalamic obesity struggle with accurate food recall, underreporting caloric intake by an average of 26%.[5] It is possible that the long-term cognitive effects of brain tumors and their treatment make food recall particularly difficult for patients with hypothalamic obesity, although underreporting is common in patients with all forms of obesity.

Hypothalamic obesity is associated with increased risk of metabolic syndrome.[6] Even children with hypothalamic obesity have been found to have impaired fasting glucose and most children with hypothalamic obesity meet criteria for metabolic syndrome. These patients often have insulin resistance and decreased insulin sensitivity. A consistent finding is increased insulin secretion, particularly an exaggerated first-phase response. In animal models, lesions of the ventromedial hypothalamus cause obesity and hyperinsulinemia that is ameliorated by vagotomy. The increased vagal efferent activity in hypothalamic obesity may directly stimulate insulin secretion from the pancreas. With the exception of bariatric surgery, currently available medical treatments have not been shown to improve glucose intolerance or metabolic syndrome in hypothalamic obesity.[4] Changes in other gut hormones are not clear; there are conflicting studies on ghrelin and peptide YY, and to our knowledge there are no studies evaluating glucagon, adiponectin, or GLP-1 levels compared with those of control participants. There are conflicting data on hyperleptinemia in patients with hypothalamic obesity.[5,7] One concern is that 2 of the studies that found hyperleptinemia in patients with hypothalamic obesity correlated leptin levels with BMI, not fat mass.[7] We suspect a role of hyperleptinemia due to both the lack of hypothalamic feedback and the stimulation of leptin production from adipocytes in chronic hyperinsulinemia.

Strategies for Diagnosis, Therapy, and/or Management

Patients may present with hypothalamic obesity at the time of brain tumor diagnosis. If a patient has obesity at diagnosis, they are at high risk of hypothalamic obesity. While obesity is common in the United States population, the presence of obesity at diagnosis may also signal abnormal weight gain over the preceding months. Most patients develop hypothalamic obesity as a result of treatment, typically surgery or radiation.[2] Surgical effects are seen immediately while radiation effects can take months to present. Presence of hypopituitarism is another risk factor for hypothalamic obesity, most likely due to the correlation with extensive hypothalamic damage. Posterior hypothalamic damage can be a marker for hypothalamic obesity risk. While not yet routinely used in clinical care, there is a published MRI scoring system that may help identify patients at high risk of developing hypothalamic obesity. The hallmark of hypothalamic obesity is rapid weight gain leading to a notable change in weight trajectory. The most rapid weight gain is typically seen in the first 6 months, highlighting the need for early diagnosis and intervention, as prevention of weight gain can be more successful than weight loss.

Medical treatments have not been very successful in treating hypothalamic obesity.[8] Octreotide, a somatostatin analogue that decreases insulin secretion, was one of the first medications tried for hypothalamic obesity, but its use in a randomized controlled trial failed to cause weight loss. Additional studies have used metformin alone or in combination but did not result in significant weight loss, although metformin may help slow the rate of weight gain. Perhaps due to its safety profile and the prevalence of metabolic syndrome/prediabetes, metformin is commonly prescribed to patients with hypothalamic obesity; 31% of patients (27 of 87) in the International Registry of Hypothalamic Obesity Disorders reported use of metformin for weight loss.[8] Low-carbohydrate diets are often recommended in clinical practice despite a lack of robust supporting evidence.[9]

GLP-1 is an incretin that enhances release of insulin in response to hyperglycemia, decreases the rate of gastric emptying, and increases satiety. At pharmacologic dosages, GLP-1 crosses the blood brain barrier and has direct effects on GLP-1 receptors in the brain. GLP-1 receptors are expressed in numerous brain regions outside of the hypothalamus, particularly the brainstem. GLP-1 receptor agonists are increasingly used for treatment of obesity; the US FDA has granted approval for liraglutide (2020) and semaglutide (2021) for chronic weight management. Due to the extrahypothalamic actions of GLP-1 receptor agonists, they are a potential pharmacotherapy for hypothalamic obesity. A randomized controlled clinical trial in children and young adults showed evidence that GLP-1 receptor agonists may slow the rate of weight gain and decrease fat mass in patients with hypothalamic obesity.[4] Unfortunately, patients treated with GLP-1 receptor agonists also showed a significant reduction in total daily energy expenditure despite simply slowing their rate of weight gain and not having significant weight loss.

Central nervous system stimulants may be helpful in treating patients with hypothalamic obesity.[9] Dexamphetamine and methylphenidate are most commonly used in attention-deficit disorder and can have a side effect of decreased appetite. Many pediatric patients with hypothalamic obesity also have attention and/or executive function deficits, warranting consideration of a stimulant. There are reports of weight stabilization and increased daytime wakefulness from dexamphetamine in patients with hypothalamic obesity. Another stimulant, phentermine, is approved for short-term treatment of obesity in adults and a phentermine/topiramate combination is approved for long-term treatment of obesity. The mechanism of action is not well understood, but most likely involves the hypothalamus. Since the degree of hypothalamic damage is variable in hypothalamic obesity, it is possible that some patients will respond to phentermine/topiramate, but studies are needed.

Oxytocin is synthesized in the hypothalamus and secreted through the posterior pituitary. Unlike other pituitary hormones, oxytocin is not routinely replaced. This neuropeptide has been shown to reduce appetite and increase energy expenditure. Oxytocin is not approved for treatment of obesity or hypopituitarism. It is typically given intranasally, and an effective dosage regimen is not yet defined. In Prader-Willi syndrome, a genetic obesity disorder with hypothalamic dysfunction, oxytocin has had variable effects on hyperphagia. An oxytocin analogue, carbetocin, was evaluated by the US FDA in 2021 for treatment of hyperphagia but was not approved due to concerns about efficacy. It is recommended that oxytocin not be used outside of clinical trials.

Bariatric surgery may be successful in patients with hypothalamic obesity.[8,10] A recent retrospective, case-control study from the Netherlands showed a mean weight loss of 22% at 5 years in patients with hypothalamic obesity.[10] While this was significantly less than weight loss in control patients, it is still clinically significant weight loss. Sleeve gastrectomy performed better than Roux-en-Y gastric bypass.[10] The International Registry of Hypothalamic Obesity Disorders found that only 8% of patients underwent bariatric surgery but it was most effective with a median 8.2 kg/m^2 decrease in BMI.[8] Patients with hypothalamic obesity who underwent gastric bypass also reported decreased hunger and cravings.

Clinical Case Vignettes

Case 1

A 9.5-year-old girl presents to her pediatrician with headaches that have been worsening for 10 days. She has decreased height velocity with steady weight gain along the 50th percentile. Head imaging shows a complex mixed cystic and solid suprasellar mass (3 × 3 × 3.4 cm) that extends superiorly, effacing the third ventricle and resulting in obstructive hydrocephalus. She is admitted to the hospital, and the tumor is resected surgically. Pathology findings are consistent with a craniopharyngioma. She is discharged on hormone replacement for panhypopituitarism, including diabetes insipidus, and a 2-week course of dexamethasone for postoperative swelling. One month later, she returns to the endocrine clinic for follow-up. Her parents report that she has experienced increased swelling and weight gain since coming home from the hospital. Her clothing size has increased from 7 to 12. She has increased hunger and is craving of sweet foods/junk foods that she never ate before. She snacks frequently throughout the day and is hungry again immediately after mealtimes. Her growth chart is shown (*see Figure*).

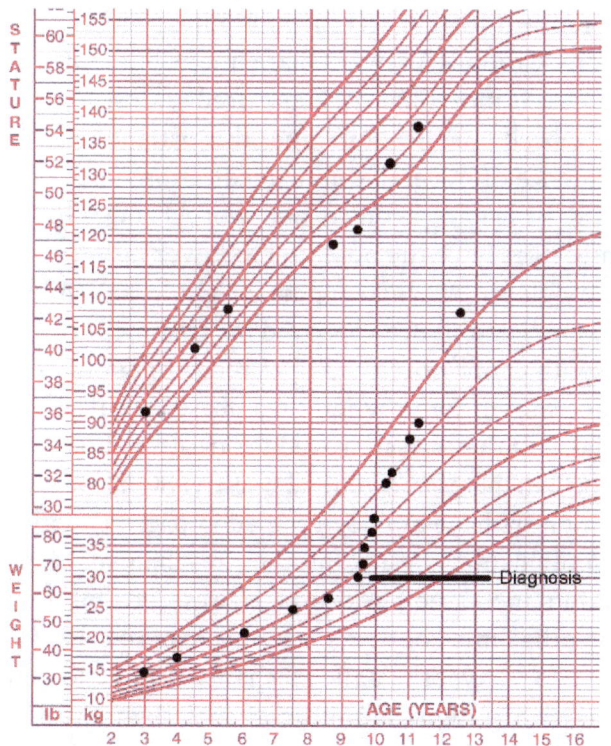

Which of the following is the most likely reason for this patient's postoperative weight gain?

A. Fluid retention due to diabetes insipidus

B. Hypothalamic obesity due to tissue damage from tumor extension

C. Increased appetite due to postoperative dexamethasone

D. Postoperative hypothalamic obesity

Answer: D) Postoperative hypothalamic obesity

This patient demonstrates the classic weight gain pattern of hypothalamic obesity due to tumor treatment with a sharp inflection point in the rate of weight gain from prediagnosis to posttreatment. Complete resection of a large tumor may increase the risk of postoperative hypothalamic obesity (Answer D). Other risk factors for hypothalamic obesity include her young age and evidence of endocrine dysfunction at diagnosis (poor growth rate). She did not have the risk factor of preoperative obesity.

Dexamethasone can increase appetite and weight gain, but the effects do not continue after the medication is discontinued (thus, Answer C is incorrect).

Hypothalamic obesity due to tumor extension is often more gradual in onset and the increased weight gain is evident pretreatment. In this patient, the rate of weight gain was steady until the time of diagnosis and intervention (thus, Answer B is incorrect).

While a small amount of weight gain caused by fluid retention is possible due to overtreatment of diabetes insipidus, a weight gain of 10 kg in 6 months cannot be explained by hypervolemia (thus Answer A is incorrect).

Early recognition of hypothalamic obesity allows for environmental and dietary interventions to decrease caloric intake and slow the rate of weight gain. A visit with a registered dietitian can help families implement daily caloric maximums and parent-guided portion sizes. This patient shows symptoms of hyperphagia such as increased interest in food and decreased satiety.

Hyperphagic symptoms should be systematically evaluated at each clinic visit to assess efficacy of interventions. Similar to patients with Prader-Willi syndrome, patients with hypothalamic obesity and hyperphagia may benefit from scheduled meals/snacks. A regular meal/snack schedule can help with anxiety around food and minimize food-seeking behaviors. For patients with food-seeking behaviors such as sneaking food and nighttime eating, environmental modification such as locking the pantry/refrigerator and not leaving food and drinks on counters can be effective. Since hyperinsulinism is common in hypothalamic obesity, a lower carbohydrate diet can be beneficial. While this has not been evaluated in a well-controlled study, several case reports demonstrate benefit, typically starting at less than 50 g of carbohydrates per day.

Case 2

A 52-year-old man is diagnosed with a craniopharyngioma after presenting to his primary care physician with concerns of decreased peripheral vision. He is treated with proton radiotherapy. Six months after radiation therapy, he develops central hypothyroidism and adrenal insufficiency, managed with levothyroxine and hydrocortisone, 8 mg/m^2 daily. He does not report symptoms of hyperphagia but does describe a 50-lb (22.6-kg) weight gain over the past 6 months. His BMI has increased from 26 kg/m^2 pretreatment to 34 kg/m^2 posttreatment. A close diet history reveals some increased snacking and decreased ability to feel full; for example, he often finishes his children's leftovers when cleaning up the kitchen. Screening labs are notable for mild mixed hyperlipidemia and a hemoglobin A$_{1c}$ value of 6.7% (50 mmol/mol).

Which of the following would be the best management strategy for this patient's weight gain?

A. Antidiabetes medication with weight-loss effects such as a GLP-1 receptor agonist

B. Bariatric surgery

C. Lifestyle modifications such as a reduced calorie diet and increased exercise

D. Reduction in his hydrocortisone dosage to 5 mg/m^2 daily

Answer: A) Antidiabetes medication with weight-loss effects such as a GLP-1 receptor agonist

This patient demonstrates evidence of hypothalamic obesity due to radiation adverse effects. Radiation can be used as adjunctive or primary therapy for craniopharyngiomas. Proton radiotherapy provides precise delivery of radiation due to a lower entrance dose and elimination of the exit dose compared with photon-beam radiotherapy. While proton radiotherapy is more targeted, treatment of suprasellar tumors still confers a risk of postradiation hypopituitarism and hypothalamic obesity. Children are more sensitive to radiation adverse effects, with about 50% of children demonstrating at least 1 pituitary hormone deficiency 4 years after treatment. Hypothalamic obesity is most commonly seen in patients who receive 51 Gy or more to the hypothalamic region.

Hypothalamic obesity is refractory to treatment and aggressive therapy is recommended to prevent further weight gain. Lifestyle modifications (Answer C) are important, but success is more likely when paired with an antiobesity medication. Since this patient has evidence of hyperglycemia, medications such as GLP-1 receptor agonists (Answer A) and SGLT-2 inhibitors have the potential to lower his hemoglobin A$_{1c}$ and support weight loss. While no medications are approved for treatment of hypothalamic obesity, GLP-1 receptor agonists have shown some benefit in a phase 2 clinical trial, and they are approved for treatment of type 2 diabetes and general obesity. SGLT-2 inhibitors have not been trialed in patients with hypothalamic obesity, but their mechanism of action, increased glucosuria, is preserved in hypothalamic obesity. These medication classes have extrahypothalamic mechanisms of action and therefore potential for efficacy in patients with hypothalamic obesity. Antidiabetes medications that increase weight gain, such as insulin and sulfonylureas, should be avoided.

There is no evidence that appropriate glucocorticoid replacement causes or worsens hypothalamic obesity, so reducing his hydrocortisone dosage (Answer D) is not indicated.

Bariatric surgery (Answer D) can be effective in treating hypothalamic obesity, but medical weight management is recommended as first-line therapy. A tertiary medical center can be necessary for patients with panhypopituitarism and hypothalamic obesity due to the increased operative and postoperative complexity of adrenal insufficiency and diabetes insipidus. We also encourage patients to follow clinicaltrials.gov, as there are several investigational drugs targeting hypothalamic obesity.

References

1. Bulow B, Attewell R, Hagmar L, Malmstrom P, Nordstrom CH, Erfurth EM. Postoperative prognosis in craniopharyngioma with respect to cardiovascular mortality, survival, and tumor recurrence. *J Clin Endocrinol Metab.* 1998;83(11):3897-3904. PMID: 9814465

2. Muller HL, Bueb K, Bartels U, et al. Obesity after childhood craniopharyngioma--German multicenter study on pre-operative risk factors and quality of life. *Klin Padiatr.* 2001;213(4):244-249. PMID: 11528558

3. Holmer H, Pozarek G, Wirfalt E, et al. Reduced energy expenditure and impaired feeding-related signals but not high energy intake reinforces hypothalamic obesity in adults with childhood onset craniopharyngioma. *J Clin Endocrinol Metab.* 2010;95(12):5395-5402. PMID: 20826582

4. Roth CL, Perez FA, Whitlock KB, et al. A phase 3 randomized clinical trial using a once-weekly glucagon-like peptide-1 receptor agonist in adolescents and young adults with hypothalamic obesity. *Diabetes Obes Metab.* 2021;23(2):363-373. PMID: 33026160

5. Shoemaker AH, Silver HJ, Buchowski M, et al. Energy balance in hypothalamic obesity in response to treatment with a once-weekly GLP-1 receptor agonist. *Int J Obes (Lond).* 2022;46(3):623-629. PMID: 34975146

6. Srinivasan S, Ogle GD, Garnett SP, Briody JN, Lee JW, Cowell CT. Features of the metabolic syndrome after childhood craniopharyngioma. *J Clin Endocrinol Metab.* 2004;89(1):81-86. PMID: 14715831

7. Roth C, Wilken B, Hanefeld F, Schroter W, Leonhardt U. Hyperphagia in children with craniopharyngioma is associated with hyperleptinaemia and a failure in the downregulation of appetite. *Eur J Endocrinol.* 1998;138(1):89-91. PMID: 9461323

8. Rose SR, Horne VE, Bingham N, Jenkins T, Black J, Inge T. Hypothalamic obesity: 4 years of the International Registry of Hypothalamic Obesity Disorders. *Obesity (Silver Spring).* 2018;26(11):1727-1732. PMID: 30296362

9. Abuzzahab MJ, Roth CL, Shoemaker AH. Hypothalamic obesity: prologue and promise. *Horm Res Paediatr.* 2019;91(2):128-136. PMID: 30884490

10. van Santen SS, Wolf P, Kremenevski N, et al. Bariatric surgery for hypothalamic obesity in craniopharyngioma patients: a retrospective, matched case-control study. *J Clin Endocrinol Metab.* 2021;106(11):e4734-e4745. PMID: 34265053

Electronic Tools to Help Patients During Their Weight-Loss Journey

Manpreet S. Mundi, MD. Division of Endocrinology, Diabetes, Metabolism, and Nutrition, Mayo Clinic, Rochester, MN; E-mail: mundi.manpreet@mayo.edu

Learning Objectives

As a result of participating in this session, learners should be able to:

- Discuss the use of electronic tools to assist in improving dietary capture.
- Review the benefits of devices such as smartwatches in terms of physical activity.

Main Conclusions

The prevalence of obesity continues to rise, with some estimates predicting that 1 in 2 adults in the United States will have obesity by 2030. The association of obesity with higher prevalence of medical conditions such as diabetes mellitus, hyperlipidemia, hypertension, obstructive sleep apnea, and cancer will have devastating implications for health care resources. Although we have a plethora of treatment options for managing obesity, including state-of-the art lifestyle modification programs, medications, endoscopic procedures, and bariatric surgery, implementation of these strategies can be quite resource-intensive. Additionally, patient adherence can be low, leading to suboptimal results, especially for programs that include intensive lifestyle modifications. To manage the high volume of patients in a cost- and resource-effective manner, we must dramatically change the way in which we deliver care to patients with obesity with the use of technological aids where feasible and beneficial. These aids, such as smartphone applications, can be used to improve capture of dietary intake, which is sometimes significantly underreported through typical dietary recall conducted in the clinical setting. Similarly, patients often overreport their physical activity levels, and accuracy is improved significantly with the use of devices with built-in accelerometers. Technological aids such as virtual visits, smartphone applications, and web-based programs can be used to augment standard cognitive behavioral therapy in an effort to improve results while reducing the time allocated by providers per patient.

Significance of the Clinical Problem

Despite significant efforts to raise awareness and develop novel treatment options, the prevalence of obesity continues to rise. Without significant changes in these trends, it is estimated that by 2030, close to 1 in 2 adult Americans will have obesity or have a BMI of 30 kg/m^2 or greater with the prevalence being higher than 50% in 29 states.[1] More alarming is the projection that close to 1 in 4 adults will have severe obesity or a BMI of 35 kg/m^2 or greater. This has devastating implications for health care, as obesity is associated with more than 60 comorbid medical conditions and increases the risk of at least 12 different types of cancer.[2] Fortunately, we have a plethora of treatment options available, including several medications approved by the US FDA with indications for weight loss, endoscopic procedures, and bariatric surgeries. Despite the availability of these modalities, we would all agree that their success is dependent on a strong foundation of lifestyle modification. Several large randomized, prospective trials have demonstrated that a combination of caloric restriction, increased activity, energy expenditure, and intensive cognitive behavior therapy can result in 5% to 7% weight loss, with some individuals achieving much better results.

Unfortunately, even though the curriculum from these large trials, such as the Diabetes Prevention Program and the Look AHEAD trial, is widely available and free to use, implementation in clinical practice has proven difficult because of several factors. The biggest limiting factors are the resources needed to effectively implement intensive lifestyle modification programs, which often require touch points with a frequency of close to once weekly for the initial weight-loss period of 3 to 6 months, followed by less frequent visits in weight maintenance periods.[3] Additionally, successful reduction in caloric intake requires accurate capture of dietary intake and accurate assessment of the caloric content and portion size of meals. Often, capture of dietary intake is conducted through self-reported recall at the time of office visits, which depends on the patient's ability to remember and willingness to report. When compared with more accurate markers such as doubly labeled water, self-reported dietary intake can be underreported by as much as 37%. Improving the accuracy of dietary recall may require ongoing interviews with trained personnel, patient education, and more accurate assessment of macronutrient composition and volume. These strategies can be quite time consuming and cost prohibitive for most clinical practices and may not overcome social and psychological determinants of underreporting.

Similarly, difficulty with assessing intensity of activity level can make it difficult for patients to achieve the 150 minutes of moderate- to vigorous-intensity activity recommended by most programs. Unfortunately, studies have noted that self-reported questionnaires are largely dependent on an individual's recall and perception of their quantity and intensity of physical activity and are thus prone to errors from recall bias, misinterpretation, and social desirability, which can be worse in patients with a higher BMI. Slootmaker et al noted that 301 adults reported a median of 340 minutes of moderate- and vigorous-intensity activity per week while the accelerometer only captured 144 minutes, an overreporting of 58%.[4] Other studies with similar design have also noted overreporting, especially of vigorous-intensity activity, in many cases by as much as double of what was actually performed.[5]

Cognitive behavioral therapy and structured lifestyle interventions (which often use frequent group or individual visits that provide nutrition and physical activity education) that rely on behavior change techniques, motivational interviewing, self-monitoring, and accountability, have been noted to increase physical activity, reduce sedentary behavior, and improve adherence to dietary interventions, resulting in significant weight loss. As an example, the Look AHEAD trial used weekly group and individual counseling sessions targeting a caloric goal of 1200 to 1800 kcal daily, along with 175 minutes of moderate-intensity activity per week for 6 months followed by less frequent visits for the next 6 months to achieve an average weight loss of 8.6% at 1 year. Unfortunately, these programs can be quite labor- and resource-intensive with limited reimbursement, making them difficult to implement for most clinical practices.

Barriers to Optimal Practice

- Accurate dietary and activity capture.
- Patient adherence to lifestyle modification.
- Cost- and resource-prohibitive intensity of therapy needed to achieve significant weight loss.
- Reimbursement for weight-loss programs.

Strategies for Diagnosis, Therapy, and/or Management

As the prevalence of obesity continues to increase, we must innovate and dramatically change the way in which we deliver care for patients with obesity, including implementation of lifestyle modifications and intensive cognitive behavioral therapy. This change initially starts with data capture, especially of dietary intake, activity level, and monitoring body weight. Transitioning away from self-reported dietary intake to point-of-consumption dietary capture can improve accuracy. Tooze et al evaluated the accuracy of dietary recall with food-frequency questionnaires and 24-hour dietary entry compared with doubly labeled water and noted that food-frequency questionnaires were associated with average underreporting of 34% in women and 30% in men.[6] Use of 24-hour entry decreased the underreporting to 17% for women and 11% for men. The authors also found that social desirability, fear of a negative evaluation, BMI, eating frequency, and variability of meals per day were factors associated with underreporting. This and other similar trials have demonstrated that although point-of-consumption dietary entry can improve accuracy, it is still dependent on the patient measuring portion sizes accurately and entering all of their food intake, which can be biased significantly by a number of factors ranging from education level and nutritional knowledge to social desirability, especially the concept that their current weight is associated with their intake. As such, we must continue to evaluate technological improvements such as imaging technology that can improve accuracy of dietary capture.

Imaging technology has been used in clinical trials in some capacity since the 1980s to better define portion sizes and caloric content of meals. Many of these studies have used a handheld device to manually capture a patient's dietary intake. More recently, use of wearable camera-assisted dietary assessment has sought to eliminate the error associated with manual image capture and further improve accuracy. In one trial, 40 ambulatory participants were asked to wear a wide-angle camera around their neck capturing an image approximately every 20 seconds.[7] The use of ongoing image capture reduced underreporting of dietary intake to 9% in men and 7% in women. Most of this improvement occurred through capture of unreported food intake and misreporting errors. These previous techniques have involved the use of a trained member of the team to analyze the captured images to assess portion sizes and percentage consumed, again requiring significant resources to implement outside of clinical trials. Advances in artificial intelligence are allowing for the development of platforms that can detect the amount of food consumed with similar accuracy to that of a dietitian analyzing images and is good to excellent when compared with the weight of the tray. Currently, these applications are being tested in the hospital setting where artificial intelligence is used to analyze before and after images to capture consumption, and they rely on knowledge of the caloric content of the meal.[8] As artificial intelligence continues to evolve, we see advancements being made towards the application of this technology to assess dietary intake for food whose caloric content has not been prespecified.

With physical activity, advancements in wearable device technology combining accelerometers with sensors continue to add the ability to monitor steps taken, distances traveled, heart rate, and energy expenditure. Additional sensors, including those that measure oxygen saturation, blood glucose, and the presence of arrhythmias, have the potential to increase safe activity for those with significant medical comorbidities. A recent trial that enrolled 40 patients with known cardiovascular disease assessed the accuracy of a consumer-grade smartwatch in measuring heart rate and energy expenditure.[9] They noted that across variable activity levels, the standard deviation of difference for energy expenditure was within the acceptable range for clinical practice at 17.5 kcal and the smartwatch tended to measure a higher value for energy expenditure by approximately 30.47 kcal. Heart rate accuracy was much better. In addition to more accurate capture, what is more intriguing is the ability of these devices to decrease sedentary behavior and increase activity. In a recent prospective trial, all participants were provided an activity tracker, with some participants being blinded while others were able to monitor their step count.[10] They also randomly assigned individuals to receive brief feedback sessions to increase activity. The combination of being able to monitor their activity combined with brief feedback sessions resulted in more than 10% increase in activity level. Another trial randomly assigning individuals to both blinding and unblinding of activity measured in a smartphone app, as well as feedback through text messages, documented similar results. Patients who were unblinded to their activity level increased their number of steps per day by 1024 compared with those who were blinded, while those who were unblinded and received feedback through text messages increased their steps by 2534.

Similar technological advancements are being made in the implementation of cognitive behavioral therapy to address many factors that lead to patient attrition. The use of virtual meetings, which reduces the need to travel for weekly meetings, has been greatly accelerated during the COVID-19 pandemic and shows similar results to in-person sessions. Virtual meetings, however, do not reduce provider resources used, as equivalent time is needed for in-person vs virtual sessions. Thus, there has been a movement to replicate many of the key components of behavioral therapy and provide them in an enhanced manner through initially web-based interface and now smartphone apps. In a clinical trial, the use of a mobile application that allows patients to enter dietary intake and activity level combined with standard cognitive behavioral therapy resulted in 3.1% more weight loss than that achieved by standard therapy alone.[11] Weight loss was even more significant in those who used the application more, which is key to efficacy of these approaches. A retrospective analysis of more than 35,000 users of a popular weight-loss smartphone app noted that 77.9% of participants lost weight to some degree, while 22.7% experienced more that 10% weight loss.[12] These investigators reported that frequency of input of body weight, exercise, and dinner along with baseline BMI were all positively correlated with the amount of weight reduction.

Clinical Case Vignettes
Case 1
A 44-year-old woman with depression and obesity complicated by type 2 diabetes presents for assistance with weight loss after recent diagnosis of diabetes.

On physical examination, her height is 68.5 in (174 cm), and weight is 202 lb (92 kg) (BMI = 30.4 kg/m^2). She has central adiposity.

In her 20s, she reports being able to maintain her weight in the range of 120 to 140 lb (54-64 kg), although she was an avid runner at the time. In her 30s, her activity level declined significantly because of knee injuries, rearing young children, and work, and her weight stabilized in the range of 160 to 180 lb (73-82 kg). In her 40s, she transitioned to a consulting position that required significantly more travel. Her weight gradually increased, and depression and diabetes were diagnosed. Bupropion was prescribed for depression, and she reports that her mood has been stable for the last 3 years. Her diabetes is managed with metformin, 500 mg twice daily, and her last hemoglobin A_{1c} measurement was 6.2% (44 mmol/mol).

She reports that although she does not capture her dietary intake, she targets between 1200 and 1500 calories per day. She describes being active at work, as well as at home with household activities such as gardening. She does not engage in any formal exercise.

Which of the following is the most appropriate next step in the management of this patient's obesity?

A. Initiation of second-line therapy for diabetes

B. Intensive lifestyle program with ongoing monitoring of dietary intake and activity level

C. Referral to psychiatry for transition to another therapy for depression

D. Very low-calorie diet targeting 600 to 800 calories per day

Answer: B) Intensive lifestyle program with ongoing monitoring of dietary intake and activity level

In this case, the initial treatment option should focus on lifestyle modification (Answer B). Patients often underreport caloric intake and overreport activity level. Starting with ongoing capture of her dietary intake through a smartphone application would be ideal, not only to ascertain her intake, but also to educate her about the caloric content of the food she is consuming. Additionally, use of an activity tracking device can assist with not only more accurate capture but also facilitate a gradual increase in activity. These efforts should be combined with an intensive lifestyle program that initially meets weekly or biweekly for 3 to 6 months followed by less frequent meetings.

Referral to psychiatry for transition to another therapy (Answer C) would not be best next step, as her depression is well controlled. Bupropion when combined with naltrexone has been shown to be an effective weight-loss agent.[13]

A caloric target of 600 to 800 calories per day (Answer D) may be too restrictive, especially in the setting of underreporting of intake. Based on predictive equations such as the Harris-Benedict equation, her caloric needs at her current weight would be approximately 2300 kcal. Thus, it would be appropriate for her to target between 1600 to 1800 calories per day combined with increased activity for weight loss. If necessary, further reduction in calories can be attempted if inadequate weight loss is achieved with that target, again keeping in mind that most individuals tend to underreport caloric intake.

Similarly, lifestyle modifications should be attempted before adding a second-line agent for diabetes (Answer A) given her current hemoglobin A_{1c} level of 6.2% (44 mmol/mol). There are many medications now approved for management of diabetes that are either weight neutral or have weight-loss properties. Some GLP-1 receptor agonists also have separate indications for weight loss and can be quite effective in reducing caloric intake.

Case 2

A 37-year-old woman with a history of bipolar disorder, posttraumatic stress disorder, tobacco use (1 pack per day), and obesity complicated by type 2 diabetes, hypertension, hyperlipidemia, and obstructive sleep apnea seeks help with weight loss. She began to gain weight in high school and weighed 210 lb (95.3 kg) by the time she graduated. Soon after graduating, she became pregnant with her son and reports that she gained 60 lb (27.2 kg) during her pregnancy, with minimal weight loss afterwards. She estimates gaining 20 to 30 lb (9.1 to 13.6 kg) with each of her 2 subsequent pregnancies and weighed close to 300 lb (136 kg) by age 30 years. She tried to lose weight through "countless" programs, including a commercial calorie-counting program, but her most successful effort was meal replacement whereby she lost 50 lb (22.7 kg) over 6 months in her early 30s.

On physical examination, her height is 66.1 in (168 cm) and weight is 317 lb (143.8 kg) (BMI = 51 kg/m²). She has increased neck circumference, acanthosis nigricans, and central adiposity.

Her diabetes is currently managed with metformin, 1000 mg twice daily, and liraglutide, 1.8 mg daily. Her last hemoglobin A_{1c} measurement was 7.9% (63 mmol/mol). She is not able to tolerate continuous positive airway pressure because she feels claustrophobic. She has longstanding posttraumatic stress disorder due to childhood trauma and feels that bipolar disorder is a misdiagnosis.

She currently eats most of her meals outside of the home. She works 2 jobs. On the way to her first job, she typically stops for breakfast at a fast-food restaurant. She then skips lunch, but usually stops for a hot dog or pretzel at a convenience store on the way to her second job. Her evening meal is usually picked up on the way home from her second job. She also reports snacking throughout the day. Her beverage of choice is soda. She does not engage in any formal exercise, but she reports being quite active at work.

Which of the following is the best next step in this patient's management?

A. Add an SGLT-2 inhibitor to improve glycemic control

B. Initiate dietary restriction targeting 800 kcal per day

C. Refer her for bariatric surgery (Roux-en-Y gastric bypass)

D. Refer her to psychiatry for evaluation of posttraumatic stress disorder/bipolar disorder followed by virtual cognitive behavioral therapy

Answer: D) Refer her to psychiatry for evaluation of posttraumatic stress disorder/bipolar disorder followed by virtual cognitive behavioral therapy

This patient's weight-loss journey should start by addressing her childhood trauma (Answer D), as that is most likely a major contributor to weight gain. A recent survey of overweight and obese individuals noted that 36.8% of participants with class III obesity (BMI ≥40 kg/m2) reported being a victim of childhood trauma.[14] Persons with a history of childhood trauma often report that weight issues began at an early age and are more likely to have weight-related comorbidities even after controlling for BMI. Victims of childhood trauma also report lower self-esteem, are more likely to feel judged by their health care provider, and are less likely to feel they are treated with respect. Thus, history of childhood trauma, whether it is physical or sexual abuse, can dramatically affect how individuals interact with their health care providers, including seeking care and being forthcoming regarding their abuse. Weight can also be protective, leading to increased failed attempts at weight loss. Therefore, in addressing weight loss, it is important to create a nonjudgmental environment that allows the patient to openly discuss contributing factors to weight gain. Providers should also solicit a history of trauma, especially in patients with weight gain at a young age, such as this patient. Patients should be referred to a provider trained in the management of trauma. Often, management will require ongoing therapy that may start with addressing mood disorders and trauma, followed by introduction of concepts focused on weight loss.

Dietary restriction (Answer B) or addition of a second-line agent for diabetes (Answer A) would not be the ideal next step in the setting of an unaddressed mood disorder and trauma history.

Bariatric surgery (Answer C) can be very beneficial for patients with class III obesity, producing significant weight loss, as well as remission of many obesity-related comorbidities such as diabetes. However, it is essential to ensure that patients are medically optimized and that mood disorders are stable and well managed before proceeding with surgery.

References

1. Ward ZJ, Bleich SN, Cradock AL, et al. Projected U.S. state-level prevalence of adult obesity and severe obesity. *N Engl J Med.* 2019;381(25):2440-2450. PMID: 31851800

2. Hurt RT, Edakkanambeth Varayil J, Mundi MS, Martindale RG, Ebbert JO. Designation of obesity as a disease: lessons learned from alcohol and tobacco. *Curr Gastroenterol Rep.* 2014;16(11):415. PMID: 25277042

3. Jensen MD, Ryan DH, Apovian CM, et al. 2013 AHA/ACC/TOS guideline for the management of overweight and obesity in adults: a report of the American College of Cardiology/American Heart Association Task Force on practice guidelines and The Obesity Society. *J Am Coll Cardiol.* 2014;63(25 Pt B):2985-3023. PMID: 24239920

4. Slootmaker SM, Schuit AJ, Chinapaw MJ, Seidell JC, van Mechelen W. Disagreement in physical activity assessed by accelerometer and self-report in subgroups of age, gender, education and weight status. *Int J Behav Nutr Phys Act.* 2009;6:17. PMID: 19320985

5. Quinlan C, Rattray B, Pryor D, et al. The accuracy of self-reported physical activity questionnaires varies with sex and body mass index. *PLoS ONE.* 2021;16(8):e0256008. PMID: 34379676

6. Tooze JA, Subar AF, Thompson FE, Troiano R, Schatzkin A, Kipnis V. Psychosocial predictors of energy underreporting in a large doubly labeled water study. *Am J Clin Nutr.* 2004;79(5):795-804. PMID: 15113717

7. Gemming L, Rush E, Maddison R, et al. Wearable cameras can reduce dietary under-reporting: doubly labelled water validation of a camera-assisted 24 h recall. *Br J Nutr.* 2015;113(2):284-291. PMID: 25430667

8. Van Wymelbeke-Delannoy V, Juhel C, Bole H, et al. A cross-sectional reproducibility study of a standard camera sensor using artificial intelligence to assess food items: The FoodIntech Project. *Nutrients.* 2022;14(1):221. PMID: 35011096

9. Falter M, Budts W, Goetschalckx K, Cornelissen V, Buys R. Accuracy of Apple Watch measurements for heart rate and energy expenditure in patients with cardiovascular disease: cross-sectional study. *JMIR MHealth UHealth.* 2019;7(3):e11889. PMID: 30888332

10. Nanda S, Hurt RT, Croghan IT, et al. Improving physical activity and body composition in a medical workplace using brief goal setting. *Mayo Clin Proc Innov Qual Outcomes.* 2019;3(4):495-505. PMID: 31993569

11. Spring B, Duncan JM, Janke E, et al. Integrating technology into standard weight loss treatment: a randomized controlled trial. *JAMA Intern Med.* 2013;173(2):105-111. PMID: 23229890

12. Chin SO, Keum C, Woo J, et al. Successful weight reduction and maintenance by using a smartphone application in those with overweight and obesity. *Sci Rep.* 2016;6:34563. PMID: 27819345

13. Khera R, Murad MH, Chandar AK, et al. Association of pharmacological treatments for obesity with weight loss and adverse events: a systematic review and meta-analysis. *JAMA.* 2016;315(22):2424-2434. PMID: 27299618

14. Mundi MS, Hurt RT, Phelan SM, et al. Associations between experience of early childhood trauma and impact on obesity status, health, as well as perceptions of obesity-related health care. *Mayo Clin Proc.* 2021;96(2):408-419. PMID: 33549259

Update on the Medical Management of Obesity

David A. D'Alessio, MD. Department of Medicine, Division of Endocrinology, Duke University Medical Center, Durham, NC; E-mail: david.d'alessio@duke.edu

Jonathan E. Campbell, PhD. Department of Medicine, Division of Endocrinology, Duke University Medical Center, Durham, NC; E-mail: jonathan.campbell@duke.edu

Learning Objectives

As a result of participating in this session, learners should be able to:

- Identify the individual characteristics that determine the appropriate weight-loss intervention.

- Develop a better understanding of the current and emerging pharmacological strategies for weight loss.

Main Conclusions

- A range of drugs that can cause weight loss is now available.

- Most agents are only modestly effective and meet the standard of clinical efficacy (>5% placebo-corrected weight loss) in half of patients.

- Recently developed injectable GLP-1 receptor agonists show more promise, with average placebo-corrected weight loss of 10% to 15%.

- Incretin-based drugs in development are likely to be even more potent.

Significance of the Clinical Problem

Obesity is a worldwide health problem that is linked to reduced life expectancy and multiple comorbidities. While the causes of the obesity epidemic are multifactorial, they involve some combination of genetic predisposition with environmental forces, which are immutable risk factors for most people. However, a desire to lose weight is one of the most common patient concerns in clinical medicine. Excessive adiposity leads to an increased risk of cardiometabolic complications, including dyslipidemia, hypertension, nonalcoholic steatosis, insulin resistance, and type 2 diabetes mellitus (T2DM). The World Health Organization has reported a 3-fold increase in the prevalence of obesity in adults in the last 50 years. Even more concerning is that the rate of obesity in children has increased nearly 5-fold during the same period, foreshadowing how if left unchecked, the current rates of obesity will continue to accelerate.

Barriers to Optimal Practice

- Lifestyle interventions, primarily diet and exercise, can lead to clinically meaningful weight loss in the short term, but success over periods longer than 1 year is limited.

- Bariatric surgery is currently the most effective mechanism to produce significant, long-term weight loss and to reverse obesity-related comorbidities. However, surgery is limited by access, scalability, and expense.

- Until recently, available drugs for weight loss had only modest efficacy (~5% placebo-corrected weight loss).

Strategies for Diagnosis, Therapy, and/or Management

The Threat of Obesity to Global Health

Obesity, defined as a BMI greater than 30 kg/m^2, now affects more than half the population of the United States. Excess weight places an enormous mechanical and psychological stress on individuals, leading to a number of daily burdens, including osteoarthritis, joint and musculoskeletal pain, impaired body image, low self-esteem, and depression. These alone greatly decrease the quality of life for individuals with obesity. Also of great concern are the numerous comorbidities associated with obesity that lead to an increased risk of death. It is generally estimated that 75% to 86% of persons with T2DM have obesity, with the increased adiposity proposed to increase inflammation, cause insulin resistance, and impair metabolic homeostasis. The combination of obesity and T2DM produces dyslipidemia, hypertension, coagulation defects, and atherosclerosis, greatly increasing the risk of cardiovascular disease.[1] Finally, obesity has been estimated to account for 10% to 20% of all cases of cancer.[2] When considered as a whole, the economic costs of chronic diseases driven by the risk factor of obesity in the United States has been estimated to be $1.72 trillion, or approximately 9% of the gross domestic product. Thus, addressing the rising prevalence of obesity is a pressing need.

Even modest reductions in body weight can have significant impacts on both health and quality of life. Compared with weight-stable individuals, patients who lose 5% to 10% of their body weight show reductions in hemoglobin A$_{1c}$ (0.5%), fasting glycemia (20 mg/dL [1.11 mmol/L]), blood pressure (5 mm Hg), and triglycerides (40 mg/dL [0.45 mmol/L]), as well as increases in HDL cholesterol (5 mg/dL [0.13 mmol/L]).[3] The improvement in these risks factors for cardiovascular disease increases in proportion to the degree of weight loss, demonstrating a linear relationship between reductions in adiposity and improvements in cardiometabolic health. Moreover, weight reductions of approximately 8% lower the risk of all obesity-related cancers by 16%.[4] Thus, even modest reductions in body weight of 5% (~10 to 15 lb [4.5 to 6.8 kg] in the majority of individuals with obesity) can have a significant effect on clinical outcomes. However, given the linear relationship between weight loss and improvements in health, a common target for weight loss proposed by various associations is 10%, with even greater losses in body weight associated with improved metabolic outcomes.

Lifestyle Interventions

Initial actions to combat obesity often start with lifestyle modifications, including reducing caloric intake through diet modifications and enhancing energy expenditure through physical activity. Diet-alone interventions have the greatest effect on weight loss, with physical activity-alone interventions often failing to produce a meaningful decrease in body weight in individuals with obesity.[5] The combination of diet and exercise comprises most nonpharmacological or nonsurgical interventions for the treatment of obesity. Intense lifestyle modifications in the setting of clinical trials, where participants often receive weekly treatment sessions designed to modify both eating and activity habits, have proven to be effective for weight loss. In this setting, patients often consume fewer calories (1200 to 2000 kcal daily, low-fat diet) and engage in 150 minutes per week of physical activity.[6] These lifestyle interventions lead to 7% reductions in body weight, sufficient to produce positive effects on cardiometabolic outcomes. However, it is important to emphasize that these changes are achieved with organized lifestyle modification programs that are biased by high attrition rates and fail to set generalizable outcomes for individuals attempting lifestyle modifications on their own. This is highlighted by the limited efficacy of the organized lifestyle modification programs when examining the long-term effects. Individuals who lose 7% of their body weight while in the program have a high likelihood of rebounding when managing their lifestyle independently, with most study participants returning to their pretrial body weight within 1 to 2 years. Based on the results of clinical trials, it seems unlikely that most individuals with obesity can maintain a reduced body weight solely with lifestyle modifications.

Surgical Interventions

Bariatric surgery is an intervention that provides effective and sustainable weight loss. Longstanding eligibility criteria for bariatric surgery are a BMI greater than 40 kg/m^2 or a BMI greater than 35 kg/m^2 in the presence of comorbidities. These criteria have been challenged in recent years with the demonstration that patients with lower BMI also benefit from surgery. For example, patients with T2DM and a BMI of 30 to 35 kg/m^2 have substantial improvements in glycemic control. Expected weight loss following bariatric surgery is between 20% to 30%, depending on starting BMI and the surgical procedure performed. A 10-year follow-up study of 573 patients undergoing Roux-en-Y gastric bypass averaged 21% weight loss 10 years following the surgery,[7] and only 3% of the participants regained to within 5% of their preoperative weight 10 years after surgery. In a randomized controlled trial of bariatric surgery compared with intensive lifestyle management, patients with T2DM who had gastric bypass or sleeve gastrectomy lost approximately 25% of starting body weight and had 2% reduction of hemoglobin A$_{1c}$, results that were 5-fold greater than in the diet and exercise group.[8] Whether these effects of bariatric surgery to improve diabetes are due to mechanisms beyond weight loss alone has been debated.[9] However, bariatric surgery is not a realistic means to have a major

effect on the obesity problem in the United States. Approximately 250,000 metabolic surgeries are performed annually in the United States, with about half being Roux-en-Y gastric bypass and half being vertical sleeve gastrectomy. Given that more than 30 million American adults have a BMI of 40 kg/m^2 or greater, performing bariatric surgery in this population is currently not feasible. This is without considering the population of the additional 100 million Americans with a BMI greater that 30 kg/m^2 who qualify as candidates for metabolic surgery. Moreover, the surgery requires a multidisciplinary team and comes with additional risks associated with an invasive procedure. Therefore, while surgical intervention for obesity is tremendously effective with proven durability, it fails to be an option for most individuals with obesity who require weight loss.

Pharmacological Interventions

Pharmacotherapy for obesity provides a mechanism to augment weight loss for individuals who do not reach clinical goals (>5% weight loss) with lifestyle modification alone. Early medications that provided weight loss were also found to increase the risk of cardiovascular disease, ultimately conferring more harm than good for overweight individuals. This led to stricter regulatory oversight, requiring current medications to demonstrate significant efficacy and pass cardiovascular safety concerns. Most antiobesity medications target appetite through neuronal networks that control food intake, which has proven to be an effective way to promote weight loss. A brief overview of current obesity drugs is presented below.

Phentermine Plus Topiramate

Approved in 2012, the combination of phentermine plus topiramate is available for persons with a BMI greater than 30 kg/m^2 or a BMI greater than 27 kg/m^2 with at least 1 weight-related comorbidity. The mechanism for phentermine involves increased norepinephrine activity in the CNS that drives a reduction in food intake. It may also act as a sympathomimetic in the periphery to increase energy expenditure. Topiramate decreases food intake through induction of taste aversion. Maximal dosage (15 mg/92 mg daily) efficacy ranges between 8.7% and 9.3% placebo-subtracted weight loss in clinical trials, with metabolic improvements in hypertension, lipids, and fasting glycemia/insulin levels. Common adverse effects include paresthesias, dizziness, constipation, insomnia, and anxiety, which are possibly mitigated with dosage titration.

Bupropion and Naltrexone

Approved is 2014, the combination of bupropion and naltrexone is available for persons with a BMI greater than 30 kg/m² or a BMI greater than 27 kg/m² with at least 1 weight-related comorbidity. Bupropion inhibits the reuptake of dopamine and norepinephrine to increase activity in the CNS and promote satiety. Naltrexone is an antagonist of the opioid receptor that inhibits the feedback loop on anorexigenic neurons that are activated by bupropion, enhancing the efficacy. Maximal dosage (360 mg/32 mg) efficacy was 4.8% placebo-subtracted weight loss in clinical trials, with significant improvements in waist circumference, adiposity, and lipids. Common adverse effects include nausea, constipation, headache, dizziness, and insomnia.

Orlistat

Approved in 1999, orlistat is available for persons with a BMI greater than 30 kg/m² or a BMI greater than 27 kg/m² with at least 1 weight-related comorbidity. It inhibits gastrointestinal lipase activity, decreasing the absorption of dietary fat by up to 30%. During a 2-year randomized, placebo-controlled trial, orlistat (120 mg, 3 times daily) produced 3.1% placebo-subtracted weight loss and led to modest improvements in waist circumference and lipids. Significant adverse effects include gastrointestinal events and deficiency in fat-soluble vitamins.

Liraglutide 3.0 mg

Approved in 2014, liraglutide 3.0 mg is available for persons with a BMI greater than 30 kg/m² or a BMI greater than 27 kg/m² with at least 1 weight-related comorbidity. Liraglutide 3.0 mg is the high-dosage option of the antidiabetes drug liraglutide (1.2/1.8 mg). It is a GLP-1 receptor agonist that activates satiety centers in the CNS to reduce food intake. In a 56-week clinical trial, liraglutide 3.0 mg produced between 4% and 5.2% reductions in placebo-subtracted weight loss. Additional improvements in waist circumference, lipids, hemoglobin A_{1c}, and blood pressure were also demonstrated in clinical trials. Liraglutide 3.0 mg has not undergone a cardiovascular outcomes trial, but liraglutide at the lower dosages (1.2/1.8 mg) has shown a 22% reduction in cardiovascular death and a 15% reduction in all-cause mortality and is approved for cardiovascular prevention in adults with T2DM. In clinical trials, liraglutide 3.0 mg produced meaningful decreases in blood pressure, LDL cholesterol, and triglycerides, along with increases in HDL cholesterol, suggesting a similar effect on cardiovascular outcomes. Adverse effects include nausea, vomiting, and gastrointestinal distress that can be potentially mitigated with dosage-titration.

Semaglutide 2.4 mg

Approved in 2021, semaglutide 2.4 mg is available for persons with a BMI greater than 30 kg/m² or a BMI greater than 27 kg/m² with at least 1 weight-related comorbidity. Semaglutide is a long-acting GLP-1 receptor agonist that is taken weekly (liraglutide is taken daily). The mechanism is similar to that of liraglutide 3.0 mg, where GLP-1 receptor agonism in the CNS promotes reduction in food intake. Clinical trials showed that semaglutide 2.4 mg produced a 10% to 15% reduction in placebo-subtracted weight loss when combined with behavioral therapy over a 68-week period.[10] Semaglutide 2.4 mg produced significant improvements in waist circumference, blood pressure, lipids, and hemoglobin A_{1c}. Cardiovascular outcomes trials are ongoing for semaglutide 2.4 mg (expected completion in 2023); however, the diabetes drug semaglutide 1.0 mg produced significant improvements in major adverse cardiac events. Common adverse effects include nausea and gastrointestinal distress that can be potentially mitigated with dosage-titration.

The Future of Metabolic Pharmacology

Tirzepatide, Eli Lilly

Tirzepatide is a multireceptor agonist for both the GLP-1 receptor and the glucose-dependent insulinotropic polypeptide receptor (GIPR). The metabolic outcomes of tirzepatide were compared with those of semaglutide 1.0 mg in a 40-week, phase-3 clinical trial in persons with T2DM.[11] Semaglutide 1.0 mg produced 6.7% reductions in body weight, while tirzepatide produced 8.5%, 11%, and 13.1% weight loss with 5-, 10-, and 15-mg doses, respectively. This resulted in greater reductions in hemoglobin A_{1c}, fasting glycemia, triglycerides, and VLDL cholesterol when comparing all doses of tirzepatide to semaglutide. All dosages of tirzepatide also produced greater reductions in waist circumference and BMI. A direct comparison to semaglutide 2.4 mg (the dosage of semaglutide used for obesity alone) has not been performed. Cardiovascular outcome trials are currently underway and are expected to be completed in 2024. The mechanism that drives weight loss in response to tirzepatide remains unresolved. There is a reduction in food intake, which has been largely attributed to GLP-1 receptor agonism. In preclinical models, GIPR agonism has been proposed to engage separate CNS networks that limit the nausea in response to GLP-1 receptor agonism. From this, it has been proposed that the combination of GIPR and GLP-1 receptor agonism may produce enhanced efficacy on food intake, but this has yet to be tested in humans. Furthermore, GIPR agonism in adipose tissue has been shown to enhance insulin sensitivity in a weight-independent manner, potentially increasing the efficacy of tirzepatide on glycemia. Adverse effects are similar to those of GLP-1 receptor agonists, with nausea and gastrointestinal distress being predominant. Dosage escalation over a 12-week period has been shown to be effective in producing a more favorable adverse effect profile.

Cagrilintide Plus Semaglutide, Novo Nordisk

Cargrilintide is a long-acting amylin analogue, given in combination with semaglutide 2.4 mg. Both are once-weekly subcutaneous injectables. In a phase 1b clinical trial, the combination of cargrilintide 2.4 mg and semaglutide 2.4 mg given for 20 weeks to overweight individuals (BMI >27 kg/m^2) produced a 17.1% reduction in body weight, compared with a 9.8% reduction for semaglutide 2.4 mg alone.[12] Native amylin is cosecreted with insulin and has been shown to reduce gastric emptying, inhibit postprandial glucagon secretion, and suppress food intake in the CNS. Amylin has also been proposed to regulate food preferences in the CNS. Given alone to individuals with obesity, high dosages of cargrilintide (4.5 mg) reduced body weight by 10.8% over a 26-week period. The mechanism that drives the additive effects on weight loss with the combination of cargrilintide and semaglutide remains unknown, but likely stems from enhanced activation of food suppression in the CNS. There were increased reports of nausea and vomiting in the combination therapy group vs the semaglutide alone group, supporting the notion of additive effects on CNS activity. Overall, adverse effects were modestly increased relative to semaglutide 2.4, supporting further pursuit of this intervention.

Glucagon Agonism

Currently, the most effective pharmacological agents for obesity primarily target the CNS to reduce food intake. The combination of reduced food intake along with interventions that enhance energy expenditure may provide additional efficacy for weight loss. Multiple interests have pursued glucagon receptor (GCGR) agonism to enhance energy expenditure. Glucagon drives numerous catabolic effects in hepatocytes, including enhanced metabolism of carbohydrates, lipids, and amino acids. There is some evidence to suggest that glucagon agonism may also enhance thermogenesis in adipose tissue. The notion that GCGR agonism also enhances endogenous glucose production is a concern for individuals with obesity who are often hyperglycemic or present with T2DM. Thus, GCGR agonism has often been paired with GLP-1 receptor agonism to mitigate the hyperglycemic effects, and in some cases, triple agonisms for the GCGR, the GLP-1 receptor, and the GIPR are being investigated. Glucagon/GLP-1 coagonism is often derived from either engineered peptides with activity at both receptors or derivatives of oxyntomodulin, a naturally occurring agonist for both receptors. There are multiple ongoing clinical trials for the glucagon/GLP-1 coagonists, with only a few published results. Many early combinations were discontinued due to unacceptable safety profiles or lack of efficacy. However, some of these compounds have provided impressive effects on weight loss. Analogue 17 (Altimmune) is a balanced glucagon/GLP-1 compound that produced 10.3% reduction in body weight over a 12-week period. Cotadutide, a separate balance glucagon/GLP-1 agonist, produced 5% reduction in body weight over a 52-week period, and LY3305677, an oxyntomodulin derivative, produced 6% reduction in body weight over a 12-week period. Thus, individual therapies have varied outcome efficacy. Combinations with GIPR agonism are also being pursued, with multiple companies investigating GLP-1/GIP/glucagon triagonists. This combination therapy has yielded impressive effects on body weight in preclinical models, with phase 1 and 2 clinical trials currently ongoing. Overall, the combination of GCGR agonism with GLP-1/GIP activity shows early promising effects on body weight and the associated metabolic outcomes.

Clinical Case Vignettes

Case 1

A 67-year-old man presents for help with weight loss. He has degenerative joint disease in both knees with limited ability to ambulate and pain that disturbs his sleep. The orthopedic surgeon who is caring for him wants him to achieve a BMI less than 35 kg/m² because evidence suggests this will decrease his risk for postoperative complications. His current weight is 273 lb (BMI = 38 kg/m²). Since his wife died 2 years ago, he has been preparing his own meals but eats at restaurants half the time. To help him qualify for surgery quickly, you choose medical management.

Which of the following options is the best choice?

A. Dulaglutide

B. Liraglutide

C. Semaglutide, injectable

D. Semaglutide, oral

E. Whatever his health insurance will cover

Answer: C) Semaglutide, injectable

Injectable semaglutide (Answer C) is the most potent medical agent available for weight loss, especially the 2.4 mg dosage. This man needs aggressive treatment to help him meet his surgeon's criteria for knee replacement. Oral semaglutide (Answer D), dulaglutide (Answer A), or liraglutide (Answer B) is unlikely to result in the 25-lb (11.3-kg) weight loss that it will take to lower his BMI to 35 kg/m². However, with injectable semaglutide, this degree of weight loss is realistic. Unfortunately, GLP-1 receptor agonists are very expensive and for long-term treatment, cost concerns are an important consideration in choosing drugs. However, for the 4 to 6 months that this man will require treatment, efficacy is probably the deciding factor (thus, Answer E is incorrect).

Case 2

A 55-year-old woman is referred for help with weight loss. Her BMI has been greater than 30 kg/m² since the birth of her third child 24 years ago, and her weight has steadily increased. Her current weight is 232 lb (105.2 kg). She has treated hypertension and stage 3 chronic kidney disease with an estimated glomerular filtration rate of 50 to 60 mL/min per 1.73 m², but no other major morbidities. She has tried multiple diets over the years with varied success, but these have ultimately not changed her long-term weight trajectory. You decide to treat her with a GLP-1 receptor agonist, and the preferred choice on her insurance formulary is liraglutide.

Which of the following adverse effects is LEAST LIKELY to occur with a course of liraglutide, 3.0 mg daily?

A. Cholelithiasis

B. Diarrhea

C. Increased heart rate

D. Nephrolithiasis

E. Vomiting

Answer: D) Nephrolithiasis

The most common adverse effects of GLP-1 receptor agonists are gastrointestinal: nausea, vomiting, and diarrhea. Patients taking liraglutide and semaglutide have also been reported to have more cholelithiasis and episodes of clinical gall bladder disease. GLP-1 receptor agonists are typically associated with an increase in heart rate of 3 to 5 beats/min, but greater increases have been reported. GLP-1 receptor agonists can cause dehydration, mostly with initiation and gastrointestinal adverse effects. This can be of a sufficient magnitude to cause acute kidney injury, but increased rates of nephrolithiasis have not been reported (thus, Answer D is correct).

References

1. Van Gaal LF, Mertens IL, De Block CE. Mechanisms linking obesity with cardiovascular disease. *Nature*. 2006;444(7121):875-880. PMID: 17167476

2. Lauby-Secretan B, Scoccianti C, Loomis D, et al; International Agency for Research on Cancer Handbook Working Group. Body fatness and cancer--viewpoint of the IARC Working Group. *N Engl J Med*. 2016;375(8):794-798. PMID: 27557308

3. Wing RR, Lang W, Wadden TA, et al; Look AHEAD Research Group. Benefits of modest weight loss in improving cardiovascular risk factors in overweight and obese individuals with type 2 diabetes. *Diabetes Care*. 2011;34(7):1481-1486. PMID: 21593294

4. Look AHEAD Research Group, Yeh H-C, Bantle JP, et al. Intensive weight loss intervention and cancer risk in adults with type 2 diabetes: analysis of the Look AHEAD Randomized Clinical Trial. *Obesity (Silver Spring)*. 2020;28(9):1678-1686. PMID: 32841523

5. Stephens SK, Cobiac LJ, Veerman JL. Improving diet and physical activity to reduce population prevalence of overweight and obesity: an overview of current evidence. *Prev Med*. 2014;62:167-178. PMID: 24534460

6. Knowler WC, Barrett-Connor E, Fowler SE, et al; Diabetes Prevention Program Research Group. Reduction in the incidence of type 2 diabetes with lifestyle intervention or metformin. *N Engl J Med*. 2002;346(6):393-403. PMID: 11832527

7. Maciejewski ML, Arterburn DE, Van Scoyoc L, et al. Bariatric surgery and long-term durability of weight loss. *JAMA Surg*. 2016;151(11):1046-1055. PMID: 27579793

8. Schauer PR, Bhatt DL, Kirwan JP, et al; STAMPEDE Investigators. Bariatric surgery versus intensive medical therapy for diabetes - 5-year outcomes. *N Engl J Med*. 2017;376(7):641-651. PMID: 28199805

9. Yoshino M, Kayser BD, Yoshino J, et al. Effects of diet versus gastric bypass on metabolic function in diabetes. *N Engl J Med*. 2020;383(8):721-732. PMID: 32813948

10. Wilding JPH, Batterham RL, Calanna S, et al; STEP 1 Study Group. Once-weekly semaglutide in adults with overweight or obesity. *N Engl J Med*. 2021;384(11):989. PMID: 33567185

11. Frias JP, Davies MJ, Rosenstock J, et al; SURPASS-2 Investigators. Tirzepatide versus semaglutide once weekly in patients with type 2 diabetes. *N Engl J Med*. 2021;385(6):503-515. PMID: 34170647

12. Enebo LB, Berthelsen KK, Kankam M, et al. Safety, tolerability, pharmacokinetics, and pharmacodynamics of concomitant administration of multiple doses of cagrilintide with semaglutide 2.4 mg for weight management: a randomised, controlled, phase 1b trial. *Lancet*. 2021;397(10286):1736-1748. PMID: 33894838

Long-Term Follow-Up of Bariatric Surgery in Adolescents

Ilene Fennoy, MD, MPH. Department of Pediatrics, Division of Pediatric Endocrinology, Diabetes, and Metabolism, New York, NY; E-mail: lf1@cumc.columbia.edu

Learning Objectives

As a result of participating in this session, learners should be able to:

- Identify clinical implications for long-term health in adolescents with severe obesity.

- Identify the magnitude of BMI change expected from bariatric surgical procedures.

- Identify the metabolic parameters shown to improve postbariatric interventions, as well as how psychopathology problems change.

- Identify key nutritional deficiencies known to occur after bariatric surgery.

Main Conclusions

Severe obesity in adolescents is associated with comorbidities that increase in prevalence as the severity of the obesity increases. Bariatric surgery results in variable changes in BMI dependent on the specific surgical procedure performed, but it leads to an overall average decrease of -13.5 kg/m^2 (95% CI, -15.1 to -11.9 kg/m^2) 1 year after the procedure. Weight regain often occurs after bariatric surgery, but patients remain, on average, significantly below their presurgical weight.

Inconsistency exists in the reporting of comorbidities. Improvements have been shown across studies evaluating prediabetes, diabetes, dyslipidemia, and hypertension. Additionally, at least 1 report has documented biopsy-proven improvement in hepatic steatosis, and another has demonstrated improvement in kidney function for patients with abnormalities at baseline. Both pseudotumor cerebri and obstructive sleep apnea improve with weight loss after bariatric procedures in adolescents. Although health-related quality of life (HRQoL) improvements are well documented, psychiatric disorders are more variable in their response and frequently require ongoing postsurgical treatment.

Nutritional deficiencies do occur, with low values for vitamin B_{12}, iron, and vitamin D frequently identified, particularly after Roux-en-Y gastric bypass (RYGB).

Significance of the Clinical Problem

Obesity, defined as a BMI ≥95th percentile, and severe obesity, defined as a BMI ≥120% of the 95th percentile, has continued to increase among children aged 2 to 19 years, with recent data demonstrating an increase from 13.9% between 1999 and 2000 to 19.3% between 2017 and 2018. The prevalence of severe obesity increased from 3.6% to 6.1% during this same period.[1] As of 2015/2016, obesity was present in 20.6% of 12- to 19-year-olds, and severe obesity was present in 7.7% of this age group.[2] Bariatric surgery in adolescence has become an expanding intervention to address this rise in severe obesity, particularly as recent studies now demonstrate that patients with severe obesity are not always successful with lifestyle interventions.[3]

Guidelines from the American Society of Metabolic and Bariatric Surgery[4] and the American Academy of Pediatrics[5,6] support bariatric surgery as appropriate for adolescents based on the definition of severe obesity as ≥120% of the 95th percentile in a patient with comorbidities or ≥140% of the 95th percentile in a patient without comorbidities. These comorbidities include type 2 diabetes, obstructive sleep apnea, nonalcoholic fatty liver disease, idiopathic intracranial hypertension, orthopedic disease (particularly slipped capital femoral epiphysis and Blount disease), gastroesophageal reflux, and hypertension. Prevalence of these comorbidities has been shown to increase as the severity of obesity increases.[7] Adolescents with severe obesity also report low HRQoL; mental health disturbances; and disordered eating encompassing loss-of-control eating, binge eating, bulimia, and night eating syndrome.[4,5]

In the adolescent population, frequency of surgical procedures, however, has slowly increased from 0.8 per 100,000 in 2000 to 2.4 per 100,000 in 2009,[8] and recently more rapidly to 22.7 per 100,000 in 2017.[9] Sleeve gastrectomy (SG) has become the most common bariatric procedure in the United States[10] and in adolescents in New York state.[11] Outcomes have been described both in terms of weight loss and resolution of comorbidities over varied periods.

Barriers to Optimal Practice

- Limited availability of comprehensive adolescent bariatric surgery programs.
- Poor reimbursement for obesity care.
- Incomplete long-term follow-up data.

Strategies for Diagnosis, Therapy, and/or Management
Outcomes
Black et al conducted a meta-analysis in 2013 that evaluated 23 studies including a total of 637 patients, ages 12 to 19 years, with reported baseline BMIs of 52.4, 49.6, and 49.6 kg/m^2 for patients undergoing RYGB, adjustable gastric banding (AGB), and SG, respectively.[12] Four of the 23 articles had follow-up of 24 to 36 months, but the remaining studies had follow-up limited to approximately 12 months. Mean BMI change at 12 months for all procedures was −13.5 kg/m^2 (95% CI, −15.1 to −11.9 kg/m^2). Mean BMI change was −17.2 kg/m^2 (95% CI, −20.1 to −14.3 kg/m^2) for RYGB; −14.1 kg/m^2 (95% CI, −17.3 to −11.7 kg/m^2) for SG; and −10.5 kg/m^2 (95% CI, −11.8 to −9.1 kg/m^2) for AGB.[12] This early meta-analysis described inconsistency in reporting of comorbidity definitions and resolution in the various studies, and only 1 study reported on significant numbers of patients with comorbidities in which dyslipidemia was moderately improved.

More recently, Pedroso et al provided a systematic literature review and meta-analysis through 2016 of weight-loss outcomes in adolescents and adults younger than 21 years from 24 studies spanning follow-up periods of 6, 12, 24, and 36 months postoperatively.[13] This study reviewed 1928 patients, of whom 1010 had AGB, 139 had SG, and 779 had RYGB. The observed mean change in BMI at 6 months was −5.4 kg/m^2 (95% CI, −3.0 to −7.8 kg/m^2) for AGB, −11.5 kg/m^2 (95% CI, −8.8 to −14.2 kg/m^2) for SG, and −18.8 kg/m^2 (95% CI, −10.9 to −26.6 kg/m^2) for RYGB. At 24 months, nadir BMI was −11.69 kg/m^2 (95% CI, −10.33 to −13.04 kg/m^2) for AGB and −27.63 kg/m^2 (95% CI, −21.56 to −33.70 kg/m^2) for RYGB, with patients in both groups showing weight regain by 36 months such that BMI change from baseline was −10.34 kg/m^2 (95% CI, −6.95 to −13.94 kg/m^2) for AGB and −15.00 kg/m^2 (95% CI, −13.50 to −16.50 kg/m^2) for RYGB. No data were reported for SG at 24 months, but 12-month and 36-month data were similar, with mean BMI change of −13.05 kg/m^2 (95% CI, −9.68 to −16.42 kg/m^2) for SG at 12 months and −13.00 kg/m^2 (95% CI, −11.00 to −15.00 kg/m^2) at 36 months. Comorbidities were not addressed in this review.

One author has published 1-year biopsy outcome data on the effect of bariatric surgery in nonalcoholic steatohepatitis and hepatic fibrosis. In this study, 20 participants had SG with baseline liver biopsy and repeated biopsy at 12 months.[14] Using histological criteria for grading steatosis, inflammation and portal inflammation, ballooning, and fibrosis, the authors were able to demonstrate improvement in all markers of nonalcoholic liver disease in association with the SG procedure compared with a similar number of patients undergoing treatment with intragastric weight-loss devices and 53 nonsurgical weight-loss patients. Only patients who underwent SG experienced significant weight loss, with a decline in weight and BMI of 21.5% and 20.6%, respectively, at 12 months.

Several authors have evaluated pediatric patients with pseudotumor cerebri who underwent bariatric surgery. Follow-up was of 6 to 18 months' duration with a very small number of patients reported as case reports. Sugerman et al described 3 adolescents who underwent gastroplasty or gastric bypass with resolution of pseudotumor cerebri 1 year after surgery.[15] Chandra et al described 1 patient with resolution 6 months after RYGB associated with 43% excess weight loss[16] and Hoang et al described 3 patients, 2 of whom had resolution 18 months after SG.[17]

Bariatric surgery has also been reported to relieve obstructive sleep apnea in adolescents. Kaar et al identified 81 patients (mean age 16.9 years), of whom 54% had obstructive sleep apnea based on an apnea hypopnea index of 5 or greater.[18] Only 23 were available for follow-up, of whom 66% had remission 5 months after surgery. Resolution of sleep apnea was not associated with amount of weight loss during the first year after surgery, but it was associated with lower presurgical weight. Similar results were found by Kalra et al in reviewing data of adolescents who underwent RYGB with a mean decrease in BMI of 19 kg/m^2 6 months after surgery.[19] All 10 patients evaluated postoperatively demonstrated improvement or resolution of obstructive sleep apnea.

Data have accumulated regarding 3-year outcomes for both RYGB and SG. In 2015,

Inge et al reported 3-year outcomes of RYGB and SG in 242 adolescents from 5 centers in the United States.[20] Mean BMI was 53 kg/m^2 with a mean decrease of –15 kg/m^2 (95% CI, –16 to –13 kg/m^2) overall at 3 years. The mean BMI decrease was –15 kg/m^2 (95% CI, –17 to –14 kg/m^2) in the RYGB group and –13 kg/m^2 (95% CI, –15 to –11 kg/m^2) in the SG group. At 3 years, only 26% of the patients still had obesity. However, 2% of those undergoing RYGB and 4% of those undergoing SG had regained above baseline weight at 3 years. Comorbidities also demonstrated improvement. Of the 96 patients with hypertension, 74% had resolution by 3 years and only 4 incident cases occurred among the 98 patients with normal blood pressure at baseline. Of 171 patients with dyslipidemia, 66% had resolution by 3 years without lipid-lowering medications and only 3 incident cases occurred among the 39 patients without lipid abnormalities at baseline. Nineteen of 20 patients with type 2 diabetes demonstrated remission at 3 years with a mean hemoglobin A_{1c} value of 5.3% (34 mmol/mol) and fasting blood glucose of concentration of 88 mg/dL (4.9 mmol/L). Prediabetes, defined as a hemoglobin A_{1c} value of 5.7% or greater (≥39 mmol/mol) and less than 6.5% (<48 mmol/mol) or fasting blood glucose concentration of 100 mg/dL or greater (≥5.6 mmol/L) and less than 126 mg/dL (<7.0 mmol/L) occurred in 19 patients at baseline. Prediabetes resolved in 76% of these patients at 3 years with 1 incident case occurring. Thirty-six of 212 patients (17%) had abnormal kidney function at baseline, with 19 of 22 patients demonstrating resolution at 3 years. Ferritin concentrations were low at baseline in 11 of 225 patients (5%) and were low at 3 years in 98 of 171 patients (57%), with a significant increase in low concentrations in patients who underwent either RYGB or SG. Vitamin B_{12} showed a similar significant trend, with 1 of 222 patients (<1%) having low values at baseline and 13 of 160 patients (8%) having low values at 3 years. Low albumin, folate, and vitamin D at baseline demonstrated no significant change at 3 years. Prevalence of high transferrin concentrations at baseline significantly increased in patients undergoing RYGB but not in patients undergoing SG.

In a nationwide Swedish study of adolescents aged 13 to 18 years who underwent bariatric surgery (RYGB), 81 patients were matched against a control group receiving conventional therapy and against adults aged 35 to 45 years undergoing RYGB.[21] Patients were evaluated 5 years after surgery. Control patients entered the conventional weight-loss program within 1 month of the bariatric surgery date and were evaluated 5 years later. Baseline BMI was greater in both adolescent and adult surgical patients compared with BMI in the control group. At 5 years, mean BMI was -13.1 kg/m^2 (95% CI, -14.5 to -11.8) in adolescents, -12.7 kg/m^2 (95% CI, -13.7 to -10.9) in adults, and $+3.3$ kg/m^2 (95% CI, $+1.1$ to $+4.8$) in the control group. Seventy-two percent and 76% of adolescent and adult surgical patients, respectively, reached a BMI less than 35 kg/m^2. Only 7% of the control group achieved a BMI less than 35 kg/m^2. Thirty-seven percent of adolescents and 40% of adults no longer had obesity, with only 3% of the control group achieving this status. Most surgical patients achieved 20% or greater weight loss (69% of adolescents and 85% of adults) while 69% of control patients gained weight. Nadir weight occurred at 2 years with similar weight regain by 5 years in both adolescents and adults, approximating a 10% rise over nadir BMI.

This Swedish study reported improvement in multiple metabolic parameters.[21] Measurements of glucose homeostasis at 5 years in the surgical group demonstrated remission of type 2 diabetes at 5 years in all patients who had diabetes at study initiation. At baseline, 27% of the surgical groups had prediabetes, which resolved in 86% at 5 years, and 2 new cases developed. The control group demonstrated a 5-year prevalence of prediabetes of 16% with 1 new case reported. Dyslipidemia prevalence decreased in surgical patients from 69% to 15%, while the control group manifested a 5-year prevalence of 73%. The prevalence of elevated C-reactive protein, alanine aminotransferase, and blood pressure decreased in the surgical group and was persistent or increased in the control group.

Nutritional disorders of vitamin B$_{12}$, iron deficiency, and vitamin D insufficiency increased in the surgical group compared with the control group.

HRQoL was also evaluated in this Swedish study using the SF-36 short form and the Obesity Related Problem Scale.[21] The physical summary component of the SF-36 showed improvement among adolescents in the domains of physical role functioning, general health-related perceptions and physical functioning. The physical role functioning domain was better in the surgical group than in the control group. Surgical patients also had improvement in weight-related psychosocial problems. Further exploration of mental health issues in this cohort has demonstrated similar proportions of patients prescribed psychiatric drugs before and after surgery compared with the control group.[22] Although treatment for mental health and behavioral disorders did not differ before surgery, the surgical group received more specialized therapy for a mental health disorder after surgery compared with the control group. Self-esteem and binge-eating improved in surgical patients, whereas mood did not. Binge eating was not related to degree of weight loss.[22] Zeller reported similar findings in a cohort of 14 adolescents undergoing RYGB with improvements in HRQoL overall, but with similar proportions remitting or requiring ongoing psychiatric support 6 years after surgery.[23]

A systematic review of bariatric surgery procedures in adolescents documented consistent improvement in HRQoL at 2 years across multiple studies irrespective of surgical procedure.[24] Physical functioning most consistently improved, with less effectiveness demonstrated for emotional and mental health functioning. Depressive symptoms were most improved at 6 to 9 months with some deterioration thereafter.[24]

Loss-of-control eating is reported to be more common in obese and overweight adolescents,[25] with eating disorders being prevalent among adolescents before bariatric surgery.[26] Higher measures of loss-of-control eating are associated with less successful weight loss.[27] However, a decrease in loss-of-control eating has been associated with weight-loss interventions both in a systematic review involving 20 of 21 studies using behavioral, pharmacotherapy, and surgical interventions over variable periods,[27] as well as in the Teen-LABS study. In the Teen-LABS study, prevalence of loss-of-control eating over 6 years after bariatric surgery declined from 32.4% presurgically to 7.9% 1 year after surgery, with a rise to 14.5% 4 years after surgery, then a decline to 11.5% 6 years after surgery.[28]

In an 8-year follow-up of 58 of 74 patients undergoing RYGB, Inge et al reported outcomes of patients who had surgery at a mean age of 17 years with a mean presurgery BMI of 58.5 kg/m². [29] At follow-up, mean BMI was 41.7 kg/m². The prevalence of hypertension decreased from 47% to 16%, dyslipidemia from 86% to 38%, and type 2 diabetes from 16% to 2%. Mild anemia was present in 46%, hyperparathyroidism in 45%, and low vitamin B_{12} in 16%.

Conclusion

Currently, data regarding long-term follow-up of bariatric surgery in adolescents beyond 5 years are limited to patients who underwent RYBG. The 3-year outcome data available for SG, the most common procedure currently performed, are not as robust as the outcome data for bypass surgery. From the weight-loss point of view, despite a greater than 10 kg/m² BMI decline, most patients still have obesity after bariatric surgery, although metabolic abnormalities and HRQoL substantially improve. Nutritional deficiencies noted at baseline for vitamin D, albumin, and folate were noted to be unchanged at 3 years by Inge et al, with vitamin B_{12} deficiency increasing after both SG and RYGB. Deficiencies of iron, vitamin B_{12}, and vitamin D have been described 5 years after RYGB. In another study, anemia, low vitamin B_{12}, and hyperparathyroidism have been reported 8 years after RYGB. Mental health problems remain in patients after bariatric surgery and require ongoing intervention. Although outcomes reported to date are favorable for both weight loss and comorbidity resolution 3 to 5 years after bariatric surgery, additional data are needed for outcomes at longer time points and with consistent reporting across comorbidities.

Clinical Case Vignettes
Case 1

A 10-year-old boy with a history of weight problems since age 5 or 6 years presents for weight-loss management. His height is 59.0 in (149.8 cm), and weight is 163.8 lb (74.3 kg) (BMI = 33.1 kg/m² [149% of the 95th percentile]). Screening for obesity comorbidities documents that he has low HDL cholesterol. Abdominal ultrasonography shows an enlarged, echogenic liver.

Which of the following interventions is most likely to successfully help this patient lose weight?

A. Lifestyle interventions

B. Bariatric surgery

Answer: B) Bariatric surgery

With respect to lifestyle interventions (Answer A), Barlow et al recently demonstrated minimal weight loss at 3 months in patients with severe obesity (>120% of the 95th percentile) compared with those with modest obesity (110% of the 95th percentile), followed by significant weight gain at 12 months in patients with severe obesity compared with weight returning to just below baseline in those with modest obesity.[3] This is in stark contrast to bariatric surgery interventions (Answer B) that result in significant weight loss at 12 months.

Case 1 (continued)

The patient participates in lifestyle interventions over the next 3 years, during which time he is noted to gain weight. His BMI is 47.8 kg/m² at age 14 years. He is referred to an adolescent bariatric surgery program. Dyslipidemia and an enlarged, echogenic liver persist, but liver enzyme levels are normal. The patient now has mild systolic hypertension (blood pressure = 132/73 mm Hg

[94th percentile; 78th percentile for age and height]). He undergoes vertical SG.

How much change in BMI is expected by 1 year after surgery?

A. −6 kg/m²
B. −13 kg/m²
C. −18 kg/m²
D. −23 kg/m²

Answer: B) −13 kg/m²

Average BMI change after SG is approximately −13 kg/m² (95% CI, −11 to −17 kg/m²) (Answer B),[11,12] whereas AGB results in a smaller degree of weight loss and RYGB results in a greater degree of weight loss.[11,12,14]

Case 1 (continued)

One year after bariatric surgery, his BMI is 30.5 kg/m².

Three to 5 years after bariatric surgery, his BMI would be expected to fall into which of the following ranges?

A. 35-40 kg/m²
B. >40 kg/m²
C. 30-35 kg/m²
D. <30 kg/m²

Answer: C) 30-35 kg/m²

Patients usually reach their nadir weight 1 to 2 years after bariatric procedures, with some rebound thereafter.[12,14] In this patient, baseline BMI was 47.8 kg/m² with a BMI decline of −17 kg/m² at 1 year. Given the rebound that usually occurs and the data suggesting BMI at 3 years is near the BMI at 1 year, one might expect his BMI to be approximately 30 to 35 kg/m² (Answer C) at 3 years.

Case 2

An 8.9-year-old old girl with a history of progressive obesity since age 3 to 4 years presents for weight management. Her height is 58.6 in (149 cm), and weight is 128.5 lb (58.3 kg) (BMI = 26.9 kg/m² [123% of the 95th percentile]). She has a history of Chiari 1 malformation status post suboccipital decompression at age 6 years, migraine headaches, pseudotumor cerebri, obstructive sleep apnea, chronic abdominal pain of unknown origin, anxiety, and obsessive-compulsive behavior. Despite ongoing dietary intervention, family therapy, and psychologic counseling, her weight continues to rise, and she undergoes bariatric surgery at age 10 years. Weight loss after surgery is excellent, with her BMI declining to 16.23 kg/m² (34th percentile) 1 year after surgery.

Which of the following comorbidities would be expected to have resolved at 1 year with successful weight loss?

A. Anxiety and obsessive-compulsive behavior
B. Obstructive sleep apnea
C. Pseudotumor cerebri
D. A and C
E. B and C
F. All of the above

Answer: E) B and C

Both pseudotumor cerebri (Answer C) and obstructive sleep apnea (Answer B) have been demonstrated to resolve[16] or improve in the first year after surgery.[15-18] Mental health issues persist in a significant number of patients and may require ongoing psychiatric intervention.

Case 2 (continued)

Given her BMI of 16.93 kg/m² (34th percentile), should one be concerned that she has developed an eating disorder?

A. Yes
B. No

Answer: B) No

Eating disorders are associated with obesity and are common in patients presenting for bariatric surgery.[26] However, their prevalence typically decreases postsurgically and, when they remain, they are associated with poor weight loss.[27]

References

1. QuickStats: prevalence of obesity* and severe obesity† among persons aged 2-19 years - National Health and Nutrition Examination Survey, 1999-2000 through 2017-2018. *MMWR Morb Mortal Wkly Rep.* 2020;69(13):390. PMID: 32240130

2. Hales CM, Fryar CD, Carroll MD, Freedman DS, Ogden CL. Trends in obesity and severe obesity prevalence in US youth and adults by sex and age, 2007-2008 to 2015-2016. *JAMA.* 2018;319(16):1723-1725. PMID: 29570750

3. Barlow SE, Durand C, Salahuddin M, Pont SJ, Butte NF, Hoelscher DM. Who benefits from the intervention? Correlates of successful BMI reduction in the Texas Childhood Obesity Demonstration Project (TX-CORD). *Pediatr Obes.* 2020;15(5):e12609. PMID: 31944617

4. Pratt JSA, Browne A, Browne NT, et al. ASMBS pediatric metabolic and bariatric surgery guidelines, 2018. *Surg Obes Relat Dis.* 2018;14(7):882-901. PMID: 30077361

5. Armstrong SC, Bolling CF, Michalsky MP, Reichard KW, Section on Obesity, Section on Surgery. Pediatric metabolic and bariatric surgery: evidence, barriers, and best practices. *Pediatrics.* 2019;144(6):e20193223. PMID: 31656225

6. Bolling CF, Armstrong SC, Reichard KW, Michalsky MP. Metabolic and bariatric surgery for pediatric patients with severe obesity. *Pediatrics.* 2019;144(6):e20193224. PMID: 31656226

7. Kelly AS, Barlow SE, Rao G, et al. Severe obesity in children and adolescents: identification, associated health risks, and treatment approaches: a scientific statement from the American Heart Association. *Circulation.* 2013;128(15):1689-1712. PMID: 24016455

8. Kelleher DC, Merrill CT, Cottrell LT, Nadler EP, Burd RS. Recent national trends in the use of adolescent inpatient bariatric surgery: 2000 through 2009. *JAMA Pediatr.* 2013;167(2):126-132. PMID: 23247297

9. Bouchard ME, Tian Y, Linton S, et al. Utilization trends and disparities in adolescent bariatric surgery in the United States 2009-2017. *Child Obes.* 2021 [Online ahead of print] PMID: 34647817

10. English WJ, DeMaria EJ, Hutter MM, et al. American Society for Metabolic and Bariatric Surgery 2018 estimate of metabolic and bariatric procedures performed in the United States. *Surg Obes Relat Dis.* 2020;16(4):457-463. PMID: 32029370

11. Humayon S, Altieri MS, Yang J, Nie L, Spaniolas K, Pryor AD. Recent trends of bariatric surgery in adolescent population in the state of New York. *Surg Obes Relat Dis.* 2019;15(8):1388-1393. PMID: 31262649

12. Black JA, White B, Viner RM, Simmons RK. Bariatric surgery for obese children and adolescents: a systematic review and meta-analysis. *Obes Rev.* 2013;14(8):634-644. PMID: 23577666

13. Pedroso FE, Angriman F, Endo A et al. Weight loss after bariatric surgery in obese adolescents: a systematic review and meta-analysis. *Surg Obes Relat Dis.* 2018;14(3):413-422. PMID: 29248351

14. Manco M, Mosca A, De Peppo F, et al. The benefit of sleeve gastrectomy in obese adolescents on nonalcoholic steatohepatitis and hepatic fibrosis. *J Pediatr.* 2017;180:31-37.e2. PMID: 27697327

15. Sugerman HJ, Sugerman EL, DeMaria EJ, et al. Bariatric surgery for severely obese adolescents. *J Gastrointest Surg.* 2003;7(1):102-108. PMID: 12559191

16. Chandra V, Dutta S, Albanese CT, et al. Clinical resolution of severely symptomatic pseudotumor cerebri after gastric bypass in an adolescent. *Surg Obes Relat Dis.* 2007;3(2):198-200. PMID: 17324634

17. Hoang KB, Hooten KG, Muh CR. Shunt freedom and clinical resolution of idiopathic intracranial hypertension after bariatric surgery in the pediatric population: report of 3 cases. *J Neurosurg Pediatr.* 2017;20(6):511-516. PMID: 28960170

18. Kaar JL, Morelli N, Russell SP, et al. Obstructive sleep apnea and early weight loss among adolescents undergoing bariatric surgery. *Surg Obes Relat Dis.* 2021;17(4):711-717. PMID: 33478907

19. Kalra M, Inge T, Garcia V, et al. Obstructive sleep apnea in extremely overweight adolescents undergoing bariatric surgery. *Obesity Res.* 2005;13(7):1175-1179. PMID: 16076986

20. Inge TH, Courcoulas AP, Jenkins TM, et al; Teen-LABS Consortium. Weight loss and health status 3 years after bariatric surgery in adolescents. *N Engl J Med.* 2015;374(2):113-123. PMID: 26544725

21. Olbers T, Beamish AJ, Gronowitz E, et al. Laparoscopic Roux-en-Y gastric bypass in adolescents with severe obesity (AMOS): a prospective, 5-year, Swedish nationwide study. *Lancet Diabetes Endocrinol.* 2017;5(3):174-183. PMID: 28065734

22. Jarvholm K, Bruze G, Peltonen M, et al. 5-year mental health and eating pattern outcomes following bariatric surgery in adolescents: a prospective cohort study. *Lancet Child Adolesc Health.* 2020;4(3):210-219. PMID: 31978372

23. Zeller MH, Pendery EC, Reiter-Purtill J, et al. From adolescence to young adulthood: trajectories of psychosocial health following Roux-en-Y gastric bypass. *Surg Obes Relat Dis.* 2017;13(7):1196-1203. PMID: 28465159

24. White B, Doyle J, Colville S, Nicholls D, Viner RM, Christie D. Systematic review of psychological and social outcomes of adolescents undergoing bariatric surgery, and predictors of success. *Clin Obes.* 2015;5(6):312-324. PMID: 26541244

25. He J, Cai Z, Fan X. Prevalence of binge and loss of control eating among children and adolescents with overweight and obesity: an exploratory meta-analysis. *Int J Eat Disord.* 2017;50(2):91-103. PMID: 28039879

26. Kim RJ, Langer JM, Baker AW, Filter DE, Williams NN, Sarwer DB. Psychosocial status in adolescents undergoing bariatric surgery. *Obes Surg.* 2008;18(1):27-33. PMID: 18085345

27. Moustafa AF, Quigley KM, Wadden TA, Berkowitz RI, Chao AM. A systematic review of binge eating, loss of control eating, and weight loss in children and adolescents. *Obesity Res.* 2021;29(8):1259-1271. PMID: 34227229

28. Goldschmidt AB, Khoury J, Jenkins TM, et al. Adolescent loss-of-control eating and weight loss maintenance after bariatric surgery. *Pediatrics.* 2018;141(1):e20171659. PMID: 29237801

29. Inge TH, Jenkins TM, Xanthakos SA, et al. Long-term outcomes of bariatric surgery in adolescents with severe obesity (FABS-5+): a prospective follow-up analysis. *Lancet Diabetes Endocrinol.* 2017;5(3):165-173. PMID: 28065736

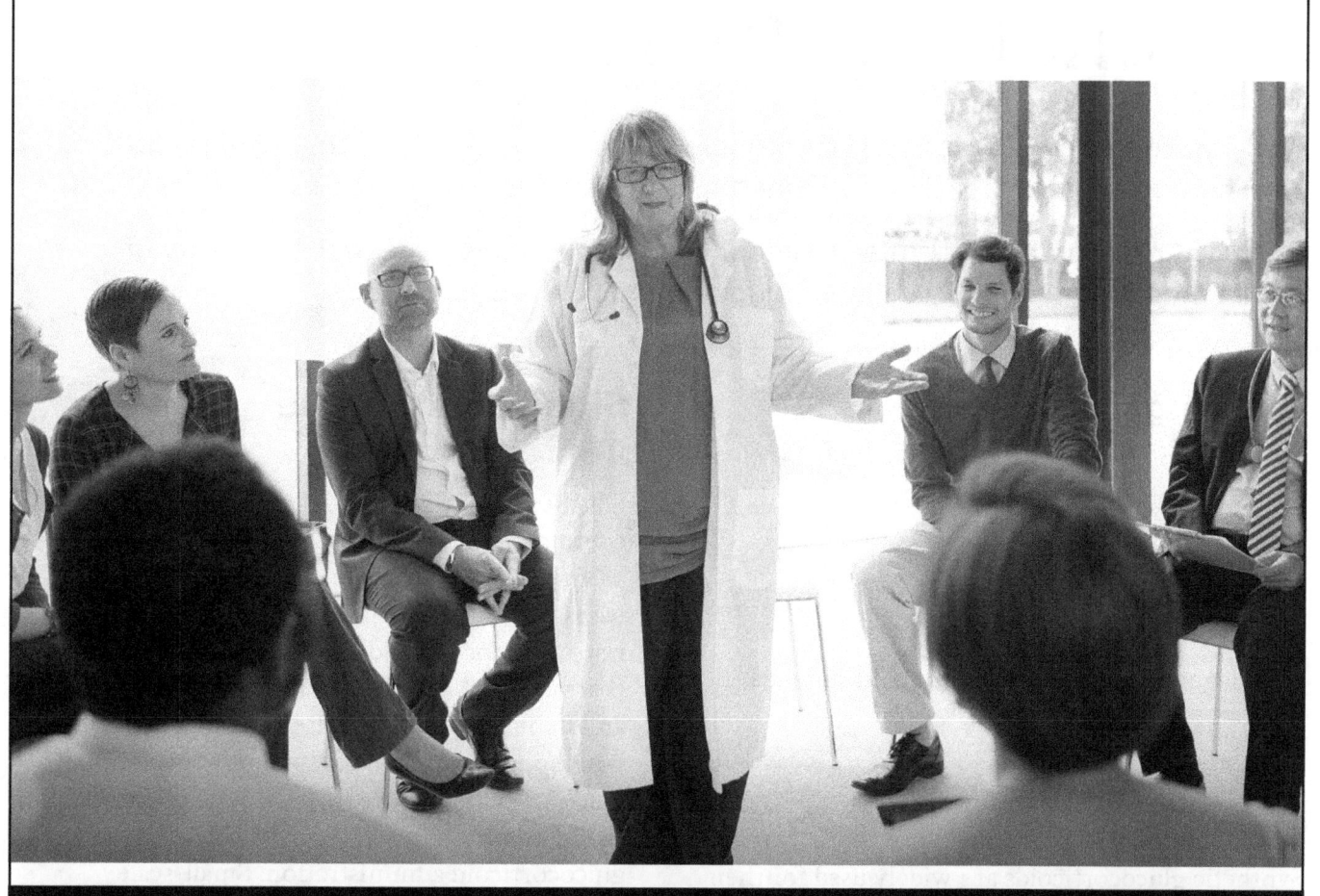

ADRENAL

Glucocorticoid-Induced Adrenal Insufficiency

Alessandro Prete, MD. Institute of Metabolism and Systems Research, University of Birmingham, Birmingham, United Kingdom; E-mail: a.prete@bham.ac.uk

Wiebke Arlt, MD, DSc. Institute of Metabolism and Systems Research, University of Birmingham, Birmingham, United Kingdom; E-mail: w.arlt@bham.ac.uk

Learning Objectives

As a result of participating in this session, learners should be able to:

- Identify patients at higher risk of glucocorticoid-induced adrenal insufficiency (AI).

- Diagnose and treat glucocorticoid-induced AI.

Main Conclusions

Synthetic glucocorticoids are widely used for their antiinflammatory and immunosuppressive actions. A possible unwanted effect of glucocorticoid treatment is the suppression of the hypothalamic-pituitary-adrenal (HPA) axis, which can lead to AI. Factors affecting the risk of glucocorticoid-induced AI include the duration of glucocorticoid therapy, mode of administration, glucocorticoid dosage and potency, and concomitant drugs that interfere with glucocorticoid metabolism. Signs and symptoms of AI can be vague and nonspecific and can overlap with those of iatrogenic Cushing syndrome and the underlying disorder for which glucocorticoids are prescribed. Glucocorticoid therapy should not be completely stopped until recovery of adrenal function is verified. When glucocorticoid-induced AI is diagnosed or suspected, patient education is essential to improve clinical outcomes.

Significance of the Clinical Problem

Glucocorticoid-induced AI is among the most common causes of cortisol deficiency.[1,2] In the adult population, 0.5% to 1.8% are long-term users of oral glucocorticoids, and the absolute risk of glucocorticoid-induced AI in this group is around 50%.[3] Inhaled glucocorticoids are also an established cause of HPA-axis suppression, with approximately 8% of patients developing glucocorticoid-induced AI.[3] HPA-axis suppression is also common following intraarticular glucocorticoid administration. Small-scale studies have shown that up to half of patients can develop some degree of biochemical HPA-axis suppression in the first 2 months following injection, but robust data regarding the duration and clinical consequences of HPA-axis suppression in these patients are lacking.[3] Glucocorticoid-induced AI is also possible following use of topical glucocorticoids, but evidence is mostly anecdotal.

A mismatch exists between the high prevalence of "biochemical" glucocorticoid-induced AI and the reporting of its "clinical" consequences, suggesting potential underdiagnosis and lack of awareness among clinicians. Considering the widespread use of glucocorticoids across multiple medical specialties, the number of patients potentially exposed to harm is staggering, and the lack of a consensus regarding management of glucocorticoid-induced AI contributes to suboptimal clinical outcomes.

Barriers to Optimal Practice

- Low specificity of signs and symptoms of glucocorticoid-induced AI.
- Lack of tools to accurately stratify patients according to their risk of developing glucocorticoid-induced AI.
- Lack of consensus on how to assess adrenal function in patients with suspected glucocorticoid-induced AI.

Strategies for Diagnosis, Therapy, and/or Management

The risk of developing glucocorticoid-induced AI is difficult to predict on an individual basis. The glucocorticoid formulation used, dosage, treatment duration, and time of administration during the day can affect this risk; there is a great degree of overlap.[1] Nonetheless, considering the various contributing factors can help clinicians establish the individualized risk for each patient (*Figure 1*). It is important to note, however, that high-quality evidence is limited.[1]

Systemic glucocorticoids, especially those with longer half-life and higher potency, are more likely to cause glucocorticoid-induced AI as compared with other administration routes because of the direct negative feedback on the HPA axis. Short courses of high-dosage glucocorticoids (<2 weeks) and pulse therapy (intermittent intravenous administration over a few days or weeks) are usually associated with swift recovery of adrenal function. The possible exception to this is the administration of frequently repeated short glucocorticoid courses, as regularly used in the treatment of asthma and chronic obstructive pulmonary disease and during emetogenic chemotherapy.[1]

Figure 1. Likelihood of Clinically Relevant Adrenal Suppression By Systemic and Inhaled Glucocorticoids

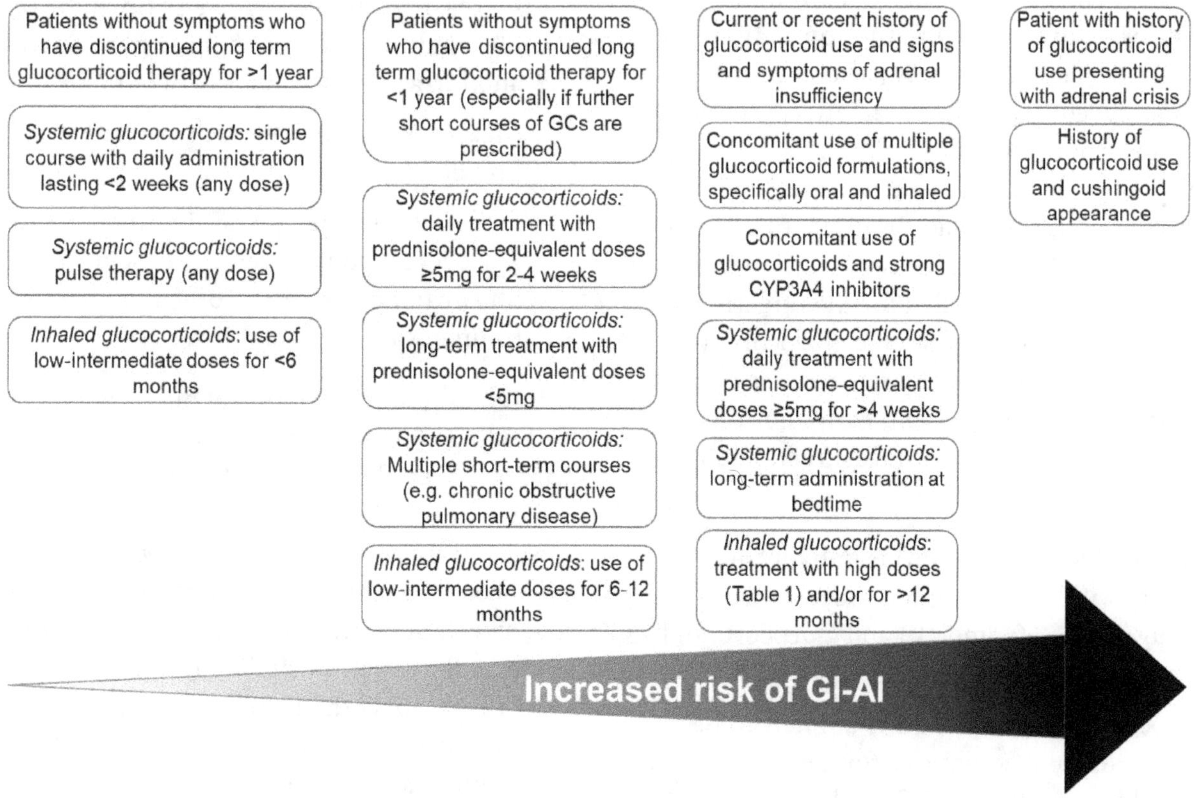

Systemic glucocorticoids include oral, intravenous, and intramuscular administration. The risk of developing glucocorticoid-induced adrenal insufficiency is a continuum, and this chart is a guide only. Clinical judgment is required to establish the risk on an individual basis.

Inhaled glucocorticoids can enter the systemic circulation via the gastrointestinal tract or direct absorption from the lungs and can exert negative feedback on the HPA axis. Patients using higher dosages for longer periods, as well as those exposed to other glucocorticoids (eg, multiple courses of rescue treatment for chronic obstructive pulmonary disease exacerbations) carry the highest risk of glucocorticoid-induced AI.[1,4]

The data regarding glucocorticoid-induced AI associated with intraarticular glucocorticoid therapy are limited and heterogeneous. Small-scale studies identified asymptomatic glucocorticoid-induced AI in up to 60% of patients in the weeks following intraarticular glucocorticoid administration; inflammatory arthropathies and repeated injections with higher dosages increase this risk.[1]

Cases of glucocorticoid-induced AI have been reported after exposure to nasal, intradermal, and transcutaneous glucocorticoid administration, but short-term administration at the recommended dosages is generally considered safe. Skin inflammation, impaired barrier function, the use of occlusive dressings, and the application to sites with higher absorption (such as mucous membranes, eyelids, and scrotum) affect the rate of systemic absorption with topical use.[1]

In patients at high risk of glucocorticoid-induced AI, glucocorticoids should not be discontinued until recovery of the HPA axis is documented. When treatment is no longer needed for the underlying disease in patients taking systemic glucocorticoids, the dosage should be gradually tapered to a dose of 5 mg prednisolone-equivalent. Early-morning serum cortisol should then be measured to guide management[1,4]:

- Glucocorticoid-induced AI is unlikely in patients with cortisol values greater than 12.7 μg/dL (>350 nmol/L) and glucocorticoids can usually be discontinued.

- Glucocorticoid-induced AI is unlikely to be relevant in basal conditions for patients with cortisol values 10.0 to 12.7 μg/dL (275 to 350 nmol/L). Daily glucocorticoids can be stopped, but the patient should be educated on stress-dose coverage (sick-day rules).

- Glucocorticoid-induced AI is possible in patients with cortisol values less than 10.0 μg/dL (<275 nmol/L). Glucocorticoids should be continued (possibly switching treatment to a replacement dosage of short-acting hydrocortisone [eg, 15 mg hydrocortisone]) and adrenal function should be reassessed over time. Repeated tests include early-morning cortisol and dynamic testing when results are indeterminate. Dynamic tests include the 250-mcg cosyntropin-stimulation test, overnight metyrapone-stimulation test, or insulin tolerance test. Patients must be educated on stress-dose coverage (sick-day rules).

HPA-axis recovery in patients with glucocorticoid-induced AI can take months to years, and 2% to 7% of patients may never recover adrenal function.[1] All patients at risk of or with established glucocorticoid-induced AI should receive adequate education. Special attention should be paid to:

- Increasing patient awareness (including over-the-counter drugs containing glucocorticoids and intraarticular glucocorticoid injections).

- Measures targeted towards adrenal crisis prevention.

- Sick-day rules (ie, the need to increase the glucocorticoid replacement dose during illness and other causes of major stress such as trauma, surgery, childbirth).

Strategies to improve clinical outcomes include providing clear information on glucocorticoid therapy, special situations that may require adjustment of the glucocorticoid replacement dosage, training on the use of injectable glucocorticoid therapy in emergency situations, and signs and symptoms of overreplacement and underreplacement, including those of adrenal crisis. Patients with glucocorticoid-induced AI should receive adequate education regardless of the estimated duration of AI/time to recovery. Patients with glucocorticoid-induced AI should wear medical alert IDs.

Clinical Case Vignettes

Important note: Cortisol cutoffs vary according to the cortisol assay used and local practices. The cortisol values reported in the following cases were measured by immunoassay (Abbott Alinity). For this immunoassay, the current cutoff used at our institution for a short 250-mcg cosyntropin-stimulation test is a 30-minute cortisol value ≥16.3 µg/dL (≥450 nmol/L).

Case 1

A 63-year-old woman is referred by her primary care physician because of an early-morning cortisol value of 1.7 µg/dL (47 nmol/L). She has a 4-month history of unintentional weight loss, muscle mass loss, and tiredness. Asthma was diagnosed at age 50 years, and she has been on regular inhaled glucocorticoids for many years.

Laboratory test results:

ACTH = 6.7 pg/mL (10-60 pg/mL) (SI: 1.47 pmol/L [2.2-13.2 pmol/L])
Serum cortisol 30 minutes after administration of 250 mcg cosyntropin = 4.0 µg/dL (SI: 110 nmol/L)

Recent pituitary MRI shows normal appearance of the hypothalamic-pituitary region.

Which of the following inhaled glucocorticoids is most commonly associated with adrenal suppression?

A. Ciclesonide

B. Extra-fine particle beclometasone dipropionate

C. Fluticasone furoate

D. Fluticasone propionate

Answer: D) Fluticasone propionate

This patient had been treated with inhaled fluticasone propionate (Answer D) for more than 5 years (initially 250 mcg daily for 2 years, then 500 mcg daily for 2 years, then 1000 mcg daily for 18 months before being tested). Most cases of glucocorticoid-induced AI in patients using inhaled glucocorticoids have been linked to fluticasone propionate. This drug has a long half-life (14.4 hours) and a strong binding affinity for the glucocorticoid receptor (18 times that of dexamethasone), which explains the high risk of HPA-axis suppression following repeated systemic absorption. Nonetheless, cases of glucocorticoid-induced AI have been associated with all the medications listed above, highlighting the importance of closely monitoring all patients treated with inhaled glucocorticoids.

Treatment with high dosages of inhaled glucocorticoids put patients at a particularly high risk of glucocorticoid-induced AI, up to 18.5% (*Table 1*).[1] It is recommended that these patients receive appropriate education, including being issued a steroid emergency card, and undergo periodic clinical assessment for signs and symptoms of glucocorticoid-induced AI.[5]

Table 1. Factors Affecting Risk of Developing Glucocorticoid-Induced Adrenal Insufficiency in Patients Receiving Inhaled Glucocorticoids

Treatment dosage	Treatment with high daily doses of inhaled glucocorticoids (regardless of treatment duration) increases the risk of glucocorticoid-induced adrenal insufficiency. High doses are: • Fluticasone propionate: >500 mcg daily (adults), >200 mcg daily (children) • Beclometasone dipropionate (standard particle inhalers): >1000 mcg daily (adults); >400 mcg daily (children) • Beclometasone dipropionate (extra-fine particle inhalers): >400 mcg daily (adults); >200 mcg daily (children) • Budesonide: >800 mcg daily (adults); 400 mcg daily (children) • Ciclesonide: >320 mcg daily (adults); >160 mcg daily (children) • Fluticasone furoate: >100 mcg daily (adults) • Mometasone furoate: >400 mcg daily (adults)
Treatment duration	Treatment for longer than 6 to 12 months (regardless of the dosage used) increases the risk of glucocorticoid-induced adrenal insufficiency
Glucocorticoid type	Fluticasone propionate carries the highest risk of causing glucocorticoid-induced adrenal insufficiency
Concomitant treatments	• Concomitant use of other exogenous glucocorticoids (including intermittent use [eg, rescue glucocorticoids in chronic obstructive pulmonary disease]) • CYP3A4 inhibitors (see *Table 3*)
Other factors (children)	• Lower BMI • Higher adherence to treatment

Partially based on information from manufactures' summaries of product characteristics, Global Initiative for Asthma (2018), British National Formulary, and British National Formulary for Children.

Case 2

An 84-year-old woman is admitted to hospital for COVID-19–related pneumonia. She collapsed at home and described symptoms of feeling lightheaded and fainting with no loss of consciousness; she has been having shortness of breath and a productive cough for a few days. Secondary AI is diagnosed during evaluation of hyponatremia:

> Random cortisol = 1.2 µg/dL (SI: 33 nmol/L)
> ACTH = 9 pg/mL (10-60 pg/mL) (SI: 1.98 pmol/L [2.2-13.2 pmol/L])
> Cortisol 30 minutes after administration of 250 mcg cosyntropin = 7.9 µg/dL (SI: 218 nmol/L)

She has a history of chronic obstructive pulmonary disease treated with beclomethasone dipropionate inhalers (800 mcg/daily) and steroid injections into the knee joint every 6 months for the last 2 years to treat osteoarthritis.

Which of the following symptoms can be found in patients with glucocorticoid-induced AI?

A. Easy bruising

B. Hypoglycemia

C. Fatigue

D. All of the above

Answer: D) All of the above

All the signs and symptoms listed can be observed in patients with glucocorticoid-induced AI (Answer D). A high degree of clinical suspicion is paramount when there is a history of glucocorticoid exposure. In fact, patients with glucocorticoid-induced AI may be asymptomatic, present with varying degrees of symptoms of cortisol deficiency and iatrogenic Cushing syndrome, or present with life-threatening adrenal crisis (*Table 2*). Importantly, signs and symptoms of cortisol deficiency and Cushing syndrome can coexist, depending on when glucocorticoids are discontinued.

Another element of interest in this case is the possible cumulative effect of intraarticular and

Table 2. Signs and Symptoms Associated With Glucocorticoid-Induced Adrenal Insufficiency and Adrenal Crisis

Iatrogenic adrenal insufficiency	Iatrogenic Cushing syndrome	Adrenal crisis
• General malaise	• Proximal muscle weakness	At least 2 of the following:
• Fatigue	• Weight gain and central obesity	• Hypotension or hypovolemic shock
• Weakness	• Disproportionate supraclavicular and dorsocervical fat pads	• Nausea or vomiting
• Dizziness (including postural dizziness)	• Facial and upper neck plethora	• Severe fatigue
• Gastrointestinal symptoms (nausea, vomiting, diarrhea, cramps, loss of appetite)	• Facial rounding	• Fever
• Weight loss	• Skin atrophy, easy bruising, red stretch marks	• Impaired consciousness (including lethargy, confusion, somnolence, collapse, delirium, coma, seizures)
• Hypotension (including postural hypotension)	• Acne	
• Headaches (usually in the morning)	• Poor wound healing	
• Arthralgias (especially in hand joints)	• Insomnia	
• Myalgias	• Increased appetite	
• Recurrent respiratory infections with slow recovery	• Irritability, impaired memory, depression	
• Alabaster-like, pale skin	• Hypertension	
• Poor linear growth (children)	• Abnormal glucose metabolism	
• Poor weight gain (children)	• Menstrual irregularities (women)	
• Hypoglycemia (more frequent in children)	• Poor linear growth (children)	
• Hyponatremia		
• Lymphocytosis		
• Eosinophilia		

inhaled glucocorticoids in causing glucocorticoid-induced AI, emphasizing the potential risks associated with their systemic absorption. Patients with glucocorticoid-induced AI were found to carry a higher risk of adrenal crisis than patients with other etiologies of adrenal insufficiency and the most common trigger was infections, as in this case.[6,7] A lack of awareness of glucocorticoid-induced AI and the presence of nonspecific signs and symptoms (which can be mistakenly attributed to other causes or to the disease for which glucocorticoids were prescribed) are likely contributors to the increased risk of life-threatening adrenal crisis in this patient population.

Case 3

A 74-year-old woman is admitted to the emergency department with collapse, vomiting, diarrhea, and hypotension.

Laboratory test results:

> Sodium = 129 mEq/L (136-142 mEq/L)
> (SI: 129 mmol/L [136-142 mmol/L])
> Plasma osmolality = 272 mOsm/kg (275-295 mOsm/kg)
> (SI: 272 mmol/kg [275-295 mmol/kg])
> Urinary sodium = 107 mEq/L (SI: 107 mmol/L)

She has been receiving steroid injections into the knee joint every 6 months for the past 2 years (methylprednisolone acetate, 40 mg), and she uses a topical steroid (betamethasone valerate, 0.1% as required) for psoriasis with psoriatic arthritis. Adrenal crisis is suspected, and measurement of random ACTH and cortisol is requested.

Which of the following is the best treatment now?

A. Bolus of intravenous hydrocortisone, 50 to 100 mg, followed by 200 mg hydrocortisone infusion/24 h + intravenous fluids

B. Bolus of intravenous hydrocortisone, 100 mg, followed by oral hydrocortisone, 20 mg 3 times daily, if the vomiting improves

C. Intravenous fluids to control the hypovolemia while awaiting ACTH and cortisol results

D. None of the above

Answer: A) Bolus of intravenous hydrocortisone, 50 to 100 mg, followed by 200 mg hydrocortisone infusion/24 h + intravenous fluids

Many cases of adrenal crisis and hospitalization for glucocorticoid-induced AI have been described, including several deaths.[1] In this case, the patient's random cortisol measurement was less than 1 µg/dL (<28 nmol/L) and her ACTH concentration was 6 pg/mL (1.32 pmol/L), suggesting secondary AI. This was later confirmed with a short 250-mcg cosyntropin test (30-minute cortisol = 11.9 µg/dL [329 nmol/L]). It is imperative to remember, however, that diagnostic measures should never delay treatment (thus, Answer C is incorrect): a patient with a suspected adrenal crisis must be promptly treated with lifesaving injectable hydrocortisone and fluid resuscitation.[5]

Continuous intravenous hydrocortisone infusion should be favored over intermittent bolus administration in the prevention and treatment of adrenal crisis during major stress (Answer A).[8,9] In fact, continuous intravenous hydrocortisone has been shown to be the only delivery mode that steadily maintains circulating cortisol in the range observed during major stress, while intermittent bolus administration of hydrocortisone results in frequent troughs with lower concentrations, thereby potentially exposing patients with adrenal insufficiency to periods of underreplacement (*Figure 2*) (thus, Answer B is incorrect).[9]

Case 4

A 63-year-old woman taking oral prednisolone for temporal giant-cell arteritis has been tapering the dosage over a 3-year period, with the aim of discontinuing treatment. While taking prednisolone, 4 mg daily, early-morning cortisol is measured 24 hours after the last dose and is documented to be 8.1 µg/dL (223 nmol/L). The patient's regimen is switched from prednisolone to twice-daily hydrocortisone (10 mg upon awakening + 5 mg at lunchtime), and a short 250-mcg cosyntropin-stimulation test is arranged. Cortisol 30 minutes after cosyntropin administration is 14.9 µg/dL (411 nmol/L).

Figure 2. Serum Cortisol Following Stress-Dose Hydrocortisone Administration and Pharmacokinetic Modeling

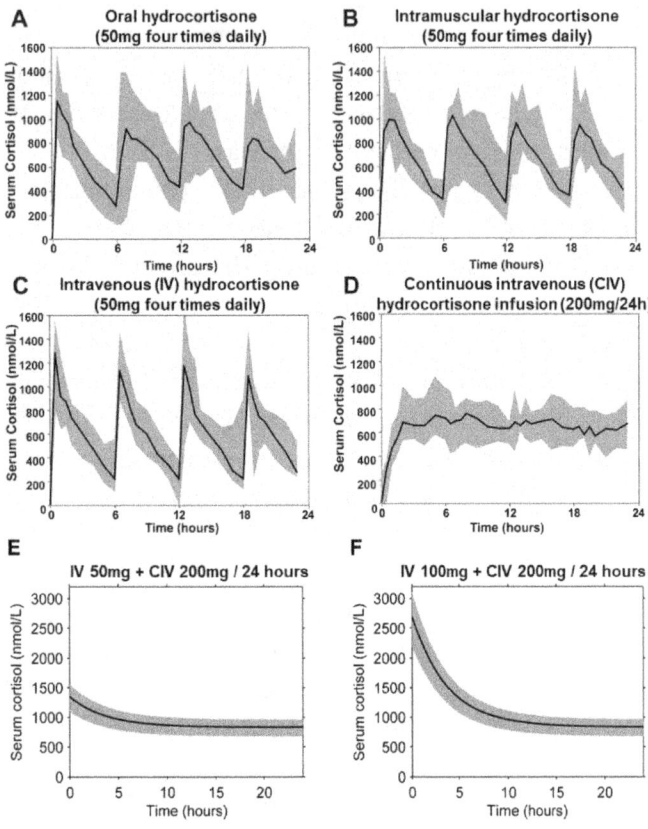

Serum cortisol (nmol/L) after hydrocortisone administered orally (*Panel A*), intramuscularly (*Panel B*), as intravenous boluses (*Panel C*), or as continuous intravenous infusion (*Panel D*). Linear pharmacokinetic modeling was used to predict the serum cortisol response to initial 50 mg (*Panel E*) and 100 mg (*Panel F*) intravenous bolus injections followed by continuous intravenous infusion of 200 mg hydrocortisone over 24 hours. Adapted from Prete A et al. *J Clin Endocrinol Metab*, 2020; 105(7) © Endocrine Society.

Which of the following is the best next step in this patient's management?

A. Continue hydrocortisone and measure early-morning cortisol in 3 months

B. Restart prednisolone, 4 mg daily, and measure early-morning cortisol in 3 months

C. Stop twice-daily hydrocortisone and discharge

D. Stop twice-daily hydrocortisone and advise stress dosing only

Answer: D) Stop twice-daily hydrocortisone and advise stress dosing only

The borderline result of the cosyntropin-stimulation test suggests that the patient has sufficient adrenal cortisol reserve in baseline conditions and is unlikely to require regular daily glucocorticoid replacement (thus, Answers A and B are incorrect).[10] The patient should be educated about hydrocortisone administration during major stress (thus, Answer D is correct and Answer C is incorrect).

Case 5

A 27-year-old woman has suspected glucocorticoid-induced AI following multiple cycles of high-dosage oral dexamethasone for relapse of Philadelphia-negative acute lymphoblastic leukemia (fatigue, hypotension, random cortisol = 4.7 μg/dL [129 nmol/L]; ACTH = <5 pg/mL [<1.10 pmol/L]). She was discharged from the hospital on twice-daily hydrocortisone (10 mg + 5 mg) 3 months ago. The patient also has a history of premature ovarian insufficiency, and her primary care physician has recently commenced oral hormone replacement therapy (estradiol, 2 mg + dydrogesterone, 10 mg). The hematology consultant requested an early-morning cortisol measurement 24 hours after the last dose of hydrocortisone (13.8 μg/dL [381 nmol/L]) and has referred the patient to the endocrinology department for further evaluation.

Which of the following is the most appropriate next step?

A. Reassess adrenal function

B. Stop hydrocortisone and discharge

C. Stop twice-daily hydrocortisone and advise stress dosing only

D. None of the above

Answer: A) Reassess adrenal function

The patient needs to stop oral hormone replacement therapy and have her adrenal function reassessed (Answer A). The estrogen component increases corticosteroid-binding globulin levels and consequently total serum cortisol. After a washout of 6 weeks from oral estradiol, the result of the short 250-mcg cosyntropin test was, in fact, abnormal:

Baseline cortisol = 4.1 µg/dL (SI: 113 nmol/L)
30-Minute cortisol = 13.0 µg/dL (SI: 358 nmol/L)

The cortisol cutoffs discussed thus far do not apply to patients treated with high-dosage oral estrogens as part of hormonal contraception (oral, intramuscular, or implant), which must be discontinued for at least 6 weeks to allow for an unambiguous assessment. Interactions between exogenous glucocorticoids and other drugs are potentially relevant for patients at risk of or with established glucocorticoid-induced AI, chiefly strong CYP3A4 inducers and inhibitors (*Table 3*). CYP3A4 is, in fact, the main pathway for the inactivation of most prescribed glucocorticoids. Strong CYP3A4 inhibitors (such as antifungal drugs, clarithromycin, and antiretrovirals) can increase the systemic exposure to glucocorticoids, leading to high risk of glucocorticoid-induced AI. Conversely, strong CYP3A4 inducers (such as carbamazepine, phenytoin, rifampicin, enzalutamide, and mitotane) increase the metabolism of glucocorticoids and can trigger symptoms of cortisol deficiency, including adrenal crisis, in patients with glucocorticoid-induced AI.

Table 3. Drug Interactions That Can Affect Patients at Risk of Glucocorticoid-Induced Adrenal Insufficiency

Drugs	Interaction mechanism with exogenous glucocorticoids	Possible consequences for patients treated with exogenous glucocorticoids
Oral estrogens	Increased corticosteroid-binding globulin levels	Increased total serum cortisol levels, which affect the interpretation of early-morning cortisol and dynamic testing
CYP3A4 inducers	Reduced systemic exposure to synthetic glucocorticoids	Increased risk of developing signs and symptoms of cortisol deficiency (including adrenal crisis) in patients with underlying glucocorticoid-induced adrenal insufficiency
CYP3A4 inhibitors	Increased systemic exposure to synthetic glucocorticoids	Increased risk of developing glucocorticoid-induced adrenal insufficiency
Megestrol acetate	Glucocorticoid activity (binds to the glucocorticoid receptor)	Increased risk of developing glucocorticoid-induced adrenal insufficiency
Medroxyprogesterone acetate (high dosages)	Glucocorticoid activity (binds to the glucocorticoid receptor)	Increased risk of developing glucocorticoid-induced adrenal insufficiency

References

1. Prete A, Bancos I. Glucocorticoid induced adrenal insufficiency. *BMJ.* 2021;374:n1380. PMID: 34253540

2. Bancos I, Hahner S, Tomlinson J, Arlt W. Diagnosis and management of adrenal insufficiency. *Lancet Diabetes Endocrinol.* 2015;3(3):216-226. PMID: 25098712

3. Broersen LH, Pereira AM, Jorgensen JO, Dekkers OM. Adrenal insufficiency in corticosteroids use: systematic review and meta-analysis. *J Clin Endocrinol Metab.* 2015;100(6):2171-2180. PMID: 25844620

4. Woods CP, Argese N, Chapman M, et al. Adrenal suppression in patients taking inhaled glucocorticoids is highly prevalent and management can be guided by morning cortisol. *Eur J Endocrinol.* 2015;173(5):633-642. PMID: 26294794

5. Simpson H, Tomlinson J, Wass J, Dean J, Arlt W. Guidance for the prevention and emergency management of adult patients with adrenal insufficiency. *Clin Med (Lond).* 2020;20(4):371-378. PMID: 32675141

6. Li D, Genere N, Behnken E, et al. Determinants of self-reported health outcomes in adrenal insufficiency: a multisite survey study. *J Clin Endocrinol Metab.* 2021;106(3):e1408-e1419. PMID: 32995875

7. Hahner S, Spinnler C, Fassnacht M, Burger-Stritt S, Lang K, Milovanovic D,et al. High incidence of adrenal crisis in educated patients with chronic adrenal insufficiency: a prospective study. *J Clin Endocrinol Metab.* 2015;100(2):407-416. PMID: 25419882

8. Bornstein SR, Allolio B, Arlt W, et al. Diagnosis and treatment of primary adrenal insufficiency: an Endocrine Society clinical practice guideline. *J Clin Endocrinol Metab.* 2016;101(2):364-389. PMID: 26760044

9. Prete A, Taylor AE, Bancos I, et al. Prevention of adrenal crisis: cortisol responses to major stress compared to stress dose hydrocortisone delivery. *J Clin Endocrinol Metab.* 2020;105(7):2262-2274. PMID: 32170323

10. Agha A, Tomlinson JW, Clark PM, Holder G, Stewart PM. The long-term predictive accuracy of the short synacthen (corticotropin) stimulation test for assessment of the hypothalamic-pituitary-adrenal axis. *J Clin Endocrinol Metab.* 2006;91(1):43-47. PMID: 16249286

Advances in the Treatment of Congenital Adrenal Hyperplasia

Adina F. Turcu, MD, MS. Division of Metabolism, Endocrinology, and Diabetes, University of Michigan, Ann Arbor, MI; E-mail: aturcu@umich.edu

Learning Objectives

As a result of participating in this session, learners should be able to:

- Describe established and upcoming therapies for patients with classic and nonclassic congenital adrenal hyperplasia (CAH).

- Implement use of traditional and novel biomarkers for monitoring disease control and guiding therapy for patients with classic and nonclassic CAH.

Main Conclusions

Treatment of CAH focuses on 2 main aspects: (1) hormonal replacement for adrenal insufficiency in classic CAH and (2) suppression of adrenal androgen excess whenever clinically relevant. Since they became available in the 1950s, glucocorticoids have been the primary tool to address both CAH treatment goals, with only a few available preparations. While sufficient for the treatment of adrenal insufficiency, glucocorticoid dosages and timing of administration required for adrenal androgen suppression are linked to numerous off-target effects. Recent developments to advance treatment of patients with CAH have focused on 2 fronts: (1) glucocorticoid delivery that closely mimics the physiologic circadian rhythm and (2) nonglucocorticoid strategies to overcome adrenal androgen excess. Examples include modified-release oral glucocorticoids and continuous subcutaneous hydrocortisone pumps; targeting ACTH excess via CRH receptor antagonists, ACTH antibodies, or ACTH receptor antagonists; and inhibiting enzymes required for androgen synthesis.

In parallel with novel therapeutic developments, growing evidence supports the use of 11-oxyandrogens as indicators of an adrenal vs gonadal source, with advantages over traditional androgens in guiding the management of patients with CAH.

Significance of the Clinical Problem

CAH is due to autosomal recessive pathogenic variants in genes encoding enzymes required for cortisol synthesis. Defects in the gene encoding steroid 21-hydroxylase (*CYP21A2*) account for most CAH cases.[1] Severe forms of 21-hydroxylase deficiency (21-OHD) result in clinically overt adrenal insufficiency and are termed "classic." Milder enzymatic defects, in which both cortisol and aldosterone synthesis are compensated, are termed "nonclassic." While classic 21-OHD affects approximately 1 in 15,000 newborns,[2] nonclassic 21-OHD is relatively common, occurring in approximately 1 in 1000 White individuals and in up to 1 in 30 individuals of certain ethnicities (eg, Ashkenazi Jewish, Hispanic, and Mediterranean).[3]

In all cases of 21-OHD, obstructed cortisol synthesis prompts ACTH elevations, which, in turn, stimulate adrenal cortical growth and steroidogenic flux. The combination of ACTH elevation and 21-OHD favors the overproduction of adrenal androgens. Clinical manifestations of adrenal androgen excess include virilization of external genitalia in girls with classic 21-OHD, premature pubarche, rapid somatic growth, advanced bone age, hirsutism, acne, irregular menses, and subfertility.[4-7] Sustained ACTH elevations also promote the expansion of adrenal rest tissue, such as testicular or ovarian adrenal rest tumors.

The 2 main treatment goals in 21-OHD are: (1) to replace insufficient hormones (glucocorticoids and mineralocorticoids, when needed) and (2) to suppress excessive production of adrenal androgens. Since their first use in the 1950s, oral glucocorticoids have been the mainstay of 21-OHD therapy. In addition to the typical daytime replacement dosing common to all forms of adrenal insufficiency, bedtime glucocorticoids are used in patients with 21-OHD to reduce the early-morning rise in ACTH and the consequent adrenal androgen excess. Supraphysiologic administration of glucocorticoids leads to obesity, dyslipidemia, hyperglycemia, and bone loss.[8-13]

Another important challenge in managing 21-OHD is the lack of reliable biomarkers to guide glucocorticoid dosing. Normalization of 17α-hydroxyprogesterone can only be achieved with excessive glucocorticoid doses and consequential iatrogenic Cushing syndrome, which is not a reasonable tradeoff. Moreover, 17α-hydroxyprogesterone, androstenedione, and testosterone correlate poorly with clinical evidence of androgen excess,[14,15] in part due to their dual adrenal and gonadal origin. DHEA-S, the major adrenal androgen precursor, is often paradoxically low in patients with poorly controlled 21-OHD.

Barriers to Optimal Practice

- Limited treatment options beyond glucocorticoids.
- Nonphysiologic administration of glucocorticoids to suppress ACTH-driven adrenal androgen excess leads to adverse effects typical of iatrogenic Cushing syndrome.
- Lack of reliable biomarkers to guide therapy.

Strategies for Diagnosis, Therapy, and/or Management

Steroid Therapy

In patients with classic 21-OHD, oral glucocorticoid regimens aim to distribute diurnal replacement doses, as in any form of adrenal insufficiency. For this purpose, short-acting hydrocortisone, administered 2 or 3 times daily, offers the lowest risk of glucocorticoid-induced adverse effects, and it is preferred in children (*Table 1*). A morning dose of an intermediate-acting glucocorticoid (prednisone or prednisolone), or even a long-acting glucocorticoid (dexamethasone), can be considered in patients who prefer to minimize medication frequency, or when adherence is challenging. To counteract adrenal androgen excess, a low dose of intermediate- or long-acting glucocorticoid can be administered at bedtime.

Table 1. Available Oral Glucocorticoids

Glucocorticoid	Relative potency	Average adrenal insufficiency replacement doses	Androgen suppression bedtime doses
Hydrocortisone	1	15 to 20 mg daily (divided in 2 to 3 doses)	*Not used for this purpose due to short half-life
Prednisolone	4	5 mg in AM	1 to 3 mg
Prednisone	4	5 mg in AM	1 to 3 mg
Dexamethasone	30	1 mg in AM	≤1 mg

To closely mimic physiologic glucocorticoid synthesis, and to minimize the adverse effects of supraphysiologic doses, modified-release glucocorticoid formulations have been developed. Plenadren (Shire Services BVBA, Belgium) is a dual-release hydrocortisone tablet with an outer immediate-release coating and an inner sustained-release core approved in Europe for once-daily administration in patients with adrenal insufficiency, but its use in patients with 21-OHD does not achieve good control of androgen excess.[16] Chronocort (Diurnal Europe B.V., The Netherlands) is a multiparticulate delayed-release hydrocortisone formulation that provides sustained drug delivery and is particularly useful for suppressing the early-morning ACTH rise in patients with 21-OHD.[17]

Further fine-tuning the delivery of glucocorticoids could theoretically be achieved with continuous intravenous or subcutaneous delivery systems, but data are limited to small studies. Like insulin pumps, such systems involve relatively complex operational logistics and add risks, including malfunction and site infections.[18,19]

Patients with nonclassic 21-OHD have compensated cortisol production and do not need replacement therapy. In women with nonclassic 21-OHD who are not interested in conceiving, oral contraceptives help reduce ovarian androgen production and increase SHBG, which lowers the fraction of bioavailable and free testosterone. Spironolactone, primarily a mineralocorticoid receptor antagonist, is also an androgen receptor antagonist at higher dosages, and it can be added to further treat hirsutism and/or acne. Spironolactone crosses the placenta, and it should not be used without reliable contraceptive methods due to feminization effects on male fetuses.

Emerging Nonglucocorticoid Therapies

Several therapeutic strategies that target adrenal androgen excess are being developed (*Table 2*). Two oral small-molecule inhibitors of the pituitary corticotropin-releasing factor type 1 (CRF1) receptors are currently in clinical trials: crinecerfont (Neurocrine Biosciences, Inc, USA) and tildacerfont (Spruce Biosciences, USA). By interrupting the signaling communication between the hypothalamus and pituitary, these agents offer an alternative to bedtime glucocorticoids to dampen the morning ACTH rise. Other strategies to reduce ACTH elevation include antiACTH monoclonal antibodies[21] and ACTH receptor antagonists,[22] but both are experimental therapies and have not yet been tested in humans.

Abiraterone acetate is a potent inhibitor of CYP17A1, an enzyme needed for both glucocorticoid and sex-hormone synthesis, and it is expressed in the adrenal glands and gonads. Abiraterone acetate effectively reduces androgen synthesis and has been shown to decrease mortality in men with castration-resistant prostate

Table 2. Novel Treatment Strategies in CAH

Treatment		Administration	Advantages	Disadvantages
Glucocorticoids	Modified-release hydrocortisone (Plenadren, Chronocort)	Twice daily	• Oral administration • Early-morning ACTH suppression	• Potential for iatrogenic Cushing syndrome
	Subcutaneous hydrocortisone infusion	Continuous	• Close replication of circadian secretory patterns for ACTH and cortisol • Potential for ultradian pulsatility replication if a real-time ACTH/cortisol monitoring is added	• Continuous device wear • Local irritation • Potential for malfunctioning • High fixed costs and complexity
Androgen biosynthetic enzyme blockage	CYP17A1 inhibitors (abiraterone acetate)	Once daily	• Highly effective • Well-tolerated	• Does not lower ACTH • Gonadal sex-steroid inhibition
CRH receptor type 1 antagonists	Crinecerfont, tildacerfont	Once daily	• Reduce ACTH secretion	• Long-term safety data are lacking

cancer.[23-25] In a study of 6 women with poorly controlled classic 21-OHD, abiraterone acetate normalized androstenedione when added to physiologic hydrocortisone and fludrocortisone.[26] Because it inhibits the production of gonadal sex steroids, abiraterone acetate is not a good option for reproductive-aged patients. Also, by posing a second block in the biosynthetic pathway of cortisol, this agent is not sensible in patients with nonclassic 21-OHD.

All therapies discussed above are adjunctive to glucocorticoid replacement. Future development of gene-based therapy[27,28] has the potential to cure 21-OHD and fully eliminate the need for glucocorticoids.

Monitoring Therapy

In women with 21-OHD, normal concentrations of testosterone and androstenedione typically indicate good disease control, although these steroids correlate poorly with clinical stigmata of hyperandrogenism. Disproportionately elevated androstenedione suggests suboptimally controlled 21-OHD. Elevated testosterone, however, can be seen in women with 21-OHD and concomitant polycystic ovary syndrome. Excessive adrenal-derived progesterone contributes to irregular menses and infertility. In preparation for conceiving, the goal of glucocorticoid therapy is to suppress serum progesterone to concentrations less than 0.6 ng/mL (<2.0 nmol/L), which is associated with higher fertility rates in women with classic 21-OHD.[29]

In men with 21-OHD, serum testosterone concentrations have little value when used in isolation. In healthy men, testosterone is produced primarily by the testes; conversely, uncontrolled 21-OHD results in larger proportions of adrenal testosterone. An androstenedione-to-testosterone ratio greater than 0.5 is suggestive of adrenal androgen excess. Excessive amounts of adrenal androgens lead to gonadotropin suppression. Normal serum testosterone concentrations along with suppressed gonadotropins in men with 21-OHD suggest abundant adrenal androgen production and low gonadal testosterone.

More than testosterone, patients with 21-OHD overproduce a set of androgens unique to the adrenal gland, called 11-oxygenated C_{19} steroids, or 11-oxyandrogens. Of these, 11β-androstenedione is the most abundant, and its downstream metabolite 11-ketotestosterone is a potent androgen, bioequivalent to testosterone.[30,31] Higher serum concentrations of 11-oxyandrogens are associated with several clinical indicators of suboptimal 21-OHD control, including larger adrenal glands, presence of testicular adrenal rest tumors, and menstrual irregularities.[32]

Serum 11-ketotestosterone assays are now offered by some commercial laboratories, and its measurement can be useful in cases with discrepant traditional biomarkers. For example, in men with 21-OHD, 11-ketotestosterone correlates inversely with testosterone, and the former can be high when testosterone is normal. In female patients with 21-OHD, 11-ketotestosterone and testosterone are positively correlated, as they are both produced primarily in the adrenal gland. In patients with either classic and nonclassic 21-OHD, 11-oxyandrogens are disproportionately higher than conventional androgens.[33,34] In contrast, androstenedione and testosterone concentrations are similar in patients with nonclassic 21-OHD and in those with hyperandrogenism of other etiologies with similar clinical presentations, including polycystic ovary syndrome.[34]

Clinical Case Vignettes
Case 1

A 29-year-old woman with nonclassic 21-OHD presents for routine follow-up. Menarche was at age 10 years. She struggles with irregular menses, acne, and facial hirsutism. All of her symptoms improved while taking oral contraceptives. However, she stopped oral contraceptives approximately 1 year ago when she got married and started trying to conceive. The couple met with a genetic counselor, and the husband's genetic testing shows no pathogenic CYP21A2 variants. The patient's only medication is a prenatal multivitamin.

Laboratory test results (obtained 7 days after her last menses):

Testosterone = 81 ng/dL (8-60 ng/dL)
(SI: 2.8 nmol/L [0.3-2.1 nmol/L])

Androstenedione = 250 ng/dL (30-200 ng/dL)
(SI: 8.7 nmol/L [1.05-6.98 nmol/L])

DHEA-S = 90 µg/dL (44-333 µg/dL) (SI: 2.44 µmol/L [1.19-9.00 µmol/L])

Progesterone = 2.0 ng/mL (≤1.0 ng/mL [follicular]; 2.0-20.0 ng/mL [luteal]) (SI: 6.36 nmol/L [≤3.2 nmol/L (follicular); 6.4-63.6 nmol/L (luteal)])

17-Hydroxyprogesterone = 1230 ng/dL (<80 ng/dL [follicular]) (SI: 37.3 nmol/L [<2.42 nmol/L])

Serum cortisol = 11.6 µg/dL (5-25 µg/dL)
(SI: 320.0 nmol/L [137.9-689.7 nmol/L])

ACTH = 61 pg/mL (10-60 pg/mL) (SI: 13.4 pmol/L [2.2-13.2 pmol/L])

Which of the following treatment options should be recommended for this patient?

A. Dexamethasone, 0.25 mg at bedtime

B. Flutamide, 250 mg daily

C. Hydrocortisone, 5 mg at bedtime

D. Prednisolone, 2 mg at bedtime

E. Spironolactone, 50 mg daily

Answer: D) Prednisolone, 2 mg at bedtime

Patients with nonclassic 21-OHD have normal production of glucocorticoids and mineralocorticoids and do not need replacement therapy for these hormones. However, to maintain normal cortisol synthesis, elevated ACTH levels are needed to overcome the defective 21-hydroxylase. The combination of elevated ACTH and 21-hydroxylase insufficiency result in overproduction of adrenal progesterone and 17α-hydroxyprogesterone, and their diversion to formation of adrenal androgens. Limited data suggest that the rates of subfertility are modest in women with nonclassic 21-OHD, but the risk of early miscarriages is lower in women taking glucocorticoids than in those who do not.[35] The goal of therapy is to suppress the early rise of ACTH to overcome adrenal progesterone and androgen excess. This goal can be achieved with a low dosage of prednisolone at bedtime (Answer D). Prednisolone is preferred over its precursor, prednisone, because the in vivo activation of prednisone at such low dosages is inconsistent.

Studies suggest that hydrocortisone once or twice daily is also associated with a decreased risk of miscarriages in women with nonclassic 21-OHD.[35] However, the mechanism of day-time hydrocortisone use in these patients is poorly understood. Because hydrocortisone is short acting (half-life of approximately 1.5 hours), the potential of bedtime dosing (Answer C) to suppress early-morning ACTH is negligible.

Bedtime dexamethasone (Answer A) is effective in suppressing the early-morning ACTH rise, although it has a higher risk of off-target adverse effects from nonphysiologic glucocorticoid exposure. In addition, unlike prednisone, prednisolone, and hydrocortisone, dexamethasone is not inactivated by the placental 11β-hydroxysteroid dehydrogenase type 2, and it can suppress the fetal hypothalamic-pituitary-adrenal axis. Dexamethasone has been used in the first trimester of pregnancy in women at risk for having a baby girl with classic 21-OHD to prevent virilization. Prenatal treatment with dexamethasone is controversial, as the maternal and fetal risks are considered by many to outweigh the benefits.[36] In this vignette, the patient's partner had no identified *CYP21A2* pathogenic variants, so prenatal treatment with dexamethasone does not deserve consideration.

Spironolactone (Answer E) is a mineralocorticoid receptor antagonist, and, at high dosages, is also an androgen receptor antagonist. Spironolactone can be used in women with hyperandrogenism of various causes. However, spironolactone crosses the placenta and can cause feminization of a male fetus. Hence, in reproductive-aged women, spironolactone must be used in conjunction with a reliable contraceptive method.

Flutamide (Answer B) is a nonsteroidal androgen receptor antagonist that has been used in castration-resistant prostate cancer. Its adverse effects include hepatotoxicity, and it is not considered safe during pregnancy.

Case 2

A 61-year-old woman with classic congenital adrenal hyperplasia due to 21-OHD presents to establish care after recently relocating. Her medical history also includes type 2 diabetes mellitus, osteoporosis, dyslipidemia, obesity, obstructive sleep apnea, anxiety, and insomnia. She currently takes hydrocortisone, 10 mg in the morning and 5 mg at 2 PM, and dexamethasone, 0.25 mg at bedtime. She is particularly concerned about diffuse alopecia and facial hirsutism.

Laboratory test results:

ACTH = 190 pg/mL (10-60 pg/mL) (SI: 41.8 pmol/L [2.2-13.2 pmol/L])

17-Hydroxyprogesterone = 4210 ng/dL (<51 ng/dL [postmenopausal]) (SI: 127.6 nmol/L [<1.55 nmol/L])

Testosterone = 92 ng/dL (8-60 ng/dL) (SI: 3.2 nmol/L [0.3-2.1 nmol/L])

DHEA-S = <15 μg/dL (15-157 μg/dL) (SI: <0.41 μmol/L [0.41-4.25 μmol/L])

Which of the following treatment options should be considered next?

A. Add spironolactone, 25 mg daily

B. Enroll in a clinical trial of a corticotropin-releasing factor type 1 (CRF-1) receptor antagonist

C. Increase bedtime dexamethasone dosage to 0.5 mg nightly

D. Stop dexamethasone and add abiraterone acetate

E. B or D

Answer: E) Enroll in a clinical trial of a corticotropin-releasing factor type 1 (CRF-1) receptor antagonist (B) or stop dexamethasone and add abiraterone acetate (D)

Abiraterone (Answer D) is a potent inhibitor of CYP17A1 (17α-hydroxylase/17,20-lyase), an enzyme required for both cortisol and androgen synthesis. Abiraterone acetate improves survival in patients with castration-resistant prostate cancer,[23] and it was approved by the US FDA for this indication in 2018. In a small, open-label study of women with classic 21-OHD, abiraterone acetate administered once daily along with hydrocortisone replacement decreased circulating androgen levels.[26] As patients with classic 21-OHD already require full replacement doses of glucocorticoids, the concern about interference with cortisol synthesis by abiraterone is irrelevant. Abiraterone also blocks the synthesis of gonadal sex steroids, but this concern is limited to reproductive-aged women and not to postmenopausal women.

Preliminary data from clinical trials show that CRF-1 receptor antagonists (Answer B) effectively reduce ACTH and 17-hydroxyprogesterone in patients with uncontrolled classic 21-OHD.[37] By directly blocking ACTH production, such nonsteroidal oral CRF-1 receptor antagonists offer promising therapeutic advantages over supraphysiologic doses and times of administration of glucocorticoids.

In this patient, increasing the bedtime dose of dexamethasone (Answer C) further enhances the risk of adverse effects, many of which the patient already experiences (worsening hyperglycemia, osteoporosis, sleep disturbances).

Spironolactone (Answer A) is a mineralocorticoid and androgen receptor inhibitor. Adding spironolactone to the regimen of a patient with androgen excess is a reasonable option, but the antiandrogenic effects are relatively modest and begin to occur at dosages of at least 100 mg daily.[38]

Case 3

A 34-year-old man with classic CAH due to 21-OHD is seen for infertility. He and his wife have been trying to conceive for about a year. He has small bilateral testicular adrenal rest tumors, which have been stable according to recent ultrasonography.

His medications include hydrocortisone, 10 mg in the morning and 10 mg at 2 PM, and prednisolone, 2 mg at bedtime.

On physical examination, the patient is well virilized. His blood pressure is 102/75 mm Hg, and pulse rate is 90 beats/min. His height is 68 in (173 cm), and weight is 192 lb (87.1)

(BMI = 29.2 kg/m^2). Testicular volume is approximately 26 mL bilaterally, and testes are heterogeneous and firm.

Laboratory test results:

Serum total testosterone = 393 ng/dL (300-900 ng/dL) (SI: 13.6 nmol/L [10.4-31.2 nmol/L])
LH = <0.20 mIU/mL (1.0-9.0 mIU/mL) (SI: <0.20 IU/L [1.0-9.0 IU/L])
FSH = <0.20 mIU/mL (1.0-13.0 mIU/mL) (SI: <0.20 IU/L [1.0-13.0 IU/L])
ACTH = 135 pg/mL (10-60 pg/mL) (SI: 29.7 pmol/L [2.2-13.2 pmol/L])
17-Hydroxyprogesterone = 4100 ng/dL (<220 ng/dL) (SI: 124.2 nmol/L [<6.67 nmol/L])
Androstenedione = 2200 ng/dL (65-210 ng/dL) (SI: 76.8 nmol/L [2.27-7.33 nmol/L])
DHEA-S = 66 µg/dL (65-334 µg/dL) (SI: 1.79 µmol/L [1.76-9.05 µmol/L])

Which of the following is the best next step in this patient's management?

A. Measure gonadotropins and 11-ketotestosterone

B. Measure serum 17-hydroxyprogesterone

C. Recommend fertility evaluation for the patient's wife, as his testosterone concentration is normal

D. Refer for surgery for testicular adrenal rest tumor removal

Answer: A) Measure gonadotropins and 11-ketotestosterone

Although this man with classic 21-OHD has a normal testosterone concentration, he most likely has hypogonadotropic hypogonadism due to suppression of the hypothalamic-pituitary-gonadal axis by adrenal androgen excess. Testosterone and androstenedione are secreted by the gonads and by the adrenal glands. In men with 21-OHD, a testosterone-to-androstenedione ratio less than 2 is suggestive of suboptimal disease control. 11α-Hydroxyandrostenedione and its bioactive peripheral metabolite, 11-ketotestosterone, are produced in large amounts in patients with uncontrolled 21-OHD. 11-Ketotestosterone correlates inversely with testosterone in men with classic 21-OHD—the excess adrenal androgens suppress gonadotropins and, consequently, gonadal testosterone. Thus, the best next step is to measure gonadotropins and 11-ketotestosterone (Answer A). While in healthy reproductive-aged men, the adrenal contribution to the pool of circulating testosterone is negligible, the adrenal component might be significant in men with uncontrolled CAH, as in this case, making testosterone an unreliable biomarker (thus, Answer C is incorrect).

Serum 17-hydroxyprogesterone (Answer B) is useful for the diagnosis of CAH, but its role in monitoring therapy is limited. A serum 17-hydroxyprogesterone value in the normal range typically indicates glucocorticoid overtreatment and risk for associated adverse effects.[39]

Testicular adrenal rest tumors develop in up to 50% of adolescent boys and men with poorly controlled classic 21-OHD.[13] These tumors contribute to male infertility via mass effect, Sertoli-cell and cell damage, and blood flow interruptions. Intensified glucocorticoid treatment can be helpful in reducing the size of testicular adrenal rest tumors and restoring fertility, particularly if initiated before permanent fibrosis develops. Surgical removal can be offered to alleviate pain if intensified glucocorticoid therapy fails, but restoration of fertility is uncommon.[40] This patient had small and stable testicular adrenal rest tumors, so surgical removal (Answer D) is not indicated.

References

1. Speiser PW, White PC. Congenital adrenal hyperplasia. *N Engl J Med.* 2003;349(8):776-788. PMID: 12930931

2. Therrell BL Jr, Berenbaum SA, Manter-Kapanke V, et al. Results of screening 1.9 million Texas newborns for 21-hydroxylase-deficient congenital adrenal hyperplasia. *Pediatrics.* 1998;101(4 Pt 1):583-590. PMID: 9521938

3. Speiser PW, Dupont B, Rubinstein P, Piazza A, Kastelan A, New MI. High frequency of nonclassical steroid 21-hydroxylase deficiency. *Am J Hum Genet.* 1985;37(4):650-667. PMID: 9556656

4. Stikkelbroeck NM, Hermus ARMM, Braat DDM, Otten BJ. Fertility in women with congenital adrenal hyperplasia due to 21-hydroxylase deficiency. *Obstet Gynecol Surv.* 2003;58(4):275-284. PMID: 12665708

5. Cabrera MS, Vogiatzi MG, New MI. Long term outcome in adult males with classic congenital adrenal hyperplasia. *J Clin Endocrinol Metab.* 2001;86(7):3070-3078. PMID: 11443169

6. Reisch N, Flade L, Scherr M, et al. High prevalence of reduced fecundity in men with congenital adrenal hyperplasia. *J Clin Endocrinol Metab.* 2009;94(5):1665-1670. PMID: 19258407

7. Claahsen-van der Grinten HL, Otten BJ, Hermus ARMM, Sweep FCGJ, Hulsbergen-van de Kaa CA. Testicular adrenal rest tumors in patients with congenital adrenal hyperplasia can cause severe testicular damage. *Fertil Steril.* 2008;89(3):597-601. PMID: 17543962

8. Horrocks PM, London DR. Effects of long term dexamethasone treatment in adult patients with congenital adrenal hyperplasia. *Clin Endocrinol (Oxf).* 1987;27(6):635-642. PMID: 2843311

9. Young MC, Hughes IA. Dexamethasone treatment for congenital adrenal hyperplasia. *Arch Dis Child.* 1990;65(3):312-314. PMID: 2334212

10. El-Maouche D, Collier S, Prasad M, Reynolds JC, Merke DP. Cortical bone mineral density in patients with congenital adrenal hyperplasia due to 21-hydroxylase deficiency. *Clin Endocrinol (Oxf).* 2014. PMID: 24862755

11. Falhammar H, Filipsson Nystrom H, Wedell A, Brismar K, Thoren M. Bone mineral density, bone markers, and fractures in adult males with congenital adrenal hyperplasia. *Eur J Endocrinol.* 2013;168(3):331-341. PMID: 23211577

12. Arlt W, Willis DS, Wild SH, et al; United Kingdom Congenital Adrenal Hyperplasia Adult Study Executive (CaHASE). Health status of adults with congenital adrenal hyperplasia: a cohort study of 203 patients. *J Clin Endocrinol Metab.* 2010;95(11):5110-5121. PMID: 20719839

13. Finkielstain GP, Kim MS, Sinaii N, et al. Clinical characteristics of a cohort of 244 patients with congenital adrenal hyperplasia. *J Clin Endocrinol Metab.* 2012;97(12):4429-4438. PMID: 22990093

14. Speiser PW, Dupont J, Zhu D, et al. Disease expression and molecular genotype in congenital adrenal hyperplasia due to 21-hydroxylase deficiency. *J Clin Invest.* 1992;90(2):584-595. PMID: 1644925

15. Krone N, Braun A, Roscher AA, Knorr D, Schwarz HP. Predicting phenotype in steroid 21-hydroxylase deficiency? Comprehensive genotyping in 155 unrelated, well defined patients from southern Germany. *J Clin Endocrinol Metab.* 2000;85(3):1059-1065. PMID: 10720040

16. Quinkler M, Miodini Nilsen R, Zopf K, Ventz M, Oksnes M. Modified-release hydrocortisone decreases BMI and HbA1c in patients with primary and secondary adrenal insufficiency. *Eur J Endocrinol.* 2015;172(5):619-626. PMID: 25656494

17. Mallappa A, Sinaii N, Kumar P, et al. A phase 2 study of Chronocort, a modified-release formulation of hydrocortisone, in the treatment of adults with classic congenital adrenal hyperplasia. *J Clin Endocrinol Metab.* 2015;100(3):1137-1145. PMID: 25494662

18. Merza Z, Rostami-Hodjegan A, Memmott A, et al. Circadian hydrocortisone infusions in patients with adrenal insufficiency and congenital adrenal hyperplasia. *Clin Endocrinol (Oxf).* 2006;65(1):45-50. PMID: 16817818

19. Nella AA, Mallappa A, Perritt AF, et al. A phase 2 study of continuous subcutaneous hydrocortisone infusion in adults with congenital adrenal hyperplasia. *J Clin Endocrinol Metab.* 2016;101(12):4690-4698. PMID: 27680873

20. Turcu AF, Auchus RJ. Novel treatment strategies in congenital adrenal hyperplasia. *Curr Opin Endocrinol Diabetes Obes.* 2016;23(3):225-232. PMID: 27032061

21. Gehrand AL, Phillips J, Malott K, Raff H. A long-acting neutralizing monoclonal ACTH antibody blocks corticosterone and adrenal gene responses in neonatal rats. *Endocrinology.* 2019;160(7):1719-1730. PMID: 31166572

22. Sanders K, Mol JA, Kooistra HS, Galac S. Melanocortin 2 receptor antagonists in canine pituitary-dependent hypercortisolism: in vitro studies. *Vet Res Commun.* 2018;42(4):283-288. PMID: 30187173

23. de Bono JS, Logothetis CJ, Molina A, et al. Abiraterone and increased survival in metastatic prostate cancer. *N Engl J Med.* 2011;364(21):1995-2005. PMID: 21612468

24. Ryan CJ, Smith MR, de Bono JS, et al. Abiraterone in metastatic prostate cancer without previous chemotherapy. *N Engl J Med.* 2013;368(2):138-148. PMID: 23228172

25. Ryan CJ, Smith MR, Fizazi K, et al. Abiraterone acetate plus prednisone versus placebo plus prednisone in chemotherapy-naive men with metastatic castration-resistant prostate cancer (COU-AA-302): final overall survival analysis of a randomised, double-blind, placebo-controlled phase 3 study. *Lancet Oncol.* 2015;16(2):152-160. PMID: 25601341

26. Auchus RJ, Buschur EO, Chang AY, et al. Abiraterone acetate to lower androgens in women with classic 21-hydroxylase deficiency. *J Clin Endocrinol Metab.* 2014;99(8):2763-2770. PMID: 24780050

27. Perdomini M, Dos Santos C, Goumeaux C, Blouin V, Bougneres P. An AAVrh10-CAG-CYP21-HA vector allows persistent correction of 21-hydroxylase deficiency in a Cyp21(-/-) mouse model. *Gene Ther.* 2017;24(5):275-281. PMID: 28165447

28. Naiki Y, Miyado M, Horikawa R, et al. Extra-adrenal induction of Cyp21a1 ameliorates systemic steroid metabolism in a mouse model of congenital adrenal hyperplasia. *Endocr J.* 2016;63(10):897-904. PMID: 27432820

29. Casteras A, De Silva P, Rumsby G, Conway GS. Reassessing fecundity in women with classical congenital adrenal hyperplasia (CAH): normal pregnancy rate but reduced fertility rate. *Clin Endocrinol (Oxf).* 2009;70(6):833-837. PMID: 19250265

30. Rege J, Turcu AF, Kasa-Vubu JZ, et al. 11-Ketotestosterone is the dominant circulating bioactive androgen during normal and premature adrenarche. *J Clin Endocrinol Metab.* 2018;103(12):4589-4598. PMID: 30137510

31. Pretorius E, Africander DJ, Vlok M, Perkins MS, Quanson J, Storbeck KH. 11-Ketotestosterone and 11-ketodihydrotestosterone in castration resistant prostate cancer: potent androgens which can no longer be ignored. *PloS One.* 2016;11(7):e0159867. PMID: 27442248

32. Turcu AF, Mallappa A, Elman MS, et al. 11-Oxygenated androgens are biomarkers of adrenal volume and testicular adrenal rest tumors in 21-hydroxylase deficiency. *J Clin Endocrinol Metab.* 2017;102(8):2701-2710. PMID: 28472487

33. Turcu AF, Nanba AT, Chomic R, et al. Adrenal-derived 11-oxygenated 19-carbon steroids are the dominant androgens in classic 21-hydroxylase deficiency. *Eur J Endocrinol.* 2016;174(5):601-609. PMID: 26865584

34. Turcu AF, El-Maouche D, Zhao L, et al. Androgen excess and diagnostic steroid biomarkers for nonclassic 21-hydroxylase deficiency without cosyntropin stimulation. *Eur J Endocrinol.* 2020;183(1):63-71. PMID: 32487778

35. Bidet M, Bellanne-Chantelot C, Galand-Portier MB, et al. Fertility in women with nonclassical congenital adrenal hyperplasia due to 21-hydroxylase deficiency. *J Clin Endocrinol Metab.* 2010;95(3):1182-1190.

36. Miller WL, Witchel SF. Prenatal treatment of congenital adrenal hyperplasia: risks outweigh benefits. *Am J Obstet Gynecol.* 2013;208(5):354-359. PMID: 23123167

37. Auchus RJ, Sarafoglou K, Fechner PY, et al. Crinecerfont lowers elevated hormone markers in adults with 21-hydroxylase deficiency congenital adrenal hyperplasia. *J Clin Endocrinol Metab.* 2022;107(3):801-812. PMID: 34653252

38. Cumming DC. Use of spironolactone in treatment of hirsutism. *Cleve Clin J Med.* 1990;57(3):285-287. PMID: 2357784

39. Silva IN, Kater CE, Cunha CF, Viana MB. Randomised controlled trial of growth effect of hydrocortisone in congenital adrenal hyperplasia. *Arch Dis Child.* 1997;77(3):214-218. PMID: 9370898

40. Claahsen-van der Grinten HL, Otten BJ, Takahashi S, et al. Testicular adrenal rest tumors in adult males with congenital adrenal hyperplasia: evaluation of pituitary-gonadal function before and after successful testis-sparing surgery in eight patients. *J Clin Endocrinol Metab.* 2007;92(2):612-615. PMID: 17090637

Hypercortisolism: A Challenging Disease to Diagnose and Manage

Ricardo R. Correa, MD, EdD. Division of Endocrinology, Diabetes, and Metabolism, Department of Medicine, University of Arizona College of Medicine Phoenix and Phoenix VAMC, Phoenix, AZ; E-mail: riccorrea20@gmail.com

Katherine A. Araque, MD, MSCR. University of Arizona College of Medicine, Phoenix, AZ; E-mail: Katherine.araque.md@gmail.com

Learning Objectives

As a result of participating in this session, learners should be able to:

- Perform the appropriate hormonal workup in the assessment of hypercortisolism.

- Demonstrate an accurate clinical approach to the diagnosis of Cushing syndrome.

Main Conclusions

Hypercortisolism, or Cushing syndrome, can be a challenging diagnosis for clinicians to make. It requires some level of expertise from the physician and the possibility of repeating tests several times. For example, in the evaluation of endogenous Cushing syndrome, the guideline algorithm recommends documenting a positive result for 2 of 3 tests to diagnose hypercortisolism. Currently available tests include 24-hour urinary free cortisol measurement, late-night or bedtime salivary cortisol measurement, and the 1-mg dexamethasone-suppression test (DST).[1]

In contrast, when adrenal hypercortisolism is suspected, the most accurate test to detect adrenal secretion of cortisol is the 1-mg DST.[2] Improving understanding of the utility of current hypercortisolism diagnostic tests could enhance the ability of clinicians to confidently recommend next steps in management. Part of the problem in the diagnosis of Cushing syndrome is that there are numerous pitfalls in hormonal diagnostic assays that often preclude an early and correct diagnosis. For example, it is well established that cortisol measurements by immunoassays can be thwarted by cross-reactivity with other adrenal steroids (eg, cortisone) and other interferences inherent to binding-protein concentrations.[3]

Surgical resection continues to be first-line therapy for patients with hypercortisolism unless precluded by comorbidities. Medical treatment is usually reserved for patients with persistent or recurrent disease not amenable to curative surgical resection or when the clinical condition precludes surgery. Medical treatment is classified in various categories: (1) medications that directly affect the ACTH-secreting corticotroph adenoma, (2) steroidogenesis inhibitors, and (3) glucocorticoid receptor antagonists. Finally, a third-line option in some patients is the use of radiation.

The presentation of hypercortisolism varies from patient to patient and sometimes only 1 sign or symptom is present or the characteristics develop very quickly. This complicates the diagnosis and is considered an uncommon presentation of the disease.

Significance of the Clinical Problem

ACTH-dependent Cushing syndrome is a rare disorder caused by an ACTH-secreting pituitary adenoma or other ectopic ACTH-secreting tumor leading to endogenous hypercortisolism. ACTH-independent Cushing syndrome is usually caused by an adrenal adenoma or, in rare cases, by an adrenocortical carcinoma.[1,2] Signs and symptoms can overlap with many other comorbidities such as obesity, metabolic syndrome, alcohol dependence, or depression. Optimal clinical outcomes require a detail-oriented diagnosis, management of comorbidities, and careful treatment selection. Clinical judgment, index of suspicion, and laboratory and imaging results allow for early diagnosis and guide management.[3] Despite the advancement of disease awareness, education for early recognition, availability of laboratory testing, and newer imaging modalities, the mean time to diagnosis is 38 months for patients with an ACTH-secreting pituitary adenoma, 14 months for patients with an ectopic ACTH-secreting tumor, and 30 months for adrenal Cushing syndrome. Moreover, the time to early diagnosis has not improved for recently treated patients in comparison with the timelines in studies published before 2000.[4] Ultimately, we need better education for nonendocrine and endocrine practitioners in pattern recognition of this condition and the development of a more sensitive and specific test to detect hypercortisolism.

Barriers to Optimal Practice

- Physicians' lack of awareness and insufficient early recognition of the disease.

- Lack of simple and effective biochemical screening approaches and reliance on a combination of the recommended diagnostic tests because of varying sensitivity and specificity.

- Inconsistent patient access to multidisciplinary teams, recommended laboratory tests, or imaging modalities.

Strategies for Diagnosis, Therapy, and/or Management

Endogenous Cushing syndrome has a variable clinical presentation.[5] Biochemical screening and diagnostic tests include: (1) late-night or bedtime salivary cortisol measurement (≥2 tests), (2) overnight 1-mg DST or low-dose 2-day DST, and (3) 24-hour urinary free cortisol measurement (≥2 tests). Current guidelines advocate a combination of the described tests accounting for clinical judgment, index of suspicion, and local test availability.[3]

After endogenous Cushing syndrome is confirmed, increased plasma ACTH measurements (>20 pg/mL [>4.4 pmol/L]) suggest ACTH-dependent Cushing syndrome, while values between 10 and 20 pg/mL (2.2 and 4.4 pmol/L) can also be seen in patients with ACTH-independent Cushing syndrome. Values less than 5 pg/mL (<1.1 pmol/L) are exclusively seen in ACTH-independent Cushing syndrome.

A summary of the recommended testing modalities to distinguish between Cushing disease and an ectopic ACTH-secreting tumor are as follows (*Figure*):

- Inferior petrosal vein sampling (IPSS): IPSS is the gold standard procedure to rule out ectopic ACTH production, particularly when there are discordant findings from noninvasive localization tests (pituitary MRI, corticotropin-releasing hormone (CRH)–stimulation test, 8-mg DST). IPSS is an invasive procedure that measures ACTH in pituitary vs peripheral venous drainage. A basal ACTH inferior petrosal sinus-to-peripheral ratio of 2 or greater or of 3 or greater after stimulation suggests Cushing disease. Prolactin measurements may improve diagnostic accuracy.[6]

Figure. Algorithm of Recent Consensus on Diagnosis and Management of Cushing Syndrome[3]

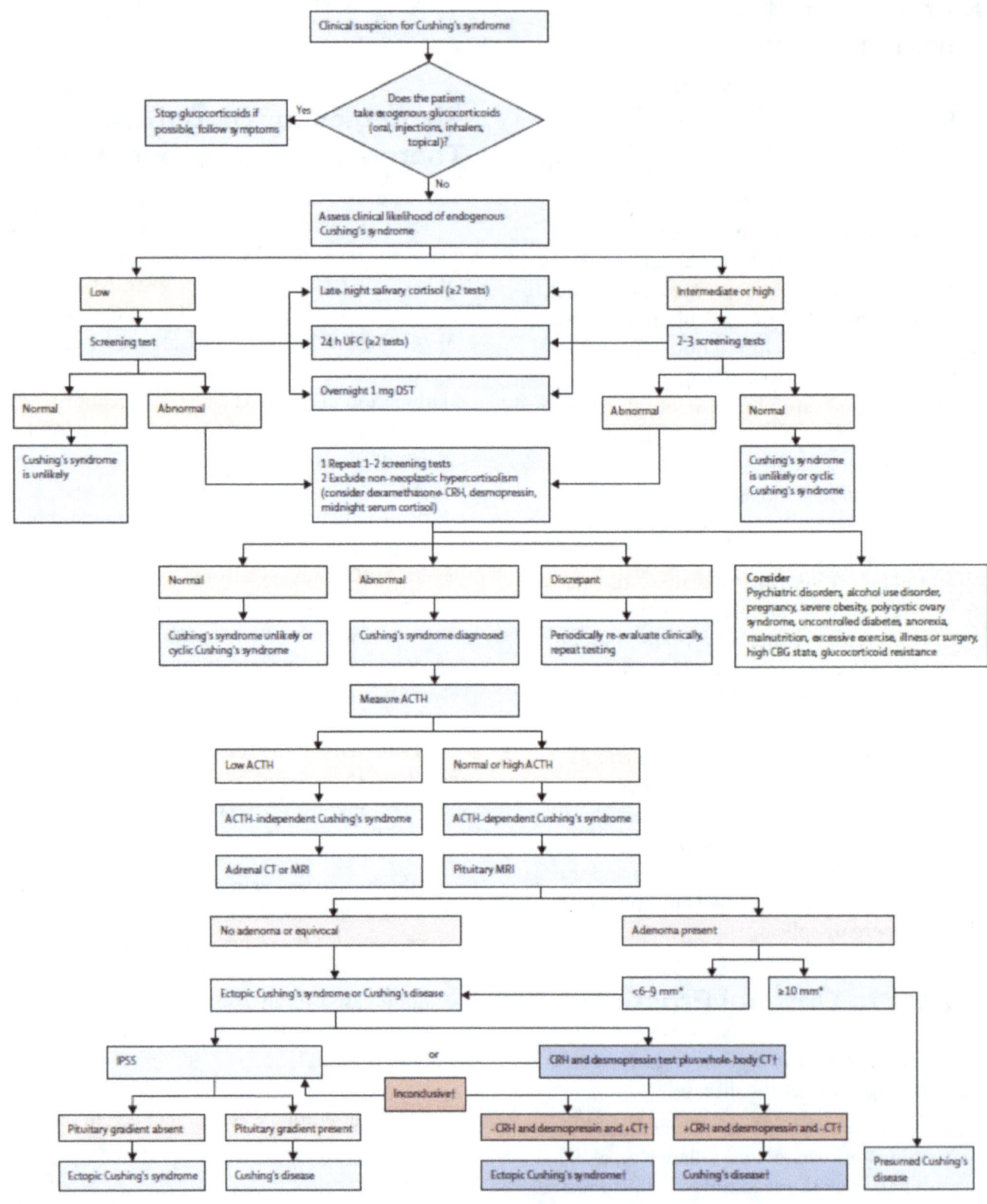

- Ovine CRH-stimulation test: Increased plasma ACTH of 35% or more from mean baseline to 15 to 30 minutes and increased serum cortisol concentrations of 20% or more from mean baseline to 30 to 45 minutes after CRH suggest Cushing disease.[7] Additional protocols with CRH or desmopressin administration can aid the confirmation Cushing disease.[8,9]

- High-dose (8-mg) DST: Serum cortisol suppression greater than 69% is observed in 77% of patients with Cushing disease. This test has variable accuracy.

- Pituitary MRI: Dedicated protocols to optimize the detection of pituitary microadenomas that may not be captured by 1.5T MRI are used. Examples of these protocols include spoiled gradient recalled acquisition echo with 1-mm slice intervals, fluid attenuation inversion recovery, T1-weighted turbo spin echo sequences, and use of 3T and 7T magnets. Pituitary adenomas smaller than 6 mm require IPSS, while adenomas 10 mm or larger may not need IPSS if there is agreement with additional biochemical localization test results. For 6- to 9-mm lesions, additional research is required; however, most experts in a recent consensus guideline advocated IPSS to confirm the diagnosis in this situation.[3]

Biochemical localization studies must be performed while the patient is hypercortisolemic. When results of noninvasive tests suggest Cushing disease, IPSS does not need to be performed.[10] Clinical presentation in combination with the described test results determines diagnosis and management. In cases where testing is suggestive of ectopic ACTH-secreting tumors, combination of anatomical (CT and/or MRI) and functional (^{68}Ga-DOTATATE) imaging aids tumor localization.

After biochemical confirmation of ACTH-independent Cushing syndrome, CT with adrenal protocol is the best next diagnostic step (*Figure*).

Treatment Modalities

The first-line treatment option for Cushing syndrome is surgery. Treatment of cortisol-induced comorbidities should also be high priority. Medical treatment is usually reserved for patients with persistent or recurrent disease not amenable to curative surgical resection or when the clinical condition precludes surgery. Radiotherapy is reserved for patients with persistent or recurrent Cushing disease after transsphenoidal surgery. Bilateral adrenalectomy is used in selected patients with persistent or recurrent Cushing disease who do not respond to medical therapy.

Pharmacologic treatments for Cushing syndrome are classified in various categories: (1) medications that directly affect the ACTH-secreting corticotroph adenoma (only for Cushing disease), (2) steroidogenesis inhibitors, and (3) glucocorticoid receptor antagonists (*Table*).

Clinical Case Vignettes

Case 1

A 38-year-old woman seeks evaluation for a 30-lb (14-kg) weight gain during the past year. She walks for 30 minutes daily and follows a healthy diet. Medical history is relevant for type 2 diabetes mellitus treated with metformin. Over the past 6 months, her hemoglobin A_{1c} level has increased from 6.5% to 8.0% (48 to 64 mmol/mol). Glipizide has been added to her treatment plan.

On physical examination, her blood pressure is 150/90 mm Hg, pulse rate is 75 beats/min, temperature is 98.4°F (37°C), and respiratory rate is 18 breaths/min. Her height is 65 in (165 cm), and weight is 220 lb (100 kg) (BMI = 36.6 kg/m²). She has erythematous, rounded facies, and prominent fat deposition in the supraclavicular area.

Laboratory test results (after fasting 8 hours):

> Hemoglobin A_{1c} = 9.0% (4.0%-5.6%) (75 mmol/mol [20-38 mmol/mol])
> Sodium = 137 mEq/L (136-142 mEq/L) (SI: 137 mmol/L [136-142 mmol/L])
> Potassium = 3.3 mEq/L (3.5-5.0 mEq/L) (SI: 3.3 mmol/L [3.5-5.0 mmol/L])

Table. Summary of Pharmacologic Medical Treatment Options for Cushing Syndrome

Agent	Mechanism of Action	Dosage	Common adverse events	FDA approval
Adrenal steroidogenesis inhibitors				
Ketoconazole	CYP11B1, CYP17 inhibitor; requires acid for biological activity	400 to 1600 mg daily every 8 to 12 hours	Hepatic dyscrasia, gastrointestinal distress, male hypogonadism, drug interactions	No
Levoketoconazole	CYP11B1, CYP17, and CYP21A2 inhibitor	150 to 600 mg every 12 hours	Nausea, headache, peripheral edema, hypertension	No
Metyrapone	CYP11B1 inhibitor; variable access	500 mg to 6 g daily every 6 to 8 hours	Gastrointestinal distress, hirsutism, hypertension, hypokalemia	No
Mitotane	Adrenolytic	250 mg to 8 g daily divided every 6 to 8 hours	Gastrointestinal distress, central nervous system toxicity, gynecomastia, low white blood cell count, high free T_4, transaminitis, high corticosteroid-binding globulin, drug interactions, teratogenic	Adrenocortical cancer
Etomidate	CYP11B1 inhibitor	Intravenous; validated intensive care unit protocols	Myoclonus, thrombophlebitis, hypnotic effects	No
Osilodrostat	CYP11B1 inhibitor	Starting dosage of 1 mg twice daily in patients of Asian descent Starting dosage of 2 mg twice daily in patients of nonAsian descent Maximum dosage: unlimited Most patients require 4 to 14 mg total daily dose	Nausea, headache, adrenal insufficiency, QT prolongation, hirsutism	Yes
Medications that target the pituitary tumor				
Pasireotide	Somatostatin analogue (SSTR5); affinity for SSTR1, 2, 3, and 5, but particularly for SSTR5	600 to 900 mcg subcutaneous every 12 hours or LAR 10 to 30 mg intramuscularly every 28 days	Hyperglycemia, bradycardia, QTc prolongation, transaminitis, cholelithiasis, hypopituitarism Drug interactions (cyclosporin, bromocriptine)	Yes
Cabergoline	Dopamine agonist (DR2)	1.5 to 7.0 mg weekly (divided into 2 doses twice a week)	Transaminitis, cardiac valvular fibrosis, hypertension, gastrointestinal distress, headaches, behavioral abnormalities	Yes
Retinoic acid/ isotretinoin NOT CONSENSUS GUIDELINES	POMC downregulation	Retinoic acid, 10 to 80 mg daily, and isotretinoin, 20 to 80 mg daily	Liver injury, conjunctival irritation, mucositis, arthralgia, transient diarrhea	No
R-roscovitine NOT CONSENSUS GUIDELINES	Selective inhibitor of the cyclin-dependent kinase 2 (CDK-2)/cyclin E signaling pathway	400 mg twice daily, 4 days per week	Teratogenic, gastrointestinal distress, hypokalemia	No
Glucocorticoid receptor antagonists				
Mifepristone	Glucocorticoid and progesterone receptor antagonist	300 to 1200 mg daily (but do not exceed 20 mg/kg per day)	Adrenal insufficiency, hypokalemia, vaginal bleeding, QTc prolongation, drug interactions	Yes, in patients with type 2 diabetes mellitus or glucose intolerance
Relacorilant NOT CONSENSUS GUIDELINES	Glucocorticoid receptor antagonist	100 to 400 mg daily	Back pain, headaches, peripheral edema, gastrointestinal distress, dizziness	No

Calcium = 8.8 mg/dL (8.2-10.2 mg/dL)
     (SI: 2.2 mmol/L [2.1-2.6 mmol/L])
Glucose = 187 mg/dL (70-99 mg/dL)
     (SI: 0.04 mmol/L [3.9-5.5 mmol/L])
Creatinine = 0.8 mg/dL (0.6-1.1 mg/dL)
     (SI: 70.7 μmol/L [53.0-97.2 μmol/L])
Total cholesterol = 300 mg/dL (<200 mg/dL)
     (SI: 7.77 mmol/L [<5.18 mmol/L]
TSH = 1.2 mIU/L (0.5-5.0 mIU/L)
Estimated glomerular filtration rate = >60 mL/min
     per 1.73 m^2 (>60 mL/min per 1.73 m^2)

Which of the following is the most appropriate next diagnostic step?

A. Measure late-night salivary cortisol

B. Measure morning ACTH

C. Measure random serum cortisol

D. Perform adrenal CT

E. Perform pituitary MRI

Answer: A) Measure late-night salivary cortisol

Late-night salivary cortisol concentrations (Answer A) are thought to correlate with level of free circulating plasma cortisol. An increase in blood cortisol is reflected by a change in the salivary cortisol concentration within a few minutes. Several factors may lead to false-positive results:

- Disruption of normal circadian rhythm in patients with depression or in shift workers

- Licorice, chewing tobacco, contamination from bleeding gums/recent tooth brushing, or cigarette smoking may cause elevated late-night cortisol

- Use of exogenous steroid-containing lotions or oral gels

- Stress immediately before collection

Neither measuring ACTH (Answer B) nor random serum cortisol (Answer C) is a screening test for hypercortisolism. After hypercortisolism is diagnosed, ACTH can be measured to determine whether it is ACTH-dependent or independent. Depending on the result, the Endocrine Society guideline algorithm indicates whether to perform

adrenal CT (Answer D) or pituitary MRI (Answer E), but neither is a first step in diagnosis.

Case 2

A 34-year-old man with a history of superior sagittal venous thrombosis, recurrent deep venous thrombosis (treated with apixaban), hypertension, type 2 diabetes mellitus, 70-lb (31.8-kg) weight gain over 5 months, and fatty liver is referred for additional workup.

Laboratory test results:

Urinary free cortisol = 220 μg/24 h (4-50 μg/24 h)
     (SI: 607.2 nmol/d [11-138 nmol/d])
Repeated measurement = 200 μg/24 h
     (SI: 552 nmol/d)
Late-night salivary cortisol (by liquid
     chromatography/mass spectrometry) = 0.42 μg/dL
     (<0.13 μg/dL) (SI: 11.59 nmol/L [<3.6 nmol/L])
Repeated measurement = 0.53 μg/dL
     (SI: 14.62 nmol/L)
ACTH = 60 pg/mL (10-60 pg/mL) (SI: 13.2 pmol/L
     [2.2-13.2 pmol/L])
8-mg DST = serum cortisol suppression by 87% with
     therapeutic dexamethasone levels

Pituitary 1.5T MRI reveals no pituitary adenoma.

Which of the following is the best next step?

A. Dexamethasone/CRH-stimulation test

B. DST (1 mg)

C. IPSS

D. Repeated pituitary MRI

Answer: C) IPSS

This patient has ACTH-dependent endogenous hypercortisolemia with negative findings on MRI. Localization with an 8-mg DST is suggestive of Cushing disease. Due to incongruence between the 2 reported noninvasive localization tests, the next step is to perform IPSS (Answer C). IPSS is the gold standard invasive test in the evaluation of ACTH-dependent Cushing syndrome.

This patient already underwent 2 screening tests and had positive results, thus confirming the diagnosis of hypercortisolism. There is therefore no need to do a 1-mg DST (Answer B).

Repeating the MRI (Answer D) would not yield any more information because the patient already had a recent MRI that did not identify an adenoma.

Case 2 (Continued)

IPSS is performed during hypercortisolemia (*see Table*):

Which of the following is the best next step?

A. Another IPSS
B. Chest CT
C. ^{68}Ga-DOTATATE scan
D. Transsphenoidal surgery

Answer: D) Transsphenoidal surgery

Prolactin measurement during IPSS can improve diagnostic accuracy and decrease the chance of false-negative results. A baseline prolactin inferior petrosal sinus-to-peripheral (IPS/P) ratio (ipsilateral to the dominant post-CRH ACTH IPS/P ratio) of 1.8 or greater suggests successful catheterization during the procedure. A basal

ACTH inferior petrosal sinus-to-peripheral (IPS/P) ratio of 2 or greater or of 3 or greater after stimulation suggests Cushing disease. The best next step is transsphenoidal surgery (Answer D). This patient underwent transsphenoidal surgery, and the pathology report described a 2-mm adenoma in the right lobe of the pituitary. Biochemical remission was subsequently achieved. The findings during transsphenoidal surgery confirmed that the patient had pituitary hypercortisolism.

There is no need to repeat IPSS (Answer A) or to evaluate the patient for ectopic hypercortisolism with a chest CT (Answer B) or ^{68}Ga-DOTATATE scan (Answer C).

Case 3

A 37-year-old woman without comorbidities presents to the emergency department with acute psychosis that rapidly evolves to depression with suicidal ideation and anorexia. Upon further interview, the patient reports weakness when walking upstairs, alopecia, and secondary

Time (min) ACTH	Right petrosal	Left petrosal	Peripheral	Right petrosal-to-peripheral ratio	Left petrosal-to-peripheral ratio
–5	260.3 pg/mL (SI: 57.3 pmol/L)	78.5 pg/mL (SI: 17.3 pmol/L)	27.0 pg/mL (SI: 5.9 pmol/L)	9.64	2.90
0	4766.3 pg/mL (SI: 1048.6 pmol/L)	211.7 pg/mL (SI: pmol/L)	28.6 pg/mL (SI: 6.3 pmol/L)	166.65	7.40
3	6218.3 pg/mL (SI: 1368.0 pmol/L)	433.7 pg/mL (SI: 46.6 pmol/L)	24.7 pg/mL (SI: 5.4 pmol/L)	251.75	17.55
5	10,650.2 pg/mL (SI: 2343.0 pmol/L)	687.3 pg/mL (SI: 151.2 pmol/L)	41.4 pg/mL (SI: 9.1 pmol/L)	257.25	16.60
10	9391.8 pg/mL (SI: 2066.2 pmol/L)	682.6 pg/mL (SI: 150.2 pmol/L)	63.0 pg/mL (SI: 13.9 pmol/L)	149.07	10.83

Time (min) prolactin	Right petrosal	Left petrosal	Peripheral	Right petrosal-to-peripheral ratio	Left petrosal-to-peripheral ratio
–5	631.4 ng/mL (SI: 27.5 nmol/L)	145.0 ng/mL (SI: 6.3 nmol/L)	66.5 ng/mL (SI: 2.9 nmol/L)	9.49	2.18
0	719.1 ng/mL (SI: 31.3 nmol/L)	165.1 ng/mL (SI: 7.2 nmol/L)	67.4 ng/mL (SI: 2.9 nmol/L)	10.66	2.44
3	735.2 ng/mL (SI: 32.0 nmol/L)	107.5 ng/mL (SI: 4.7 nmol/L)	62.8 ng/mL (SI: 2.7 nmol/L)	11.70	1.71
5	662.8 ng/mL (SI: 28.8 nmol/L)	75.4 ng/mL (SI: 3.3 nmol/L)	63.0 ng/mL (SI: 2.7 nmol/L)	10.52	1.19
10	787.6 ng/mL (SI: 34.2 nmol/L)	68.0 ng/mL (SI: 3.0 nmol/L)	62.2 ng/mL (SI: 2.7 nmol/L)	12.66	1.09

amenorrhea. She has been taking valproic acid, 600 mg daily; risperidone, 3 mg daily; sertraline, 100 mg daily; diazepam, 5 mg daily; vitamin B$_{12}$, 100 mcg daily; vitamin D, 1000 IU daily; and calcium, 1000 mg daily.

On physical examination, her blood pressure is 130/80 mm Hg. She has a rounded face, abdominal adiposity, muscle atrophy of the limbs, and spontaneous bruising of the lower limbs.

Laboratory workup (after 8 hours of fasting):

Plasma glucose = 82 mg/dL (70-99 mg/dL)
(SI: 4.6 mmol/L [3.9-5.5 mmol/L])
White blood cell count = 4896/μL (4500-11,000/μL)
(SI: 4.89 × 10⁹/L [4.5-11.0 × 10⁹/L])
Hematocrit = 42.6% (35%-45%) (SI: 0.426 [0.35-0.45])
Sodium = 141 mEq/L (136-142 mEq/L)
(SI: 141 mmol/L [136-142 mmol/L])
Potassium = 2.5 mEq/L (3.5-5.0 mEq/L)
(SI: 2.5 mmol/L [3.5-5.0 mmol/L])
Creatinine = 0.54 mg/dL (0.6-1.1 mg/dL)
(SI: 47.7 μmol/L [53.0-97.2 μmol/L])
Serum cortisol (8 AM) = 20.7 μg/dL (5-25 μg/dL)
(SI: 571.1 nmol/L [137.9-689.7 nmol/L])
Cortisol after 1-mg DST = 20.2 μg/dL
(SI: 557.3 nmol/L)
Late-night salivary cortisol = 0.55 μg/dL
(<0.13 μg/dL) (SI: 15.2 nmol/L [<3.6 nmol/L])
Repeated measurement = 0.52 μg/dL
(SI: 14.3 nmol/L)
Urinary free cortisol = 600 μg/24 h (4-50 μg/24 h)
(SI: 1656 nmol/d [11-138 nmol/d])
Repeated measurement = 550 μg/24 h
(SI: 1518 nmol/d)

Which of the following is the best next step?

A. ACTH measurement
B. Adrenal CT
C. Pituitary MRI
D. Repeated 1-mg DST with dexamethasone measurement

Answer: A) ACTH measurement

After the diagnosis of endogenous Cushing syndrome is established, serum ACTH is measured as a first step (Answer A) to determine the cause.

Patients with evidence of hypercortisolism and elevated ACTH levels should undergo additional testing, usually with pituitary MRI (Answer C). Further testing after pituitary MRI may include IPSS, CRH and desmopressin testing, and whole-body CT.

Patients with low serum ACTH concentrations should undergo adrenal imaging with CT (Answer B) and/or MRI to identify unilateral masses with adjacent and contralateral atrophy or bilateral disease.

This patient already has documented elevated urinary free cortisol and late-night salivary cortisol, satisfying 2 of 3 screening tests necessary to diagnose hypercortisolism. Cortisol after 1-mg DST was elevated too. She has hypercortisolism, so there is no need to repeat a 1-mg DST (Answer D).

References

1. Carroll TB, Findling JW. The diagnosis of Cushing's syndrome. *Rev Endocr Metab Disord.* 2010;11(2):147-153. PMID: 20821267

2. Biller BM, Grossman AB, Stewart PM, et al. Treatment of adrenocorticotropin-dependent Cushing's syndrome: a consensus statement. *J Clin Endocrinol Metab.* 2008;93(7):2454-2462. PMID: 18413427

3. Fleseriu M, Auchus R, Bancos I, et al. Consensus on diagnosis and management of Cushing's disease: a guideline update. *Lancet Diabetes Endocrinol.* 2021;9(12):847-875. PMID: 34687601

4. Rubinstein G, Osswald A, Hoster E, et al. Time to diagnosis in Cushing's syndrome: a meta-analysis based on 5367 patients. *J Clin Endocrinol Metab.* 2020;105(3):dgz136. PMID: 31665382

5. Nieman LK, Biller BM, Findling JW, et al. The diagnosis of Cushing's syndrome: an Endocrine Society clinical practice guideline. *J Clin Endocrinol Metab.* 2008;93(5):1526-1540. PMID: 18334580

6. Sharma ST, Raff H, Nieman LK. Prolactin as a marker of successful catheterization during IPSS in patients with ACTH-dependent Cushing's syndrome. *J Clin Endocrinol Metab.* 2011;96(12):3687-3694. PMID: 22031511

7. Nieman LK, Oldfield EH, Wesley R, Chrousos GP, Loriaux DL, Cutler GB Jr. A simplified morning ovine corticotropin-releasing hormone stimulation test for the differential diagnosis of adrenocorticotropin-dependent Cushing's syndrome. *J Clin Endocrinol Metab.* 1993;77(5):1308-1312. PMID: 8077325

8. Tsagarakis S, Tsigos C, Vasiliou V, et al. The desmopressin and combined CRH-desmopressin tests in the differential diagnosis of ACTH-dependent Cushing's syndrome: constraints imposed by the expression of V2 vasopressin receptors in tumors with ectopic ACTH secretion. *J Clin Endocrinol Metab.* 2002;87(4):1646-1653. PMID: 11932296

9. Ritzel K, Beuschlein F, Berr C, et al. ACTH after 15 min distinguishes between Cushing's disease and ectopic Cushing's syndrome: a proposal for a short and simple CRH test. *Eur J Endocrinol.* 2015;173(2):197-204. PMID: 25953828

10. Frete C, Corcuff J-B, Kuhn E, et al. Non-invasive diagnostic strategy in ACTH-dependent Cushing's syndrome. *J Clin Endocrinol Metab.* 2020;105(10):dgaa409. PMID: 32594169

Pheochromocytoma and Paraganglioma: Diagnosis and Perisurgical Management

Annika M. A. Berends, MD. Department of Endocrinology, University Medical Center Groningen, University of Groningen, Groningen, The Netherlands; E-mail: m.a.berends@umcg.nl

Michiel N. Kerstens, MD, PhD. Department of Endocrinology, University Medical Center Groningen, University of Groningen, Groningen, The Netherlands; E-mail: m.n.kerstens@umcg.nl

Learning Objectives

As a result of participating in this session, learners should be able to:

- Describe the main steps in the diagnostic workup of a pheochromocytoma or sympathetic paraganglioma (PPGL).

- Illustrate the optimal approach to the perioperative management of patients with a PPGL with respect to preoperative evaluation, surgical approach, and perioperative medical treatment.

- Identify drugs that can be given safely and drugs that should be avoided in patients with PPGL.

Main Conclusions

- Liquid chromatography/tandem mass spectrometry is the preferred assay method for measurement of metanephrines.

- A pheochromocytoma is unlikely in a patient with an adrenal tumor that has an unenhanced attenuation value on CT less than 10 Hounsfield units (HU).

- Genetic testing should be offered to all patients with a new diagnosis of PPGL, regardless of age.

- Management of PPGL is complex and requires a multidisciplinary team of dedicated specialists in centers with broad expertise.

- Surgical resection of a PPGL is a high-risk procedure for which optimal pretreatment with antihypertensive drugs, preferably α-adrenergic blockade, is required in combination with state-of-the-art surgical procedures and anesthetic techniques.

Significance of the Clinical Problem

PPGLs are rare chromaffin-cell tumors originating in the adrenal medulla (pheochromocytomas) and sympathetic paraganglia (paragangliomas), which share the capacity to synthesize and release catecholamines. If not recognized or treated in a timely manner, patients with PPGL are at risk to develop fatal cardiovascular complications from the excessive amounts of circulating catecholamines, which may result in myocardial infarction, cardiomyopathy, arrhythmias, cerebrovascular disease, or hypertensive emergencies with multiorgan failure. Another cause of mortality is related to metastatic disease. Most PPGLs are benign, but approximately 15% are metastatic, and metastases are present at the initial diagnosis in 10% to 30% of cases.[1]

Diagnosis of PPGL can be challenging for several reasons. Symptoms and signs are highly variable, which may impede early recognition. Importantly, PPGLs belong to the group of orphan diseases and, as such, the pretest probability of this disease is low. Biochemical confirmation is based on the demonstration of increased levels of metanephrines in plasma or urine. Reliable assessment of metanephrines requires advanced laboratory techniques, which are not always available. Even when using a robust assay with high specificity, the positive predictive value is limited because of the low pretest probability of PPGL. Therefore, selecting patients with an estimated higher risk of PPGL is important to improve the positive predictive value of biochemical testing.[1] Measurement of metanephrines is recommended in the following clinical scenarios or patients:

- Patients with signs and symptoms of PPGL

- Patients with a history of cardiovascular events (including Takotsubo cardiomyopathy) with suggestive signs or symptoms of PPGL

- When an adrenal incidentaloma is identified if the unenhanced attenuation value is 10 HU or greater

- Patients who are lean (BMI <25 kg/m^2) with type 2 diabetes

- Patients with history of PPGL or are a known carrier of a germline pathogenic variant in one of the PPGL susceptibility genes

- Patients who have features suggesting genetically determined or syndromic PPGL (eg, medullary thyroid carcinoma, multiple café-au-lait spots)[1]

About 40% of PPGL cases are hereditary with an autosomal dominant pattern of inheritance. In fact, PPGLs have the highest rate of heritability of all solid tumors in humans. Targeted next-generation sequencing should be offered to all patients with a new diagnosis of PPGL, regardless of age. It is worth considering repeated next-generation sequencing in patients who tested negative in the past, as the number of newly identified susceptibility genes is still growing.[1]

Surgery is the only curative treatment option for benign PPGL, but it should only be performed in centers with a multidisciplinary management team with sufficient expertise. During surgery, a patient is exposed to several stimuli that may evoke an uncontrolled and massive release of catecholamines from the PPGL into the circulation. This surge may result in potentially life-threatening cardiovascular complications ("pheo crisis"). Hazardous stimuli can be either mechanical (eg, endotracheal intubation, incision, peritoneal insufflation, tumor manipulation) or pharmacological (eg, metoclopramide, some neuromuscular-blocking agents). Over the years, the perioperative mortality rate has dropped significantly from approximately 40% in the early days to 0% to 3% when performed in a center with extensive expertise. Major developments in PPGL management that most likely have contributed to this notable improvement in surgical outcomes are advancements in medical imaging allowing precise tumor localization, introduction of minimally invasive surgery, optimization of presurgical treatment care, and refinement of anesthetic techniques.[2]

Barriers to Optimal Practice

- Due to the low incidence of PPGL, the diagnosis is often delayed and expertise in its management is not widely available. In addition, the rarity of this disease is a barrier to conducting well-controlled clinical trials.

- There is insufficient awareness that measurement of metanephrines should be considered when an adrenal incidentaloma is found.

- There is no uniformly accepted definition of hemodynamic instability, which impedes comparative research to establish optimal perisurgical management.

- The perisurgical risk of a patient with PPGL is difficult to predict, as determinants of hemodynamic instability during surgical resection are largely unknown.

Strategies for Diagnosis, Therapy, and/or Management

Biochemical Diagnosis of PPGL

Measurement of the O-methylated metabolites of catecholamines (ie, free metanephrines) in either plasma or 24-hour urine is considered to be the cornerstone for the biochemical diagnosis of PPGL. Caffeine, cigarette smoking, and alcohol intake should be withheld for approximately 24 hours before testing to avoid false-positive results. Sample collection for plasma metanephrines should be done after at least 20 minutes of supine rest. Laboratory methods for assessment of metanephrines differ in diagnostic performance. Liquid chromatography–tandem mass spectrometry has the highest sensitivity (98%-100%) and specificity (94%-96%) and is virtually unaffected by analytical interference.[3] Liquid chromatography with electrochemical detection has good sensitivity (95%-100%), but it might be affected by analytical interference from medications such as acetaminophen, α-methyldopa, sulfasalazine, and sotalol. Immunoassays for metanephrines demonstrate insufficient diagnostic performance and should preferably not be used. Apart from analytical interference, which is assay dependent, pharmacodynamic interference by medications causing falsely elevated plasma or urinary metanephrines should also be considered. Such interference is independent from the assay applied and can be encountered with drugs such as antidepressants, phenoxybenzamine, MAO-inhibitors, sympathomimetics, and levodopa. Withdrawal of these medications might be considered when initial testing yields a positive result.

Imaging of PPGL

In the diagnostic workup of PPGL, biochemical confirmation is followed by imaging studies to locate the tumor. Cross-sectional imaging by contrast-enhanced CT or MRI is usually sufficient to visualize the tumor. The addition of functional imaging studies, however, improves the sensitivity and specificity, in particular for demonstrating multifocal disease or metastases. Moreover, functional imaging studies can be used to evaluate the possibility of peptide-receptor radionuclide therapy. Several radiotracers are available, and the optimal choice depends on tumor genotype, biology, size, and biochemical phenotype. The European Association of Nuclear Medicine and the Society of Nuclear Medicine and Molecular Imaging have recently proposed a clinical algorithm for nuclear imaging investigations of PPGL (*Table 1*).[4]

Table 1. Proposed Clinical Algorithm for Nuclear Imaging Investigations in Patients With Pheochromocytoma and Paraganglioma.[4]

Diagnosis	First choice	Second choice	Third choice (if ^{18}F-DOPA or ^{68}Ga-SSA is not available)
Pheochromocytoma (sporadic)	^{18}F-DOPA or ^{123}I-MIBG	^{68}Ga-SSA	^{18}F-FDG
Inherited pheochromocytoma (except SDHx): NF1/RET/VHL/MAX	^{18}F-DOPA	^{123}I-MIBG or ^{68}Ga-SSA	^{18}F-FDG
Head and neck paraganglioma (sporadic)	^{68}Ga-SSA	^{18}F-DOPA	^{111}In-SSA/^{99m}Tc-SSA
Extraadrenal sympathetic and/or multifocal and/or metastatic and/or SDHx mutation	^{68}Ga-SSA	^{18}F-FDG and ^{18}F-DOPA	^{18}F-FDG and -^{123}I-MIBG or ^{18}F-FDG and ^{111}In-SSA/^{99m}Tc-SSA

The algorithm can be proposed as per the clinical situation. This algorithm should be practically adapted in each institution and evolve with time. Abbreviations: ^{123}I-MIBG, iodine-123-labeled metaiodobenzylguanidine; ^{18}F-FDA, fluorine-18-labeled fluorodopamine; ^{18}F-DOPA, fluorine-18-labeled fluorodihydroxyphenylalanine; ^{18}F-FDG, fluorine-18-labeled fluorodeoxyglucose; ^{68}Ga-SSA, gallium-68-labeled somatostatin analogue; ^{111}In-SSA, indium-111-labeled somatostatin analogue; ^{99m}Tc-SSA, technetium-99-labeled somatostatin analogue. Adapted with permission from Taïeb D et al. *Eur J Nucl Med Mol Imaging*, 2019;46(10) © Springer-Verlag GmbH Germany, part of Springer Nature.

Genetics of PPGL

PPGL has the highest known heritability rate among all solid tumors in humans; almost 40% of PPGLs are hereditary. Genetic testing should therefore be offered to patients with a new diagnosis of PPGL. Lack of family history of PPGL does not preclude the presence of a germline pathogenic variant. Next-generation sequencing is the preferred technique to analyze all relevant genes in a single testing panel. It is important to engage patients in shared decision-making before genetic testing.[1] Currently, more than 20 different causative germline variants have been identified. Based on their transcriptional profile, PPGLs have been divided into 2 clusters. Cluster 1, or the pseudohypoxia subgroup, includes pathogenic variants in genes encoding the succinate dehydrogenase complex (*SDHx* [ie, *SDHA*, *SDHAF2*, *SDHB*, *SDHC*, *SDHD*), *VHL*, *EPAS1*, *FH*, *MDH2*, or *EGLN1* (*PHD2*). These pathogenic variants stabilize hypoxia-inducible factor 1α and 2α, which in turn activate genes that induce angiogenesis, metabolism, and proliferation. Cluster 2, or the kinase signaling subgroup, includes pathogenic variants in the *RET* protooncogene, *NF1*, *MAX*, and *TMEM127*. In addition, 30% to 40% of sporadic PPGLs have somatic driver variants in cluster 1 genes (eg, *VHL*, *EPAS1*) or cluster 2 genes (eg, *NF1*, *RET*). Cluster 3 genes have been identified as a separate group of somatic variants resulting in increased expression of genes in the Wnt signaling pathway. These include genes include *CSDE1* and *MAML3*.[5] Germline pathogenic variants in PPGL susceptibility genes demonstrate an autosomal dominant inheritance pattern. In the case of *SDHD*, *SDAF2*, and *MAX* variants, there is maternal imprinting. Thus, the disease is only manifest when the pathogenic variant is paternally inherited. *SDHx* variants are the most prevalent (20%-30% of cases of PPGL), with the highest frequency in *SDHB* (9%-10%) and *SDHD* (2%-9%). The risk of metastatic PPGL is also highest in cluster 1 tumors. In particular, development of metastatic PPGL is most often seen in patients with *SDHB* (~25%) and *SDHA* variants (~12%).[6]

Perisurgical Management

Treatment of PPGL requires a multidisciplinary team of dedicated specialists in centers that have extensive experience in managing these complex patients. Minimally invasive adrenalectomy (including the laparoscopic transperitoneal, posterior retroperitoneal, and lateral retroperitoneal technique) is currently the preferred surgical approach for most pheochromocytomas. Laparoscopic surgery was found to be safe and resulted in a shorter duration of surgery, shorter hospital stay, and lower complication rate, including less blood loss, when compared with open adrenalectomy.[1] Bleeding complications, however, should not be neglected with the laparoscopic approach (reported frequency of approximately 4%). Lateral transperitoneal adrenalectomy and posterior retroperitoneoscopic adrenalectomy have been evaluated in 2 relatively small randomized controlled trials, demonstrating either no difference or superiority of the posterior approach with respect to perioperative and recovery outcomes. Open adrenalectomy is advised as the primary approach in case of large (usually >6 cm) or invasive PPGL.[1]

Another important aspect of presurgical management is medical treatment to provide symptom relief and control of hypertension. For this purpose, α-adrenergic receptor blockers are often considered the treatment of choice. Table 2 displays the proposed presurgical oral treatment options for patients with PPGL.[2] Instead of orally administered medications, there are also some intravenous alternatives that could be considered in specific cases (*Table 3*).[2] Tachycardia frequently occurs in patients with PPGL, either as a direct consequence of catecholamines or as an adverse effect of α-adrenergic receptor blockers. Tachycardia is effectively treated with either selective or nonselective β-adrenergic receptor blockers. An important point to keep in mind when starting β-adrenergic receptor blockers is that these drugs should only be started after a patient is already receiving α-adrenergic receptor blockade for several days. Otherwise, a crisis could be provoked due to unopposed stimulation of the α-adrenergic receptors. It is usually advised to give intravenous saline during the last 24 hours prior to surgery. The hypothesis underlying this practice is that high sodium should reduce the risk of preoperative orthostatic hypotension and postoperative hypotension. Supportive evidence for this is limited and based on only a few retrospective studies.

In general, the anesthetic management aims to provide optimal hemodynamic stability during PPGL surgery and the postoperative stage. Intraarterial blood pressure measurement is essential, as it allows for real-time monitoring of hemodynamic fluctuations and frequent blood sampling. Urine output monitoring via urinary bladder catheterization is routinely performed, and placement of a central venous catheter is strongly recommended for central venous pressure measurement and administration of vasoactive agents and fluid management. Transesophageal echocardiography might be considered for more optimal real-time monitoring of intravascular volume status and early detection of myocardial wall motion abnormalities.[7] Blood pressure should be kept within safe limits during surgery. There is, however, no consensus with respect to the exact blood pressure threshold values that require intervention by the anesthesiologist and no clear agreement on the definition of hemodynamic instability. In the PRESCRIPT study, these thresholds were defined as a mean arterial pressure less than 60 mm Hg and a

Table 2. Suggested Presurgical Oral Treatment of Patients With PPGL[2]

Drug	Starting dosage	Incremental dose steps*	Dose range	Comments
Phenoxybenzamine or Doxazosin ER	10 mg daily 4 mg daily	20 mg 4 mg	10-140 mg 4-56 mg	Preferably started at least 7 to 14 days prior to surgery, also in case of normotension; doses higher than starting dose are administered twice daily
Nifedipine ER or amlodipine or Metyrosine	30 mg daily 5 mg daily 250 mg 3 times daily	30 mg 5 mg 250-500 mg	30-90 mg 5-10 mg 750-2000 mg	Add-on to α-adrenergic receptor blockade in case of persistent hypertension (blood pressure supine >130/80 mm Hg, systolic blood pressure upright >110 mm Hg)
Metoprolol ER or Propranolol or Atenolol	50 mg daily 20 mg 3 times daily 25 mg daily	50 mg 20 mg 25 mg	50-200 mg 20-240 mg 25-100 mg	Add-on in case of tachycardia (heart rate supine >80 beats/min, heart rate upright >100 beats/min); preferably started after sufficient preparation with α-adrenergic receptor blockade (≥3 to 4 days)
High-sodium chloride diet and Saline, 0.9% intravenously	≥15 g 2 L/24 h	... ...	... ...	Restoration of intravascular volume depletion; prevention of preoperative orthostatic hypotension and postoperative hypotension Diet should be started >7 to 14 days before surgery Intravenous saline should be started 24 hours before surgery

*Dosage adjustments preferably every 2 to 4 days at the discretion of the clinician and guided by the response of blood pressure and/or heart rate

If supine blood pressure is greater than 160/100 mm Hg 24 hours before planned surgery, consider postponing surgery. Surgery is usually performed in the morning, and the last dose of each oral drug should preferably be administered the evening before surgery. In case surgery begins after 12 AM, the last dose of each oral drug should be administered at 7 AM the day of surgery. Only the administration of 0.9% saline should be continued during surgery. Adapted from Berends AMA et al. J Clin Endocrinol Metab, 2020; 105(9) © Endocrine Society.

Table 3. Suggested Intravenous Treatment of Hypertension and Tachyarrhythmia in Case of PPGL Crisis or During Surgery[2]

Indication	Drug	Dosage	Onset of action	Duration of action (after discontinuation)
Hypertension				
Step 1[a]	Magnesium sulfate[b]	Loading dose: 40-60 mg/kg followed by infusion of 1-4 g/h	Immediate	30 min
Step 2	Phentolamine[c]	Bolus: 2.5-5 mg at 1 mg/min, repeated every 3-5 min 2.5-5 mg at 1 mg/min, repeated every 3 to 5 min	1-2 min	10-30 min
		Continuous: 100 mg in 500 mL of 5% dextrose 20-100 mg/h	1-5 min	5-11 h
	or			
	Urapidil	Bolus: initial dose, 25-50 mg orolus: initial dose: 25-50 mg	1-5 min	15-30 min, may exceed 12 h after prolonged infusion
		Continuous: 10-15 mg/h		
Step 3	Nicardipine	Starting dose: 5 mg/h, increased by 2.5 mg/h every 5 min (if needed), maximum dose 15 mg/h	2-4 min	5-15 min
	or			
	Clevidipine	Starting dose: 1-2 mg/h, increase by doubling the dose every 90 seconds (if needed), maximum dose 32 mg/h	Immediate	2-3 min
Step 4	Sodium nitroprusside	Starting dose: 0.5-1.5 mcg/kg per min, dosage range: 0.5-4 mcg/kg per min; stop administration if no results are achieved after 10 min of infusion, maximal dose for 10 min only	2-5 min	5-10 min
	or			
	Nitroglycerine	Infusion adjusted according to response within the range of 10-200 mcg/min[d]		
Tachyarrhythmias				
Step 1	Esmolol[e]	Bolus: 500 mcg/kg in 1 min, repeat bolus after 5 min (if needed)	1-5 min	15-30 min
		Continuous: 25-100 mcg/kg per min, increase infusion rate to 300 mcg/kg per min (if needed)		
Step 2	Amiodarone	Loading dose (bolus): 5 mg/kg, followed by infusion of 15 mcg/kg per min	1-30 min	1-3 h
	or			
	Lidocaine	Loading dose (bolus): 1 mg/kg, repeat after 5-10 min (if needed)	<2 min	15-20 min
		Continuous: 2-4 mg/min (1-2 mg/mL), maximum 300 mg/h		

Suggested steps need to be individualized based on comorbidity.

[a] Check for adequate pain treatment and depth of anesthesia.

[b] Also prevention and treatment of tachyarrhythmias.

[c] In case of norepinephrine-producing tumor, 2 mg before tumor manipulation.

[d] Tachyphylaxis can occur after a continuous infusion greater than 24 hours.

[e] In case of epinephrine- or dopamine-producing tumor, 20 mg before tumor manipulation.

Adapted from Berends AMA et al. *J Clin Endocrinol Metab*, 2020; 105(9) © Endocrine Society.

systolic blood pressure greater than 160 mm Hg.[8] The number of vasoactive agents and volume therapy (infusion of fluids, predominantly intravenous saline, to correct hypotension) required to maintain the blood pressure within these limits may vary substantially among patients. Blood pressure levels alone are therefore insufficient to evaluate hemodynamic stability during PPGL resection. To overcome this problem, a hemodynamic instability score has been developed consisting of 3 components (hemodynamic variables including blood pressure and heart rate, volume therapy, and vasoactive agents), which provides a tool to quantify the degree of intraoperative hemodynamic instability.[9]

Clinical Case Vignettes

Case 1

A 51-year-old woman with chronic hypertension, palpitations, and intermittent headaches is evaluated for the presence of a pheochromocytoma. She follows a diet rich in fruits and vegetables. She has no family history of pheochromocytoma.

On physical examination, her blood pressure is 176/105 mm Hg and pulse rate is 88 beats/min. BMI is 22 kg/m^2.

Laboratory test results:

> Serum creatinine = 1.4 mg/dL (0.6-1.1 mg/dL)
> (SI: 125.0 µmol/L [53.0-97.2 µmol/L])
> Plasma normetanephrine = 220 pg/mL (<165 pg/mL)
> (SI: 1.20 nmol/L [<0.90 nmol/L])
> Plasma metanephrine = 108 pg/mL (<99 pg/mL)
> (SI: 0.55 nmol/L [<0.50 nmol/L])
> 3-Methoxytyramine = <0.04 nmol/L (<0.04 nmol/L)

Which of the following is correct regarding biochemical analysis for PPGL?

A. Plasma metanephrines are not affected by age or sex

B. PPGL can be safely excluded when the plasma metanephrine elevation is less than 2 times the upper normal limit

C. Renal insufficiency may increase the plasma metanephrine concentration

D. The plasma metanephrine concentration is affected by ingestion of certain food products

Answer: C) Renal insufficiency may increase the plasma metanephrine concentration

Clinical manifestations of PPGL are highly variable and are related to the amounts, proportions, and secretion patterns of catecholamines (ie, episodic or continuous). In a prospective cohort of patients with (n = 245) and without (n =1820) PPGL (participants in whom metanephrines had been determined), it was demonstrated that only 19% of patients with PPGL presented with the classic triad of headache, palpitations, and sweating.[10] In the same study, a score system was developed to estimate PPGL risk. The likelihood was increased with a symptom score of 3 or greater, where 1 point was assigned to each of 7 features (ie, BMI <25 kg/m^2, heart rate ≥85 beats/min, pallor, sweating, palpitations, tremor, nausea), with a negative point for obesity. The patient in this case had a symptom score of at least 3, so further evaluation for PPGL was justified.

The interpretation of plasma or urinary metanephrine measurement is optimized when using sex- and age-specific reference intervals (thus, Answer A is incorrect).[11] Negative test results virtually exclude PPGL, the exception being very small or nonsecreting tumors. Elevations of any plasma metabolite greater than 2 times the upper reference limit or increases in 2 or more metabolites are very rare in the absence of PPGL but occur in more than 80% of patients with PPGL (thus, Answer B is incorrect).[1]

Catecholamine-rich foods may increase the plasma or urine concentration of 3-methoxytyramine, but they do not affect the plasma or urine concentration of metanephrine (thus, Answer D is incorrect).

A common problem in clinical practice is the presence of kidney impairment. Plasma levels of free metanephrines are frequently elevated in patients with stage 3 chronic kidney disease (or worse) and in those on long-term dialysis treatment (thus, Answer C is correct). In addition,

PPGL is frequently suspected in patients with chronic kidney disease, as both conditions share similar signs and symptoms such as hypertension, blood pressure swings, palpitations, and pulmonary edema. Optimized reference intervals for plasma metanephrines in patients with chronic kidney disease have been established.[12]

Case 2

A 65-year-old man with obesity is admitted to the thoracic surgery department for coronary artery bypass grafting the following day. The thoracic surgeon asks for advice on the finding of a tumor in the right adrenal gland, which was demonstrated 6 months earlier on CT of the thorax and has not been evaluated. The adrenal tumor measures 2.1 × 2.6 cm, has sharp margins, and has an unenhanced attenuation value of 8 HU. The patient does not report any symptoms suggestive of PPGL and has hypertension controlled with an ACE inhibitor and a β-adrenergic blocker.

Which of the following is the best advice for the thoracic surgeon?

A. Continue with coronary artery bypass grafting after informing the anesthesiologist about the presence of the adrenal incidentaloma

B. Measure plasma metanephrines and postpone coronary artery bypass grafting

C. Start doxazosin, 8 mg once daily, and continue with coronary artery bypass grafting as planned

Answer: A) Continue with coronary artery bypass grafting after informing the anesthesiologist about the presence of the adrenal incidentaloma

The median reported frequency of pheochromocytoma in adrenal incidentalomas is 7% (range, 1.4%-14%), although this figure is probably an overestimation, as pheochromocytoma is a rare disease. A recent nationwide study in the Netherlands demonstrated an incidence rate for pheochromocytoma of 0.46 per 100,000 person years. This patient had a symptom score less than 3, and the low

unenhanced attenuation value of the adrenal tumor also predicts a very low pheochromocytoma risk. In a meta-analysis, it was shown that a precontrast HU value less than 10 had a sensitivity of 99% for excluding pheochromocytoma.[13] To find 1 pheochromocytoma with a density less than 10 HU, it was estimated that 1232 patients would have to be screened by measuring metanephrines. A limitation of this meta-analysis, however, is that all of the included studies were retrospective in design.

In general, it is probably prudent to measure metanephrines in any patient with an adrenal incidentaloma before undergoing surgery. This decision should be balanced, however, against the risk and inconvenience of postponing surgery, as results of metanephrine measurement are often not available within a day after blood sampling. In this case, information on the very small risk of a pheochromocytoma provided the anesthesiologist the opportunity to take precautionary measures and be prepared for the unlikely event of hemodynamic instability occurring during coronary artery bypass grafting (thus, Answer A is correct and Answers B and C are incorrect). Apart from the absence of a clear indication for starting doxazosin, a further drop in already well-controlled blood pressure carries the risk of inducing cardiac ischemia in a patient with coronary artery disease.

Case 3

A 35-year-old man is referred by the clinical geneticist because of the recent finding of a pathogenic variant in the *SDHB* gene identified on family screening. He feels well, has no concerns, and is normotensive. His father was the index patient in whom the *SDHB* variant was first detected after resection of a PPGL at age 62 years.

Which of the following tests is NOT indicated as part of the initial workup of an asymptomatic carrier of an *SDHB* pathogenic variant?

A. 24-Hour ambulatory blood pressure monitoring

B. Examination by a urologist

C. Measurement of plasma metanephrines

D. MRI of the head and neck and thoracic, abdominal, and pelvic regions

E. PET with ^{68}Ga-DOTATATE

Answer: B) Examination by a urologist

Apart from PPGL, including head and neck paragangliomas, patients with *SDHx* germline pathogenic variants are also at increased risk for renal cell carcinoma and gastrointestinal stromal tumors. A recently issued consensus statement on initial screening and follow-up of asymptomatic *SDHx* variant carriers recommends initial screening with 24-hour ambulatory blood pressure monitoring (Answer A), symptom questionnaire, measurement of plasma metanephrines (Answer C), and MRI of the head and neck and thoracic, abdominal, and pelvic regions (Answer D).[14] In addition, asymptomatic adults who carry an *SDHx* variant should have a baseline PET (Answer E). The expert panel did not reach consensus on the optimal PET tracer to be used for this purpose, but it did refer to the recent EANM-SNMMI guideline, which recommends the use of ^{68}Ga-DOTA-somatostatin analogue PET as the first-choice functional imaging modality (*Table 1*). For screening purposes, examination by a urologist does not have additional value, as renal cell carcinoma is best diagnosed by imaging (thus, Answer B is correct).

Follow-up consists of annual measurement of blood pressure, measurement of plasma metanephrines, and symptom questionnaire. MRI of the aforementioned regions should be repeated every 2 to 3 years. Recommended follow-up in children is similar, except for measurement of metanephrines every 2 years. The first tumor screening should be performed between age 6 and 10 years for asymptomatic carriers of *SDHB* variants and between 10 and 15 years in asymptomatic

carriers of *SDHA*, *SDHC*, and *SDHD* variants (only in case of parental inheritance for *SDHD* carriers).

Case 4

A 45-year-old man presents to the outpatient clinic for evaluation of an incidentally found adrenal mass on ultrasonography performed for abdominal pain for which no cause was eventually established. Other than abdominal pain, the patient has no concerns. Biochemical analysis confirms the diagnosis of a pheochromocytoma. CT reveals a right adrenal mass measuring 2.1 × 2.5 × 3.0 cm, with no evidence for locally invasive or metastatic disease. The patient is referred to the endocrine surgeon for adrenalectomy.

Which of the following additional examinations should be performed preoperatively?

A. Ambulatory blood pressure monitoring

B. Electrocardiography

C. Echocardiography

D. A and B

E. B and C

F. A and C

G. All of the above

Answer: G) All of the above

Preoperative evaluation of a patient with PPGL should include detailed history taking, physical examination, electrocardiography (Answer B), echocardiography (Answer C), and 24-hour ambulatory blood pressure monitoring (Answer A). Thus, the best answer is "all of the above" (Answer G). Examination of cardiac function should be performed in every patient regardless of physical performance, clinical picture, tumor size, cardiovascular risk factors, or age. A smaller tumor size (<3 cm) does not protect against the occurrence of cardiovascular complications, and it has been shown that there is no relationship between tumor size and the rate of perisurgical complications. The clinical picture of catecholamine-induced cardiomyopathy is often atypical, and this disorder might also develop in a patient at a young age in the absence of cardiovascular risk factors. Notably, preoperative abnormalities on electrocardiography or echocardiography are associated with an increased risk for cardiac complications.[15]

Case 4 (continued)

Nifedipine, 30 mg once daily, is started. Supine blood pressure is 152/85 mm Hg, and it drops to 140/75 mm Hg after 3 minutes in the upright position. Pulse rate is 88 beats/min. Laboratory measurements demonstrate normal electrolytes and normal kidney function. Electrocardiography shows a sinus rhythm of 70 beats/min with no abnormalities. Transthoracic echocardiography reveals a left ventricular ejection fraction of 58%, stroke volume of 90 mL, and normal diastolic and valvular function with no additional strain pattern visible.

Which of the following is the preferred next step in this patient's management?

A. Administer no pretreatment

B. Increase the nifedipine dose to 60 mg once daily

C. Start doxazosin 4 mg once daily

D. Start metoprolol, 50 mg once daily

E. Start metyrosine, 250 mg 3 times daily

Answer: C) Start doxazosin 4 mg once daily

Table 2 displays an overview of the suggested presurgical oral treatment of patients with PPGL.[2] In general, α-adrenergic receptor blockers are advised as the treatment of first choice. There is longstanding experience with these agents, and their use is a good example of targeted therapy, as these drugs specifically block the overstimulation of the α receptors by catecholamines. These drugs are started at least 7 to 14 days before surgery in a stepwise manner until blood pressure targets are achieved. Either a competitive, selective α1 receptor blocker (eg, doxazosin [Answer C], prazosin, or terazosin), or a noncompetitive, nonselective α1 and α2 receptor blocker (ie, phenoxybenzamine) may be

given orally. Doxazosin has been studied more extensively than either prazosin or terazosin. Compared with doxazosin, phenoxybenzamine has a longer duration of action and causes more reflex tachycardia due to the irreversible receptor binding and blockade of the presynaptic α2 receptor, respectively. A practical disadvantage of phenoxybenzamine is the relatively high cost and its limited availability in several countries. In a recently published meta-analysis, there were no differences found between groups with respect to overall morbidity and mortality. There is only one randomized controlled trial on this topic (the PRESCRIPT study).[8] In this study, no differences were found in the total duration of blood pressure outside a predefined target range. There was, however, less hemodynamic instability during surgery after pretreatment with phenoxybenzamine. Furthermore, there were no differences between groups with respect to postoperative hypotension, duration of hospital stay, perioperative complications, or adverse events.

β-adrenergic receptor blockers (Answer D) should only be started after a patient is already receiving α-adrenergic receptor blockade for several days. Otherwise, a crisis could be provoked due to unopposed stimulation of the α-adrenergic receptors.

There are a few alternative drugs for α-receptor blockers, such as calcium channel blockers (Answer B) and metyrosine (Answer E). Calcium channel blockers are most often used as an add-on drug to α-receptor blockers if blood pressure control is not achieved sufficiently. These drugs inhibit the catecholamine-mediated calcium influx in vascular smooth muscle cells, thereby reducing vasoconstriction. Calcium channel blockers do not cause tachycardia and have only a moderate effect on preload reduction, which could be an advantage in case of coexisting heart failure. Presurgical monotherapy with oral calcium channel blockers has been described, but they should probably be used in only selected patients. Another suggested preparation drug is metyrosine (α-methyl-para-tyrosine), which significantly reduces circulating catecholamine levels through inhibition of tyrosine hydroxylase, the key enzyme catalyzing the rate-limiting step in catecholamine biosynthesis. In general, metyrosine should be prescribed as an add-on drug to α-adrenergic blockade, since monotherapy has been shown to be less effective. Compared with α-receptor blockers and calcium channel blockers, metyrosine has some disadvantages: it is expensive, has limited availability, and has several adverse effects such as depression, anxiety, and somnolence. Of notice, the absence of hypertension does not preclude the occurrence of cardiovascular complications, and normotensive patients therefore also require adequate medical pretreatment. The level of evidence supporting pretreatment in patients with PPGL is moderate and mainly based on observational studies and expert opinion. There are no randomized placebo-controlled trials on this topic.

Several investigators have recently questioned the need for presurgical treatment, especially with α-adrenergic receptor blockade.[16] The few available comparative studies suggesting that these drugs could be omitted safely are without exception small-sized, retrospective in design, and flawed by several methodological shortcomings. The debate about the clinical value of presurgical α-receptor blockade can only be resolved by a well-designed randomized controlled trial. Until then, it is advised to follow the Endocrine Society's guideline that all patients with a functional PPGL, regardless of tumor size, degree of catecholamine production, or blood pressure should undergo pretreatment (thus, Answer A is incorrect).[1,3]

Case 5

A 70-year-old woman with pheochromocytoma is admitted to the hospital. Surgery is scheduled in 2 weeks. She has been experiencing nausea and vomiting, which has compromised her adherence to doxazosin, 4 mg twice daily. On physical examination, her blood pressure is 140/80 mm Hg, and pulse rate is 75 beats/min with a normal sinus rhythm. She would like a prescription for antiemetic treatment.

How should this patient be advised regarding antiemetic treatment?

A. Data regarding safety of antiemetic therapy are conflicting

B. Metoclopramide is superior to ondansetron

C. Most antiemetic agents should only be given after sufficient α-adrenergic receptor blockade has been achieved

D. No antiemetic medication is safe to use preoperatively

Answer: C) Most antiemetics should only be given after sufficient α-adrenergic receptor blockade has been achieved

Several antiemetic medications have been suggested to elicit a pheochromocytoma crisis, either by direct or indirect stimulation of catecholamine release. Importantly, frequently prescribed antiemetics such as metoclopramide and other dopamine receptor antagonists are contraindicated in this setting. Table 4 displays an overview of the drugs that should be avoided and those drugs that can be given safely in patients with PPGL. Most of these observations are based on case reports. It is, however, best to avoid these drugs or to only introduce them after sufficient α-adrenergic receptor blockade has been achieved (Answer C).

Case 6

A 56-year-old man is admitted to the hospital because of cardiogenic shock. Physical examination shows a strongly fluctuating blood pressure, ranging from addition 112/70 mm Hg to 193/95 mm Hg, pulse rate of 60 beats/min, sinus rhythm, and peripheral oxygen saturation (SpO_2) of 90% on room air. He is noted to have mild nonpitting bilateral ankle edema. He has a history of coronary artery disease and has been taking enalapril, metoprolol, acetylsalicylic acid, and a statin. Electrocardiography shows ST elevations, and serum levels of cardiac-specific troponins are increased. Transthoracic echocardiography is notable for a diffusely dyskinetic left ventricle,

Table 4. Overview of Medications That Can Be Safely Used and Potential Precipitants of Adverse Outcomes During Perioperative Anesthesia in Patients With PPGL[2]

Sedative-hypnotic agents used for anesthetic induction/maintenance	
Inhalation agents	
Safe	**Comments**
Sevoflurane	
Isoflurane	
Enflurane	
Nitrous oxide	
Not safe	**Comments**
Halothane	Arrhythmogenic, sensitizing the myocardium to circulating catecholamines
Desflurane	Used without incident in some cases; however, not recommended, can induce sympathomimetic effects
Intravenous agents	
Safe	**Comments**
Propofol	
Etomidate	
Dexmedetomidine	
Not safe	**Comments**
Ketamine	Sympathomimetic effects
Thiopental (thiopentone)	Used without incident in some cases; however, not recommended, can precipitate hypertensive crises, linked to histamine-releasing properties
Neuromuscular-blocking agents	
Safe	**Comments**
Rocuronium	
Vecuronium	
Not safe	**Comments**
Succinylcholine (suxamethonium)	Can precipitate a hypertensive crisis and severe cardiac arrhythmias
Pancuronium	Histamine release, thereby causing severe pressor response
Atracurium Tobucurarine Mivacurium	Cause histamine release, thereby provoking catecholamine release, associated with severe arterial hypertension and ventricular arrhythmias
Cisatracurium	Adverse reactions linked to histamine-releasing properties, thereby provoking catecholamine release

Sedative-hypnotic agents used for anesthetic induction/maintenance	
Anxiolytic agents	
Safe	**Comments**
Midazolam	No anxiolytic agent is superior
Lorazepam	
Diazepam	
Analgesic agents	
Safe	**Comments**
Fentanyl	
Sufentanil	
Alfentanil	
Remifentanil	
Not safe	**Comments**
Morphine Hydromorphone Pethidine*	These opioids cause histamine release, thereby provoking catecholamine release
Antiemetic agents	
Safe	**Comments**
Ondansetron	
Not safe	**Comments**
Metoclopramide Chlorpromazine Prochlorperazine	D2 receptor antagonists: cause indirect but potent release of catecholamines by stimulation of presynaptic D2 receptors
Domperidone	Can induce hypertensive crisis
Droperidol Haloperidol	Severe hypertension due to increased catecholamine efflux
Cisapride	Can stimulate catecholamine release from PPGL cells through activation of serotonin type 4 receptors
Miscellaneous	
Not safe	**Comments**
Ephedrine	Sympathomimetic effects, stimulates catecholamine release from PPGL
Atropine	Inhibits cardiac vagus and potentiates chronotropic effects of catecholamines

*Pethidine is also known as meperidine, isonipecaine, lidol, operidine, pethanol, and piridosal.

Adapted from Berends AMA et al. *J Clin Endocrinol Metab*, 2020; 105(9) © Endocrine Society.

consistent with the diagnosis of Takotsubo cardiomyopathy with a reduced ejection fraction of 15%. Coronary angiography reveals no significant coronary stenosis. Cardiac ischemia is mainly attributed to coronary spasms. An underlying diagnosis of pheochromocytoma is suspected and confirmed by additional biochemical testing and CT that demonstrates a 3.5-cm right adrenal mass. The patient is transferred to the intensive care unit for hemodynamic stabilization.

Which of the following is the best treatment recommendation?

A. Bolus of phentolamine intravenously

B. Bolus of sodium nitroprusside intravenously

C. Continuous administration of esmolol intravenously

D. Continuous administration of urapidil intravenously

E. Doxazosin orally twice daily

F. Emergency resection of the pheochromocytoma

G. No additional treatment is feasible given the strong blood pressure swings

Answer: D) Continuous administration of urapidil intravenously

Pharmacotherapy is the mainstay of medical stabilization in case of a pheochromocytoma crisis, and emergency resection of a pheochromocytoma (Answer F) should be avoided given the associated high perioperative morbidity and mortality.

Control of hypertension should be the initial treatment goal here, preferably achieved through medication that has rapid onset with a relatively short duration of action, thereby enabling effective dosage titration. There are no evidence-based recommendations with respect to the preferred medical management of a pheochromocytoma crisis. Several drugs have been described in the literature (*Table 3*). In view of the patient's medical history of coronary artery disease, urapidil (Answer D) should be the preferred option. Urapidil is a competitive α1-adrenergic receptor antagonist with central agonistic action at serotonin 5-HT1A receptors and it does not cause reflex tachycardia.

Phentolamine (Answer A) is contraindicated in patients with coronary artery disease because it can induce reflex tachycardia.

Sodium nitroprusside (Answer B) may reduce coronary perfusion and induce intracoronary steal due to a strong decline in mainly diastolic arterial pressure, which is undesirable in case of heart failure and concomitant coronary artery spasm.

A β1 selective adrenergic receptor blocker, such as esmolol (Answer C), should be given in case of tachyarrhythmia after achievement of sufficient α-adrenergic receptor blockade.

References

1. Lenders JWM, Kerstens MN, Amar L, et al. Genetics, diagnosis, management and future directions of research of phaeochromocytoma and paraganglioma: a position statement and consensus of the Working Group on Endocrine Hypertension of the European Society of Hypertension. *J Hypertens.* 2020;38(8):1443-1456. PMID: 32412940

2. Berends AMA, Kerstens MN, Lenders JWM, Timmers HJLM. Approach to the patient: perioperative management of the patient with pheochromocytoma or sympathetic paraganglioma. *J Clin Endocrinol Metab.* 2020;105(9):dgaa441. PMID: 32726444

3. Lenders JWM, Duh Q-Y, Eisenhofer G, et al; Endocrine Society. Pheochromocytoma and paraganglioma: an Endocrine Society clinical practice guideline. *J Clin Endocrinol Metab.* 2014;99(6):1915-1942. PMID: 24893135

4. Taïeb D, Hicks RJ, Hindié E, et al. European Association of Nuclear Medicine Practice Guideline/Society of Nuclear Medicine and Molecular Imaging Procedure Standard 2019 for radionuclide imaging of phaeochromocytoma and paraganglioma. *Eur J Nucl Med Mol Imaging.* 2019;46(10):2112-2137. PMID: 31254038

5. Berends AMA, Eisenhofer G, Fishbein L, et al. Intricacies of the molecular machinery of catecholamine biosynthesis and secretion by chromaffin cells of the normal adrenal medulla and in pheochromocytoma and paraganglioma. *Cancers (Basel).* 2019;11(8):1121. PMID: 31390824

6. Amar L, Pacak K, Steichen O, et al. International consensus on initial screening and follow-up of asymptomatic SDHx mutation carriers. *Nat Rev Endocrinol.* 2021;17(7):435-444. PMID: 34021277

7. Naranjo J, Dodd S, Martin YN. Perioperative management of pheochromocytoma. *J Cardiothorac Vasc Anesth.* 2017;31(4):1427-1439. PMID: 28392094

8. Buitenwerf E, Osinga TE, Timmers HJLM, et al. Efficacy of α-blockers on hemodynamic control during pheochromocytoma resection: a randomized controlled trial. *J Clin Endocrinol Metab.* 2020;105(7):2381-2391. PMID: 31714582

9. Buitenwerf E, Boekel MF, van der Velde MI, et al. The haemodynamic instability score: development and internal validation of a new rating method of intra-operative haemodynamic instability. *Eur J Anaesthesiol.* 2019;36(4):290-296. PMID: 30624247

10. Geroula A, Deutschbein T, Langton K, et al. Pheochromocytoma and paraganglioma: clincial feature-based disease probability in relation to catecholamine biochemistry and reason for disease suspicion. *Eur J Endocrinol.* 2019;181(4):409-420. PMID: 31370000

11. Eisenhofer G, Peitzsch M, Kaden D, et al. Reference intervals for LC-MS/MS measurements of plasma free, urinary free and urinary acid-hydrolyzed deconjugated normetanephrine, metanephrine and methoxytyramine. *Clin Chim Acta.* 2019;490:46-54. PMID: 30571948

12. Pamporaki C, Prejbisz A, Małecki R, et al. Optimized reference intervals for plasma free metanephrines in patients with CKD. *Am J Kidney Dis.* 2018;72(6):907-909. PMID: 30146420

13. Buitenwerf E, Berends AMA, van Asselt ADI, et al. Diagnostic accuracy of computed tomography to exclude pheochromocytoma: a systematic review, meta-analysis, and cost analysis. *Mayo Clin Proc.* 2019;94(10):2040-2052. PMID: 31515105

14. Amar L, Pacak K, Steichen O, et al. International consensus on initial screening and follow-up of asymptomatic SDHx mutation carriers. *Nat Rev Endocrinol.* 2021;17(7):435-444. PMID: 34021277

15. Shen J, Yu R. Perioperative management of pheochromocytoma: the heart of the issue. *Minerva Endocrinol.* 2013;38(1):77-93. PMID: 23435444

16. Groeben H, Walz MK, Nottebaum BJ, et al. International multicentre review of perioperative management and outcome for catecholamine-producing tumours. *Br J Surg.* 2020;107(2):e170-e178. PMID: 31903598

Below the Tip of the Iceberg: Just How Much Aldosterone Is Out There?

Martin Reincke, MD. Medizinische Klinik und Poliklinik IV, Munich University Hospital, Munich, Germany; E-mail: martin.reincke@med.uni-muenchen.de

Learning Objectives

As a result of participating in this session, learners should be able to:

- Describe the prevalence of and populations at risk for endocrine hypertension.

- Describe the target population that should be screened for primary aldosteronism (PA).

- Order appropriate tests to diagnose and subtype PA.

- Initiate individualized treatment depending on PA subtype.

Main Conclusions

PA, also called Conn syndrome, is a common cause of secondary hypertension associated with high cardiovascular morbidity and mortality. PA remains underdiagnosed because it does not have a specific, easily identifiable feature and clinicians are often unaware of the disease. The causes of PA can be a unilateral aldosterone-producing adrenal adenoma (APA) or bilateral idiopathic adrenal cortex hyperplasia (BAH). However, advances in molecular histopathology challenge this traditional concept of PA as a binary disease. The classic hypokalemic form occurs more frequently in the case of APA, whereas the normokalemic form is mostly observed in patients with BAH. PA screening is required in patients with refractory hypertension, younger patients with hypertension, patients with arterial hypertension and hypokalemia, patients with arterial hypertension and obstructive sleep apnea, and patients with arterial hypertension and adrenal incidentaloma. Screening is performed using the sensitive, but not specific, aldosterone-to-renin ratio (ARR). The diagnosis requires confirmatory testing in most patients, using tests such as the saline-loading test or the captopril challenge test. Subtype differentiation is carried out by means of CT imaging of the adrenal glands in combination with, as a gold standard, adrenal venous sampling to distinguish between unilateral and bilateral aldosterone production. Patients with PA have an increased risk of stroke, myocardial infarction, atrial fibrillation, and renal insufficiency compared with patients who have essential hypertension. Early diagnosis and appropriate targeted therapy are critically important. Adrenalectomy is indicated for patients with unilateral PA. In patients with BAH, therapy with spironolactone (starting dosage 25 mg daily, up-titrated according to blood pressure, hypokalemia, and renin concentration) should be initiated.

Significance of the Clinical Problem

Once considered rare, PA is now thought to be the most common secondary endocrine form of hypertension. The introduction of ARR as a screening tool and its application to a widening population of patients with hypertension have led to a marked increase in the detection of PA. Most studies report PA prevalence rates between 5% and 15%, with most affected patients being normokalemic. Recent studies have suggested that autonomous aldosterone secretion could be even more frequent than currently accepted in patients with hypertension. Variability in prevalence rates reported in different studies is explained by the use of different diagnostic methods and cutoffs.

Aldosterone excess in persons with PA is associated with deleterious effects on the heart, vessels, brain, and kidney, which are partly independent of elevated blood pressure determined by hyperaldosteronism. These effects result in disproportionate degrees of organ damage for a given blood pressure and lead to left ventricular hypertrophy, diastolic dysfunction, heart failure, increased intima media thickening, arterial stiffness, arterial wall inflammation, stroke, renal hyperfiltration, albuminuria, and glomerulosclerosis. In terms of metabolic effects, aldosterone excess causes decreased insulin secretion and insulin resistance leading to diabetes mellitus, lower serum calcium and higher urinary calcium excretion leading to hyperparathyroidism, increased prevalence of osteoporosis and risk of bone fractures, and sleep apnea through fluid retention.

Barriers to Optimal Practice

- The patient groups for whom screening is recommended account for approximately 50% of the hypertensive population. However, currently fewer than 1% of patients with PA are screened and treated during their lifetime.

- Subtyping using imaging and adrenal venous sampling is driven by the intention to identify suitable candidates for unilateral adrenalectomy. Adrenal venous sampling is complex, costly, and not widely available.

- The 2 subtypes of PA, unilateral and bilateral forms, represent extremes of a spectrum of histomorphological and biochemical phenotypes and are not totally distinct.

Asymmetric bilateral primary aldosteronism with some lateralization is common, and this poses challenges in diagnosis and treatment.

Strategies for Diagnosis, Therapy, and/or Management

Introduction

PA is defined as hypertension caused by disproportionately high aldosterone secretion with consequent low plasma renin and increased ARR. PA is the most common cause of endocrine arterial hypertension: recent data indicate a prevalence of 5.8% in unselected hypertensive patients in primary care, 6% to 12% in patients in hypertensive outpatient clinics, and up to 30% in patients with resistant hypertension.[1]

Compared with essential hypertension, PA is associated with increased morbidity and mortality, even when patients have the same blood pressure. This underscores the importance of a timely diagnosis of the affected patients, as there is an excellent long-term prognosis after adequate therapy. A recently published meta-analysis showed a decrease in mortality, which started to become noticeable 5 to 7 years after initiation of therapy, especially in the group of patients who underwent unilateral adrenalectomy. Mortality decreased below that of patients with essential hypertension.[2]

Diagnosing PA is a 3-part process: screening, confirmatory testing, and subtyping. The 2 most common causes of PA are APAs (accounting for approximately one-third of cases), which can be treated surgically by means of unilateral adrenalectomy, and BAH (accounting for approximately two-thirds of cases), which can be treated with mineralocorticoid receptor antagonists. Rare causes are unilateral aldosterone-producing carcinomas and familial forms of the disease caused by germline pathogenic variants (familial hyperaldosteronism [FH] I-IV).

In recent years, important new articles on the diagnosis and treatment of PA have been published.

Diagnosis

Who should be screened? According to the Endocrine Society guidelines, groups at risk for PA should be screened, which applies to up to 50% of hypertensive patients.[3] Screening is recommended for patients with the following:

- Blood pressure >150/100 mm Hg on 3 different days
- Therapy-resistant hypertension (3 antihypertensive agents, including a diuretic)
- Controlled hypertension on ≥4 antihypertensive drugs
- Hypertension and hypokalemia
- Hypertension and adrenal incidentaloma
- Hypertension and sleep apnea
- Hypertension and positive family history of early-onset hypertension or cerebrovascular event occurring at younger than 40 years
- First-degree relatives with PA

Screening

Patients are screened using the ARR. In some settings, renin activity has been replaced by renin concentration because of its rapidity and reproducibility. Plasma aldosterone measurement using radioimmunoassay is also being gradually replaced by much more precise mass spectrometry.

Note: To achieve a high level of reliability when screening using ARR, care should be taken to ensure a liberal salt intake, to compensate for any hypokalemia that may be present, and to take into consideration antihypertensive drugs that potentially interfere with the renin-angiotensin-aldosterone system.

In particular, β-adrenergic blockers and mineralocorticoid receptor antagonists lead to false-positive or false-negative screening results due to their influence on renin secretion. A recently published meta-analysis, which included 10 studies on a total of 4110 patients, showed that the sensitivity of ARR varies between 10% and 100% and the specificity ranges from 70% to 100%. These results suggest that ARR has a limited ability to identify patients with PA.[4]

Confirmatory Testing

Since ARR as a screening test has limited sensitivity and specificity, most patients with a positive screening test should be further evaluated with confirmatory testing. The principle of a dynamic confirmation test is used here, which is intended to demonstrate the lack of aldosterone suppressibility.

Note: The intravenous saline-load test, captopril challenge test, oral saline-load test, and fludrocortisone-suppression test are available as confirmation tests. These tests have similar diagnostic accuracies, but they differ in adverse effects and feasibility.

The diagnostic algorithm allows the confirmatory test to be bypassed in certain situations: patients with high plasma aldosterone (>20 ng/dL [>555 pmol/L]), low renin, and spontaneous hypokalemia can proceed directly to subtype differentiation.[3,5] Very recently, a study involving 240 patients undergoing the saline-infusion test assessed discordance between automated immunoassay and mass spectrometry–based measurements of plasma aldosterone. Plasma aldosterone measured by immunoassays were respectively 86% and 58% higher than by mass spectrometry. Discordance was noted in 16% to 32% of patients, who by adrenal venous sampling were classified as having BAH. Discordance was eliminated by plasma purification to remove interferents. These findings raise concerns about the validity of automated immunoassay-based diagnosis of PA.[6]

To simplify the diagnosis, the use of a so-called prediction score has been investigated several times. Recently, an Italian working group was able to create a flow chart and score with various parameters (sex, antihypertensive drugs, potassium, end-organ damage, renin, aldosterone) with which 22.8% of all confirmatory tests could be bypassed.[7]

Subtyping

The rate of incidentaloma increases with age, so that bilateral adrenal venous sampling is recommended for subtype differentiation.[3] The details of the adrenal vein catheter protocol (sequential vs simultaneous withdrawal or cosyntropin-stimulated vs unstimulated withdrawal) differ among centers. Adrenal venous sampling is a costly and invasive procedure and is very rarely associated with severe adverse effects (hemorrhage). It requires a high level of expertise and is therefore not widely available. Imaging of the adrenal glands is always performed to not only visualize adrenal morphology, but also as a planning tool to visualize adrenal vein anatomy. Imaging also rules out the very rare adrenal carcinoma. Some older studies were able to show that adrenal venous sampling leads to more accurate lateralization than imaging (sensitivity 95% vs 78%; specificity 100% vs 75%).[8,9] A more recent European randomized controlled study of 200 patients with PA (SPARTACUS trial) showed no significant difference in the clinical and biochemical outcome when the therapeutic decision for adrenalectomy was based on adrenal venous sampling or CT[10]; however, this result has not been confirmed in most other studies. In a retrospective data analysis of a large multicenter cohort that included 18 centers, there were again indications of inferiority of CT-based decision-making vs adrenal venous sampling–based diagnostics.[11,12] In additional studies, the discrepancy of CT vs catheter-based diagnostics could be demonstrated several times, so taken together, adrenal venous sampling remains firmly anchored as the preferred test in the differential diagnosis of PA.

Note: Adrenal venous sampling continues to be the gold standard in the differential diagnosis of PA and paves the way for subtype-specific therapy: adrenalectomy for APA and mineralocorticoid receptor antagonist treatment for BAH.

The guidelines recommend proceeding directly to adrenalectomy in certain situations (young age with pronounced clinical signs, adrenal mass in imaging).[3] Various scores can predict

unilateral disease with a high specificity of 89% to 100%.[13-15] To simplify the diagnostic flow, "prediction scores" based on steroid profiling or clinical parameters were also examined. Several studies have demonstrated a difference in the secretion of the hybrid steroids 18-hydroxycortisol and 18-oxocortisol between patients with PA vs primary hypertension, but also between the PA subtypes.[16] A Japanese working group was able to show that the 18-oxocortisol values in patients with unilateral APAs were significantly higher than in patients with BAH (diagnostic sensitivity 83%, specificity 99%).[17] The authors proposed that by measuring 18-oxocortisol in their diagnostic model, mineralocorticoid receptor antagonist therapy could be started directly in 43% of patients with bilateral disease without the need for adrenal venous sampling. Subsequently, another European study demonstrated a reduced ability of 18-hydroxycortisol and 18-oxocortisol to discriminate between the 2 subtypes. Mass spectrometry measurement of 12 different steroids led to correct subtype classification in 80% of patients with PA.[18] Although some of the steroids used were different, these study findings suggest that peripheral blood steroid profiling may make adrenal venous sampling unnecessary in the future in patients with bilateral disease.

Modified criteria from confirmatory testing are also useful in subtype differentiation. Various studies have shown that subtype differentiation is possible based on results of the saline-infusion test using a score.[19,20] The addition of clinical parameters (age, potassium, adrenal mass) may increase the discriminatory ability of the saline-infusion test.[21] Recently, Burello et al validated prediction models for PA subtype diagnostics in a large study using machine learning.[22]

A high expression of CXCR4 (CXC chemokine receptor type 4) in APA could be demonstrated, correlating with the expression of CYP11B2 (aldosterone synthase). In one study, the specific CXCR4 tracer ^{68}Ga-pentixafor PET-CT showed a stronger uptake in patients with known APA.[23] Functional imaging using ^{11}C-metomidate PET-CT also represents a promising method for noninvasive subtype differentiation, as recently published case reports suggest.[24,25] The ^{11}C-metomidate labels CYP11B2 activity in the adrenal cortex. However, other studies show limited suitability, so further analyses appear necessary.[26]

Therapy

Current data suggest that adrenalectomy is superior to mineralocorticoid receptor antagonist therapy in terms of mortality, cardiovascular and metabolic risk, kidney function, and quality of life.[27-29] Patients with PA who are treated with mineralocorticoid receptor antagonists have a higher risk of atrial fibrillation than patients with essential hypertension, while adrenalectomized patients no longer have an increased risk.[30] A large population-based study was able to demonstrate a reduced risk of diabetes mellitus in adrenalectomized patients vs the risk in patients with essential hypertension, while patients treated with medication showed an increased risk.[29] The PASO study recently defined the criteria for surgical cure.[10] The complete clinical cure represents the postoperative normalization of blood pressure; complete biochemical cure represents normalization of serum potassium and ARR. In the PASO study, 37% of 700 patients studied met criteria for complete clinical cure, while 94% had complete biochemical remission. A recent nomenclature consensus workshop (HISTALDO, histopathology of primary aldosteronism) supported use of CYP11B2 (aldosterone synthase)-based immunohistochemistry for classification of adrenal histopathology lesions in PA.[31] It distinguished classic histopathologic findings (APA, dominant aldosterone-producing nodules) from nonclassic ones (multiple aldosterone-producing micronodules, diffuse adrenal hyperplasia). A prospective study over 3 years in 60 adrenalectomized patients[32] showed that APA or dominant aldosterone-producing nodes were associated with higher initial aldosterone and ARR values and a higher probability of postoperative remission (97.6% vs 66.7% [$P = .002$]) compared with observations in patients with nonclassic histopathology. Patients with nonclassic histopathology showed a higher absolute aldosterone concentration in the vein of the (unresected) contralateral adrenal gland during adrenal venous sampling.

Prior to adrenalectomy, therapy with MR antagonists should be initiated to compensate for hypokalemia and control blood pressure. After adrenalectomy, follow-up is necessary to verify biochemical and clinical remission of PA. Medical therapy with mineralocorticoid receptor antagonists is recommended to treat BAH. Drug therapy can also be prescribed for patients who cannot undergo operation for medical reasons or who decline to do so. A study by Hundemer et al compared cardiovascular outcomes among 3 groups: 205 patients with unilateral disease who underwent adrenalectomy, 602 patients with BAH who received medical treatment, and more than 40,000 patients with primary hypertension.[33] Despite similar blood pressure control, patients treated with mineralocorticoid receptor antagonists had a significantly higher risk of cardiovascular events than patients who underwent adrenalectomy, while patients who underwent adrenalectomy had a significantly lower risk than patients with primary hypertension. However, patients who experienced renin normalization induced by mineralocorticoid receptor antagonist therapy had a similar cardiovascular risk to that of patients who underwent adrenalectomy. A similar conclusion was reached by another study showing that the increased risk of atrial fibrillation in drug-treated patients with PA was associated with renin suppression.[34] This illustrates the importance of adequate dosing of mineralocorticoid receptor antagonists.

Note: Mineralocorticoid receptor antagonists should be gradually titrated: the starting dosage of spironolactone is 25 to 50 mg daily. The aim is to normalize blood pressure, serum potassium levels, and renin levels. In addition, care should be taken to restrict salt intake.

Summary

PA is the most common cause of endocrine arterial hypertension, affecting 6% of the hypertensive population, most of whom are undiagnosed. The diagnostic workup continues to consist of a 3-step process: screening using ARR, confirmatory testing, and subtyping (with CT and adrenal venous sampling). To simplify the diagnosis, so-called prediction scores are increasingly used. Steroid profiling from peripheral blood (using liquid chromatography–mass spectrometry) could reduce the need for adrenal venous sampling in patients with bilateral disease. Functional imaging is also a promising method for noninvasive subtype differentiation. Adrenalectomy offers the potential for a cure by eliminating aldosterone excess, leading to improved patient outcomes. In the case of drug therapy, mineralocorticoid receptor antagonists should be dosed adequately: the aim is to normalize blood pressure, potassium levels, and renin levels.

Clinical Case Vignettes

Case 1

A 44-year-old woman presents with an 8-year history of arterial hypertension. Her height is 67 in (170 cm), and weight is 181 lb (82 kg) (BMI = 28.3 kg/m²). She has tried many antihypertensive medications, but her blood pressure has become increasingly unresponsive in recent years. Currently, she takes candesartan, 8 mg twice daily; chlortalidone, 25 mg daily; and amlodipine, 5 mg twice daily. Her office blood pressure is 170/99 mm Hg and automated ambulatory blood pressure monitoring reading is 161/95 mm Hg without night dipping.

Laboratory test results:

> Serum creatinine, normal
> Serum potassium = 3.8 mEq/L (SI: 3.8 mmol/L)
>   (on a low-salt diet)
> Serum sodium = 144 mEq/L (SI: 144 mmol/L)

Which of the following is the most likely pretest probability for PA in this patient?

A. <5%

B. 5%-10%

C. 10%-15%

D. >15%

Answer: D) >15%

This patient has resistant hypertension, as defined by the American Heart Association and European Society of Cardiology classification, and she should be screened for PA according to all guidelines. The pretest probability for such a patient in most studies between 15% and 30% (Answer D).

Case 2

A 33-year-old man with recent-onset grade 2 WHO hypertension has been evaluated for primary aldosteronism. His height is 69 in (175 cm), and weight is 165 lb (75 kg) (BMI = 24.4 kg/m²). He has spontaneously hypokalemia (lowest potassium concentration, 2.6 mEq/L [2.6 mmol/L]), and he does not currently take any antihypertensive drugs.

His biochemical workup shows the following hormone levels:

> Plasma aldosterone = 455 ng/dL (50-200 ng/dL)
>   (SI: 12,622 pmol/L [1387-5548 pmol/L])
> Plasma renin = <2 pg/mL (3-40 pg/mL)
>   (SI: <0.05 pmol/L [0.07-0.95 pmol/L])
> ARR = 152 (<20)

These values are similar to those documented 1 week earlier. Abdominal CT without contrast shows a 1.5-cm adrenal mass with a density of 5 Hounsfield units. The contralateral adrenal gland is normal in appearance.

Which of the following diagnostic procedures is most appropriate?

A. Adrenal MRI

B. Adrenal venous sampling

C. Confirmatory testing using saline-infusion test

D. No diagnostic testing; the patient can be directly referred for right adrenalectomy

Answer: D) No diagnostic testing; the patient can be directly referred for right adrenalectomy

This young patient has a pronounced form of PA. According to guideline recommendations, he does not need confirmatory testing (Answer C) because of the severe biochemical phenotype. He also does not need adrenal venous sampling (Answer B) because he is younger than 35 years and the right adrenal nodule is suggestive of a fat-rich adenoma (Hounsfield units <10). Adrenal MRI (Answer A) is not superior to adrenal CT in localizing adrenal adenomas in patients with PA. Thus, the patient can be referred directly for right adrenalectomy (Answer D).

Case 3

A 55-year-old man with recent-onset grade 2 WHO hypertension has been diagnosed with PA based on an elevated ARR and nonsuppressed aldosterone in response to intravenous saline loading. Abdominal CT demonstrates a 3.5-cm adrenal mass in the left adrenal gland and a 1.5-cm right adrenal lesion. The patient undergoes bilateral simultaneous unstimulated adrenal venous sampling (*see Table*).

Which of the following interpretations is most appropriate?

A. The adrenal venous sampling procedure is technically successful for both adrenal glands, in terms of selectivity index

B. The results suggest lateralization to the right adrenal vein

C. The results suggest contralateral suppression in the left adrenal vein

D. The results suggest probable cortisol secretion in the left adrenal vein

E. All of the above

Answer: E) All of the above

Answers A through D are all correct. The selectivity index (ratio of cortisol right and left adrenal / cortisol peripheral vein) is greater than 2.0, which suggests selective catheterization. There is strong lateralization to the right side (ratio aldosterone/cortisol right adrenal vein / ratio aldosterone/cortisol left adrenal vein of 296 [>4.0 indicate lateralization]). The contralateral aldosterone/cortisol ratio is below the peripheral aldosterone/cortisol ratio, and the absolute aldosterone concentration in the right adrenal vein (400 ng/dL [11,096 pmol/L]) is minimally higher than in the periphery (320 ng/dL [8877 pmol/L]). The large adrenal mass on the right side, however, and the high cortisol concentration in the left adrenal vein could suggest cortisol cosecretion. A 1-mg dexamethasone-suppression test should be performed to rule this out.

Source	Cortisol	Aldosterone	Selectivity index adrenal veins	Lateralization index
Right adrenal vein	35 μg/dL (SI: 965.6 nmol/L)	14,500 ng/dL (SI: 402,230 pmol/L)	7	414
Peripheral vein	15 μg/dL (SI: 413.8 nmol/L)	320 ng/dL (SI: 8877 pmol/L)		21
Left adrenal vein	277 μg/dL (SI: 7641.9 nmol/L)	400 ng/dL (SI: 11,096 pmol/L)	18	1.4

References

1. Yang Y, Reincke M, Williams TA. Prevalence, diagnosis and outcomes of treatment for primary aldosteronism. *Best Pract Res Clin Endocrinol Metab.* 2020;34(2):101365. PMID: 31837980

2. Meng Z, Dai Z, Huang K, et al. Long-term mortality for patients of primary aldosteronism compared with essential hypertension: a systematic review and meta-analysis. *Front Endocrinol (Lausanne).* 2020;11:121. PMID: 32210920

3. Funder JW, Carey RM, Mantero F, et al. The management of primary aldosteronism: case detection, diagnosis, and treatment: an Endocrine Society Clinical Practice Guideline. *J Clin Endocrinol Metab.* 2016;101(5):1889-1916. PMID: 26934393

4. Hung A, Ahmed S, Gupta A, et al. Performance of the aldosterone to renin ratio as a screening test for primary aldosteronism: a systematic review and meta-analysis. *J Clin Endocrinol Metab.* 2021;106(8):2423-2435. PMID: 34008000

5. Wang K, Hu J, Yang J, et al. Development and validation of criteria for sparing confirmatory tests in diagnosing primary aldosteronism. *J Clin Endocrinol Metab.* 2020;105(7):dgaa282. PMID: 32449927

6. Eisenhofer G, Kurlbaum M, Peitzsch M, et al. The saline infusion test for primary aldosteronism: implications of immunoassay inaccuracy. *J Clin Endocrinol Metab.* 2021 [Online ahead of print] PMID: 34963138

7. Burrello J, Amongero M, Buffolo F, et al. Development of a prediction score to avoid confirmatory testing in patients with suspected primary aldosteronism. *J Clin Endocrinol Metab.* 2020;106(4):e1708-e1716. PMID: 33377974

8. Young WF, Stanson AW, Thompson GB, Grant CS, Farley DR, van Heerden JA, Role for adrenal venous sampling in primary aldosteronism. *Surgery.* 2004;136(6):1227-1235. PMID: 15657580

9. Nwariaku FE, Miller BS, Auchus R, et al. Primary hyperaldosteronism: effect of adrenal vein sampling on surgical outcome. *Arch Surg.* 2006;141(5):497-502. PMID: 16702522

10. Dekkers T, Prejbisz A, Schultze Kool LJ, et al; SPARTACUS Investigators. Adrenal vein sampling versus CT scan to determine treatment in primary aldosteronism: an outcome-based randomised diagnostic trial. *Lancet Diabetes Endocrinol.* 2016;4(9):739-746. PMID: 27325147

11. Williams TA, Lenders JWM, Mulatero P, et al; Primary Aldosteronism Surgery Outcome (PASO) Investigators. Outcomes after adrenalectomy for unilateral primary aldosteronism: an international consensus on outcome measures and analysis of remission rates in an international cohort. *Lancet Diabetes Endocrinol.* 2017;5(9):689-699. PMID: 28576687

12. Williams TA, Burrello J, Sechi LA, et al. Computed tomography and adrenal venous sampling in the diagnosis of unilateral primary aldosteronism. *Hypertension.* 2018;72(3):641-649. PMID: 29987100

13. Riester A, Fischer E, Degenhart C, et al. Age below 40 or a recently proposed clinical prediction score cannot bypass adrenal venous sampling in primary aldosteronism. *J Clin Endocrinol Metab.* 2014;99(6):E1035-E1039. PMID: 24601689

14. Kupers EM, Amar L, Raynaud A, Plouin P-F, Steichen O. A clinical prediction score to diagnose unilateral primary aldosteronism. *J Clin Endocrinol Metab.* 2012;97(10):3530-3537. PMID: 22918872

15. Sze WCC, Soh LM, Lau JH, et al. Diagnosing unilateral primary aldosteronism - comparison of a clinical prediction score, computed tomography and adrenal venous sampling. *Clin Endocrinol (Oxf).* 2014;81(1):25-30. PMID: 24274335

16. Mulatero P, di Cella SM, Monticone S, et al. 18-Hydroxycorticosterone, 18-hydroxycortisol, and 18-oxocortisol in the diagnosis of primary aldosteronism and its subtypes. *J Clin Endocrinol Metab.* 2012;97(3):881-889. PMID: 22238407

17. Satoh F, Morimoto R, Ono Y, et al. Measurement of peripheral plasma 18-oxocortisol can discriminate unilateral adenoma from bilateral diseases in patients with primary aldosteronism. *Hypertension.* 2015;65(5):1096-1102. PMID: 25776074

18. Eisenhofer G, Dekkers T, Peitzsch M, et al. Mass spectrometry-based adrenal and peripheral venous steroid profiling for subtyping primary aldosteronism. *Clin Chem.* 2016;62(3):514-524. PMID: 26787761

19. Nagano H, Kono T, Saiga A, et al. Aldosterone reduction rate after saline infusion test may be a novel prediction in patients with primary aldosteronism. *J Clin Endocrinol Metab.* 2020;105(3):dgz092.

20. Hashimura H, Shen J, Fuller PJ, et al. Saline suppression test parameters may predict bilateral subtypes of primary aldosteronism. *Clin Endocrinol (Oxf).* 2018;89(3):308-313. PMID: 29873811

21. Kocjan T, Janez A, Stankovic M, Vidmar G, Jensterle M. A new clinical prediction criterion accurately determines a subset of patients with bilateral primary aldosteronism before adrenal venous sampling. *Endocr Pract.* 2016;22(5):587-594. PMID: 26789347

22. Burrello J, Burrello A, Pieroni J, et al. Development and validation of prediction models for subtype diagnosis of patients with primary aldosteronism. *J Clin Endocrinol Metab.* 2020;105(10):dgaa379. PMID: 32561919

23. Heinze B, Fuss CT, Mulatero P, et al. Targeting CXCR4 (CXC chemokine receptor type 4) for molecular imaging of aldosterone-producing adenoma. *Hypertension.* 2018;71(2):317-325. PMID: 29279316

24. Burton TJ, Mackenzie IS, Balan K, et al. Evaluation of the sensitivity and specificity of (11)C-metomidate positron emission tomography (PET)-CT for lateralizing aldosterone secretion by Conn's adenomas. *J Clin Endocrinol Metab.* 2012;97(1):100-109. PMID: 22112805

25. O'Shea PM, O'Donoghue D, Bashari W, et al.,= (11) C-Metomidate PET/CT is a useful adjunct for lateralization of primary aldosteronism in routine clinical practice. *Clin Endocrinol (Oxf).* 2019;90(5):670-679. PMID: 30721535

26. Soinio, M., et al., Functional imaging with 11C-metomidate PET for subtype diagnosis in primary aldosteronism. *Eur J Endocrinol.* 2020;183(6):539-550. PMID: 33055298

27. Hundemer GL, Curhan GC, Yozamp N, Wang M, Vaidya A. Renal outcomes in medically and surgically treated primary aldosteronism. *Hypertension.* 2018;72(3):658-666. PMID: 29987110

28. Velema MS, de Nooijer AH, Burgers VWG, et al. Health-related quality of life and mental health in primary aldosteronism: a systematic review. *Horm Metab Res.* 2017;49(12):943-950. PMID: 29202493

29. Wu VC, Chueh S-CJ, Chen L, et al; TAIPAI Study Group. Risk of new-onset diabetes mellitus in primary aldosteronism: a population study over 5 years. *J Hypertens.* 2017;35(8):1698-1708. PMID: 28661412

30. Rossi GP, Maiolino G, Flego A, et al; PAPY Study Investigators. Adrenalectomy lowers incident atrial fibrillation in primary aldosteronism patients at long term. *Hypertension.* 2018;71(4):585-591. PMID: 29483224

31. Williams TA, Gomez-Sanchez CE, Rainey WE, et al. International histopathology consensus for unilateral primary aldosteronism. *J Clin Endocrinol Metab.* 2021;106(1):42-54. PMID: 32717746

32. Meyer LS, Handgriff L, Lim JS, et al. Single-center prospective cohort study on the histopathology, genotype, and postsurgical outcomes of patients with primary aldosteronism. *Hypertension.* 2021;78(3):738-746. PMID: 34024122

33. Hundemer GL, Curhan GC, Yozamp N, Wang M, Vaidya A. Cardiometabolic outcomes and mortality in medically treated primary aldosteronism: a retrospective cohort study. *Lancet Diabetes Endocrinol.* 2018;6(1):51-59. PMID: 29129576

34. Hundemer GL, Curhan GC, Yozamp N, Wang M, Vaidya A. Incidence of atrial fibrillation and mineralocorticoid receptor activity in patients with medically and surgically treated primary aldosteronism. *JAMA Cardiol.* 2018;3(8):768-774. PMID: 30027227

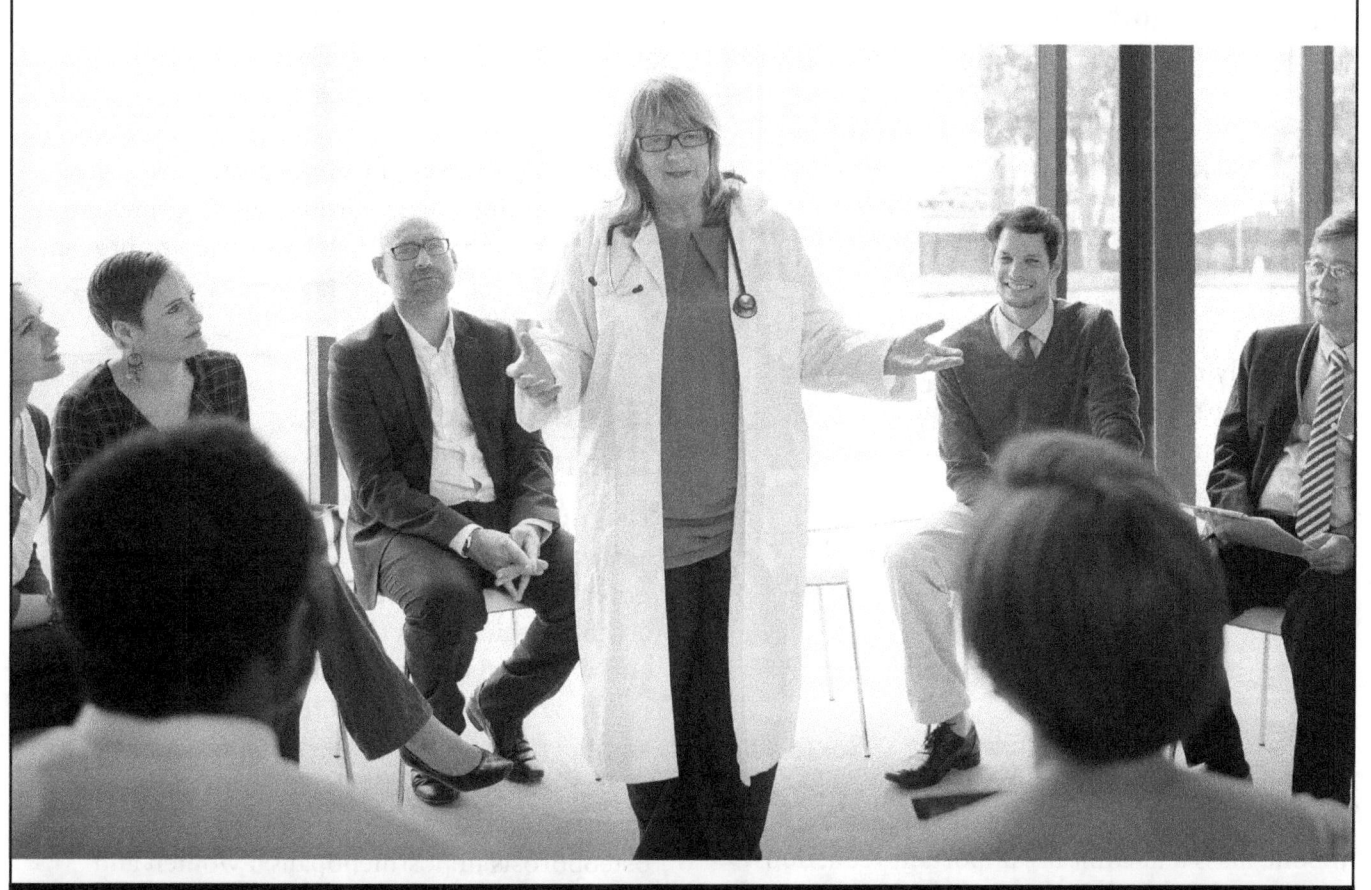

BONE AND MINERAL METABOLISM

Denosumab Discontinuation

Bente L. Langdahl, MD, PhD, DMSc. Endocrinology and Internal Medicine, Aarhus University Hospital, Aarhus, Denmark; E-mail: bente.langdahl@aarhus.rm.dk

Learning Objectives

As a result of participating in this session, learners should be able to:

- Explain and discuss the pathophysiology underlying the rebound increase in bone turnover and bone loss following discontinuation of denosumab.

- Apply the current guidelines regarding follow-on treatment in patients discontinuing denosumab.

Main Conclusions

Denosumab is an effective treatment of osteoporosis that leads to substantial increases in bone mass and clinically important reductions in fracture risk with few adverse effects. Most patients should continue treatment; however, some patients may need to discontinue treatment due to comorbidities or adverse effects. Furthermore, some patients want to discontinue treatment because of normal or near-normal bone mineral density (BMD) and absence of fractures after years on treatment. Unlike bisphosphonates, but like most other pharmacological treatments, denosumab has no continuing effect after it is discontinued. Due to the accumulation of receptor activator of nuclear factor kappaB ligand (RANKL) and possibly osteoclasts during treatment with denosumab, a rebound activation of bone resorption is observed in patients who discontinue denosumab after more than 1 to 2 years of treatment. This can partly be prevented by the administration of bisphosphonates, primarily zoledronate. Patients need frequent monitoring with measurement of C-telopeptide of type I collagen (CTX) and, in some cases, multiple administrations of zoledronate during the first year after denosumab discontinuation to prevent bone loss.

Significance of the Clinical Problem

Denosumab is a fully human IgG2 monoclonal antibody that neutralizes RANKL and thereby potently decreases osteoclast recruitment and activity, which leads to reduced bone turnover and increased bone mineral density.[1] Denosumab reduces the risk of new vertebral fractures by 70% and the risk of hip and nonvertebral fractures by 40% and 20%, respectively, in postmenopausal women and is approved for the treatment of osteoporosis in postmenopausal women and men and treatment of glucocorticoid-induced osteoporosis. Furthermore, the risk of adverse effects is low and a positive benefit-to-risk ratio over 10 years has been demonstrated in postmenopausal women with osteoporosis.[2] Denosumab is therefore a potent antiresorptive treatment of osteoporosis; however, unlike bisphosphonates, denosumab's effect is not maintained after discontinuation, as bone resorption increases rapidly leading to bone loss (the rebound phenomenon).[3] This increase in bone resorption increases fracture risk, especially vertebral fractures. Post hoc analyses of data from the FREEDOM trial (phase 3 pivotal fracture trial) demonstrated that discontinuation of denosumab treatment was associated with an increased risk of vertebral and multiple vertebral fractures compared with risk in women discontinuing placebo and that the risk was higher among women with prior vertebral fractures, longer duration of therapy, and more prominent BMD loss at the hip after discontinuation.[4] Other studies have suggested that younger age and chronic kidney disease may also be risk factors for vertebral fractures after discontinuation of denosumab.[5]

Physicians should consider the issues associated with discontinuation of denosumab when making the decision to initiate denosumab. Denosumab treatment has many benefits, including prominent and continuing increases in BMD and easy administration, which supports adherence. However, the patient and the physician should also be aware of the challenges associated with denosumab's discontinuation.[5]

Barriers to Optimal Practice

- Lack of knowledge among physicians and patients about the rebound phenomenon when denosumab is discontinued.

- Limited availability or reimbursement of measuring CTX or bone turnover markers in general or as frequently as is needed to optimally manage patients in the first year following denosumab discontinuation.

- Logistical challenges in the administration of zoledronate in general practitioner practices and/or lack of resources in the hospital setting to see all patients discontinuing denosumab.

Strategies for Diagnosis, Therapy, and/or Management

Denosumab Discontinuation

Bone turnover markers increase rapidly 6 months after the last denosumab injection and remain elevated until slowly decreasing to baseline levels after 1 to 2 years.[3] BMD is lost and returns to or even below pretreatment levels.[3] There is speculation whether the increase in bone turnover following denosumab discontinuation is modified by treatment with bisphosphonates prior to denosumab therapy; however, only observational data are available. Pretreatment with bisphosphonates appears to be associated with a diminished increase in bone turnover markers in patients with osteoporosis who discontinue denosumab when compared with bone turnover markers in patients without bisphosphonate exposure. However, no studies have found an effect of prior bisphosphonate treatment on BMD loss following denosumab discontinuation.

Longer duration of denosumab treatment is associated with a more pronounced rebound in bone resorption and subsequent bone loss after denosumab withdrawal. Therefore, duration of denosumab treatment should be considered when interpreting the studies investigating the rebound phenomenon and measures should be taken to prevent or diminish this. A number of studies have investigated the effects of other antiresorptive drugs after denosumab discontinuation. The effects of alendronate after denosumab were assessed in the DAPS study (Denosumab Adherence Preference Satisfaction). Alendronate for 1 year after 1 year of denosumab therapy maintained the BMD gained with denosumab.[6]

Prevention of the Rebound Phenomenon After Short-Term Denosumab Treatment

Several studies have investigated the effects of zoledronate use after short-term denosumab treatment. In general, zoledronate is more effective in maintaining BMD when denosumab has only been given for a few years. An observational study of 11 women who received zoledronate after discontinuation of denosumab for 2 years reported minimal loss of BMD gained during denosumab treatment at all skeletal sites. Similarly, a retrospective observational study of 18 postmenopausal women who received zoledronate after denosumab for 1.5 years on average showed preservation of BMD gained during the denosumab treatment period. Furthermore, the initial results of the DATA-HD Extension trial indicated that a single dose of zoledronate maintains the BMD gains achieved with a combination of teriparatide and denosumab for 9 months followed by denosumab alone for 9 months at all skeletal sites. A randomized controlled trial investigated the efficacy of a single intravenous infusion of zoledronate in 57 postmenopausal women who had been treated with denosumab for a mean duration of 2.4 years and had achieved BMD in the osteopenic range. At 24 and 36 months, BMD at the lumbar spine and femoral neck was maintained. Patients treated with zoledronate had small but significant increases in procollagen type 1 aminoterminal propeptide and CTX during the first year but stabilization thereafter.[7] Based on these results, it seems that the rebound phenomenon after treatment with denosumab for up to 2.5 years can be controlled by administration of bisphosphonates, with most of the evidence focused on the use of zoledronate.

Prevention of the Rebound Phenomenon After Long-Term Denosumab

Several studies have investigated the effects of antiresorptive drugs after discontinuation of denosumab following more than 2.5 years of treatment. Small observational studies and case reports seem to indicate that selective estrogen receptor modulators and oral bisphosphonates do not prevent bone loss following discontinuation of long-term denosumab treatment.[5] Most studies show that zoledronate is less effective in preventing BMD loss when the denosumab treatment period exceeds 2.5 years compared with a shorter duration of denosumab therapy. In a case series of 6 women receiving a single infusion of 5 mg zoledronate after 7 years of denosumab, a partial preservation of the BMD gained during denosumab treatment was observed at the spine, while a complete loss of the bone gain was noted at the hip 2 years after zoledronate infusion.[8] An observational study of 120 postmenopausal women with osteoporosis treated for 2 to 5 years with denosumab who received a single infusion of 5 mg zoledronate 6 months after the last denosumab injection found that 66% of the BMD gained with denosumab was retained at the spine and 49% was retrained at the hip 2 years after denosumab discontinuation. The bone loss occurred within the first 18 months after zoledronate infusion.[9]

The effect of bisphosphonates on the rebound phenomenon was speculated to be better if given when the increase in resorption was already evident. To investigate this further, we conducted the ZOLARMAB study, a randomized controlled trial evaluating zoledronate treatment after discontinuation of long-term denosumab.[10] The study included 61 postmenopausal women and elderly men who had received denosumab for a mean duration of 4.6 years. The patients were randomly assigned to receive a single 5-mg zoledronate infusion either 6 months after the last denosumab injection (6-month group, n = 20), 9 months after (9-month group, n = 20), or when bone turnover markers were increased (observation group, n = 21). Patients in the 2 latter groups were monitored monthly and promptly received an infusion of zoledronate if CTX increased substantially (50% above the range for postmenopausal women and elderly men) or if they sustained a fragility fracture. Twelve months after the initial zoledronate infusion, BMD had decreased significantly at the lumbar spine, total hip, and femoral neck in all 3 groups without differences between groups. The decline in BMD was more rapid in the 9-month group and in the observation group, which may at least in theory result in a higher fracture risk. Two women, both in the 9-month group, experienced a vertebral fracture. In addition, 10 patients in the 6-month group needed retreatment with zoledronate 6 or 12 months after the initial treatment compared with 5 patients in each of the 2 other groups. Based on these findings, we concluded that treatment with zoledronate, regardless of timing, did not fully prevent BMD loss in patients with osteopenia who had been treated with denosumab for 4.6 years.[10]

Similar to the findings in the ZOLARMAB study, an observational study of 20 postmenopausal women who received a single 5-mg infusion of zoledronate after discontinuing denosumab when bone turnover markers exceeded the upper limit of the premenopausal reference ranges also found a secondary increase in bone turnover markers after an initial decrease following zoledronate administration. This suggests that a single infusion of zoledronate may not be sufficient to completely control bone turnover in all patients discontinuing long-term denosumab treatment.

The rapid reversal of the beneficial skeletal effects of denosumab attributed to a transient increase in bone turnover overriding pretreatment status has commonly been described as the "rebound phenomenon." It has been postulated that osteoclast precursors remaining dormant during the treatment period retain their activity and/or that a high RANKL-to-osteoprotegerin ratio ensues after denosumab is cleared from the patient's circulation. Although the exact pathophysiology of the rebound phenomenon is yet to be fully elucidated, the clinical data reviewed above suggest that denosumab discontinuation results in increased bone turnover and bone loss and in an augmented fracture risk compared with continuation of the drug. This observation gives rise to the following questions related to clinical practice:

- What is the optimal treatment duration with denosumab for patients at high risk for fracture?

- What should be done after denosumab discontinuation?

- How should vertebral fractures be managed that occur after denosumab discontinuation?

Optimal Duration of Denosumab Treatment in Patients at High Risk for Fracture

The goal of osteoporosis treatment is to achieve an acceptable level of fracture risk. As increase in BMD is a very strong mediator of fracture risk reduction on treatment, BMD has been suggested as a possible treatment target. Hip BMD between –2.5 and –1.5 has been proposed by different working groups and societies. However, a BMD-only–based concept is not universally embraced and more data are needed. In addition, it is important to remember that the concept of a limited duration of treatment for osteoporosis was developed based on the retention of bisphosphonates in bone and therefore cannot automatically be applied to denosumab or other treatments. The decision about treatment duration should be individualized and should, in addition to fracture-free period and BMD, also include an evaluation of additional risk factors of a high fracture-risk profile. These risk factors are mainly linked to prevalent osteoporotic fractures and concomitant comorbidities (eg, continuous use of glucocorticoids or aromatase inhibitors, diabetes, inflammatory diseases, frailty, etc). In patients considered to be at high risk for fracture, the efficacy and safety profile of denosumab allows for long-term treatment, with existing data supporting a duration of up to 10 years. Regarding serious adverse effects, the FREEDOM study investigating denosumab for up to 10 years reported 2 atypical femur fractures and 13 cases of osteonecrosis of the jaw.

Pending data on longer treatment duration from registries, decisions regarding treatment beyond 10 years should be individualized, as is the case with most medical treatments beyond the first few years. These considerations also underscore the importance of a careful assessment of the indications to start denosumab treatment in the first place, especially in younger patients, who may be at higher risk of fractures or bone loss following discontinuation.

Regarding elective dental procedures where treatment discontinuation is demanded by the dentist, it is suggested to perform the procedure approximately 5 months after the last denosumab injection and resume treatment as soon as the lesion is healed. This suggestion is based on expert opinion only.

Optimal Treatment Strategy After Denosumab Discontinuation

Current evidence regarding use of raloxifene and risedronate to prevent the rebound phenomenon is not convincing and therefore the following will focus on the use of potent bisphosphonates. Current data suggest that the duration of denosumab treatment is an important determinant of the extent of the rebound phenomenon, which may have potential implications for the type and duration of subsequent treatment with bisphosphonates. Very little data are available to help define the optimal timing of initiation of oral bisphosphonates in relation to denosumab discontinuation. Most of the few studies available describe initiation of oral bisphosphonates 6 months after the last denosumab injection. The European Calcified Tissue Society position statement on denosumab discontinuation[5] suggests performing DXA 6 months after the last denosumab injection and starting treatment with an oral bisphosphonate, preferably alendronate, at that time. Measuring bone turnover markers 3 months after initiating the oral bisphosphonate is recommended to monitor adherence and efficacy.

Regarding bisphosphonate treatment, an adequate response is defined as a CTX level below the mean in healthy premenopausal women, the exact values depending on the assays. This recommendation is supported by data from the ReoLaus cohort in which patients with stable BMD at the spine after 1 year had mean CTX values close to the premenopausal mean, significantly lower than the mean CTX level in patients who lost BMD. In patients with adequate response and low fracture risk, treatment with an oral bisphosphonate can be continued for 1 to 2 years (ie, the estimated time of the rebound upregulation of bone turnover). It is, however, recommended to continue the assessment of bone turnover markers, initially after another 3 months and if stable, every 6 months to ensure that they remain within the lower half of the premenopausal reference range. At 1 to 2 years, a reevaluation including DXA should be performed and the decision to discontinue oral bisphosphonate treatment should align with current guidelines, keeping in mind that 1 to 2 years of treatment with bisphosphonates most likely has not led to sufficient accumulation of bisphosphonates in the bone to prevent future bone loss and therefore age- and/or menopause-related bone loss is likely to resume.

In patients with gastrointestinal intolerability of oral bisphosphonates, inadequate response to oral bisphosphonates, or a long duration of denosumab treatment, the European Calcified Tissue Society position statement recommends administering zoledronate intravenously. The timing of this infusion is of great importance. In the ZOLARMAB study, we found very rapid increases in CTX and rapid bone loss in patients with delayed infusions of zoledronate (9 to 12 months after the last denosumab injection). In addition, case series have reported multiple vertebral fractures at very early time points after 1 missed denosumab injection. The current recommendation is therefore to initiate treatment with zoledronate 6 months after the last denosumab injection and to monitor the effect with measurement of bone turnover markers, for example, at 3 and 6 months after the zoledronate infusion. If bone turnover markers are increased (ie, above the mean found in age- and gender-matched cohorts) repeated infusion of zoledronate should be considered. If bone turnover markers are not available for monitoring a patient, a pragmatic approach could be giving a second infusion of zoledronate 6 months after the first infusion. Similar to oral bisphosphonates, and in cases of otherwise low fracture risk, the duration of zoledronate treatment should be tailored to the duration of increased bone turnover, although as mentioned above, the optimal duration of zoledronate treatment may be adjusted when more data become available.

Management of Vertebral Fractures Occurring After Denosumab Discontinuation

No data currently support the optimal management of vertebral fractures occurring after denosumab discontinuation. The fractures seem to be caused by the high bone turnover and/or the rapid bone loss that most likely also comprises an element of deterioration of bone microarchitecture. Quickly counteracting the increased bone turnover is therefore important, and since denosumab is a very potent antiresorptive agent with the ability to suppress bone turnover markers in a matter of days, prompt reinitiation of denosumab treatment may be the best solution. Alternatively, a combination of denosumab with an osteoanabolic agent (eg, teriparatide) can be prescribed to stimulate bone formation and at the same time avoid the transient but rapid decrease in BMD, especially at cortical sites, reported with teriparatide subsequent to denosumab therapy. This is why monotherapy with teriparatide after denosumab should be discouraged at the present time. Indeed, the combination of denosumab with teriparatide, although currently off-label in most countries, has been shown to be highly effective in improving BMD. However, the combination treatment period should be followed by a potent antiresorptive therapy (ie, zoledronate) to consolidate BMD gains. Moreover, novel data report that romosozumab following denosumab for 1 year also results in BMD gains, although more modest than with romosozumab treatment in treatment-naïve patients. Vertebroplasty has been identified as a potential precipitating risk factor for subsequent vertebral fractures and should therefore be avoided in this situation.

Summary and Conclusion

Discontinuation of denosumab following at least 2 denosumab injections carries a significant risk of a rebound effect, manifesting as rapidly increasing bone resorptive activity, considerable loss of the bone mass gained during denosumab treatment, and an augmented risk for (multiple) vertebral fractures. To limit the consequences of this phenomenon, it is currently recommended to continue denosumab therapy or to prescribe a potent bisphosphonate when denosumab is discontinued (*see Figure*). The rebound phenomenon depends on the duration

of treatment with denosumab. In patients with low fracture risk and a shorter duration of denosumab treatment (ie, up to 2.5 years), the rebound phenomenon can probably be controlled by treatment with alendronate for 1 to 2 years. If treatment with alendronate is not possible, zoledronate can be given once and repeated if bone turnover is inappropriately high after 3 to 6 months. Patients who have been treated with denosumab for a longer period (ie, more than 2.5 years) or who are still at high risk for fracture should receive zoledronate. Bone turnover markers can provide clinical guidance on the timing and duration of zoledronate treatment. Patients who experience vertebral fractures after stopping denosumab need prompt treatment to reduce the high bone turnover.

Figure. Osteoporosis Management With Denosumab

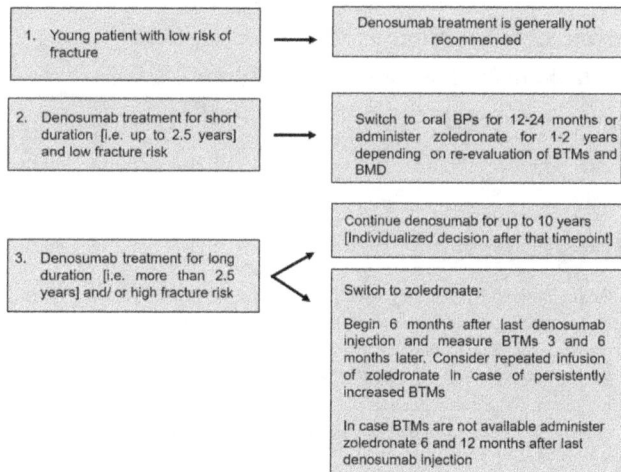

Abbreviations: BPs, bisphosphonates; BTMs, bone turnover markers.

Reprinted from Tsourdi E, Zillikens MC, Meier C et al. *J Clin Endocrinol Metab*, 2021; 106(1) © Endocrine Society.

Clinical Case Vignettes
Case

A 70-year-old woman is diagnosed with osteoporosis. Alendronate is initiated, but she develops upper gastrointestinal adverse effects and her regimen is switched to denosumab after a few months. She responds well and has increases in BMD at the spine and hip of 12.9%

and 7.6%, respectively, after 6 years of treatment. She is doing well, with no fractures and no adverse effects, but her BMD T-scores are still low: –3.4 at the spine and –3.8 at the hip. The patient has heard about patients discontinuing bisphosphonate treatment and would like to discontinue denosumab.

Which of the following is the best recommendation?

A. Continue denosumab

B. Discontinue denosumab and monitor CTX

C. Give alendronate for 1 to 2 years and monitor CTX; give zoledronate if CTX is uncontrolled

D. Give zoledronate for 1 to 2 years and monitor CTX; repeat zoledronate if CTX is uncontrolled

E. Give zoledronate 6 and 12 months after the last denosumab injection

Answers: A) Continue denosumab or D) Give zoledronate for 1 to 2 years and monitor CTX; repeat zoledronate if CTX is uncontrolled

I recommended continuing denosumab; however, the patient was determined to discontinue, and she did not want another parentally administrated treatment. She was therefore started on alendronate 6 months after the last denosumab injection. Bone turnover markers, CTX, and procollagen type 1 aminoterminal propeptide increased from unmeasurable levels at the time of alendronate initiation to 150% to 200% above the premenopausal reference range after 6 months. BMD at the spine and hip decreased by 2.6% and 20.4%, respectively. The patient then accepted zoledronate treatment.

Continuing denosumab (Answer A) or giving zoledronate for 1 to 2 years and monitoring CTX (repeating administration of zoledronate if CTX is uncontrolled) (Answer D) are the recommended options. However, giving alendronate for 1 to 2 years and monitoring CTX (and giving zoledronate if CTX is uncontrolled) (Answer C) and giving zoledronate 6 and 12 months after the last denosumab injection (Answer E) would also reduce the rebound phenomenon but probably less effectively than Answer D.

References

1. Cummings SR, San Martin J, McClung MR, et al; FREEDOM Trial. Denosumab for the prevention of fractures in postmenopausal women with osteoporosis. *N Engl J Med.* 2009;361(8):756-765. PMID: 19671655

2. Ferrari S, Lewiecki EM, Butler PW, et al. Favorable skeletal benefit/risk of long-term denosumab therapy: a virtual-twin analysis of fractures prevented relative to skeletal safety events observed. *Bone.* 2020;134:115287. PMID: 32092479

3. Bone HG, Bolognese MA, Yuen CK, et al. Effects of denosumab treatment and discontinuation on bone mineral density and bone turnover markers in postmenopausal women with low bone mass. *J Clin Endocrinol Metab.* 2011;96(4):972-980. PMID: 21289258

4. Cummings SR, Ferrari S, Eastell R, et al. Vertebral fractures after discontinuation of denosumab: a post hoc analysis of the randomized placebo-controlled FREEDOM trial and its extension. *J Bone Miner Res.* 2018;33(2):190-198. PMID: 29105841

5. Tsourdi E, Zillikens MC, Meier C, et al. Fracture risk and management of discontinuation of denosumab therapy: a systematic review and position statement by ECTS. *J Clin Endocrinol Metab.* 2021 [online ahead of print]. PMID: 33103722

6. Freemantle N, Satram-Hoang S, Tang ET, et al; DAPS Investigators. Final results of the DAPS (Denosumab Adherence Preference Satisfaction) study: a 24-month, randomized, crossover comparison with alendronate in postmenopausal women. *Osteoporos Int.* 2012;23(1):317-326. PMID: 21927922

7. Anastasilakis AD, Papapoulos SE, Polyzos SA, Appelman-Dijkstra NM, Makras P. Zoledronate for the prevention of bone loss in women discontinuing denosumab treatment. A prospective 2-year clinical trial. *J Bone Miner Res.* 2019;34(12):2220-2228. PMID: 31433518

8. Reid IR, Horne AM, Mihov B, Gamble GD. Bone loss after denosumab: only partial protection with zoledronate. *Calcif Tissue Int.* 2017;101(4):371-374. PMID: 28500448

9. Everts-Graber J, Reichenbach S, Ziswiler HR, Studer U, Lehmann T. A single infusion of zoledronate in postmenopausal women following denosumab discontinuation results in partial conservation of bone mass gains. *J Bone Miner Res.* 2020;35(7):1207-1215. PMID: 31991007

10. Sølling AS, Harsløf T, Langdahl B. Treatment with zoledronate subsequent to denosumab in osteoporosis: a randomized trial. *J Bone Miner Res.* 2020;35(10):1858-1870. PMID: 32459005

Using the Best Available Evidence to Personalize Osteoporosis Treatment

E. Michael Lewiecki, MD. University of New Mexico Health Sciences Center, Albuquerque, NM; E-mail: mlewiecki@gmail.com

Micol S. Rothman, MD. University of Colorado School of Medicine, Aurora, CO; E-mail: micol.rothman@cuanschutz.edu

Learning Objectives

As a result of participating in this session, learners should be able to:

- Assess fracture risk and tailor medication choice accordingly.

- Identify strategies for treatment sequence with osteoporosis medications.

- Recognize the onset and offset of treatment effects of different osteoporosis medications.

Main Conclusions

Many clinical practice guidelines address the management of patients with osteoporosis.[1-4] These guidelines are often developed by societies or organizations that focus on specific patient populations using divergent approaches to analyzing and interpreting the medical evidence, with or without consideration of cost-effectiveness, and with differing views on inclusion of expert opinion. Guidelines that rely exclusively on data derived from large, randomized, placebo-controlled clinical trials are scientifically rigorous but tend to be restrictive, complex, and lacking the flexibility needed to address the needs of some patients. Many or most patients seen in clinical practice would not qualify for participation in the clinical trials supporting the approval of the medications used to treat them,[5] casting into doubt the applicability of the studies for some patients. Guidelines developed by experts interpreting the best available medical evidence may be simpler, more intuitive, and easier to apply in clinical practice, but are open to criticism that they are overly subjective and based on a lower level of evidence. The application of any guideline for making decisions for individual patients must consider all available clinical information. Individual fracture risk should be examined when making treatment decisions. Additionally, prior medication exposure and duration of treatment, as well as patient preference, must be taken into account when thinking about future therapies.

Significance of the Clinical Problem

Osteoporosis is a common disorder characterized by low bone density and poor bone quality resulting in increased risk of fractures. Despite the availability of excellent tools to assess fracture risk and approved medications that reduce fracture risk, most patients at risk for fractures are not being treated.[6] The large treatment gap is now recognized as a global crisis in the care of patients with osteoporosis.[7]

Barriers to Optimal Practice

Many factors contribute to the treatment gap, including fear of medication adverse effects, poor understanding of the balance of benefits and risks with treatment, inadequate communication skills to quantify risk, lack of appreciation of the potentially serious consequences of fractures, failure to recognize that a prior fracture is due to osteoporosis, reductions in reimbursement for bone density testing (in the United States) resulting in the closure of many office-based DXA facilities, conflicting clinical practice guidelines, limited available time for physician-patient encounters, and competing health care priorities.

Strategies for Diagnosis, Therapy, and/or Management

Many strategies to reduce the treatment gap have been proposed,[8] including technology-enabled collaborative learning, the prototype of which is Bone Health TeleECHO.[9] Tools and algorithms have been developed to help patients and providers alike better quantify the risks and benefits of osteoporosis therapy. However, providers must recognize that there is not a "one size fits all" answer for many patients. At times, more than 1 visit and a variety of materials may be needed for patients to understand their diagnosis of osteoporosis and feel comfortable with initiation of medication. Clinical judgment, patient preference, and other factors are key aspects of managing complex cases of osteoporosis.

Clinical Case Vignettes

Case 1

A 54-year-old man with a history of lung transplant for chronic obstructive pulmonary disorder 1 year ago presents after DXA shows a lowest T-score of –3.1 in the lumbar spine. He had been treated with prednisone bursts prior to his lung transplant, has had several episodes of rejection that required pulse doses of steroids, and remains on a prednisone dosage of 10 mg daily. He reports no fractures, but old chest x-rays suggest prior compression fractures. Workup for secondary causes, including vitamin D measurement, reveals no additional abnormalities other than a low morning testosterone concentration of 250 ng/dL (8.7 nmol/L).

Which of the following treatments would best reduce this patient's future risk of vertebral fracture?

A. Calcium and vitamin D, weight-bearing exercise as tolerated, and steroid taper (discuss with transplant team)

B. Subcutaneous teriparatide

C. Weekly oral alendronate

D. Weekly testosterone injections

Answer: B) Subcutaneous teriparatide

This patient has severe osteoporosis with very high fracture risk. Prevention of further compression fractures could be crucial to protect his lung function. Pharmacologic therapy is indicated (thus, Answer A is incorrect).

Given his low testosterone level, he should be worked up for true hypogonadism. However, even if further workup indicates he would benefit from testosterone replacement, there are no data regarding the effect of testosterone on fracture risk (thus, Answer D is incorrect). Endocrine Society guidelines suggest that hypogonadal men who are at high risk of fracture be treated with an agent with fracture-proven efficacy and that testosterone should only be given "in lieu of a bone drug" if serum levels are below 200 ng/dL (<6.9 nmol/L) on more than 1 occasion with symptoms of androgen deficiency and if the fracture risk is borderline-high.[10]

An 18-month, randomized, head-to-head trial in 414 patients comparing teriparatide (Answer B) to alendronate (Answer C) in patients with glucocorticoid-induced osteoporosis showed larger gains in spine bone mineral density (7.2% vs 3.4%) and lower rates of vertebral compression fracture (0.6 vs 6.1%) in the teriparatide-treated group.[11] Although oral alendronate is a reasonable choice if teriparatide is not financially feasible, is contraindicated, or is otherwise not desired by the patient, the strongest data for secondary fracture prevention in this scenario would be with teriparatide. The American College of Rheumatology guidelines suggest alendronate for first-line therapy based on cost, while other guidelines from Europe advocate for teriparatide as first-line therapy in a patient at high risk.[12] Note that other anabolic agents (abaloparatide and romosozumab) are not US FDA-approved for osteoporosis in men at this time.

Case 2

A 67-year-old woman with a history of a Colles fracture at age 63 years was treated with denosumab for 4 years. On the advice of her oral surgeon, she stopped denosumab before having a tooth extraction 10 month ago and has not resumed treatment since then. She returns for follow-up after a recent hospitalization for multiple painful vertebral compression fractures. She has normal kidney function and no history of cardiovascular disease or malignancy.

Which of the following should NOT be advised?

A. Administer intravenous zoledronic acid

B. Consult with interventional radiology for kyphoplasty

C. Resume denosumab now

D. Start anabolic therapy with teriparatide, abaloparatide, or romosozumab

Answer: B) Consult with interventional radiology for kyphoplasty

There has been much recent discussion of how and when to stop/bridge denosumab if needed or desired. First, it must be emphasized that there is no role for a drug holiday with denosumab. After stopping denosumab, treatment effect will be rapidly lost if another agent is not started. The properties of bisphosphonates are unique in that they are slowly released from the bone, providing continuing protection for variable amounts of time after administration is stopped.[13] This does

not exist for any other osteoporosis therapy. We know that stopping denosumab can lead to rapid rise in bone turnover markers, rapid decrease in bone mineral density, return of fracture risk to baseline, and possible increase in the risk of multiple vertebral fractures.[14] Ideally, there would have been discussion with the oral surgeon *before* the tooth extraction to discuss the possibilities of a short delay of therapy, changing to an alternative medication, or performing extraction without delaying or stopping denosumab.

When patients present with vertebral fracture in the setting of stopping denosumab, kyphoplasty has not been shown to be beneficial and may, in fact, lead to further compression fractures (therefore, Answer B is correct, as this step should NOT be advised now).[15]

It is crucial for this patient to resume some type of osteoporosis therapy; however, there are multiple options as outlined in the remaining answer choices. If the patient has done well on denosumab, resumption of this medication (Answer C) is reasonable. If she cannot commit to resuming therapy every 6 months, giving intravenous zoledronic acid (Answer A) could also be an option considering its antifracture benefits and ease of administration. Although there are concerns about bone loss when switching from denosumab to an anabolic agent,[16] given this patient's compression fractures and possible need for ongoing dental work, anabolic therapy (Answer D) could be an option as well. This would perhaps be best done in combination with antiresorptive therapy.[15]

Case 3

A 56-year-old woman presents after recently stopping menopausal hormone therapy with patch estradiol and daily progestin. She has been on this therapy since the onset of menopausal symptoms in her early 50s. To her knowledge, she has never had a fracture. She is not having hot flashes or other bothersome menopausal symptoms, but she worries about bone loss because her mother had a hip fracture at age 78 years. Recent DXA shows

T-scores of –2.1 in the spine and –1.8 in the femoral neck. She wants to know how best to mitigate bone loss in the setting of stopping estrogen.

Which of the following statements is most correct?

A. A bisphosphonate could provide skeletal benefit

B. If spine imaging shows a previously unrecognized vertebral fracture, she should resume estrogen

C. She should avoid weight training due to her low spine bone mineral density

D. Stopping estrogen will most likely decrease serum C-telopeptide, a marker of bone turnover

Answer: A) A bisphosphonate could provide skeletal benefit

This patient's current fracture risk is likely low. However, if imaging were to show compression fractures, a more aggressive option should be considered (thus, Answer B is incorrect).

Since she has stopped menopausal hormone therapy without symptoms, returning to this option would not be advised at this time. However, studies looking at bone mineral density and bone turnover markers confirm a rapid return to high bone turnover marker levels, a different profile than that observed after stopping long-term bisphosphonate therapy, where a slow rise of bone turnover markers can be expected.[17,18] Therefore, stopping estrogen would likely lead to an increase in serum C-telopeptide (thus, Answer D is incorrect).

In a healthy patient with osteopenia and no known fractures, weight training is not contraindicated (thus, Answer C is incorrect).

The latest Endocrine Society guidelines for postmenopausal osteoporosis suggest starting alternative treatments when estrogen is stopped in women with osteoporosis,[13] but this does not cover women at lower risk, such as this patient. However, bisphosphonates can benefit postmenopausal women with osteopenia.[19,20] Given this patient's concerns based on family history, bisphosphonate therapy (Answer A) could be an attractive option.[21]

References

1. Eastell R, Rosen CJ, Black DM, Cheung AM, Murad MH, Shoback D. Pharmacological management of osteoporosis in postmenopausal women: an Endocrine Society clinical practice guideline. *J Clin Endocrinol Metab.* 2019;104(5):1595-1622. PMID: 30907953

2. Cosman F, de Beur SJ, LeBoff MS, et al; National Osteoporosis Foundation. Clinician's guide to prevention and treatment of osteoporosis. *Osteoporos Int.* 2014;25(10):2359-2381. PMID: 25182228

3. Camacho PM, Petak SM, Binkley N, et al. American Association of Clinical Endocrinologists and American College of Endocrinology clinical practice guidelines for the diagnosis and treatment of postmenopausal osteoporosis - 2016--executive summary. *Endocr Pract.* 2016;22(9):1111-1118. PMID: 27643923

4. Qaseem A, Forciea MA, McLean RM, Denberg TD, et al; Clinical Guidelines Committee of the American College of Physicians. Treatment of low bone density or osteoporosis to prevent fractures in men and women: a clinical practice guideline update from the American College of Physicians. *Ann Intern Med.* 2017;166(11):818-839. PMID: 28492856

5. Dowd R, Recker RR, Heaney RP. Study subjects and ordinary patients. *Osteoporos Int.* 2000;11(6):533-536. PMID: 10982170

6. Miller PD. Underdiagnosis and undertreatment of osteoporosis: the battle to be won. *J Clin Endocrinol Metab.* 2016;101(3):852-859. PMID: 26909798

7. Khosla S, Shane E. A crisis in the treatment of osteoporosis. *J Bone Miner Res.* 2016;31(8):1485-1487. PMID: 27335158

8. Khosla S, Cauley JA, Compston J, et al. Addressing the crisis in the treatment of osteoporosis: a path forward. *J Bone Miner Res.* 2017;32(3):424-430. PMID: 28099754

9. Lewiecki EM, Boyle JF, Arora S, Bouchonville MF 2nd, Chafey DH. Telementoring: a novel approach to reducing the osteoporosis treatment gap. *Osteoporos Int.* 2017;28(1):407-411. PMID: 27439373

10. Watts NB, Adler RA, Bilezikian JP, et al; Endocrine Society. Osteoporosis in men: an Endocrine Society clinical practice guideline. *J Clin Endocrinol Metab.* 2012;97(6):1802-1822. PMID: 22675062

11. Saag KG, Shane E, Boonen S, et al. Teriparatide or alendronate in glucocorticoid-induced osteoporosis. *N Engl J Med.* 2007;357(20):2028-2039. PMID: 18003959

12. Rothman MS, Olenginski TP, Stanciu I, Krohn K, Lewiecki EM. Lessons learned with Bone Health TeleECHO: making treatment decisions when guidelines conflict. *Osteoporos Int.* 2019;30(12):2401-2406. PMID: 31471665

13. Eastell R, Rosen CJ, Black DM, Cheung AM, Murad MH, Shoback D. Pharmacological management of osteoporosis in postmenopausal women: an Endocrine Society* clinical practice guideline. *J Clin Endocrinol Metab.* 2019;104(5):1595-1622. PMID: 30907953

14. Anastasilakis AD, Polyzos SA, Makras P, Aubry-Rozier B, Kaouri S, Lamy O. Clinical features of 24 patients with rebound-associated vertebral fractures after denosumab discontinuation: systematic review and additional cases. *J Bone Miner Res.* 2017;32(6):1291-1296. PMID: 28240371

15. Tsourdi E, Zillikens MC, Meier C, et al. Fracture risk and management of discontinuation of denosumab therapy: a systematic review and position statement by ECTS. *J Clin Endocrinol Metab.* 2020;dgaa756. PMID: 33103722

16. Leder BZ, Tsai JN, Uihlein AV, et al. Denosumab and teriparatide transitions in postmenopausal osteoporosis (the DATA-Switch study): extension of a randomised controlled trial. *Lancet.* 2015;386(9999):1147-1155. PMID: 26144908

17. Greenspan SL, Emkey RD, Bone HG, Wet al. Significant differential effects of alendronate, estrogen, or combination therapy on the rate of bone loss after discontinuation of treatment of postmenopausal osteoporosis. A randomized, double-blind, placebo-controlled trial. *Ann Intern Med.* 2002;137(11):875-883. PMID: 12458987

18. Wasnich RD, Bagger YZ, Hosking DJ, et al;Early Postmenopausal Intervention Cohort Study Group. Changes in bone density and turnover after alendronate or estrogen withdrawal. *Menopause.* 2004;11(6 Pt 1):622-630. PMID: 15545790

19. Reid IR, Brown JP, Burckhardt P, et al. Intravenous zoledronic acid in postmenopausal women with low bone mineral density. *N Engl J Med.* 2002;346(9):653-661. PMID: 11870242

20. Quandt SA, Thompson DE, Schneider DL, Nevitt MC, Black DM, Fracture Intervention Trial Research G. Effect of alendronate on vertebral fracture risk in women with bone mineral density T scores of -1.6 to -2.5 at the femoral neck: the Fracture Intervention Trial. *Mayo Clin Proc.* 2005;80(3):343-349. PMID: 15757015

21. Rothman MS, Olenginski TP, Stanciu I, Krohn K, Lewiecki EM. Lessons learned with Bone Health TeleECHO: making treatment decisions when guidelines conflict. *Osteoporos Int.* 2019;30(12):2401-2406. PMID: 31471665

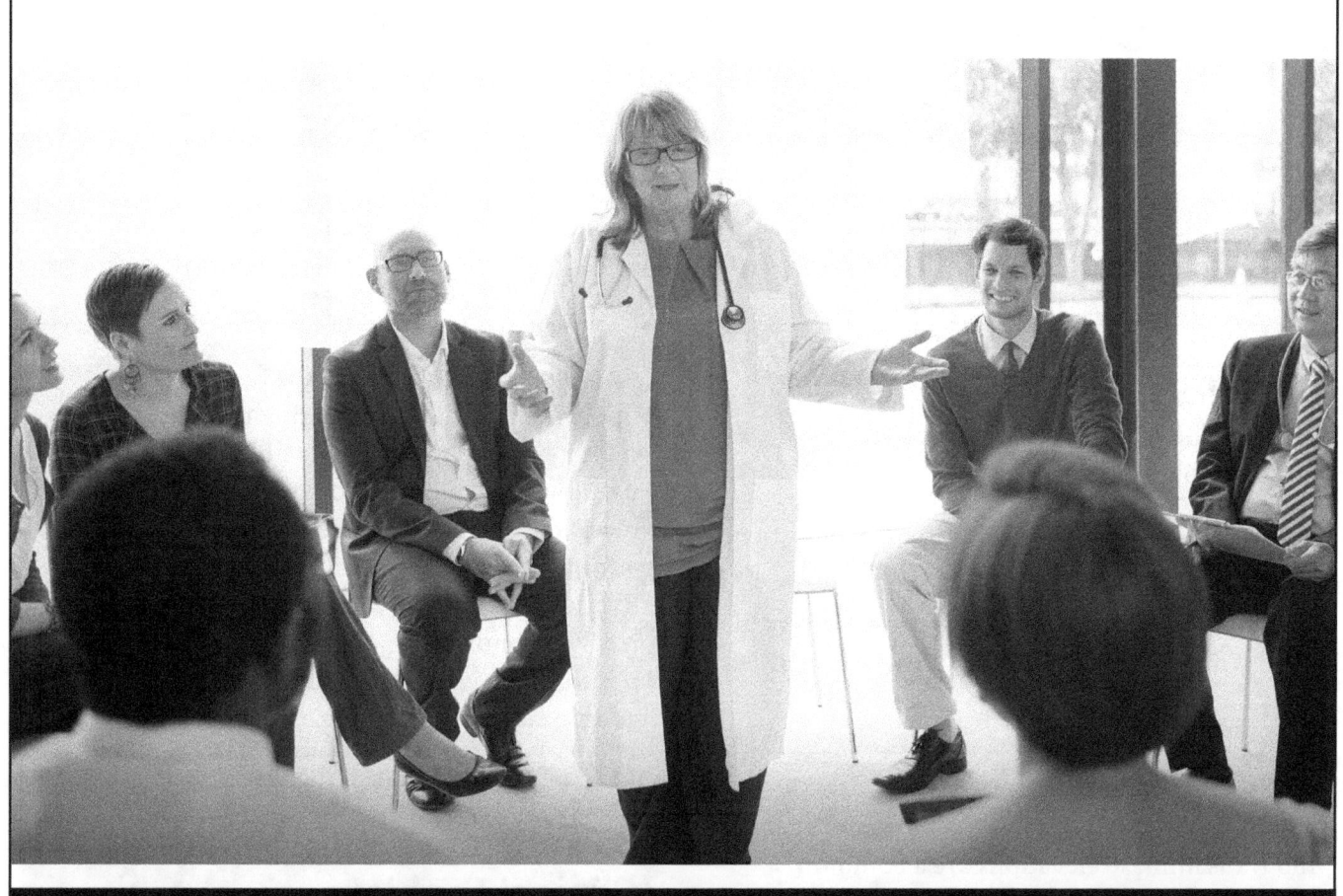

CARDIOVASCULAR
ENDOCRINOLOGY

Choosing Cholesterol-Lowering Medications in Patients With Liver Disease

Savitha Subramanian, MD. Department of Medicine, Division of Metabolism, Endocrinology, and Nutrition, University of Seattle, Seattle, WA; E-mail: ssubrama@uw.edu

Learning Objectives

As a result of participating in this session, learners should be able to:

- Appropriately stratify risk and manage patients with dyslipidemia in the setting of liver disease.

- Initiate appropriate lipid-lowering therapy in patients with liver function test abnormalities.

Main Conclusions

Mild transaminase elevations are a common occurrence in persons with nonalcoholic/metabolic fatty liver disease (NAFLD or recently referred to as MAFLD), where hepatic steatosis is associated with metabolic dysfunction such as insulin resistance, metabolic syndrome, and type 2 diabetes mellitus. Statin therapy is indicated for treatment of cardiovascular risk reduction in patients with NAFLD. Statin therapy decreases LDL-cholesterol levels and can improve transaminitis.[1] Ezetimibe may also be used to lower LDL cholesterol, but cardiovascular benefits in this population are still unknown. Fibrates can be used to treat moderate hypertriglyceridemia and are safe and usually well tolerated in patients with NAFLD. However, evidence that treatment of dyslipidemia with any lipid-lowering agent improves histology or liver-related outcomes in patients with steatohepatitis is currently lacking.

Dyslipidemia is also described in patients with other liver disorders such as cholestatic liver disease. Lipoprotein X is an abnormal lipoprotein particle containing free cholesterol often observed in acquired cholestatic liver dysfunction. Skin xanthomas may arise and marked hypercholesterolemia occurs in persons with lipoprotein X. Treatment of the underlying liver dysfunction, often requiring liver transplant, resolves abnormal lipoprotein X. Dyslipidemia that occurs after liver transplant should be promptly addressed with appropriate lipid-lowering therapy.

Significance of the Clinical Problem

Dyslipidemia is a common occurrence in individuals with NAFLD, and it drives cardiovascular risk. NAFLD is increasing in prevalence and is currently estimated to affect nearly 25% of adults worldwide and is the leading cause of liver disease. It is closely associated with other metabolic disorders such as obesity and type 2 diabetes, and its prevalence is much higher in persons with these conditions. An atherogenic dyslipidemia is often observed; NAFLD is now considered a cardiovascular risk factor, and risk mitigation strategies are essential. However, individuals with NAFLD often have elevated liver enzymes, and there is still clinician hesitancy in starting and/or continuing lipid-lowering therapy, especially statins. Additionally, guidelines on lipid management in NAFLD are lacking.

The liver has a central role in cholesterol metabolism, including cholesterol biosynthesis, storage, and excretion. Therefore, liver disease can affect cholesterol levels, depending on the type of liver injury (eg, parenchymal, cholestatic, or mixed). Hypercholesterolemia, with a relative increase of free cholesterol, is an early and peculiar metabolic alteration in cholestatic liver disease. Lipoprotein composition and metabolism are altered, and an anomalous lipoprotein called lipoprotein X is present. Very high cholesterol levels (>1000 mg/dL [>25.90 mmol/L]) levels can occur. This condition is often underrecognized in clinical practice.

Barriers to Optimal Practice

- Hesitancy using appropriate lipid-lowering medication in the setting of transaminitis associated with NAFLD and NASH.

- Recognition of the underlying etiology leading to dyslipidemia in liver disease.

Strategies for Diagnosis, Therapy, and/or Management

Lipid Disorders in NAFLD

Diagnosis
Atherogenic dyslipidemia characterized by mild to moderate hypertriglyceridemia with low HDL cholesterol and increased small dense LDL particles is commonly observed.

Treatment
Cardiovascular morbidity and mortality are increased in patients with NAFLD. Metabolic derangements are the primary contributor to increased cardiovascular risk in these individuals. NAFLD is associated with increased risk of fatal and nonfatal cardiovascular events, as well as other cardiac complications, such as cardiomyopathy, cardiac valvular calcification, and cardiac arrhythmias. This increased risk is independent of traditional cardiovascular risk factors and is proportional to the severity of liver disease.[2] In individuals with type 2 diabetes and NALFD, atherogenic dyslipidemia is associated with

moderate-to-advanced liver fibrosis compared with what is observed in those without diabetes. Therefore, dyslipidemia of NAFLD should be addressed in a timely manner by initiating statin therapy.[3]

The liver has a central role in lipoprotein metabolism, as it is involved in the synthesis and/ or clearance of all lipoproteins.[4] Hepatocytes, a major site of cholesterol metabolism, are a main target of statins. Alanine aminotransferase elevations occur independently of statins in patients with NAFLD. Several studies have established the safety of statins in patients with a baseline elevation in liver enzymes. Statins decrease hepatic transaminases in NAFLD. Risk of statin-induced hepatotoxicity is not increased in individuals with NAFLD or NASH, and serious liver injury from statin therapy is very rare in clinical practice. Statins should be avoided in patients with decompensated cirrhosis, as there are very few safety data. Periodic monitoring of serum alanine aminotransferase levels does not detect or prevent serious liver injury due to statin use and is therefore *not recommended*.[5] Ezetimibe is also associated with LDL-cholesterol reductions in NAFLD; improvements in liver function have also been observed. Effects on steatosis and NAFLD activity score appear to be mixed. A post hoc analysis of the IMPROVE-IT study showed that patients classified as being at high risk for liver fibrosis using the NAFLD fibrosis score showed greater reductions in recurrent cardiovascular disease with simvastatin and ezetimibe compared with those classified as being at low risk. PCSK9 inhibitors show promise in decreasing intrahepatic fat in patients with NAFLD but further evidence is needed.

Lipid Disorders in Other Liver Diseases

Cholestatic Liver Disease
The liver converts cholesterol to bile acids and removes free cholesterol via biliary excretion. Cholestatic liver disease (primary biliary cirrhosis or primary sclerosing cholangitis) due to impaired bile flow results in accumulation of bile acids and other metabolites in the liver and

systemic circulation. In the setting of cholestatic liver disease, a unique, abnormal lipoprotein with similar density to LDL but without its surface protein apolipoprotein B appears in the circulation.[6] These lipoproteins contain only phospholipid and unesterified cholesterol and are referred to as lipoprotein X. In cholestasis, there is impaired bile flow; it is believed that these lipoprotein-like lipoprotein X particles are due to reflux of biliary lipoproteins into the systemic circulation due to cholestasis.

Extreme cholesterol elevations can occur and result in artifactual abnormalities in electrolytes (hyponatremia) and hyperviscosity. Xanthomas can develop in the palms on occasion. Neuropathic symptoms can occur because of large xanthomas. Such striking cholesterol elevations are reflective of significant liver dysfunction, and hypercholesterolemia resolves only after liver dysfunction resolves.

Statins, ezetimibe, and fibrates have all been shown to be safe in patients with cholestatic liver disease but are of limited benefit when serum cholesterol levels are markedly elevated. Blood filtering using plasma exchange can be used as a temporizing measure to decrease cholesterol levels; only correction of underlying liver pathology (often with liver transplant) results in complete reversal of lipid abnormalities. Lipoprotein X is not believed to be atherogenic. It is estimated, however, that about 10% of patients with primary biliary cirrhosis have a significant risk of cardiovascular disease and should be treated with medications to reduce that risk.

Dyslipidemia After Liver Transplant

Dyslipidemia is common following liver transplant, occurring in more than 60% of transplant recipients. Posttransplant dyslipidemia is commonly observed in patients with higher BMI or type 2 diabetes before transplant; it can also develop in the absence of these comorbid conditions. Use of immunosuppressant medications, including calcineurin inhibitors and mTOR inhibitor sirolimus, increase the risk of dyslipidemia. Lipids should be regularly assessed in liver transplant recipients.

Liver transplant recipients have increased cardiovascular risk, especially those with features of the metabolic syndrome or diabetes. Liver graft steatosis can occur. Statins are mostly safe to use in the posttransplant setting. Calcineurin inhibitors and several statins are metabolized by cytochrome P450 3A4, and concurrent use of higher dosages may increase the risk of statin-associated myopathy.[7]

Time point	Total cholesterol	Triglycerides	HDL cholesterol	LDL cholesterol	Fasting plasma glucose	Hemoglobin A$_{1c}$	AST	ALT
5 years ago	253 mg/dL (SI: 6.55 mmol/L)	293 mg/dL (SI: 3.31 mmol/L)	41 mg/dL (SI: 1.06 mmol/L)	153 mg/dL (SI: 3.96 mmol/L)	106 mg/dL (SI: 5.88 mmol/L)	5.6% (38 mmol/mol)	22 U/L (SI: 0.37 µkat/L)	61 U/L (SI: 1.02 µkat/L)
5 years ago (atorvastatin, 10 mg daily, started)	274 mg/dL (SI: 7.10 mmol/L)	275 mg/dL (SI: 3.11 mmol/L)	40 mg/dL (SI: 1.04 mmol/L)	179 mg/dL (SI: 4.64 mmol/L)	130 mg/dL (SI: 7.22 mmol/L)	6.2% (44 mmol/mol)	26 U/L (SI: 0.43 µkat/L)	47 U/L (SI: 0.78 µkat/L)
3 years ago	196 mg/dL (SI: 5.08 mmol/L)	377 mg/dL (SI: 4.26 mmol/L)	36 mg/dL (SI: 0.93 mmol/L)	85 mg/dL (SI: 2.20 mmol/L)	143 mg/dL (SI: 7.94 mmol/L)	6.8% (51 mmol/mol)	23 U/L (SI: 0.38 µkat/L)	64 U/L (SI: 1.07 µkat/L)
Most recent	181 mg/dL (SI: 4.69 mmol/L)	422 mg/dL (SI: 4.77 mmol/L)	39 mg/dL (SI: 1.01 mmol/L)	...	150 mg/dL (SI: 8.33 mmol/L)	7.1% (54 mmol/mol)	47 U/L (SI: 0.78 µkat/L)	86 U/L (SI: 1.44 µkat/L)

Abbreviations: ALT, alanine aminotransferase; AST, aspartate aminotransferase.

Reference ranges: fasting glucose, 70-99 mg/dL (SI: 3.9-5.5 mmol/L); hemoglobin A$_{1c}$, 4.0%-5.6% (20-38 mmol/mol); ALT, 10-40 U/L (SI: 0.17-0.67 µkat/L); AST, 20-48 U/L (SI: 0.33-0.80 µkat/L).

Clinical Case Vignettes

Case 1

A 44-year-old woman is referred for management of dyslipidemia and gradually increasing elevated liver enzymes first noted about 5 years ago. At that time, atorvastatin (10 mg daily) was initiated, and she has continued this regimen.

Laboratory test results are shown in the Table (previous page).

She followed up with her primary care provider for a few years. Recently, her hemoglobin A_{1c} level has increased, type 2 diabetes has been diagnosed, and metformin has been initiated at a dosage of 500 mg twice daily. She reports a weight gain of 15 lb (6.8 kg) in the past 18 months. Her weight continues to increase, and physical activity levels have dropped. Abdominal ultrasonography obtained as part of the evaluation for elevated liver enzymes reveals hepatic steatosis. Her most recent hemoglobin A_{1c} level is 7.5% (58 mmol/mol).

There is a family history of premature atherosclerotic cardiovascular disease in her mother, and many family members have type 2 diabetes. She does not drink more than 1 alcoholic beverage a week. She is commercially insured through her employer.

She is concerned about her liver test results and seeks your recommendation.

Which of the following is the best next step?

A. Discontinue atorvastatin and start fenofibrate

B. Increase the atorvastatin dosage to 40 mg daily

C. Increase the metformin dosage to 1000 mg twice daily

D. Start intermittent scanned glucose monitoring

Answer: C and D): Increase the metformin dosage to 1000 mg twice daily (C) and start intermittent scanned glucose monitoring (D)

This patient has a history of mild liver transaminase elevations, which have recently worsened. Low-intensity atorvastatin is safe and has been effective in lowering this woman's LDL cholesterol. However, recent elevation in aspartate aminotransferase and alanine aminotransferase levels are likely a reflection of recent-onset diabetes corresponding to weight gain. There is no indication to discontinue atorvastatin (Answer A) at this time. Although increasing the atorvastatin dosage to 40 mg daily (Answer B) is not necessarily wrong, it is not the best option, as she had good LDL-cholesterol lowering on the dosage of 10 mg daily. Statins are not good triglyceride-lowering agents.

Instead, maximizing metformin therapy (Answer C) is a better option due to rising hemoglobin A_{1c} values.

Additionally, intermittent scanned continuous glucose monitoring (Answer D), if covered by insurance, is acceptable. This patient specifically came to clinic requesting use of intermittent scanned continuous glucose monitoring. She incorporated lifestyle efforts and was able to decrease her hemoglobin A_{1c} level to 6.1% (43 mmol/mol). Liver transaminase levels decreased to what was observed 7 years prior.

Therefore, both Answers C and D are correct.

Case 2

A 24-year-old man with a diagnosis of primary sclerosing cholangitis is referred from hepatology for management of very high cholesterol levels and bumps on his elbows and palms.

Laboratory test results:

Total cholesterol = 1382 mg/dL (<200 mg/dL [optimal]) (SI: 35.79 mmol/L [<5.18 mmol/L])

Triglycerides = 141 mg/dL (<150 mg/dL [optimal]) (SI: 1.59 mmol/L [<1.70 mmol/L])

LDL cholesterol = 1347 mg/dL (<100 mg/dL [optimal]) (SI: 34.89 mmol/L [mmol/L])

HDL cholesterol = 7 mg/dL (>60 mg/dL [optimal]) (SI: 0.18 mmol/L [>1.55 mmol/L])

Serum sodium = measurements range from 129 to 133 mEq/L (129 to 133 mmol/L)

Alanine aminotransferase = 255 U/L (10-40 U/L) (SI: 4.26 µkat/L [0.17-0.67 µkat/L])

Aspartate aminotransferase = 298 U/L (20-48 U/L) (SI: 4.98 µkat/L [0.33-0.80 µkat/L])

Total bilirubin = 6.0 mg/dL (0.3-1.2 mg/dL) (SI: 102.6 µmol/L [5.1-20.5 µmol/L])

Which of the following is the best next step in this patient's care?

A. Refer for LDL apheresis

B. Refer for therapeutic plasma exchange

C. Start colesevelam

D. Start pravastatin

E. None of the above

Answer: E) None of the above

In cholestatic liver disease, lipoprotein X (LDL-like particles lacking apolipoprotein B on the surface) can be present in the circulation, occurring in up to 45% of patients. Extreme cholesterol elevations can occur with resultant artifactual abnormalities in electrolytes (hyponatremia) and hyperviscosity. Xanthomas can occur in the palms.

While statins (Answer D) seem to be safe in individuals with cholestatic liver disease, it is highly unlikely statins will result in significant LDL-cholesterol reduction in a patient with such marked hypercholesteremia.

Colesevelam (Answer C) is a bile acid resin with only modest cholesterol-lowering ability.

LDL apheresis (Answer A), which physically removes LDL particles (by virtue of the presence of apolipoprotein B on LDL) from the blood, will not clear lipoprotein X, which lacks apolipoprotein B on its surface.

Plasma exchange (Answer B) can be useful in decreasing cholesterol levels, but it is a temporizing measure.

This patient underwent orthotopic liver transplant, which normalized lipid levels:

Total cholesterol = 219 mg/dL (SI: 5.67 mmol/L)
Triglycerides = 178 mg/dL (SI: 2.01 mmol/L)
LDL cholesterol = 155 mg/dL (SI: 4.01 mmol/L)

Therefore, the best answer is none of the above (Answer E).

Case 3

A 62-year-old woman is referred from hepatology. She underwent liver transplant for NASH-related cirrhosis. At the 1-year postliver transplant biopsy, macrovesicular steatosis was noted, and she was subsequently referred for treatment options. Her history is notable for hypertension and type 2 diabetes (managed with lifestyle efforts) prior to transplant, as well as longstanding hyperlipidemia with intolerance to statins. Multiple statins were tried over the years with significant muscle adverse effects. There is also a history of possible transient ischemic attack 3 years before transplant.

Currently, her immunosuppression regimen includes tacrolimus. She also takes ezetimibe without issues. Metformin was recently added due to rising hemoglobin A_{1c} values.

Laboratory test results are shown in the Table.

Which of the following therapies should be added at this time?

A. Bempedoic acid

B. Evolocumab

C. Icosapent ethyl

D. Fenofibrate

Time point	Total cholesterol	Triglycerides	HDL cholesterol	LDL cholesterol	Hemoglobin A_{1c}
Pretransplant (started ezetimibe, 10 mg daily)	190 mg/dL (SI: 4.92 mmol/L)	82 mg/dL (SI: 0.93 mmol/L)	59 mg/dL (SI: 1.53 mmol/L)	115 mg/dL (SI: 2.98 mmol/L)	6.2% (44 mmol/mol)
1 year after transplant (continued ezetimibe, 10 mg daily, added metformin)	195 mg/dL (SI: 5.05 mmol/L)	430 mg/dL (SI: 4.86 mmol/L)	54 mg/dL (SI: 1.40 mmol/L)	141 mg/dL (SI: 3.65 mmol/L)	6.6% (49 mmol/mol)
After transplant; most recent measurements (continued, ezetimibe, 10 mg daily)	252 mg/dL (SI: 6.53 mmol/L)	357 mg/dL (SI: 4.03 mmol/L)	63 mg/dL (SI: 1.63 mmol/L)	118 mg/dL (SI: 3.06 mmol/L)	6.7% (50 mmol/mol)

Reference range: hemoglobin A_{1c}, 4.0%-5.6% (20-38 mmol/mol).

Answer: B) Evolocumab

Evolocumab (Answer B) is a PCSK9 inhibitor that can be used in individuals at high risk for atherosclerotic cardiovascular disease (such as this woman) who have not reached their LDL-cholesterol targets. In this patient with type 2 diabetes, hypertension, and history of transient ischemic attack, the LDL-cholesterol goal is less than 70 mg/dL (<1.81 mmol/L). Addition of a PCSK9 inhibitor is an appropriate next step. Icosapent ethyl (Answer C) is also beneficial in patients at high cardiovascular risk when it is added to statin therapy; monotherapy benefit is unclear.

Bempedoic acid (Answer A) is a new agent that acts in the same cholesterol biosynthesis pathway as statins. It targets ATP-citrate lyase (an enzyme that is upstream of HMG-CoA reductase), upregulates LDL receptors, and therefore lowers LDL cholesterol. Bempedoic acid is converted into an active drug by a specific isozyme that is not present in skeletal muscle and can be used in patients with statin intolerance due to muscle adverse effects. LDL-cholesterol reduction of approximately 18% to 28% is observed (36% to 46% when used in combination with ezetimibe). However, safety in liver transplant recipients is unknown.

Fenofibrate (Answer D) is an effective triglyceride-lowering agent; however, there are very limited data on use in liver transplant recipients and there is lack of proven cardiovascular benefit to justify addition at this time.

This patient started PCSK9 inhibitor therapy with excellent response:

Total cholesterol = 139 mg/dL (SI: 3.60 mmol/L)
Triglycerides = 311 mg/dL (SI: 3.51 mmol/L)
LDL cholesterol = 16 mg/dL (SI: 0.41 mmol/L)
HDL cholesterol = 61 mg/dL (SI: 1.58 mmol/L)

References

1. Speliotes EK, Balakrishnan M, Friedman LS, and Corey KE. Treatment of dyslipidemia in common liver diseases. *Clin Gastroenterol Hepatol.* 2018;16(8):1189-1196. PMID: 29684459

2. Targher G, Corey KE, Byrne CD. NAFLD, and cardiovascular and cardiac diseases: factors influencing risk, prediction and treatment. *Diabetes Metab.* 2021;47(2):101215. PMID: 33296704

3. Amor AJ, and Perea V. Dyslipidemia in nonalcoholic fatty liver disease. *Curr Opin Endocrinol Diabetes Obes.* 2019;26(2):103-108. PMID: 30694825

4. Nemes K, Aberg F, Gylling H, Isoniemi H. Cholesterol metabolism in cholestatic liver disease and liver transplantation: from molecular mechanisms to clinical implications. *World J Hepatol.* 2016;8(22):924-932. PMID: 27574546

5. Bays H, Cohen DE, Chalasani N, Harrison SA, The National Lipid Association's Statin Safety Task Force. An assessment by the Statin Liver Safety Task Force: 2014 update. *J Clin Lipidol.* 2014;8(Suppl 3):S47-S57. PMID: 24793441

6. Brandt EJ, Regnier SM, Leung EK, et al. Management of lipoprotein X and its complications in a patient with primary sclerosing cholangitis. *Clin Lipidol.* 2015;10(4):305-312. PMID: 26413163

7. Kellick KA, Bottorff M, Toth PP; The National Lipid Association's Safety Task Force. A clinician's guide to statin drug-drug interactions. *J Clin Lipidol.* 2014;8(Suppl 3):S30-S46. PMID: 24793440

Update on Genetic Causes of Hypercholesterolemia: What's New in the Evaluation and Treatment of These Hard-to-Treat Patients

Marc-Andre Cornier, MD. Division of Endocrinology, Diabetes, and Metabolic Diseases, Medical University of South Carolina, Charleston, SC; E-mail: cornier@musc.edu

Learning Objectives

As a result of participating in this session, learners should be able to:

- Recognize and initiate an appropriate evaluation of patients with hypercholesterolemia.

- Provide individualized goals for treatment of hypercholesterolemia.

- Explain different medical treatment options for cholesterol lowering.

- Be aware of other treatment options such as new pharmacologic therapies and LDL apheresis and recognize when to refer patients to a lipid disorders specialist.

Main Conclusions

Severe hypercholesterolemia usually has a genetic cause such as familial hypercholesterolemia (FH) and is associated with premature atherosclerotic cardiovascular disease (ASCVD). Aggressive, early treatment is warranted and necessary to prevent ASCVD. Combination medical therapy is typically necessary to adequately reduce the total cholesterol burden. The new PCSK9 modulating therapies offer novel mechanisms to substantially lower LDL cholesterol in these otherwise difficult-to-treat patients. Finally, in some patients, LDL apheresis is necessary and should be considered.

Significance of the Clinical Problem

It was not until the turn of the 20th century that cholesterol was identified as a key component of atherosclerosis and that feeding cholesterol to rodents was shown to produce atherosclerosis. It was not until the 1930s, though, that the genetic link between high cholesterol and coronary heart disease (CHD) was identified and described as FH. This disorder was later known to be consistent with heterozygous FH and was associated with significantly elevated cholesterol levels and increased risk for premature ASCVD. In the 1950s, the biosynthetic pathways of cholesterol were further understood.[1] LDL cholesterol was identified, and high levels were determined to be associated with higher risk for CHD.[2] It was not until the seminal work of Brown and Goldstein in the 1970s that the LDL receptor was identified and that a defect in the LDL-receptor gene was discovered to be the primary defect responsible for FH.[3] We now know that there are many different pathogenic variants in the LDL-receptor gene, and depending on the site of the variant, patients with homozygous FH are unable to produce any functional receptors or are able to produce low levels of normally active LDL receptors. We also know that patients with heterozygous FH have about half the normal amount of normally functional LDL receptors.

ASCVD remains a major cause of death in the United States and around the world. Cholesterol is at the core of atherosclerosis development and is one of the major modifiable risk factors. Individuals with severe hypercholesterolemia due to a genetic cause are at greatly increased risk for premature ASCVD because of a high cumulative burden of cholesterol. Current guidelines recommend that any individual with an LDL-cholesterol concentration greater than 190 mg/dL (>4.92 mmol/L) should be treated aggressively.[4]

Severe hypercholesterolemia can occur in isolation, as seen in the different forms of FH, or it can be associated with other lipid abnormalities such as concomitantly elevated triglycerides and/or low HDL cholesterol such as in familial combined hyperlipidemia and dysbetalipoproteinemia. These disorders are also associated with a greatly increased risk for ASCVD.

Isolated severe hypercholesterolemia is generally consistent with FH. Approximately 1 in 1 million persons is homozygous and has extremely high cholesterol levels with LDL-cholesterol concentrations often reaching greater than 600 mg/dL (>15.54 mmol/L). If untreated, these individuals develop significant tendinous xanthomas and are at risk for ASCVD and death at a very young age (before 20 years). More than 1600 pathogenic variants in the gene encoding the LDL receptor have been documented. The prevalence of heterozygous FH is as high as 1 in 200 to 300 persons depending on the population, rendering FH as one of the most common serious genetic disorders. Untreated patients with heterozygous FH typically have LDL-cholesterol levels in the range of 200 to 300 mg/dL (5.18 to 7.77 mmol/L) and can also develop xanthomas. They are at increased risk for premature ASCVD events before the fourth and fifth decades of life.

PCSK9 is an important regulator of LDL-receptor degradation because binding of PCSK9 to the LDL receptor results in degradation of the receptor, thereby preventing recycling of the receptor. Individuals with elevated PCSK9 levels due to gain-of-function pathogenic variants in gene encoding PCSK9 may also have severe hypercholesterolemia clinically similar to that observed in patients with FH. Individuals with loss-of-function pathogenic variants in the gene encoding PCSK9 are associated with increased LDL-receptor function, very low levels of LDL cholesterol, and very low incidence of ASCVD. This knowledge has led to new treatment options for lowering LDL cholesterol, including inhibitors of PCSK9 by monoclonal antibodies and inhibition of the production of PCSK9.

Severe hypercholesterolemia can occur in the setting of mixed hyperlipidemias, which is also associated with premature ASCVD. Familial combined hyperlipidemia is the most common genetic disorder of mixed hyperlipidemia occurring in up to 1 in 250 persons. While a specific gene variant has not been identified, affected individuals have increased production of apolipoprotein B–containing lipoproteins. Familial dysbetalipoproteinemia is due to a genetic variation in apolipoprotein E (the E2 isoform). This is associated with reduced clearance of remnant particles (chylomicron and VLDL remnants) and leads to planar and tuberous xanthomas and premature ASCVD if untreated. "Metabolic dyslipidemia" is the most common cause of mixed hyperlipidemia associated with other features of the metabolic syndrome, but it is generally associated with more modest elevations in cholesterol.

Barriers to Optimal Practice

- Lack of effectiveness of available treatment options.
- Adverse effects of currently available treatment options.
- Cost of therapies.

Strategies for Diagnosis, Therapy, and/or Management

Diagnosis

Persons with homozygous FH typically have LDL-cholesterol levels greater than 600 mg/dL (>15.54 mmol/L) and have a family history that suggests both parents have heterozygous FH. Such patients must be identified at a young age and treated aggressively. Genetic testing can be done, but not all of the more than 1600 pathogenic variants are identified by clinically available genetic testing. As such, negative results on genetic testing does not exclude the diagnosis. Patients with heterozygous FH should be suspected in the setting of an LDL-cholesterol concentration greater than 160 mg/dL (>4.14 mmol/L) in children or greater than 190 mg/dL (>4.92 mmol/L) in adults. Most affected adults have an LDL-cholesterol level greater than 220 mg/dL (>5.70 mmol/L). FH should also be suspected in the setting of the following physical examination findings: (1) tendon xanthomas at any age (most commonly in the Achilles tendon and finger extensor tendons; (2) corneal arcus in patients younger than 45 years; and (3) xanthelasmas in patients younger than 20 to 25 years.

Different criteria have been established to help make the clinical diagnosis of FH:

1. Dutch or World Health Organization diagnostic criteria. Diagnosis of heterozygous FH is certain when the point total is greater than 8, probable when 6 to 8, and possible when 3 to 5:

   a. Family history:

      - First-degree relative with known premature (men <55 years, women <60 years) cardiovascular disease (1 point)

      - First-degree relative with known LDL-cholesterol concentration greater than the 95th percentile for age and sex, and/or with tendon xanthomata and/or arcus cornealis, or children younger than 18 years with an LDL-cholesterol concentration greater than the 95th percentile for age and sex (2 points)

   b. Clinical history:

      - Patient has premature (men <55 years, women <60 years) CAD (2 points) or other cardiovascular disease (1 point)

   c. Physical examination:

      - Tendon xanthomata (6 points)

      - Arcus cornealis at an age younger than 45 years (4 points)

   d. Laboratory analysis:

      - LDL cholesterol >330 mg/dL (>8.55 mmol/L) (8 points)

      - LDL cholesterol 250-329 mg/dL (>6.48-8.52 mmol/L) (5 points)

      - LDL cholesterol 190-249 mg/dL (>4.92-6.45 mmol/L) (3 points)

      - LDL cholesterol 155-189 mg/dL (>4.01-4.89 mmol/L) (1 points)

      - HDL cholesterol and triglycerides are normal

      - DNA analysis: functional pathogenic variant present in the LDL-receptor gene (8 points)

2. Simon Broome Register Diagnostic Criteria for heterozygous FH:

   a. Definite FH is defined as:

      - Total cholesterol >260 mg/dL (6.73 mmol/L) or LDL cholesterol >155 mg/dL (>4.01 mmol/L) in a child younger than 16 years or total cholesterol >290 mg/dL (>7.51 mmol/L) or LDL cholesterol >190 mg/dL (>4.92 mmol/L) in an adult PLUS tendon xanthomas in the patient or in a first- or second-degree relative

        OR

- DNA-based evidence of an *LDLR* pathogenic variant or familial defective apolipoprotein B$_{100}$

b. Possible FH is defined as:

- Total cholesterol >260 mg/dL (>6.73 mmol/L) or LDL cholesterol >155 mg/dL (>4.01 mmol/L) in a child younger than 16 years or total cholesterol >290 mg/dL (>7.51 mmol/L) or LDL cholesterol >190 mg/dL (>4.92 mmol/L) in an adult

- And at least 1 of the following:

  ◦ Family history of myocardial infarction at age younger than 50 years in second-degree relative or younger than 60 years in first-degree relative

  ◦ Family history of elevated cholesterol values >290 mg/dL (>7.51 mmol/L) in an adult first- or second-degree relative or >260 mg/dL (>6.73 mmol/L) in a child or sibling younger than 16 years

It is also important to also consider secondary causes of hypercholesterolemia in these patients, including hypothyroidism, nephrotic syndrome, cholestatic liver disease, medications, and diet.

Treatment Goals

The primary treatment goal is to reduce the risk of ASCVD-related events. Current joint guidelines published by the American College of Cardiology and the American Heart Association in 2018 have established that all individuals with an LDL-cholesterol value greater than 190 mg/dL (>4.92 mmol/L) should be treated with a high-intensity statin (atorvastatin, 40/80 mg or rosuvastatin, 20/40 mg) to lower LDL cholesterol by at least 50%.[4] Secondary goals for primary prevention are to lower LDL-cholesterol levels to less than 100 mg/dL (<2.59 mmol/L). Other

ASCVD risk factors should also be aggressively managed, including hypertension, cigarette smoking, and unhealthy lifestyle.

In patients with mixed hyperlipidemia, the primary goal is to treat the hypercholesterolemia to reduce the ASCVD risk as discussed above. Triglycerides should be targeted in patients with severe elevations, (>400 or 500 mg/dL [>4.52 or 5.65 mmol/L]) with a primary goal of reducing the risk of pancreatitis. Consideration should be given to prescribing icosapent ethyl to further reduce ASCVD risk in patients with hypertriglyceridemia and known ASCVD or in patients with diabetes and multiple ASCVD risk factors.

Treatment Options

Medical Therapy

Medical therapy with high-intensity statins is the standard of care and cornerstone of treatment with a goal of reducing LDL cholesterol by 50% or more.[4] Patients who are homozygous and most patients who are heterozygous, however, need more LDL-cholesterol lowering than can be achieved by statin therapy alone. Multiple drugs are usually necessary and often may not be sufficient. Other medical treatment options to consider include PCSK9 inhibitors, ezetimibe, bempedoic acid, inclisiran, bile acid sequestrants, and niacin. In patients who are homozygous, lomitapide and evinacumab are possible options.

Statins are the gold standard therapy due to the number of clinical trials that have shown benefit in patients with and without FH. Recent evidence suggests that combination therapy with ezetimibe or PCSK9 inhibitors confers further risk reduction.[5-7] There is less evidence in support of other treatment options such as combination therapy with bile acid sequestrants. More recently, there have been 2 trials with negative outcomes regarding the addition of niacin to statin therapy.

Two PCSK9 inhibitors, alirocumab and evolocumab, have now been approved in the United States for the treatment of heterozygous FH[8,9] and should be considered as an important treatment option for those patients who do not respond adequately to statins +/- ezetimibe. These agents lower LDL cholesterol 60%, on average, beyond maximally tolerated statin therapy. These agents have also been approved for the treatment of homozygous FH with LDL-cholesterol lowering 20% to 40% beyond maximally tolerated statin therapy.[10] Inclisiran is small interfering RNA that inhibits translation of PCSK9 and thus the production of PCSK9. It was recently approved for use in Europe and the United States to treat heterozygous FH. It is dosed at baseline, 3 months, and then every 6 months thereafter as a subcutaneous injection. Inclisiran reduces LDL-cholesterol levels by 50% to 55%, on average, beyond maximally tolerated statin therapy.[11] Bempedoic acid, an inhibitor of adenosine triphosphate citrate lyase upstream from HMG-CoA reductase in the cholesterol synthesis pathway, is also approved for the treatment of heterozygous FH. It is taken orally at a dosage of 180 mg daily and results in 15% to 27% LDL-cholesterol lowering depending on other background therapy.

Lomitapide and evinacumab are also approved for the treatment of homozygous FH. Lomitapide is a microsomal triglyceride transfer protein inhibitor that is taken orally at a dosage of 5 to 60 mg daily. Lomitapide has been shown to reduce LDL cholesterol by up to 40% in those who can tolerate it. Fat in the diet must be restricted to prevent diarrhea. Because it inhibits VLDL secretion, triglycerides can accumulate in the liver, leading to hepatotoxicity. Evinacumab is a monoclonal antibody against ANGPTL3, which is dosed as a monthly intravenous infusion. Evinacumab has been shown to reduce LDL cholesterol by 45% to 50%.

Apheresis

LDL apheresis, the direct removal of cholesterol, has been shown to prolong survival. Apheresis should be considered in patients at high risk such as those with known ASCVD whose condition has been refractory to medical therapy and/or those intolerant to medical therapy. LDL apheresis only temporarily removes LDL particles and thus must be repeated on a regular basis, generally every 1 to 2 weeks. Some patients are able to extend the frequency of apheresis with newer medical therapies. Because of the frequent need for vascular access, many, if not most, patients require fistulas. Successful treatment of patients with LDL apheresis requires a well-coordinated team of experienced personnel.[12]

Nonlipid Treatments

Lifestyle modification, including cigarette smoking cessation, increased physical activity, and reduced saturated fat intake should be recommended to all patients with hypercholesterolemia. Secondary causes of hyperlipidemia should also be treated if present. Hypertension and diabetes should be aggressively treated. Antiplatelet therapy with low-dosage aspirin should be considered.

Clinical Case Vignettes
Case 1

A 45-year-old woman is referred for evaluation and management of hyperlipidemia. She was otherwise healthy until she had a transient ischemic attack and myocardial infarction with stent placement 2 years ago. Atorvastatin, 80 mg daily, was started after her myocardial infarction for "high" cholesterol, but she developed significant muscle aches on this treatment. Her cardiologist then tried rosuvastatin, 20 mg daily, but she again developed muscle aches. She has been able to tolerate pravastatin, 20 mg daily. She has not had any further ASCVD events to this point. She also takes clopidogrel, carvedilol, lisinopril, and sertraline. Her other medical problems include hypertension and depression. Her family history is notable for her father having a myocardial infarction in his 40s and her brother undergoing coronary artery bypass graft surgery in his early 50s. She does not smoke cigarettes, tries to eat a diet low in saturated fat, and walks 2 miles every day.

Physical examination findings are unremarkable except for the presence of arcus cornealis.

Laboratory test results (sample drawn while fasting):

Total cholesterol = 247 mg/dL (SI: 6.40 mmol/L)
Triglycerides = 100 mg/dL (SI: 1.13 mmol/L)
LDL cholesterol = 175 mg/dL (SI: 4.53 mmol/L)
HDL cholesterol = 52 mg/dL (SI: 1.35 mmol/L)
Complete metabolic panel, normal

Question 1. What should this patient's primary LDL-cholesterol goal be?

A. LDL cholesterol <100 mg/dL (<2.59 mmol/L)

B. LDL cholesterol <70 mg/dL (<1.81 mmol/L)

C. LDL-cholesterol reduction >50%

D. Lowest LDL-cholesterol level she can tolerate

Answer: C) LDL-cholesterol reduction >50%

Based on current guidelines, the primary goal would be to treat this patient with high-intensity statin therapy with a goal of reducing her LDL cholesterol by 50% or more (Answer C). Unfortunately, she has been unable to tolerate high-intensity statin therapy. In addition, a more aggressive LDL-cholesterol goal aiming for concentrations lower than 70 mg/dL (<1.81 mmol/L) (Answer B) is a reasonable secondary goal in light of her known clinical ASCVD. An LDL-cholesterol goal less than 100 mg/dL (<2.59 mmol/L) (Answer A) is not aggressive enough. While potentially practical, aiming for the lowest LDL-cholesterol level she can tolerate (Answer D) is not specific or aggressive enough and is not supported by any guidelines.

Question 2. What are the treatment options?

A. Add a PCSK9 inhibitor

B. Add ezetimibe

C. Retry atorvastatin or rosuvastatin at a lower dosage

D. Try a different more effective statin such as simvastatin or pitavastatin

E. All of the above

Answer: E) All of the above

All of these options are reasonable to consider and try (Answer E). Maximizing statin therapy should first be tried. This could be done by increasing the dosage of the current treatment (pravastatin), trying a different higher-potency statin such as simvastatin or pitavastatin (Answer D), or retrying atorvastatin or rosuvastatin at a lower dosage (Answer C). It would also be reasonable to try combination therapy with an agent such as ezetimibe (Answer B), bempedoic acid, or a bile acid sequestrant in addition to maximized statin therapy. Finally, PCSK9 inhibitors (Answer A) are also approved for the treatment of heterozygous FH in patients who have not achieved control on maximally tolerated statin therapy. These agents are the most likely to achieve good control of severe hypercholesterolemia. Aggressive medical therapy may also help prevent the need for LDL apheresis. Apheresis might be a good option if this patient's LDL cholesterol cannot be controlled with aggressive medical therapy and/or she continues to have recurrent ASCVD events. Before the approval of PCSK9 inhibitors, apheresis was more commonly used as a way to control the overall cholesterol burden to which these patients are exposed.

Case 2

A 56-year-old man with a complex medical history recently moved to the area and seeks your help. He was diagnosed with "homozygous FH" and significant coronary artery disease and has been treated with LDL apheresis. He was first diagnosed 15 years ago, although he knew that his cholesterol was very high since age 30 years. He has had multiple stents and myocardial infarctions and is status post coronary artery bypass graft surgery before apheresis was started. He has had LDL-cholesterol levels in the range of 500 to 600 mg/dL (12.95 to 15.54 mmol/L) and has xanthomas of the knuckles, as well as the Achilles tendons. He has a very strong family history of heart disease in both parents and knows of family members who have cholesterol levels greater than 300 mg/dL (>7.77 mmol/L). He has been intolerant to statins because of myopathy. Colesevelam led to significant gastrointestinal adverse effects, niacin led to intolerable flushing, and ezetimibe caused muscle aches. He finally started LDL apheresis 4 years ago, which has helped reduce the occurrence of new ASCVD events. He has had more trouble with angina, however, since moving to a higher altitude.

Question 1. What should this patient's LDL-cholesterol goal be?

A. LDL cholesterol <150 mg/dL (<3.9 mmol/L)
B. LDL cholesterol <100 mg/dL (cholesterol 2.6 mmol/L)
C. LDL-cholesterol reduction >50%
D. Lowest LDL-cholesterol level he can tolerate
E. Treatment with statin therapy is primary goal

Answer: D) Lowest LDL-cholesterol level he can tolerate

Based on current guidelines, the primary goal would be to treat this patient with high-intensity statin therapy to reduce his LDL cholesterol by 50% or more. However, he has persistent ASCVD. As such, his LDL cholesterol should be treated as aggressively as he can tolerate (thus, Answer D is correct and Answers A, B, C, and E are incorrect).

Question 2. What are the treatment options?

A. Add evinacumab
B. Add lomitapide
C. Add a PCSK9 inhibitor
D. Continue LDL apheresis
E. All of the above

Answer: E) All of the above

All of these options are reasonable to consider and try (Answer E). At this time, LDL apheresis (Answer D) should be continued, as he has had persistent disease and apheresis has helped reduce event rates. It would also be reasonable, though, to add medical therapy to see if the frequency of apheresis could be reduced. All 3 listed medical treatment options are approved for patients with homozygous FH. While all of these agents are associated with a high cost, they are much less expensive than frequent apheresis.

PCSK9 inhibitors (Answer C) are approved for the treatment of homozygous FH with LDL-cholesterol lowering of 20% to 30%.

Lomitapide (Answer B) has been shown to lower LDL cholesterol up to 40% at higher dosages, but it can be difficult to tolerate.

Evinacumab (Answer A) lowers LDL cholesterol 45% to 50% as a monthly intravenous infusion.

Combinations of these newer agents have not been studied.

References

1. Bloch K. The biological synthesis of cholesterol. *Science*. 1965;150(3692):19-28. PMID: 5319508

2. Gofman JW, Glazier F, Tamplin A, Strisower B, De Lalla O. Lipoproteins, coronary heart disease, and atherosclerosis. *Physiol Rev*. 1954;34(3):589-607. PMID: 13185756

3. Goldstein JL, Brown MS. Familial hypercholesterolemia: identification of a defect in the regulation of 3-hydroxy-3-methylglutaryl coenzyme A reductase activity associated with overproduction of cholesterol. *Proc Natl Acad Sci U S A*. 1973;70(10):2804-2808. PMID: 4355366

4. Grundy SM, Stone NJ, Bailey AL, et al. 2018 AHA/ACC/AACVPR/AAPA/ABC/ACPM/ADA/AGS/APhA/ASPC/NLA/PCNA guideline on the management of blood cholesterol: a report of the American College of Cardiology/American Heart Association Task Force on Clinical Practice Guidelines. *J Am Coll Cardiol*. 2019;73(24):e285-e350. PMID: 30423393

5. Cannon CP, Blazing MA, Giugliano RP, et al. Ezetimibe added to statin therapy after acute coronary syndromes. *N Engl J Med*. 2015;372(25):2387-2397. PMID: 26039521

6. Sabatine MS, Giugliano RP, Keech AC, et al; FOURIER Steering Committee and Investigators. Evolocumab and clinical outcomes in patients with cardiovascular disease. *N Engl J Med*. 2017;376(18):1713-1722. PMID: 28304224

7. Schwartz GG, Step PG, Szarek M, et al; ODYSSEY OUTCOMES Committees and Investigators. Alirocumab and cardiovasular outcomes after acute coronary syndrome. *N Engl J Med*. 2018;379(22):2097-2107. PMID: 30403574

8. Raal FJ, Stein EA, Dufour R, et al; RUTHERFORD-2 Investigators. PCSK9 inhibition with evolocumab (AMG 145) in heterozygous familial hypercholesterolaemia (RUTHERFORD-2): a randomised, double-blind, placebo-controlled trial. *Lancet*. 2015;385(9965):331-340. PMID: 25282519

9. Kastelein JJP, Ginsberg HN, Langslet G, et al. ODYSSEY FH I and FH II: 78 week results with alirocumab treatment in 735 patients with heterozygous familial hypercholesterolaemia. *Eur Heart J*. 2015;36(43):2996-3003. PMID: 26330422

10. Raal FJ, Honarpour N, Blom DJ, et al; TESLA Investigators. Inhibition of PCSK9 with evolocumab in homozygous familial hypercholesterolaemia (TESLA Part B): a randomised, double-blind, placebo-controlled trial. *Lancet*. 2015;385(9965):341-350. PMID: 25282520

11. Ray KK, Landmesser U, Leiter LA, et al. Inclisiran in patients at high cardiovasular risk with elevated LDL cholesterol. *N Engl J Med*. 2017;376(15):1430-1440. PMID: 28306389

12. Heigl F, Hettich R, Eder B, Arendt R. Lipoprotein apheresis standard for apheresis competence centers--an updated synthesis and amendment to pre-existing standards. *Atheroscler Suppl*.2013;14(1):57-65. PMID: 23357142

PCSK9 Inhibitors: Basic Biology to Clinical Outcomes

Connie B. Newman, MD, MACP. Department of Medicine, Division of Endocrinology, Diabetes and Metabolism, New York University Grossman School of Medicine, New York, NY; Email: connie.newman@nyulangone.org

Learning Objectives

As a result of participating in this session, learners should be able to:

- Describe the mechanism of action of medications that reduces LDL cholesterol (LDL-C) by targeting proprotein convertase subtilisin/kexin type 9 (PCSK9).

- Explain the indications, dosing, efficacy, and safety of medications that reduce the synthesis or inhibit the action of PCSK9.

- Appropriately prescribe PCSK9 inhibitors and small interfering RNA (siRNA) to reduce LDL-C and manage excess cardiovascular risk.

Main Conclusions

PCSK9 binds to and escorts LDL receptors to the hepatic lysosome, where the receptor is degraded. Pathogenic gain-of-function variants in the *PCSK9* gene are associated with higher LDL-C; loss-of-function variants are associated with low LDL-C and decreased risk of atherosclerotic cardiovascular disease (ASCVD). Medications targeting PCSK9 to lower LDL-C include monoclonal antibodies to PCSK9 (alirocumab, evolocumab) and a novel siRNA (inclisiran).

Alirocumab and evolocumab inhibit binding of PCSK9 to the LDL receptor, thus increasing LDL-receptor recycling, which clears LDL-C. Inclisiran, which is approved in the United Kingdom, Europe, and United States, degrades PCSK9 mRNA, reducing PCSK9 synthesis. Alirocumab and evolocumab are administered subcutaneously once or twice monthly. Inclisiran is administered subcutaneously 3 times the first year and twice annually thereafter. Alirocumab and evolocumab are indicated as adjunct to diet alone or with other lipid-lowering therapies to lower LDL-C in adults with ASCVD or primary hyperlipidemia, including heterozygous familial hypercholesterolemia and homozygous familial hypercholesterolemia, and to reduce risk of myocardial infarction and stroke in adults with ASCVD. Evolocumab is approved for pediatric patients with homozygous familial hypercholesterolemia who are 10 years or younger. Inclisiran has an indication for LDL-C reduction in adults taking statins who have heterozygous familial hypercholesterolemia or clinical ASCVD. Effects of inclisiran on cardiovascular disease are being studied. Available data show that the main adverse effects for the monoclonal antibodies and inclisiran are injection site reactions. A monoclonal antibody or the siRNA, alone or in addition to statin therapy, reduces LDL-C by 50% or more. Very low LDL-C levels have been observed in persons taking alirocumab or evolocumab. The cardiovascular benefit of lowering LDL-C below 25 mg/dL (<0.65 mmol/L) has not been established, although randomized controlled trials show that levels below 15 mg/dL (<0.39 mmol/L) are not harmful.

Medications targeting PCSK9 are useful, with or without other lipid-lowering therapies, for reducing LDL-C in patients with familial hypercholesterolemia or ASCVD. Inclisiran is a novel advanced therapy with the potential (if affordable) to change the treatment paradigm for hypercholesterolemia.

Significance of the Clinical Problem

Elevated LDL-C is the root cause of atherosclerosis, and it increases the risk of ischemic heart disease, which is the number 1 cause of mortality in the United States (Centers for Disease Control report 2019 https://www.cdc.gov/nchs/data/nvsr/nvsr70/nvsr70-08-508.pdf).[1] Globally, ischemic heart disease was the leading cause of death, followed by stroke, in 2019 (World Health Organization https://www.who.int/news-room/fact-sheets/detail/the-top-10-causes-of-death).[2] However, in low-income countries, neonatal conditions were the number 1 cause of death in 2019, followed by lower respiratory infections, ischemic heart disease, and stroke (World Health Organization https://www.who.int/news-room/fact-sheets/detail/the-top-10-causes-of-death).[2]

In numerous randomized controlled trials with a median duration of 4 years, statins have been shown to reduce LDL-C and cardiovascular morbidity and mortality in adults with ASCVD, diabetes mellitus, hypertension, previous stroke, or transient ischemic attack, and kidney disease (except end-stage kidney disease), as well as in persons without ASCVD or any of these disorders.[3,4] Statins do not reduce ASCVD in adults with congestive heart failure or in those on dialysis. When added to statin therapy, nonstatin medications such as ezetimibe (which has data showing ASCVD risk reduction), bile acid sequestrants, and bempedoic acid further lower LDL-C (*Table*). However, patients taking statins or statins plus any of the above nonstatin medications who have an LDL-C concentration above 70 mg/dL (>1.81 mmol/L), or in certain cases above 55 mg/dL (>1.42 mmol/L), may still have excess ASCVD risk.[5] The development of medications targeting PCSK9 has advanced our ability to reduce LDL-C to low levels (25 to 50 mg/dL [0.65 to 1.30 mmol/L]) and potentially further reduce ASCVD (as shown by randomized controlled trials of monoclonal antibodies to PCSK9).

Barriers to Optimal Practice

- Insufficient knowledge of the benefits of PCSK9 inhibitors.
- Cost of medication; lack of coverage by some insurance plans.
- Poor adherence.
- Fear of adverse effects.
- Fear of injections.

Strategies for Diagnosis, Therapy, and/or Management

Management of LDL-C With Medications Targeting PCSK9

This chapter will describe the biology of PCSK9, effects of new medications targeting PCSK9 on lipids, lipoproteins, and ASCVD; safety concerns; and approved indications and dosages in the United States. Medication cost will be covered briefly.

Biology of PCSK9

PCSK9 is a protein that binds to hepatic LDL receptors and inhibits LDL-receptor recycling by escorting the LDL receptor to the hepatic lysosome, where the LDL receptor is degraded.[6,7] Inhibition of the binding of PCSK9 to the LDL receptor, or reduction in PCSK9 synthesis through interference with PCSK9 mRNA, increases the recycling of hepatic LDL receptors, which increases the number of LDL receptors to clear LDL-C, thus reducing LDL-C levels in the circulation.

Genetic variants in the *PCSK9* gene that increase PCSK9 function are associated with heterozygous familial hypercholesterolemia.[8] However, PCSK9 variants are associated with fewer than 1% of cases of familial hypercholesterolemia. About 80% to 90% of persons with familial hypercholesterolemia have loss-of-function variants in the LDL-receptor gene and 5% to 10% have genetic variants in the gene encoding the apolipoprotein B receptor.

Persons with *PCSK9* loss-of-function variants have lifelong low levels of LDL-C and reduced risk of ASCVD.[9] In one study, African American participants with loss-of-function heterozygous *PCSK9* variants had lower LDL-C levels (by 35 mg/dL [0.91 mmol/L]) and the risk of coronary heart disease was reduced by 49%.[10] White participants with loss-of-function heterozygous *PCSK9* variants were found to have reduced LDL-C levels (by 13 mg/dL [0.34 mmol/L]) and an 18% lower risk of coronary heart disease.

Medications targeting PCSK9 approved for use in the United States, Europe, and other countries are monoclonal antibodies to PCSK9 and a novel siRNA:

- Human monoclonal antibodies directed against PCSK9 (evolocumab and alirocumab) inhibit the binding of PCSK9 to the LDL receptor. This increases the recycling of LDL receptors and results in lower plasma LDL-C. The LDL receptor on the surface of the hepatocyte binds to LDL, forming a complex that enters the liver through endocytosis. The LDL receptor is separated from LDL in the lysosome where LDL is broken down into amino acids (from apolipoprotein B), cholesterol, and free fatty acids. Cholesterol may be excreted (in an unesterified form or after conversion into bile acids) via the bile or incorporated into VLDL in the liver.

- A double-stranded siRNA (inclisiran) directs the catalytic breakdown of PCSK9 mRNA, thus reducing the synthesis of PCSK9. Lower levels of PCSK9 in the liver increase the recycling of LDL receptors, which increase LDL uptake into the liver and excretion of cholesterol via the bile, as described previously. Inclisiran is approved for use in the United States, Europe, and other countries. Inclisiran is conjugated on the sense strand with triantennary N-acetylgalactosamine to increase uptake by hepatocytes. After inclisiran doses of 284 mg on day 1 and day 90, mean serum PCSK9 levels have been shown to be reduced by 75% at day 120 and 69% at day 180.[11]

Effect on Lipids and Lipoproteins

In randomized controlled trials, evolocumab and alirocumab alone and in statin-treated adults reduce LDL-C by about 50% to 60%.[12,13]

Several randomized controlled trials comparing inclisiran with placebo have demonstrated that inclisiran given on days 1, 30, 270, and 540 reduced LDL-C by about 50% in patients taking statins. ORION-10 evaluated LDL-C changes in response to inclisiran in 1561 statin-treated patients (31% women) with ASCVD (mean age, 66 years [range, 35-90 years]).[14] Subcutaneous injection of inclisiran 284 mg on days 1, 90, 270, and 540 in 781 participants reduced mean LDL-C by 51%, mean non–HDL-C by 47%, and mean apolipoprotein B by 45%. The *Figure* shows inclisiran's effects on LDL-C compared with placebo in the randomized controlled trial ORION-11.

Effects on ASCVD

Large randomized, placebo-controlled ASCVD outcomes trials of alirocumab (ODYSSEY OUTCOMES)[12] in statin-treated patients with acute coronary syndrome and trials of evolocumab (FOURIER)[13] in statin-treated patients with ASCVD demonstrated a relative risk reduction in ASCVD events of 15% and absolute reduction of 1.6% and 2.0%, respectively, in the PCSK9 inhibitor treatment groups. The median duration of follow-up was 2.8 years in ODYSSEY OUTCOMES and 2.2 years in FOURIER. The mean LDL-C concentrations in ODYSSEY OUTCOMES in an on-treatment analysis were 38 mg/dL (0.98 mmol/L), 42 mg/dL (1.09 mmol/L), and 53 mg/dL (1.37 mmol/L) at 4, 12, and 48 months, respectively. In FOURIER, the mean LDL-C concentration was 30 mg/dL (0.78 mmol/L) at 4 months.

A prespecified analysis of FOURIER found that evolocumab significantly reduced ASCVD risk in participants with and without diabetes, did not increase the risk of new-onset diabetes, and did not worsen glycemia.[15] In addition, a prespecified analysis of ODYSSEY OUTCOMES showed that the absolute reduction in ASCVD events in participants assigned to alirocumab was

2-fold greater in those with diabetes than in those without diabetes, and the risk of new diabetes was not increased.[16]

The effect of inclisiran on cardiovascular events in patients with ASCVD is being studied in ORION-4.

Safety

The main adverse events in patients taking alirocumab and evolocumab are injection site reactions characterized by itching, swelling, and/or erythema. Hypersensitivity reactions such as angioedema are rare. Impaired cognitive function had been suggested in early trials, but was not shown in the EBBINHAUS study,[17] which involved a subgroup analysis of the FOURIER cardiovascular disease outcomes trial.

Statins increase the risk of newly diagnosed diabetes, especially in patients with risk factors for diabetes, by an estimated 0.2% per year depending upon the population.[18] The mechanism is not known. Genetic studies have shown 10% to 29% higher risk of new diabetes in persons with loss-of-function variants in the *PCSK9* gene.[19-21] Nevertheless, new-onset diabetes has not been detected in FOURIER (evolocumab)[15] or ODYSSEY OUTCOMES (alirocumab).[16] However, diabetes was not detected as an adverse event of statins until about 20 years after approval when multiple large trials of a median duration of 4 years were completed.[22] Whether there is an increased risk of diabetes associated with long-term treatment with PCSK-9 inhibitors that begins in adulthood is unknown.[23]

Inclisiran may cause injection site reactions, as shown in the analysis of ORION-9, -10, and -11, which were placebo-controlled trials with a duration of 18 months.[24] While there was a small increase in bronchitis (4.3% inclisiran vs 2.7% placebo), there was no evidence of differences in liver function tests, creatine kinase, or platelet count. More long-term data are needed, and an ongoing cardiovascular disease outcomes trial will provide more information about safety.

Indications

Indications for evolocumab and alirocumab in the United States:

- As adjunct to diet alone or in combination with other LDL-C–lowering therapies in adults with primary hyperlipidemia, including heterozygous familial hypercholesterolemia, to reduce LDL-C. Evolocumab is indicated for patients with heterozygous familial hypercholesterolemia who are 10 years and older.

- As adjunct to other LDL-C–lowering therapies in adults with homozygous familial hypercholesterolemia to reduce LDL-C. Evolocumab is indicated for patients with homozygous familial hypercholesterolemia who are 10 years and older.

- To reduce the risk of myocardial infarction and stroke in adults with established cardiovascular disease. Evolocumab also has an indication for reduction in risk of coronary revascularization in adults with cardiovascular disease; alirocumab also has an indication for reduction in risk of unstable angina requiring hospitalization.

Indication for inclisiran in the United States:

- As adjunct to diet and maximally tolerated statin therapy for the treatment of adults with heterozygous familial hypercholesterolemia or clinical ASCVD who require additional lowering of LDL-C. The effect on cardiovascular morbidity and mortality has not been determined.

Indication for inclisiran in Europe:

- For adults with primary hypercholesterolemia (familial hypercholesterolemia and nonfamilial hypercholesterolemia) or mixed dyslipidemia as adjunct to diet, in combination with a statin alone or a statin with other lipid-lowering therapies. Inclisiran is also indicated alone or in combination with other lipid-lowering therapies for patients who do not tolerate statins or for whom a statin is contraindicated.

Dosages

Alirocumab and evolocumab may be administered subcutaneously every 2 weeks or every month; dosages are shown in the Table. For patients with an inadequate LDL-C response, the dosage of alirocumab may be increased from 75 mg to 150 mg every 2 weeks. Similarly, for patients who do not have an adequate LDL-C response at 12 weeks, the dosage of evolocumab may be increased from 140 mg every 2 weeks to 420 mg every month. For patients with homozygous familial hypercholesterolemia on apheresis, the dosage of evolocumab may be initiated at 420 mg every 2 weeks.

Evolocumab can be administered via a prefilled autoinjector, or prefilled syringe, every 2 weeks, or a single-use body infusor with a prefilled cartridge. Alirocumab is available in prefilled injection pens.

Inclisiran is given as 284 mg subcutaneously in a single prefilled syringe at 3 months and 6 months after the initial dose and subsequently every 6 months.

Estimates of Cost

This information was accessed January 29, 2022, from websites of Regneron, Amgen, Novartis, England's National Health Service, and others.

The annual cost of alirocumab and evolocumab without insurance is about $5800 (reduced from an initial cost of $14,000) in the United States. Insurance companies may require preclearance, which may require the prescriber to document that other lipid-lowering medications have failed. About 75% of Medicare prescriptions for evolocumab cost patients less than $50 a month, and the cost is even lower in patients who are eligible for the low-income subsidy plan. Most patients with Medicaid coverage pay $10 a month, and others pay less than $50 a month. Insurance plans vary in their coverage of evolocumab. Amgen has a no-cost plan (Amgen Safety Net Foundation) for patients who do not have insurance or cannot afford the medicine.

Alirocumab is covered by most Medicare Part D plans with a copay. Regeneron has a $25 copay plan for alirocumab for eligible patients with insurance not funded by a government plan. Regeneron also has a patient assistance program for patients without health or prescription insurance who meet income restrictions. Patients prescribed alirocumab who are covered by Medicare may qualify for the low-income subsidy plan.

In England, the list price for 1 pack of inclisiran, 284 mg, costs close to £2000. A population health agreement between the manufacturer of inclisiran (Novartis) and England's National Health Service and NHS Improvement has been reached. Under this

Table. Nonstatin LDL-C–Lowering Medications

Medication	Mechanism of action	Dosage for LDL-C reduction	Estimated LDL-C reduction
Ezetimibe	Binds to Nieman Pick N1L1 receptor; prevents gastrointestinal absorption of cholesterol	10 mg orally daily	15% to 20%
Alirocumab	Monoclonal antibody to PCSK9; prevents LDL receptor degradation by inhibition of PCSK9	75 mg to 150 mg subcutaneously every 2 weeks or 300 mg every 4 weeks	56% to 61% on top of statin
Evolocumab	Monoclonal antibody to PCSK9; prevents LDL receptor degradation by inhibition of PCSK9	140 mg subcutaneously every 2 weeks or 420 mg subcutaneously every month (or every 2 weeks as needed)	63% to 71% on top of statin
Inclisiran	Small interfering RNA that directs breakdown of mRNA for PCSK9	284 mg subcutaneously initial dose, at 3 months, and then every 6 months	52% on top of statin
Cholestyramine	Bile acid sequestrant; reduces cholesterol pool	8 to 16 g orally daily, divided doses	12% to 25%
Colesevelam	Bile acid sequestrant; reduces cholesterol pool	1250 to 1875 mg orally twice daily	15% to 18%
Bempedoic acid	ATP citrate lyase inhibitor; inhibits cholesterol synthesis	180 mg orally daily	17% on top of statin

Figure. Mean Percentage Change from Baseline in LDL-C in Patients With ASCVD on Maximally Tolerated Statin Therapy, Assigned to Inclisiran or Placebo (ORION-11)

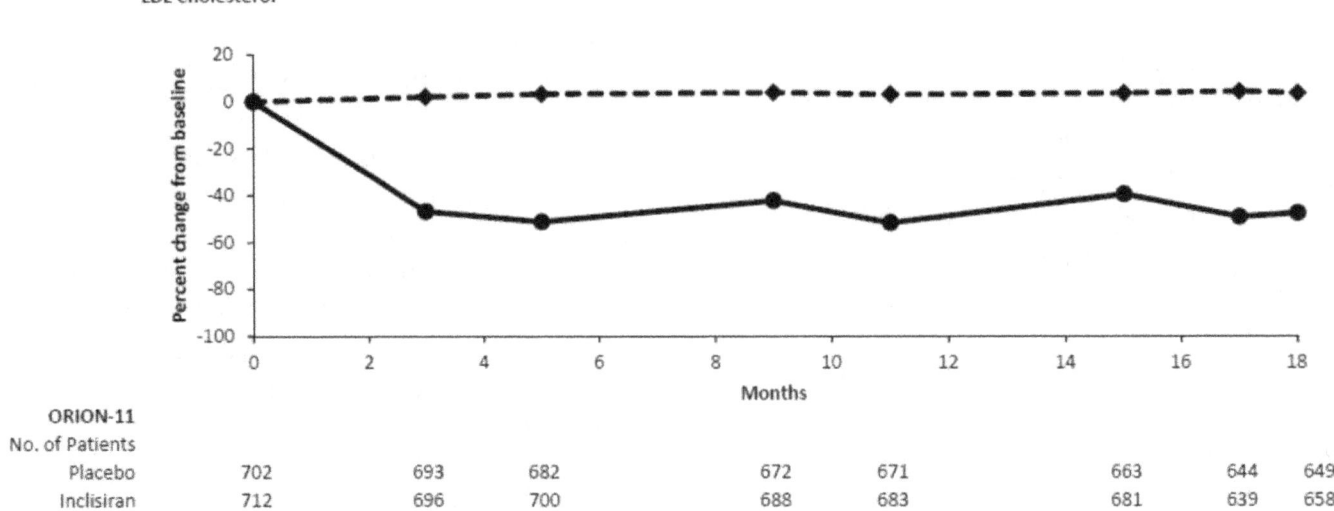

ORION-11
No. of Patients

Placebo	702	693	682		672	671		663	644	649
Inclisiran	712	696	700		688	683		681	639	658

From US Prescribing Information. 2021. Novartis Pharmaceuticals, downloaded from FDA website January 9, 2022.

agreement, inclisiran, 284 mg, may be ordered by primary care in England at the price of £45 per pack.

The price of inclisran in the United States is not known at this time. Inclisiran is expected to cost $3250 per injection or $6500 annually for 2 doses. The first year requires 3 doses and will therefore be more expensive.

Clinical Case Vignettes

Case 1

A 68-year-old man with type 2 diabetes mellitus, hypertension controlled on valsartan, and a history of myocardial infarction describes intermittent pain in his chest accompanied by nausea that is intensified by physical activity. Current medications are atorvastatin, 80 mg daily; ezetimibe, 10 mg daily; valsartan, 80 mg daily; metformin, 2000 mg daily; semaglutide, 7 mg daily; and vitamin D, 2000 IU daily.

Laboratory test results:

Total cholesterol = 160 mg/dL (SI: 4.14 mmol/L)
LDL-C = 75 mg/dL (SI: 1.94 mmol/L)
Triglycerides = 175 mg/dL (SI: 1.98 mmol/L)
HDL-C = 50 mg/dL (SI: 1.30 mmol/L)
Hemoglobin A_{1c} = 7.2% (55 mmol/mol)

Question 1. Which of these options would be appropriate for lipid management in this patient? (may choose more than 1 answer)

A. Add bempedoic acid, 180 mg daily

B. Add evolocumab, 140 mg subcutaneously every 2 weeks

C. Add inclisiran, 284 mg subcutaneously first dose

D. Discontinue atorvastatin and start rosuvastatin, 20 mg daily

E. Recommend no change in medications

Answer: B or C) Add evolocumab, 140 mg subcutaneously every 2 weeks (B), or add inclisiran, 284 mg subcutaneously first dose (C)

This patient has type 2 diabetes and ASCVD. Despite an LDL-C concentration of 75 mg/dL (1.94 mmol/L), he is now having chest pain, most likely due to coronary ischemia. He is taking high-intensity statin therapy and ezetimibe. His symptoms indicate that he would benefit from additional reduction of LDL-C.

The most effective medications to add to statin therapy to further reduce LDL-C (by about 50%) to decrease ASCVD events are PCSK-9 inhibitors (evolocumab or alirocumab) or the siRNA inclisiran. Inclisiran has not been proven to reduce ASCVD; the clinical trial is ongoing.

Question 2. What should this patient's LDL-C target be? Why?

A. <100 mg/dL (SI: <2.59 mmol/L)

B. <70 mg/dL (SI: <1.81 mmol/L)

C. <55 mg/dL (SI: <1.42 mmol/L)

D. <40 mg/dL (SI: <1.04 mmol/L)

Answer: C) <55 mg/dL (<1.42 mmol/L)

This patient has a history of myocardial infarction, as well as multiple risk factors for ASCVD, and is now having chest pain, suggesting that LDL-C should be reduced further. The American Heart Association/American College of Cardiology guidelines from 2018 suggest that treatment of patients with ASCVD should aim to reduce LDL-C by 50%. Although goals are not specified, it is stated that patients with ASCVD and an LDL-C concentration greater than 70 mg/dL (>1.81 mmol/L) would benefit from LDL-C reduction with a statin and, if needed, by the addition of nonstatin medications. The European Society of Cardiology/European Atherosclerosis Society 2019 cholesterol management guidelines specify an LDL-C goal of less than 55 mg/dL (<1.42 mmol/L) (Answer C) for patients with ASCVD.

Case 2

A 30-year-old woman presents for evaluation and management of high cholesterol. Hypercholesterolemia was diagnosed 10 years ago. At that time, she had tendon xanthomas and the following laboratory test results:

> Total cholesterol = 290 mg/dL (SI: 7.51 mmol/L)
> LDL-C = 220 mg/dL (SI: 5.70 mmol/L)
> HDL-C = 50 mg/dL (SI: 1.30 mmol/L)
> Triglycerides = 100 mg/dL (SI: 1.13 mmol/L)

Current medications are atorvastatin, 80 mg daily; ezetimibe, 10 mg daily; and vitamin D, 2000 IU daily.

Her maternal grandfather, now deceased, had a myocardial infarction at age 45 years. Her 65-year-old mother has a history of very high cholesterol

and is taking rosuvastatin, 10 mg daily; ezetimibe, 10 mg daily; and colesevelam, 3 tablets (625 mg each) twice daily.

On physical examination, her blood pressure is 115/80 mm Hg and pulse rate is 68 beats/min. BMI is 23 kg/m², and waist circumference is 29 in (73.7 cm). There are xanthelasmas in both eyes. She has dry skin and no rash or tendinous xanthomas. Examination findings are otherwise normal.

Current lipid panel results:

> Total cholesterol = 160 mg/dL (SI: 4.14 mmol/L)
> LDL-C = 90 mg/dL (SI: 2.33 mmol/L)
> HDL-C = 50 mg/dL (SI: 1.30 mmol/L)
> Triglycerides = 100 mg/dL (SI: 1.13 mmol/L)

Other laboratory test results:

> Hemoglobin A_{1c} = 4.9% (4.0%-5.6%) (30 mmol/mol [20-38 mmol/mol])
> Creatinine = 1.0 mg/dL (0.6-1.1 mg/dL) (SI: 88.4 μmol/L [53.0-97.2 μmol/L])
> Liver function, normal

Question 1. What is the most likely diagnosis?

A. Familial combined hyperlipidemia

B. Heterozygous familial hypercholesterolemia

C. Homozygous familial hypercholesterolemia

D. Polygenic hypercholesterolemia

E. Type III hyperlipidemia

Answer: B) Heterozygous familial hypercholesterolemia

This patient has heterozygous familial hypercholesterolemia (Answer B), as demonstrated by an elevated LDL-C concentration in a young adult, normal HDL-C and triglyceride levels, the presence of tendon xanthomas at diagnosis, and family history of premature ASCVD in a second-degree relative. In addition, the patient's mother has a history of very high cholesterol and is being treated with multiple medications.

The patient has not undergone genetic testing.

Homozygous familial hypercholesterolemia (Answer C) is rare, and if untreated, affected persons develop ASCVD early and may have a myocardial infarction in their teen years.

Familial combined hyperlipidemia (Answer A) is characterized by elevations in LDL-C and triglycerides.

Polygenic hypercholesterolemia (Answer D) is the most common type of hypercholesterolemia and shares some features of heterozygous familial hypercholesterolemia. Cholesterol levels may be as high as those seen in this patient but are usually lower. Triglycerides are normal. Tendon xanthomas and xanthelasmas may be present. However, the history of premature coronary heart disease and young age at presentation suggest that this patient's diagnosis is heterozygous familial hypercholesterolemia.

Type III hyperlipidemia (Answer E), also known as dysbetalipoproteinemia, is characterized by elevations in total cholesterol, triglycerides, and LDL-C and low HDL-C concentrations.

Question 2. What is the next step for cholesterol management?

A. Add alirocumab or evolocumab

B. Add bempedoic acid

C. Discontinue ezetimibe and add a PCSK9 inhibitor

D. Switch atorvastatin, 80 mg daily, to rosuvastatin, 10 mg daily

Answer: A) Add alirocumab or evolocumab

This patient has a lifelong history of elevated LDL-C because of heterozygous familial hypercholesterolemia, and therefore LDL-C should be further reduced to below 70 mg/dL (<1.81 mmol/L). Alirocumab and evolocumab (Answer A) are monoclonal antibodies to PCSK9 and would be anticipated to reduce the LDL-C concentration from 90 mg/dL (2.33 mmol/L) to 45 to 50 mg/dL (1.17 to 1.30 mmol/L).

Ezetimibe may be continued; it reduces LDL-C by 18% to 20% and reduces the risk of ASCVD (thus, Answer C is incorrect).

Bempedoic acid (Answer B) reduces LDL-C by 17%, but its effect on cardiovascular morbidity and mortality is not known. This patient needs high-intensity statin therapy (eg, atorvastatin, 40 or 80 mg daily, or rosuvastatin, 20 mg daily), which lowers LDL-C by 50% or more. Rosuvastatin, 10 mg daily (Answer D), is a moderate-intensity statin.

Question 3. One year later, the patient's LDL-C concentration is 20 mg/dL (0.52 mmol/L) (on 2 measurements). What is the next step?

A. Continue all medications at the current dosages

B. Discontinue ezetimibe

C. Lower the dosage of atorvastatin

D. Lower the dosage of the PCSK9 inhibitor

E. Stop the PCSK9 inhibitor

Answer: A) Continue all medications at the current dosages

Clinical trials show that very low LDL-C levels (≤15 mg/dL [≤0.39 mmol/L]) are not harmful, although evidence for a benefit regarding ASCVD has not been established.[25] Prespecified analysis of ODYSSEY OUTCOMES found that in patients with ASCVD, risk did not differ in participants with LDL-C concentrations below 25 mg/dL (<0.65 mmol/L) or participants with concentrations of 25 to 50 mg/dL (0.65 to 1.30 mmol/L).[26] In ODYSSEY Outcomes, LDL-C fell below 15 mg/dL (<0.39 mmol/L) on 2 occasions in 730 patients who had been treated for a median of 6.8 months, and these patients were blindly switched from alirocumab to placebo as per the protocol.[12] However, there was no evidence that these low levels caused harm. There was no increased incidence of diabetes or neurocognitive disorders in patients treated with alirocumab. None of these participants developed hemorrhagic stroke. In the FOURIER study, 1335 patients assigned to evolocumab had LDL-C concentrations on treatment less than 15 mg/dL (<0.39 mmol/L), and 504 patients had concentrations below 10 mg/dL (<0.26 mmol/L).[27] There was no evidence that such low levels of LDL-C were unsafe. Thus, this patient should continue all medications at the current dosages (Answer A).

References

1. Xu J, Murphy SL, Kochanek KD, Arias E. Deaths: final Data for 2019. National Vital Statistics Reports. Vol 70(8). National Center for Health Statistics. 2021. DOI: https://dx.doi.org/10.15620/cdc:106058

2. World Health Organization. The top 10 causes of death. Available at: https://www.who.int/news-room/fact-sheets/detail/the-top-10-causes-of-death.

3. Cholesterol Treatment Trialists' (CTT) Collaboration, Baignet C, Blackwell L, et al. Efficacy and safety of more intensive lowering of LDL cholesterol: a meta-analysis of data from 170,000 participants in 26 randomised trials. *Lancet*. 2010;376(9753):1670-1681. PMID: 21067804

4. Collins R, Reith C, Emberson J, et al. Interpretation of the evidence for the efficacy and safety of statin therapy. *Lancet*. 2016;388(10059):2532-2561. PMID: 27616593

5. Authors/Task Force M, ESC Committee for Practice Guidelines (CPG); ESC National Cardiac Societies. 2019 ESC/EAS guidelines for the management of dyslipidaemias: lipid modification to reduce cardiovascular risk. *Atherosclerosis*. 2019;290:140-205. PMID: 31591002

*6. Horton JD, Cohen JC, Hobbs HH. PCSK9: a convertase that coordinates LDL catabolism. *J Lipid Res*. 2009;50(Suppl):S172-S177. PMID: 19020338

*7. Rosenson RS, Hegele RA, Fazio S, Cannon CP. The evolving future of PCSK9 inhibitors. *J Am Coll Cardiol*. 2018;72(3):314-329. PMID: 30012326

*8. Gidding SS, Champagne MA, de Ferranti SD, et al; American Heart Association Atherosclerosis, Hypertension, and Obesity in Young Committee of Council on Cardiovascular Disease in Young, Council on Cardiovascular and Stroke Nursing, Council on Functional Genomics and Translational Biology, and Council of Lifestyle and Cardiometabolic Health. The agenda for familial hypercholesterolemia: a scientific statement from the American Heart Association. *Circulation*. 2015;132(22):2167-2192. PMID: 26510694

9. Cohen JC, Boerwinkle E, Mosley TH Jr, Hobbs HH. Sequence variations in PCSK9, low LDL, and protection against coronary heart disease. *N Engl J Med*. 2006;354(12):1264-1272. PMID: 16554528

10. Kent ST, Rosenson RS, Avery CL, et al. PCSK9 loss-of-function variants, low-density lipoprotein cholesterol, and risk of coronary heart disease and stroke: data from 9 studies of Blacks and Whites. *Circ Cardiovasc Genet*. 2017;10(4):e001632. PMID: 28768753

*11. Leqvio (inclisiran) injection. Prescribing information. Novartis Pharmaceuticals, 2021. Accessed January 9, 2022. https://www.novartis.us/sites/www.novartis.us/files/leqvio.pdf

12. Schwartz GG, Steg PG, Szarek M, et al; ODYSSEY OUTCOMES Committees and Investigators. Alirocumab and cardiovascular outcomes after acute coronary syndrome. *N Engl J Med*. 2018;379(22):2097-2107. PMID: 30403574

13. Sabatine MS, Giugliano RP, Keech AC, et al; FOURIER Steering Committee and Investigators. Evolocumab and clinical outcomes in patients with cardiovascular disease. *N Engl J Med*. 2017;376(18):1713-1722. PMID: 28304224

14. Ray KK, Wright RS, Kallend D, et al; ORION-10 and ORION-11 Investigators. Two phase 3 trials of inclisiran in patients with elevated LDL cholesterol. *N Engl J Med*. 2020;382(16):1507-1519. PMID: 32187462

15. Sabatine MS, Leiter LA, Wiviott SD, et al. Cardiovascular safety and efficacy of the PCSK9 inhibitor evolocumab in patients with and without diabetes and the effect of evolocumab on glycaemia and risk of new-onset diabetes: a prespecified analysis of the FOURIER randomised controlled trial. *Lancet Diabetes Endocrinol*. 2017;5(12):941-950. PMID: 28927706

16. Ray KK, Colhoun HM, Szarek M, et al; ODYSSEY OUTCOMES Committees and Investigators. Effects of alirocumab on cardiovascular and metabolic outcomes after acute coronary syndrome in patients with or without diabetes: a prespecified analysis of the ODYSSEY OUTCOMES randomised controlled trial. *Lancet Diabetes Endocrinol*. 2019;7(8):618-628. PMID: 31272931

17. Giugliano RP, Mach F, Zavitz K, et al. Cognitive function in a randomized trial of evolocumab. *N Engl J Med*. 2017;377(7):633-643. PMID: 28813214

*18. Newman CB, Preiss D, Tobert JA, et al; American Heart Association Clinical Lipidology, Lipoprotein, Metabolism and Thrombosis Committee, a Joint Committee of the Council on Atherosclerosis, Thrombosis and Vascular Biology and Council on Lifestyle and Cardiometabolic Health; Council on Cardiovascular Disease in the Young; Council on Clinical Cardiology; and Stroke Council. Statin safety and associated adverse events: a scientific statement from the American Heart Association. *Arterioscler Thromb Vasc Biol*. 2018;39(2):e38-e81. PMID: 30580575

19. Ference BA, Robinson JG, Brook RD, et al. Variation in PCSK9 and HMGCR and risk of cardiovascular disease and diabetes. *N Engl J Med*. 2016;375(22):2144-2153. PMID: 27959767

20. Lotta LA, Sharp SJ, Burgess S, et al. Association between low-density lipoprotein cholesterol-lowering genetic variants and risk of type 2 diabetes: a meta-analysis. *JAMA*. 2016;316(13):1383-1391. PMID: 27701660

21. Schmidt AF, Swerdlow DI, Holmes MV, et al. PCSK9 genetic variants and risk of type 2 diabetes: a mendelian randomisation study. *Lancet Diabetes Endocrinol*. 2017;5(2):97-105. PMID: 27908689

22. Newman CB. Safety of statins and non-statins for treatment of dyslipidemia in update in the diagnosis and management of dyslipidemia. *Endocrinol Metab Clin North Am*. In press.

23. Lee J, Hegele RA. PCSK9 inhibition and diabetes: turning to Mendel for clues. *Lancet Diabetes Endocrinol*. 2017;5(2):78-79. PMID: 27939390

24. Wright RS, Ray KK, Raal FJ, et al; ORION Phase III Investigators. Pooled patient-level analysis of inclisiran trials in patients with familial hypercholesterolemia or atherosclerosis. *J Am Coll Cardiol*. 2021;77(9):1182-1193. PMID: 33663735

*25. Tobert J. LDL cholesterol: how low can we go? in update in the diagnosis and management of dyslipidemia. *Endocrinol Metab Clin North Am*. In press.

*26. Schwartz GG, Steg PG, Bhatt DL, et al; ODYSSEY OUTCOMES Committees and Investigators. Clinical efficacy and safety of alirocumab after acute coronary syndrome according to achieved level of low-density lipoprotein cholesterol: a propensity score-matched analysis of the ODYSSEY OUTCOMES Trial. *Circulation*. 2021;143(11):1109-1122. PMID: 33438437

27. Giugliano RP, Pedersen TR, Park J-G, et al; FOURIER Investigators. Clinical efficacy and safety of achieving very low LDL-cholesterol concentrations with the PCSK9 inhibitor evolocumab: a prespecified secondary analysis of the FOURIER trial. *Lancet*. 2017;390(10106):1962-1971. PMID: 28859947

* Suggested reading

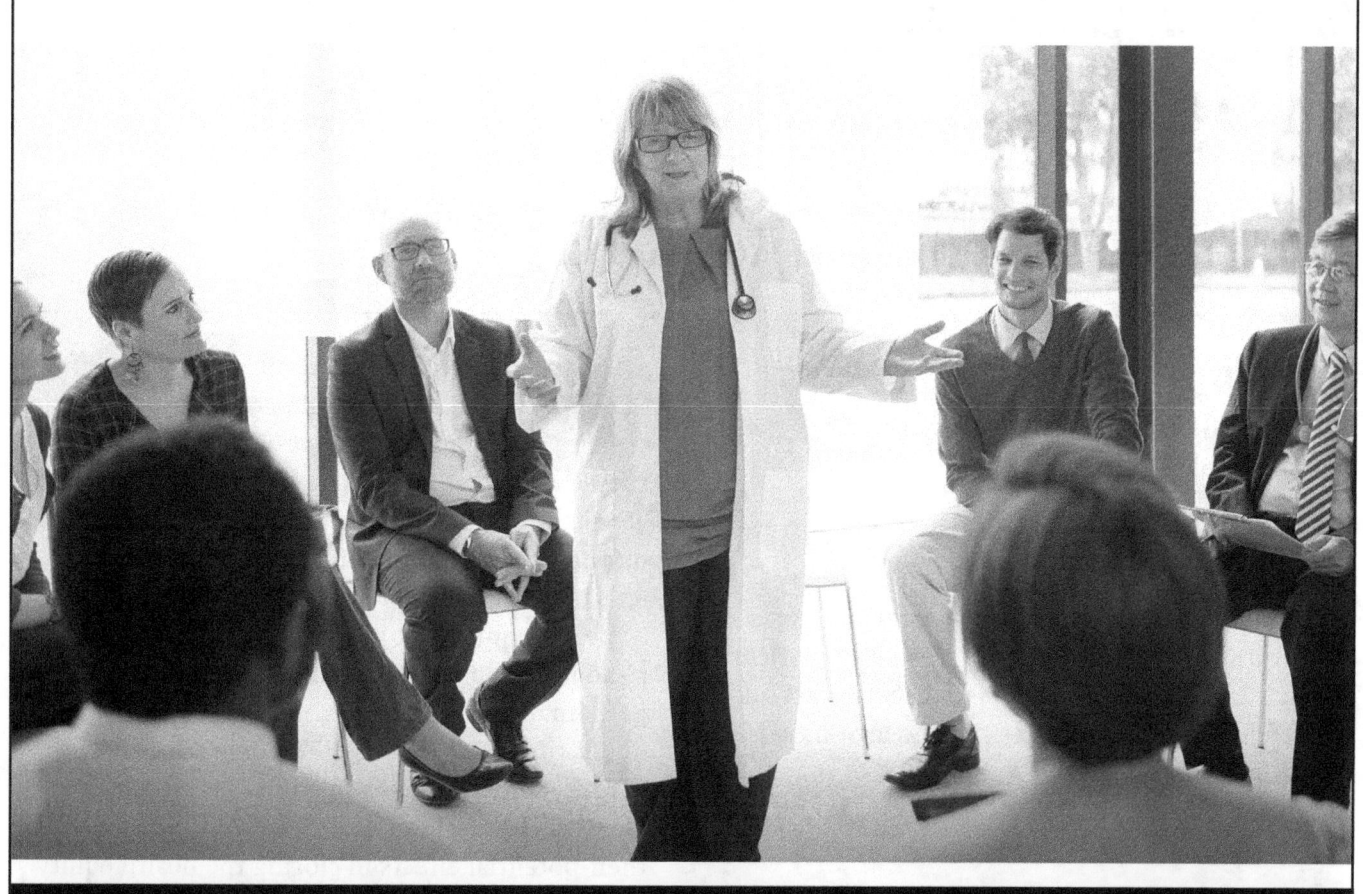

DIABETES MELLITUS AND GLUCOSE METABOLISM

Disparities in Diabetes Care and Evidence-Based Programs to Address Them

Rocio I. Pereira, MD. Division of Endocrinology, Denver Health, Denver, CO, and University of Colorado School of Medicine, Aurora, CO; E-mail: rocio.pereira@dhha.org

Learning Objectives

As a result of participating in this session, learners should be able to:

- Summarize the nature and extent of disparities in diabetes and diabetes care.

- Apply knowledge of social determinants of health (SDoH) and health equity best practices to identify patient barriers to diabetes care and refer patients to appropriate evidence-based programs.

Main Conclusions

Diabetes mellitus and its complications disproportionately affect racial and ethnic minority communities in the United States. Persons of color, including those from Black, Latino, Asian, and Native American populations, have a higher prevalence of diabetes, diabetes complications, and diabetes mortality, than those from nonLatino White populations. These disparities are not explained by biological or behavioral differences across populations, but rather are a result of SDoH and unequal treatment in the health care system due to longstanding systemic racism in our society.

Persons of color with diabetes, regardless of diabetes type, are more likely to face social barriers to obtaining health care such as food and housing insecurity, low or no access to health services, high costs of medications and diabetes technology, and provider inertia. Although many of these factors are beyond our control as clinicians, by identifying SDoH factors in our clinical practices and referring patients to evidence-based programs to address these factors, we can improve the care of racial/ethnic minority patients, thereby decreasing disparities. A solid understanding of the health effects of social factors and a working knowledge of health equity best practices will enable us to address and/or compensate for factors that perpetuate disparities.

In this session, we will become familiar with SDoH, identify the health equity best practice elements in successful interventions, and examine their potential effects in closing the health equity gap in diabetes care.

Significance of the Clinical Problem

In 2019, there were more than 460 million persons with diabetes worldwide and more than 34 million in the United States.[1] In 2017, diabetes care costs in the United States totaled $327 billion and accounted for $1 of every $4 spent on health care. Racial and ethnic minority communities in the United States have disproportionately higher rates of diabetes than nonLatino White communities.[1] Minority communities also experience higher rates of diabetes complications and higher mortality. Compared with rates of end-stage kidney disease for nonLatino white adults, rates are 1.5 times as high for Latino adults and 3 times as high for Black adults.[1] Diabetes mortality in major cities in the United States are on average twice as high for Black adults as they are for White adults.[2] Between 2013 and 2017, there were more than 7000 excess deaths among Black individuals per year due to racial inequalities in diabetes death in major US cities.[2]

Racial/ethnic disparities in diabetes, as with other health conditions, are primarily a result of social factors and SDoH, which disproportionately affect persons of color due to historic and persistent systemic racism. Persons who experience lower education access and quality, economic instability, unhealthy social and community interactions, poor neighborhoods and unhealthy built environments, and lower access to and quality of health care, also are more likely to have diabetes, higher hemoglobin A_{1c}, more frequent diabetic ketoacidosis, higher rates of diabetes complications, and higher diabetes mortality.[3] Furthermore, unequal care experienced by minority communities further increases disparities. Endocrinologists and primary care providers can start to close care disparity gaps by identifying patient-specific SDoH that adversely affect diabetes care and by referring patients to evidence-based diabetes programs. However, most clinical providers, including endocrinologists, do not have the knowledge and skills to appropriately identify and address SDoH, or sufficient familiarity with health equity best practices to incorporate these into their routine workflows.

Barriers to Optimal Practice

Clinicians caring for patients with diabetes from ethnic/racial minority groups face the following potential barriers to diabetes management:

- *Patient-level barriers:* patient social factors that affect diet, physical activity, and self-management behaviors.

- *Provider-level barriers:* clinical inertia, lack of cultural competence, and communication barriers (including language).

- *System-level barriers:* reactive instead of proactive system.

Strategies for Diagnosis, Therapy, and/or Management

The case management strategies reviewed here include assessment of SDoH factors that present barriers to diabetes self-management, referral of patients to appropriate evidence-based programs and services, and adoption of provider-specific tools and system-level interventions to improve care for individuals from racial/ethnic minority groups.

Recognition of SDoH factors that present barriers to diabetes self-management is the first step. Once these factors are recognized, the clinician can more appropriately work to address or compensate for them.

Barriers to optimal diabetes care occur at 3 different levels: patient, provider, and health system.[4] When identifying interventions to reduce diabetes care disparities within a specific medical practice, clinic, or health care organization, it is important to consider interventions at each of these levels. Health care interventions focused at any of these levels have been shown to reduce racial/ethnic disparities in diabetes outcomes.[5]

Screening for and Addressing SDoH

SDoH have typically been considered at a population and community level, but recent efforts in Canada and the United States are aimed at identifying and addressing SDoH factors in clinical settings. The Protocol for Responding to and Addressing Patient's Assets, Risks, and Experiences (PRAPARE) toolkit[6] authored by the National Association of Community Health Centers provides guidance on incorporating SDoH screening into clinical care in community health center settings. The PRAPARE patient survey collects race, ethnicity, and language (REAL) data, and assesses for food and housing insecurity, poverty, and immigrant status, among other factors. A recent review by Frier et al[7] describes emerging strategies to identify social determinant–related barriers to diabetes self-management in clinical settings. The authors note the importance of using an individualized approach and bringing relevance to the screening by considering an individual's personal circumstances and whether they perceive the SDoH issue to be a barrier to diabetes self-management. Addressing SDoH factors that present barriers to diabetes self-management can lead to improved diabetes care. This is especially relevant for minority communities that are disproportionately affected by SDoH factors.

The most important consideration when discussing SDoH with a patient is to do so in a supportive and nonjudgmental manner. Ideally, this discussion should take place after the clinician and patient have established a trusting relationship. In a clinical practice where SDoH data are available at the time of the clinical visit, clinicians should review these data and ask the patient whether the SDoH factors they are experiencing present barriers to their diabetes care. An example of this in a patient who reports having food insecurity is to ask: "Does not having enough food at home affect your diabetes management?" If yes, "In what way?" and "Do you ever skip meals?" or "What types of foods do you eat when you are running out of food at home?" Follow-up questions could tie in medication-taking behavior: "When you skip a meal, do you still inject meal-time insulin? What about long-acting insulin?" In a clinical practice where SDoH information is not available at the time of the visit, the clinician can focus SDoH questions based on the clinical situation. For instance, for a patient who is not taking prescribed medications regularly, the clinician could ask "Does the cost of your medication make it difficult for you to get it from the pharmacy regularly?" Or, in the case of a patient who reports taking their medications differently from what is prescribed, the clinician might ask: "Are you able to read the medication instructions on your medication bottles?" For a patient who has not come to clinic in the recommended amount of time, the clinician might ask "Is it difficult for you to get transportation for your clinic visits?" or "Does the cost of your visit make it difficult for you to come see me more frequently?"

Patient Interventions

Patient-level interventions to decrease disparities in diabetes care focus on supporting healthy diet and exercise habits, increasing diabetes self-management knowledge, and addressing social health barriers. Patient-level interventions can be general quality improvement initiatives or can be culturally tailored to specific racial/ethnic populations. These interventions can take place within or outside the health care system and can be implemented with in-person and/or virtual strategies.

Diabetes Self-Management Education and Support

Patient education and support services should follow national standards such as the 2022 National Standards for Diabetes Self-Management Education and Support (DSMES)[8] published by the American Diabetes Association and Association of Diabetes Care & Education Specialists.

The 2022 National Standards outline 6 evidence-based requirements for successful DSMES efforts:

1. *Support for DSMES services:* leadership support.

2. *Population and service assessment:* alignment of the intervention with the target population's needs and preferences.

3. *DSMES team:* a designated team including at least 1 DSMES quality coordinator to oversee effective implementation, evaluation, tracking, and reporting of DSMES service outcomes.

4. *Delivery and design of DSMES services:* use of a curriculum to guide evidence-based content and delivery, ensure consistency, and serve as a resource for the team; DSMES curriculum must include the following core content:

   - Pathophysiology of diabetes and treatment options

   - Healthy coping

   - Healthy eating

   - Being active

- Taking medication
- Monitoring
- Reducing risk (treating acute and chronic complications)
- Problem-solving and behavior change strategies

5. ***Person-centered DSMES:*** services should be provided over the patient's lifespan, and each patient's DSMES plan should be unique and based on the patient's concerns, needs, and priorities.

6. ***Measuring and demonstrating outcomes of DSMES services:*** ongoing continuous quality improvement strategies will measure the effect of DSMES services, and systematic evaluation of process and outcome data will be used to identify areas for improvement and to guide service optimization.

DSMES teams working in collaboration with primary care have been shown to be the most effective approach to overcoming therapeutic inertia. DSMES lowers hemoglobin A_{1c} by at least 0.6%, which is equivalent to the effect of many diabetes medications, but with no adverse effects.

Telehealth Interventions

The increased use of telehealth interventions during the COVID-19 pandemic has led to concerns for worsening health disparities for communities of color with low access to technology. A recent pooled analysis of telehealth interventions focused on improved diabetes control among Black and Latino adults with diabetes found that patient-level telehealth interventions are generally effective for these minority groups, with a mean reduction in hemoglobin A_{1c} of 0.476%.[9] Interventions in this analysis were delivered via telephone, text messaging, web-based portals, and/or virtual visits; were conducted over an average period of 9 months; and varied in intensity of contact from daily, weekly, to monthly.

Although telehealth interventions have proven benefit for minority and nonminority populations, uptake of this intervention is lower among racial/ethnic minorities. Telemedicine use has been reported to be lower for patients older than 65 years, for those who speak a language other than English, and for patients on public health insurance. The most common barriers to telemedicine service use reported were perceived lower quality of care and technological barriers.

Elements of Successful Patient-Level Interventions

Patient-level interventions that are effective in decreasing diabetes disparities use interpersonal skill and social networks such as family members, peer-support groups, interactive or one-on-one education, and community health workers.[5] Interventions that make use of community health workers are particularly effective since they are able to address multiple SDoH factors, including cultural and language barriers, lack of transportation, and trust issues. Culturally tailored interventions appear to be more effective among racial/ethnic minorities than generalized diabetes self-management training interventions.[5] However, these data are mostly limited to Black and Latino communities, since few interventions have been tested in Alaskan Native/American Indian populations. Expansion is also needed for older racial/ethnic minorities who remain understudied despite representing the fastest growing population of persons with diabetes.

Provider Interventions

Provider-level interventions are focused on decreasing clinical inertia, defined as a lack of medication intensification when intensification is clinically indicated. These interventions can include use of provider reminder systems and tools to increase use of provider guidelines such as the *Standards of Medical Care in Diabetes-2022*[10,11] authored by the American Diabetes Association, continuing medical education, computerized decision-support reminders, in-person feedback, or problem-based learning.

In-person feedback to providers has been reported to be superior to computerized decision-support in creating sustained provider behavioral change and health outcomes. Relevant to racial/ethnic minorities, who are more likely to be managed by a primary care provider rather than an endocrinologist, and more likely to have worse diabetes control than that of White individuals, primary care provider interventions resulted in hemoglobin A_{1c} control similar to that seen in a diabetes specialty clinic. Patients with higher hemoglobin A_{1c} values at baseline had the greatest reduction in hemoglobin A_{1c}.[5]

There are insufficient data on the effectiveness of provider interventions focused on provider communication, cultural competence, or shared decision-making, despite positive correlations between enhanced communication and shared decision-making and diabetes control. Similarly, there is a growing awareness of the associations between provider bias and health disparities, but there are insufficient data to conclude that programs to decrease provider bias improve care for minority populations.

Health System Interventions

Health system interventions include innovative use of health care staff (case managers, community health workers, or nonphysician clinicians) to provide improved patient services. Other interventions include use of medical assistance programs to increase patient access to newer medications and disease management systems (which identify the populations of interest; have guidelines for performance standards for care; conduct nurse care management of identified individuals, and use a health information system for tracking and monitoring).

Case management, particularly when community health workers are used for this purpose, is particularly effective in improving care for minority individuals. Community health workers can be effective in helping patients make/keep appointments with primary care providers and subspecialists, acting as an adjunct to the primary care team, and working as a nurse in case management. Nonphysician providers can be instrumental in extending the care that specialists are able to provide.

Medical assistance programs improve prescription adherence and clinical outcomes, decrease hospitalizations, and reduce hospital costs.

Health care services for persons with limited English proficiency can be improved by providing language translation and interpretation services, increasing the number of language-concordant providers on staff, and/or making medical language courses available to existing staff. Language-concordant services often, although not always, result in better clinical outcomes for patients with limited English proficiency.[12]

Clinical Case Vignettes

Case 1

A 21-year-old Black man with type 1 diabetes is seen in an endocrinology clinic for follow-up. Diabetes was diagnosed 2 years ago, and he first met you in clinic 1 year ago. He has rescheduled multiple prior visits and tells you today that he is almost out of his insulin and supplies. He requests refills for all his medications. He is on basal and bolus insulin pens but would like a more affordable alternative. He states he has no hypoglycemia, but he admits that he has not been checking his blood glucose more than once or twice weekly.

Which of the following is the best course of action for this patient's diabetes management?

A. Change insulin pens to vials and syringes and schedule a follow-up visit next month

B. Change insulin pens to NPH and regular insulin and schedule a follow-up visit next month

C. Discuss his concerns regarding his current insulin pens and order a continuous glucose monitor

D. Discuss his concerns regarding his current insulin pens and identify the barriers to attending clinic visits; develop a plan of care based on those discussions

Answer: D) Discuss his concerns regarding his current insulin pens and identify the barriers to attending clinic visits; develop a plan of care based on those discussions

The best approach is to discuss this patient's concerns regarding his current insulin pens and identify the barriers to attending clinic visits (Answer D). A plan of care can be developed based on this discussion.

Changing from insulin pens to vials and syringes (Answer A) could potentially decrease his medication costs. However, we currently do not have enough information to know if he is able to afford analogue insulins in a vial. This answer also does not address the patient's barriers to keeping clinic appointments.

Changing insulin pens to NPH and regular insulin (Answer B) potentially addresses the cost issue. However, NPH insulin does have an increased risk of hypoglycemia compared with insulin analogues, so it would be best to verify that this is the best possible choice for the patient at this time. This answer also does not address barriers to making it to clinic. Use of continuous glucose monitoring (Answer C) could make glucose monitoring easier for the patient and allow for the collection of more glucose data to inform insulin dose changes. However, it is unclear whether the patient would be able to afford a continuous glucose monitor, and this should be discussed. This answer also does not address the problem with attending clinic visits.

Upon further discussion with the patient and some research of his medication formulary, it became clear that alternative insulin analogues were covered. His prescriptions were changed to alternative analogue pens. Further conversation also reveals that the patient must ask for a day off from work every time he comes to clinic. After some discussion, it was decided that the patient would see a physician every 6 months, but he would see the endocrinology nurse practitioner in between these visits, as the nurse practitioner's schedule was more flexible and aligned with his days off.

Case 2

A 50-year-old Hispanic, Spanish-speaking woman is referred for management of type 2 diabetes. You do not speak Spanish but are able to conduct the visit with the assistance of a phone interpreter. The patient has had diabetes for more than 20 years. Her blood glucose used to be well controlled, but for the past 6 months, her values have been high (in the range of 200 to 400 mg/dL [11.1-22.2 mmol/L]). She has had no changes in her diet or exercise habits. She reports taking her medications as prescribed, and these include metformin, a weekly GLP-1 receptor agonist, and an SGLT-2 inhibitor. Her hemoglobin A_{1c} value last month was 11.0% (97 mmol/mol). Review of her medications reveals that she is not taking her medications as prescribed. When you review possible SDoH barriers with her, you learn that she only completed grade school and does not read very well. You also learn that she does not drive and relies on public transportation to get to the clinic. The ride today took her 1 hour.

Which of the following is the best course of action in this patient's care?

A. Encourage her to increase her current medications to the prescribed amounts and to start insulin

B. Encourage her to start insulin and transfer her care to a Spanish-speaking colleague

C. Refer her to a community health worker–directed DSMES program

D. Review the prescribed dosages of her medications and encourage her to start taking them appropriately

Answer: C) Refer her to a community health worker–directed DSMES program

The best strategy is to refer this patient to a community health worker–directed DSMES program (Answer C). She has multiple social barriers making it difficult to access care, including low health literacy, language barriers, and transportation barriers. These barriers can be addressed by a community health worker who can help the patient compare her list of prescribed medications with the medications she is taking, instruct her on dosages, and answer nonclinical questions.

Transferring her care to a Spanish-speaking colleague (Answer B) could help, but it may not be necessary, and will not address the barriers of low literacy and transportation needs. Language concordance between physicians and patients can improve care when it results in better communication and a more trusting relationship.

Reviewing her prescribed medications and encouraging her to take them as prescribed (Answer D) is unlikely going to improve her care if her health literacy and transportation barriers are not addressed.

Encouraging the patient to increase her current medications to the prescribed amounts and to start insulin (Answer A) is also unlikely to work if SDoH are not addressed first.

References

1. Centers for Disease Control and Prevention. National Diabetes Statistics Report. Available at: https://www.cdc.gov/diabetes/data/statistics-report/index.html. Accessed May 2022.

2. Rosenstock S, Whitman S, West JF, Balkin M. Racial disparities in diabetes mortality in the 50 most populous US cities. *J Urban Health.* 2014;91(5):873-885. PMID: 24532483

3. Hill-Briggs F, Adler NE, Berkowitz SA, et al. Social determinants of health and diabetes: a scientific review. *Diabetes Care.* 2020;44(1):258-279. PMID: 33139407

4. Chin MH, Walters AE, Cook SC, Huang ES. Interventions to reduce racial and ethnic disparities in health care. *Med Care Res Rev.* 2007;64(5 Suppl):7S-28S. PMID: 17881624

5. Peek ME, Cargill A, Huang ES. Diabetes health disparities: a systematic review of health care interventions. *Med Care Res Rev.* 2007;64(5 Suppl):101S-156S. PMID: 17881626

6. National Association of Community Health Centers and Association of Asian Pacific Community Health Organizations. PRAPARE Toolkit. Available at: https://prapare.org/. Accessed May 2022.

7. Frier A, Devine S, Barnett F, Dunning T. Utilising clinical settings to identify and respond to the social determinants of health of individuals with type 2 diabetes-a review of the literature. *Health Soc Care Community.* 2020;28(4):1119-1133. PMID: 31852028

8. Davis J, Fischl AH, Beck J, et al. 2022 National Standards for Diabetes Self-Management Education and Support. *Sci Diabetes Self Manag Care.* 2022;48(1):44-59. PMID: 35049403

9. Anderson A, O'Connell SS, Thomas C, Chimmanamada R. Telehealth interventions to improve diabetes management among black and hispanic patients: a systematic review and meta-analysis. *J Racial Ethn Health Disparities.* 2022:1-12. PMID: 35000144

10. American Diabetes Association. Introduction: standards of medical care in diabetes-2022. *Diabetes Care.* 2022;45(Suppl 1):S1-S2. PMID: 34964812

11. American Diabetes Association Professional Practice Committee, Draznin B, Aroda VR, et al. 9. Pharmacologic approaches to glycemic treatment: standards of medical care in diabetes-2022. *Diabetes Care.* 2022;45(Suppl 1):S125-S143. PMID: 34964831

12. Diamond L, Izquierdo K, Canfield D, Matsoukas K, Gany F. A systematic review of the impact of patient-physician non-English language concordance on quality of care and outcomes. *J Gen Intern Med.* 2019;34(8):1591-1606. PMID: 31147980

Time in Range: The New Hemoglobin A$_{1c}$?

Jane E. B. Reusch, MD. University of Colorado School of Medicine, Division of Endocrinology, Metabolism, Diabetes, Aurora, CO; E-mail: jane.reusch@cuanschutz.edu

Learning Objectives

As a result of participating in this session, learners should be able to:

- Describe current guidelines on glycemic targets across the spectrum of diabetes, including those for type 1 diabetes, type 2 diabetes, gestational diabetes, and drug-induced diabetes.

- Master the information generated using continuous glucose monitoring (CGM) and have a clear understanding of the following metrics: time in range (TIR), time below range (TBR), and time above range (TAR).

Main Conclusions

Metrics for assessing overall glycemic control and glucose profiles in persons with and at risk for diabetes mellitus have evolved rapidly over the last decade. We now have technology that can provide real-time CGM in easily accessible systems. These devices can be used across the lifespan and many have capabilities for remote data access. The relationship between data generated using CGM and values obtained using hemoglobin A$_{1c}$ or fingerstick blood glucose monitoring are now well established, and the correlations are very strong. Data demonstrating a clear relationship between CGM metrics, such as TIR, and diabetes complications are accumulating in the literature. As such, CGM offers real-time biofeedback to the individual with diabetes, accessible data for the clinician, which can be used in a telemedicine setting, and detailed profiles on hyperglycemia and hypoglycemia not available with blood glucose monitoring or hemoglobin A$_{1c}$ testing. This technology has been deployed in populations and was demonstrated to improve overall glycemic control. Given these benefits, what are the unanswered questions? Based on the recent American Diabetes Association and European Association for the Study of Diabetes guidance for the management of type 1 diabetes, all individuals capable of using this technology should have access to it and TIR can be considered the equivalent of hemoglobin A$_{1c}$. In contrast, in the majority of the more than 537 million people globally living with diabetes, assessment of overall glycemic control and its relationship to outcomes is still most accessibly addressed using hemoglobin A$_{1c}$ or fingerstick blood glucose monitoring. It is critical to continuously evaluate the balance among patient burden, access to education, cost-effectiveness, access to the Internet and/or smart phones, patient interface with new technology, diabetes literacy and numeracy, and the effect on quality of life and clinical outcomes. So, is TIR the new hemoglobin A$_{1c}$? Hemoglobin A$_{1c}$ still has a central role in diabetes management, and TIR and be used to assess goal-directed therapy and has added value.

Significance of the Clinical Problem

Diabetes is a common clinical condition currently affecting more than 37 million people in the United States alone, and it is defined by glucose values and/or hemoglobin A_{1c}.[1] Working with individuals living with diabetes to optimize their blood glucose values requires an investment on the part of the provider and the individual with diabetes. The evolution from urine dipstick blood glucose to the use of CGM in the last 50 years has changed the landscape and enhanced our capacity to nearly normalize blood glucose in certain individuals living with diabetes. Improvements in blood glucose control decrease microvascular complications of diabetes, including retinopathy, neuropathy, and nephropathy. Epidemiological evidence supports a significant correlation between glycemic burden over time and the most common macrovascular complications of diabetes, atherosclerotic cardiovascular disease and heart failure. As such, tools to optimize glycemic control are increasingly useful in diabetes management. The question remains, which tool and in which setting?

Guidance from primary care and subspecialty societies endorse individualized glucose targets for patients living with diabetes. These targets are based on the likelihood to benefit vs risk from more or less intensive glucose control. The most recent summary of glycemic targets is outlined in the 2022 American Diabetes Association Standards for Medical Care of Diabetes.[1] Depending on the glycemic target for a given individual, the management strategy (diet, exercise, medications), the risk of hypoglycemia, and access to care and technology, differing strategies for monitoring treatment response are warranted. For individuals with type 1 diabetes, recent-onset diabetes, younger age, long life expectancy, and fewer comorbidities, the use of newer diabetes management tools should be actively considered, as they have demonstrated improvement in glycemic control.[2,3] For individuals using agents that could increase risk of hypoglycemia, use of CGM can be exceptionally useful for risk mitigation. In contrast, for individuals at low risk for hypoglycemia whose diabetes is managed with diet and physical activity, agents without hypoglycemia risk and simple tools for achieving hemoglobin A_{1c} targets may suffice. It is also an

option to use CGM at the time of diagnosis, time of change in medical management, or as a tool to guide choice of therapy. In each of these settings, it is not the TIR alone but the comprehensive CGM profile that is most informative.

Implied in the title of this session is a bias to consider that CGM is appropriate for all. To keep this conversation balanced, we must consider the implications of this question in the clinical setting. TIR is predictive of hemoglobin A_{1c}. More to the point, 14-day CGM can generate a glucose management indicator that aligns with hemoglobin A_{1c} very well. CGM offers more information than hemoglobin A_{1c} or fingerstick blood glucose monitoring. Hemoglobin A_{1c} measures average glycemic burden and not low or high blood glucose, whereas fingerstick blood glucose detects certain patterns but may or may not capture hyperglycemia and hypoglycemia. CGM captures the full picture and provides metrics, including TIR, TBR, TAR, and glucose management indicator. Figure 1 illustrates the consensus ambulatory glucose profile report generated from a CGM download.[1,4,5] Does this increase in data available using CGM mean that clinical practice guidance should replace hemoglobin A_{1c} with TIR, or perhaps replace hemoglobin A_{1c} with CGM? The answer to this question is "no" in 2022. Either can be used to assess achievement of glycemic targets.[6] The objective for the practicing clinician is to use tools that will optimize outcomes and safety for an individual with diabetes in their clinic.

One useful strategy for determining when and in whom to use CGM is to consider who would benefit and how. Glucose is not static and glucose variability is not well characterized using either hemoglobin A_{1c} or blood glucose monitoring by fingerstick. Let's imagine different fingerstick blood glucose monitoring and CGM scenarios where an individual has a hemoglobin A_{1c} value of 7.0% (53 mmol/mol). In a scenario of an individual with all blood glucose monitoring values before meals and at bedtime in the target range, lows and highs can still be missed. Using CGM in Figure 2, an individual could have a TIR ranging from

Figure 1. Consensus Ambulatory Glucose Profile Report Generated from CGM Download

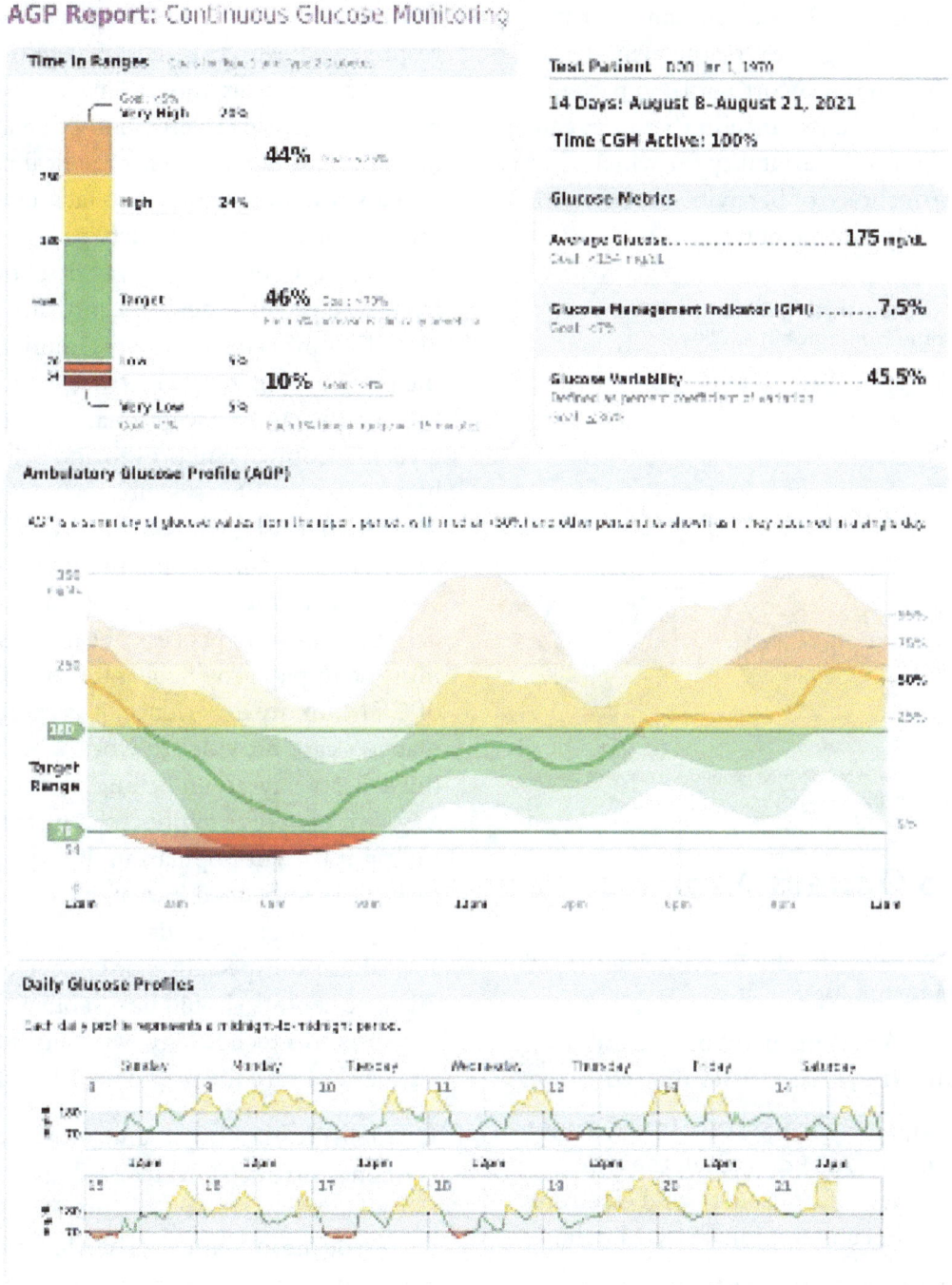

40% to 90%. For example, if a patient had a TIR of 50% and a hemoglobin A_{1c} level between 6.0% and 7.0% (42 and 53 mmol/mol), one would need to be exceptionally concerned about hypoglycemia lowering the overall glucose burden represented in the hemoglobin A_{1c}. If a patient had a TIR of 90% and a hemoglobin A_{1c} level of 7.0% (53 mmol/mol), one would expect that most of the blood glucose values not in range were above range. It is also quite possible for a patient with substantial hyperglycemia and hypoglycemia (high glycemic variability) to have excellent hemoglobin

A$_{1c}$ with dangerous glycemic profiles. This figure demonstrates with undeniable clarity that CGM offers additional insight. These data can inform medical decision-making both for the provider and the patient with diabetes. Worth noting, patients treated with insulin and noninsulin therapies can have significant glucose variability for which CGM data could inform choice of behavior modification[7] and or antihyperglycemic agent.

Figure 2. CGM Data Illustrating Different TIR Possible With Same Hemoglobin A$_{1c}$ Level

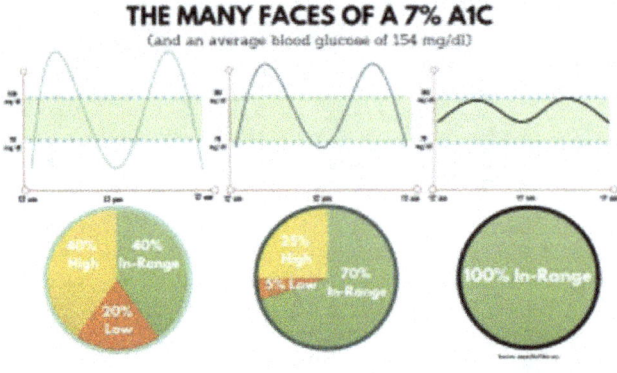

Reprinted with permission from the diaTribe Foundation resource page: https://diatribe.org/time-range.

Barriers to Optimal Practice

- Choosing the optimal patient who will benefit from CGM technology.

- Justifying CGM to third-party payers and the system within the clinic to determine coverage.

- Building adequate infrastructure for education about and use of CGM devices in the clinic, access and review of CGM data, and electronic health record documentation of CGM data.

- Implementing billing structures to support implementation of this technology.

Strategies for Diagnosis, Therapy, and/or Management

The routine use of CGM (all aspects, not just TIR) offers benefits for assessment of goal-directed therapy and clinical decision-making.

However, incorporation into a clinical practice requires setting up an infrastructure for approval, download, and interpretation of the data. A responsive health care system requires the capacity to educate the patient on the use of CGM, processes in place to efficiently download the data for review and use for medical management of diabetes, infrastructure to facilitate effective interactions with third-party payers for coverage of this technology, systems to incorporate data into the electronic health record, and standard operating procedures for communication with the patient. For the correctly selected patient, the benefit can be exceptional, both in terms of glycemic control and prevention or avoidance of hypoglycemia. Few systems outside of diabetes centers have streamlined this process to optimize care. This is a current gap in many health care systems with the proven assets for patient care driving change in process of care. A system must be in place to enable safe and effective use of CGM. In my experience, it is crucial for the diabetes care provider to work with their practice, third-party payers, and clinic staff to establish a system of care to support the use of CGM for the right patient population. If these stipulations cannot be embedded into a provider's clinical setting, partnerships with certified diabetes care and education specialists or endocrinology/diabetes centers should be established to enable access to this technology, which is now the standard of care for patients with diabetes.

1. Identification of patients most likely to benefit from CGM technology. (This is not exhaustive; please see American Diabetes Association Standards of Medical Care for Diabetes for a complete list.)[3,4]

    a. *Patients on insulin therapy:* The use of CGM and assessment of TIR, TBR, and TAR are essential for the safe management of patients living with type 1 diabetes or of patients with any type of diabetes on multiple daily insulin injections (MDI). Patients treated with MDI, insulin pump therapy (including CGM-augmented insulin pump therapy and hybrid closed-loop systems) are able to communicate with their provider using this technology for fine-tuning diabetes management and decreasing hypoglycemia. For patients treated with basal insulin alone, use of CGM and TIR, TBR, and TAR can optimize the use of additional antihyperglycemic agents to achieve glycemic targets. In these settings, TIR can be used in lieu of hemoglobin A_{1c} for assessing glycemic targets with the added value of providing information about hyperglycemia and hypoglycemia.

b. *Patients with inadequate glycemic control:* For patients who have suboptimal glycemic control on their current regimen and/or have glycemic variability, the use of CGM and TIR, TBR, and TAR can be informative for guiding medical management and choice of glucose-lowering medication.

c. *Patients in high-risk work settings:* CGM is particularly important for those operating machinery or engaging in extensive physical activity.

d. *Patients in remote settings:* Telemedicine access to the CGM-derived metrics TIR, TBR, and TAR can inform point-of-care decision-making for remote clinical decision-making.

In many health care systems, there is a stipulation that the individual using CGM technology be embedded in a clinical practice with expertise in the use of this technology.

2. Provider and patient comfort with the use of and interpretation of CGM technology.

a. Education on different CGM models, readers, report downloading, apps.

 i. Education can be obtained through certified diabetes care and education specialists, device companies, and continuing medical education sessions.

 ii. Most companies offer the educational opportunity for providers to wear devices.

b. Education on technical aspects of CGM insertion and care (as above).

c. Data downloading, reports, and decision tools.

 i. HIPAA-compliant platforms are available for provider download.

 ii. Education is available for use of the ambulatory glucose profile and other insights embedded in the reports.

d. Process of care infrastructure for CGM review and communication with the patient.

 i. Certified diabetes care and education specialists or others developing this expertise within the clinic can set up the infrastructure for initiating patients on the devices and educating patients on the processes for downloading and sharing data with the practice.

 ii. Support staff from each of the device manufacturers can be partnered with to facilitate optimal use by the patient.

 iii. Troubleshooting for alarms or sensor malfunctions can be done either by the practice or in some cases through support from the device manufacturers.

e. Cost of technology and coverage by third-party payers (need process).

 i. Third-party payers have specific rules, as do integrated health care systems such as the Veterans Health Administration and Kaiser Permanente, for eligible individuals (see above). These rules are in continuous evolution; as the evidence for benefit continues to increase, the patient populations covered continues to increase.

ii. As providers, we need to advocate for access to this technology for correctly selected patients.

3. Educational support for optimal use of technology.

a. Formal provider education is needed, analogous to electrocardiography interpretation.

i. The ambulatory glucose profile outlines the metrics that should be considered upon review of CGM beyond TIR.

ii. Algorithms have been established for the review of CGM download to guide clinical decision-making.

b. CGM download, interpretation, and communication back to the patient.

i. Within the clinical practice setting, a process of care must be established for the review of CGM, and timelines should be set up for communication with the patient.

ii. Embedding these processes into the post-visit care plan can facilitate optimal communication.

iii. When possible, remote access for CGM data can optimize review and follow-up communication with the patient.

c. Patient education on pattern recognition and thresholds for contacting provider. At each patient visit, an assessment of diabetes literacy and numeracy around CGM use and pattern recognition should be addressed. Interval visits with educators should be arranged if the patient is unable to use the device to optimally guide their decision-making.

Clinical Case Vignettes
Case 1

A 31-year-old man was diagnosed with new-onset type 1 diabetes after an episode of diabetic ketoacidosis 6 months ago. He is preparing to transition from MDI to automated insulin delivery. His current regimen consists of insulin glargine, 24 units at bedtime; meal coverage insulin-to-carbohydrate ratio of 1:10; and correction factor of 1:30 over 120 mg/dL. He does not correct at bedtime due to fear of hypoglycemia. CGM download is shown (*see image*).

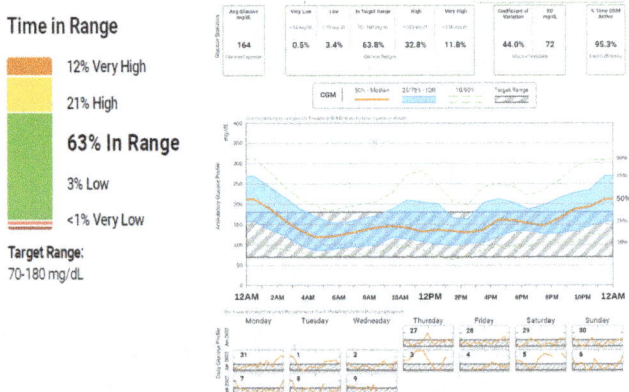

After reviewing the data, which of the following should be the first area of concern?

A. Daytime glucose profiles

B. High and very high total 33%

C. Low and very low total 3.9%

D. Nocturnal glucose profiles

Answer: D) Nocturnal glucose profiles

In review of the patient's download, there is a trend for blood glucose to drop through the night by more than 100 mg/dL (5.6 mmol/L). As such, any changes in his regimen that lower overall glucose concentrations may place the patient at risk for nocturnal hypoglycemia (Answer D). The priority in CGM review is to look for patterns that could place the patient at risk for hypoglycemia.

The Table and Figure show targets of therapy using CGM.

Table. Standardized CGM Metrics for clinical care

1.	Number of days CGM device is worn (recommend 14 days)	
2.	Percentage of time CGM device is active (recommend 70% of data from 14 days)	
3.	Mean glucose	
4.	Glucose management indicator	
5.	Glycemic variability (%CV) target ≤36%*	
6.	TAR: % of readings and time >250 mg/dL (>13.9 mmol/L)	Level 2 hyperglycemia
7.	TAR: % of readings and time 181-250 mg/dL (10.1-13.9 mmol/L)	Level 1 hyperglycemia
8.	TIR: % of readings and time 70-180 mg/dL (3.9-10.0 mmol/L)	In range
9.	TBR: % of readings and time 54-69 mg/dL (3.0-3.8 mmol/L)	Level 1 hyperglycemia
10.	TBR: % of readings and time <54 mg/dL (<3.0 mmol/L)	Level 2 hyperglycemia

CGM, continuous glucose monitoring; CV, coefficient of variation; TAR, time above range; TBR, time below range, TIR, time in range. *Some studies suggest that %CV targets (<33%) provide additional protection against hypoglycemia for those receiving insulin or sulfonylureas.

Reprinted from American Diabetes Association Professional Practice Committee; Draznin B et al. *Diabetes Care*, 2022; 45(Suppl 1); and Holt RIG et al. *Diabetes Care*, 2021; 44(11).

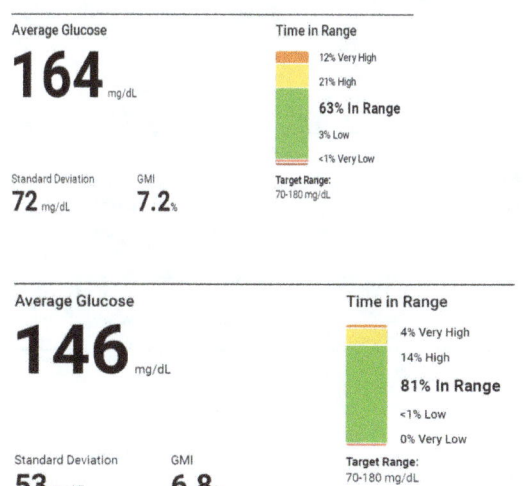

Case 2

A 92-year-old man has a 70-year history of type 1 diabetes without complications. He has been shuttered in his assisted living home during the COVID pandemic. He is now vaccinated with a booster and would like input on his diabetes management. Recent laboratory testing reveals a hemoglobin A_{1c} level of 7.8% (62 mmol/mol). He is concerned about elevated glucose values. His regimen consists of insulin glargine, 2 units in the evening, and insulin aspart, 5 units with breakfast and 2 units at lunch and dinner. He had recurrent nocturnal hypoglycemia requiring third-party assistance when on insulin glargine, 3 to 4 units daily; severe nocturnal hypoglycemia when on insulin degludec, 2 units daily; and severe nocturnal hypoglycemia when administering lunch or dinner aspart doses greater than 2 units. CGM data are shown (*see image*).

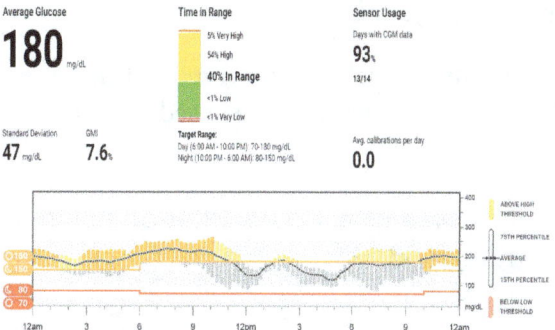

After reviewing the data, what should be the priority to discuss with this patient?

A. Achieving a TIR of at least 70%

B. Blood glucose trends before lunch and dinner

C. Postdinner and nighttime glucose elevations

D. No changes recommended at this time

Answer: D) No changes recommended at this time

The patient is not having hypoglycemia, and this is an outstanding overall result. He has a 70-plus-year history of diabetes without clinically significant complications. There is no evidence that very tight glycemic control would improve any clinically significant aspect of this patient's life. It is noted in the vignette's stem that most minor changes in insulin have previously resulted in hypoglycemia. Therefore, no changes are recommended at this time (Answer D).

Case 3

A 68-year-old woman with a 10-year history of type 2 diabetes is managed with metformin. An SGLT-2 inhibitor is added for kidney indications. CGM data are shown (*see images*).

What information from this patient's CGM is useful in decision-making?

A. Glycemic variability

B. Nocturnal blood glucose values

C. Postprandial blood glucose values

D. Helping the patient see that a change needs to be made

Answer: A) Glycemic variability

The glycemic variability observed in this patient's CGM data (Answer A) can be used to help the patient see that the SGLT-2 inhibitor may be beneficial in addressing postprandial glucose in addition to the kidney benefit it provides.

Case 3 (Continued)

Should CGM use be continued in this setting?

A. Yes

B. No

C. Only as needed

Answer: B) No

CGM is not needed in this setting (Answer B), as there appears to be no indication of risk for hypoglycemia.

68 yo female with T2DM, BDR and an eGFR = 58, A/C ratio = 98.

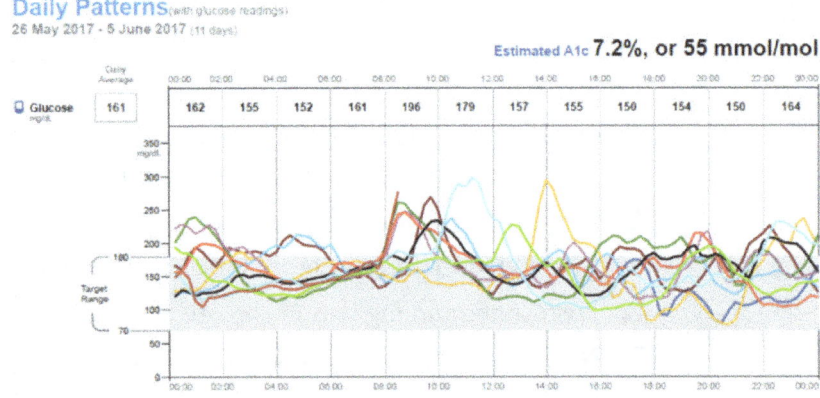

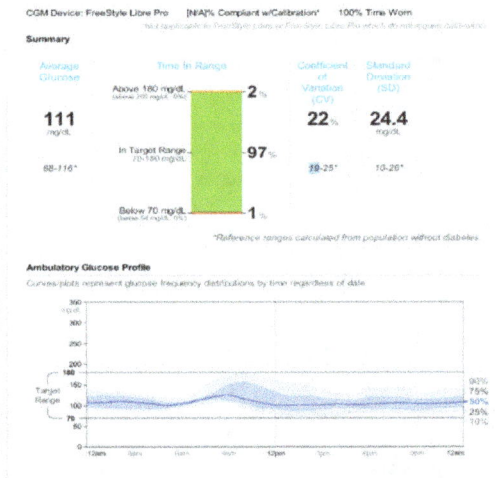

References

1. American Diabetes Association Professional Practice Committee; Draznin B, Aroda VR, et al. 6. Glycemic targets: standards of medical care in diabetes-2022. *Diabetes Care.* 2022;45(Suppl 1):S83-S96. PMID: 34964868

2. Dicembrini I, Cosentino C, Monami M, Mannucci E, Pala L. Effects of real-time continuous glucose monitoring in type 1 diabetes: a meta-analysis of randomized controlled trials. *Acta Diabetol.* 2021;58(4):401-410. PMID: 32789691

3. Holt RIG, DeVries JH, Hess-Fischl A, et al. The management of type 1 diabetes in adults. A consensus report by the American Diabetes Association (ADA) and the European Association for the Study of Diabetes (EASD). *Diabetes Care.* 2021;44(11):2589-2625. PMID: 34593612

4. American Diabetes Association Professional Practice Committee; Draznin B, Aroda VR, et al. 7. diabetes technology: standards of medical care in diabetes-2022. *Diabetes Care.* 2022;45(Suppl 1):S97-S112. PMID: 34964871

5. Carlson AL, Criego AB, Martens TW, Bergenstal RM. HbA(1c): the glucose management indicator, time in range, and standardization of continuous glucose monitoring reports in clinical practice. *Endocrinol Metab Clin North Am.* 2020;49(1):95-107. PMID: 31980124

6. Desouza CV, Holcomb RG, Rosenstock J, et al. Results of a study comparing glycated albumin to other glycemic indices. *J Clin Endocrinol Metab.* 2020;105(3):677-687. PMID: 31650161

7. Merino J, Linenberg I, Bermingham KM, et al. Validity of continuous glucose monitoring for categorizing glycemic responses to diet: implications for use in personalized nutrition. *Am J Clin Nutr.* 2022 [Online ahead of print] PMID: 35134821

Closed-Loop Insulin Delivery

Sue A. Brown, MD. Division of Endocrinology, University of Virginia, Charlottesville, VA; E-mail: sab2f@virginia.edu

Learning Objectives

As a result of participating in this session, learners should be able to:

- Explain the functionality of different automated insulin delivery (AID) systems.

- Evaluate the effect of changes to glycemic parameters on algorithmic performance in AID systems.

Main Conclusions

AID devices have demonstrated consistent improvement in glycemic outcomes for people with type 1 diabetes mellitus (T1DM).[1-4] As such, AID devices are increasingly used for glycemic control, as there remains a gap in achieving glycemic goals for many people with T1DM.[5,6] Each AID device has unique algorithms with different functionalities that are important for clinicians to understand. Current AID systems are hybrid closed-loop controllers in which the devices are intended to be used alongside carbohydrate counting to deliver meal boluses. Therefore, adjustment of carbohydrate ratios remains one of the most important parameters that affects glycemic outcomes in currently available AID systems. Adjustments to basal rates and correction factors affect some AID systems but not others. An understanding of which parameters are truly adjustable and their potential impact on algorithmic performance is relevant for optimal use of these AID systems.

Significance of the Clinical Problem

Reports suggest that people with T1DM are not meeting established glycemic targets.[5,6] A variety of tools and devices have been developed in an effort to address these deficiencies. For people with T1DM, one key advancement in the past 5 years has been the availability of AID devices. These systems consistently improve time in target range (70-180 mg/dL [3.9-10.0 mmol/L]), reduce hypoglycemia (<70 mg/dL [<3.9 mmol/L]), and often improve hemoglobin A_{1c} when compared with not using an AID device.[1-4]

These devices consist of an insulin pump, a continuous glucose monitoring (CGM) system, and an algorithm that is either embedded in the pump/device or on a phone app. These algorithms use data from both the CGM and insulin pump to "close the loop" and make insulin dosing decisions automatically based on algorithmic targets. As of February 2022, there are 4 AID systems that are currently FDA-approved in the United States, as well as other systems available outside the United States. Health care practitioners need to understand how the algorithms are configured and how individual algorithms are affected by insulin parameter adjustments. This discussion will focus on the use of the FDA-approved AID devices for clinicians to consider for optimal glycemic management in a person with T1DM.

Barriers to Optimal Practice

- It can be challenging for clinicians to efficiently analyze the significant quantity of data available with contemporary AID devices to develop optimal treatment-related decisions.

- This challenge is further compounded by the variety of algorithmic approaches to glycemic control that require an understanding of the specifics of each device.

Strategies for Diagnosis, Therapy, and/or Management

It is important to untangle the terminology related to the variety of systems available and described in the literature (*Table*). An AID system consists of 3 main components: a CGM, an insulin pump, and an algorithm connecting the devices (closed-loop system or AID). Each system can be operated in a manual mode where the AID algorithm is not activated. When CGM is not being used for insulin delivery, some studies refer to this mode as sensor-augmented pump (SAP). Systems or modes that only use CGM to decrease or suspend insulin delivery with no ability to automatically increase insulin delivery are often termed low-glucose suspend (LGS) or predictive-low glucose suspend (PLGS) systems depending on whether the CGM threshold for insulin attenuation is based on a fixed or a predictive value. This discussion focuses on AID systems that are capable of increasing and decreasing insulin automatically based on device-specific algorithmic solutions. These systems can also be referred to as AID or closed-loop control or artificial pancreas systems. Each system has a variety of inputs into the algorithm. Understanding the inputs into the algorithm is critical to determining which options can be adjusted to individualize it for a person with T1DM.[7-9] This discussion is focused on the more common use of AID devices in T1DM with commercially available options in the United States as of February 2022. The 4 AID devices discussed are the 670G, 770G, Control-IQ (C-IQ), and Omnipod 5 (OP5).

Insulin Delivery

Insulin delivery can come from several sources in an AID system: (a) user-initiated meal and correction boluses; (b) AID algorithm-initiated insulin delivery given as a microbolus every 5 minutes and constantly adjusted to meet the prevailing targets; and (c) in some systems, discrete automated boluses given periodically that are generally of a higher magnitude than the microboluses every 5 minutes.

Changing Algorithmic Targets

In general, the changing of a target will directly affect insulin delivery. The general concept of a target or target range is similar across devices: insulin will be increased if CGM is predicted to be above the prevailing target and insulin will be decreased or paused if CGM is predicted to be below the prevailing target. The algorithm targets are used to guide automated insulin delivery by the device, and some systems allow adjustment by time of day. The algorithm targets can be

Table. Types of Insulin Delivery System Configurations

CGM+ pump connection	Insulin delivery	System abbreviation	Definition	Description	Examples
Not driven by CGM	No effect on insulin	SAP	Sensor-Augmented Pump	CGM and pump not connected, operate independently	Any CGM + Any insulin pump operated separately
Driven by CGM	Only decreases insulin	LGS	Low Glucose Suspend	Suspends at a user-set threshold	630G Manual 670G (suspend on low)
		PLGS	Predictive-Low Glucose Suspend	Decreases or suspends based on predicted glucose	Basal-IQ Manual 670G (suspend before low)
Driven by CGM	Increases and decreases insulin	HCL (a type of AID)	Hybrid Closed-Loop	AID device where people are expected to bolus after meals	670G/770G Control-IQ Omnipod 5

different from the targets used for a user-requested meal or correction bolus done through the bolus calculator. Current targets are:

- 670G/770G: Fixed algorithmic target of 120 mg/dL (6.7 mmol/L). This can be changed by activating the temp target feature that raises the target to 150 mg/dL (8.3 mmol/L). Note: When a user requests a correction bolus, the target used in the bolus calculator is 150 mg/dL (8.3 mmol/L).

- C-IQ: "Normal mode" algorithmic target range of 112.5 to 160 mg/dL (6.2-8.9 mmol/L); "sleep mode": gradual tightening of target down to 112.5 to 120 mg/dL (6.2-6.7 mmol/L) over the scheduled sleep time; "exercise activity": raises target to 140 to 160 mg/dL (7.8-8.9 mmol/L). Note: when a user requests a correction bolus, the target used in the bolus calculator is 110 mg/dL (6.1 mmol/L).

- OP5: Five available algorithmic targets of 110 mg/dL (6.1 mmol/L), 120 mg/dL (6.7 mmol/L), 130 mg/dL (7.2 mmol/L), 140 mg/dL (7.8 mmol/L), or 150 mg/dL (8.3 mmol/L) that can be preprogrammed at different times of day (eg, if there is a need for a different target overnight vs daytime). The "activity" function temporarily changes the target to 150 mg/dL (8.3 mmol/L). Note: the selected algorithmic target is the same one used for user-requested correction boluses.

Meal Boluses

Adjustment of carbohydrate ratios remains a key intervention because current AID systems rely on carbohydrate counting. For this reason, they are considered hybrid closed-loop controllers (a type of AID system). Although AID systems can adjust insulin during the postprandial period to compensate for inaccurate or missed meal boluses, the systems consistently perform better when carbohydrate intake is entered as part of a meal bolus. In general, it is strongly recommended that the bolus calculator function of each system be used to ensure that insulin-on-board is considered when calculating the meal or correction bolus, thus compensating for the additional insulin delivered by the AID device.

Hypoglycemic Treatments

Because these systems can suspend insulin for prolonged periods, it is typical that a person enters a hypoglycemic episode with a lower amount of insulin-on-board. This means that fewer carbohydrates may be needed to treat an individual hypoglycemic event. This varies by individual but could be as much as 10% to 40% less carbohydrate administration (eg, 8-16 g rather than 16-24 g). AID systems generally respond well to the rebound hyperglycemia that occurs following hypoglycemic treatments, but occasionally this additional insulin can set up a recurrent hypoglycemic event later.

Exercise

Exercise remains a glycemic challenge with current AID systems. Most systems have a mechanism for setting a temporary target that can be selected by the user. Traditional methods to avoid exercise-induced hypoglycemia by ingesting carbohydrate prior to activity may result in a greater amount of insulin-on-board than desired as the AID system reacts to the rise in CGM. This can be mitigated by adjusting targets and may even require the disconnection of the pump for some types of activity. The following adjustable targets are:

- 670G/770G: Has a temp target of 150 mg/dL (8.3 mmol/L), which can be used during exercise.

- C-IQ: Has an exercise activity that increases the target to 140 to 160 mg/dL (7.8 to 8.9 mmol/L). Of note, the additional automated corrections that can occur hourly are still active during the exercise activity.

- OP5: Has an activity function the increases the target to 150 mg/dL (8.3 mmol/L).

Total Daily Insulin

Many current systems are oriented toward incorporating total daily insulin (TDI) as an important driver of algorithmic solutions. Therefore, each of the current systems tracks TDI and uses it to some degree to adjust insulin delivery. Depending on the system, TDI may be updated at different times.

- 670G/770G: Uses a running TDI over approximately 6 days with a fading memory to determine the AID parameters in effect (eg, auto basal rate and insulin sensitivity factor).

- C-IQ: An initial input for TDI is required with a new system start but then uses a rolling 6-day average for determining TDI, which has a role in modulating the automated insulin microboluses.

- OP5: Updates TDI with each pod change (eg, every 3 days) and is used to determine an adaptive basal rate.

Preset Insulin Parameters

Preset basal rates and correction factors are always relevant when the AID system is being operated in manual mode for all current systems. Preset basal rates, however, are not used during automated mode for the 670/770G and are only used for the very first system pod of OP5 to gauge the TDI. Thereafter, these systems use the TDI to determine the effective basal rate. The C-IQ system does use the preset basal rate, and its adjustment will have some influence on insulin delivery. The correction factor has no relevance for automated mode in 670G/770G, is only used for user-request boluses for OP5, and is used for both user-requested boluses and some insulin delivery calculations during AID use for C-IQ. The most relevant parameters that can be adjusted by an AID system to alter insulin delivery are:

- 670G/770G: carbohydrate ratio, duration of insulin action

- C-IQ: carbohydrate ratio, correction factor, basal rates, setting of sleep schedule

- OP5: carbohydrate ratio, setting of AID target, correction factor (only used for user-requested corrections not automated insulin delivery by the device)

Clinical Case Vignettes

Case 1

A 55-year-old man with T1DM has no complications and a recent hemoglobin A_{1c} measurement of 6.7% (50 mmol/mol). He currently uses an AID device (670G) with the summary information shown (*see Figure*). Although he is meeting glycemic targets, he requests advice on how to handle postprandial hyperglycemia after dinner. He estimates carbohydrates carefully and administers his meal bolus on time.

If a parameter change is needed, which of the following changes is the most direct way to address his postprandial hyperglycemia?

A. Decrease insulin action time to increase insulin delivery for the meal

B. Decrease the carbohydrate ratio at dinner to increase insulin delivery for the meal

C. Decrease the correction factor (insulin sensitivity factor) to increase automated insulin delivery by the algorithm

D. Increase the basal rate because that is the most direct way to affect automated insulin delivery by the algorithm

E. Lower the target of the algorithm for the postprandial dinner or overnight period

Answer: B) Decrease the carbohydrate ratio at dinner to increase insulin delivery for the meal

The carbohydrate ratio (Answer B) is the only applicable intervention in the 670G/770G systems that would directly adjust insulin effectively for a meal.

Decreasing insulin action time to increase insulin delivery for the meal (Answer A) is a consideration, as it is an adjustable parameter and programming a shorter insulin action time may help with increasing insulin delivery.

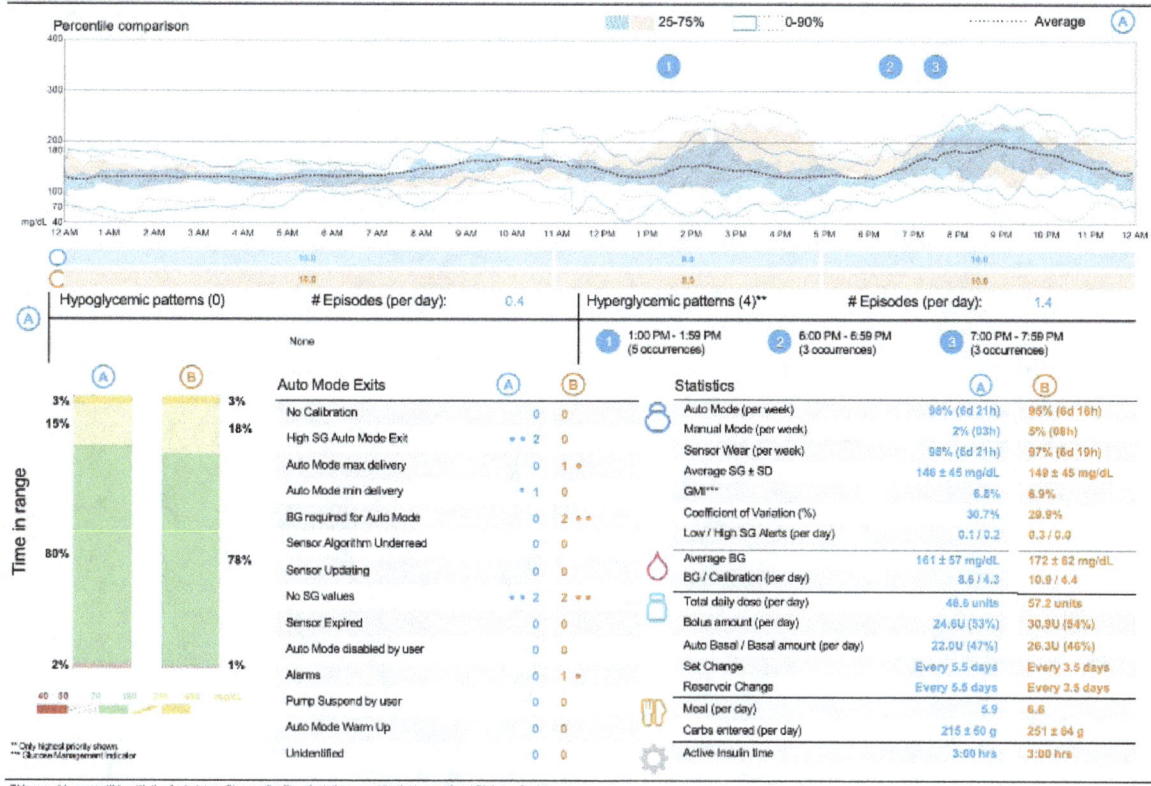

This report is compatible with the Ambulatory Glucose Profile calculations used by the International Diabetes Center

However, it is not the preferred parameter in this situation and cannot be adjusted to specific time segments.

Increasing the basal rate (Answer D) and decreasing the correction factor (insulin sensitivity factor) (Answer C) are not viable options because basal rates or correction factors cannot be adjusted when the automated mode is activated. Both are system-determined settings based on TDI.

Lowering the target of the algorithm for the postprandial dinner or overnight period (Answer E) is not feasible because the target of the algorithm itself cannot be lowered below fixed targets (120 mg/dL [6.7 mmol/L] during auto mode or 150 mg/dL [8.3 mmol/L] during temp target).

Case 2

A 21-year-old college student has T1DM without complications and a recent hemoglobin A$_{1c}$ measurement of 6.9% (52 mmol/mol). He currently uses an AID device (C-IQ). The Figure shows a day when he experienced hypoglycemia while moving items between apartments. He required several hypoglycemic treatments and was eating throughout the day. He misses occasional meal boluses, including on the day shown in the Figure, and is not using exercise mode. He asked for your advice on strategies to avoid hypoglycemia during this type of activity.

Which of the following would be a reasonable initial adjustment for this type of activity?

A. Decrease the basal rate

B. Increase insulin action time to decrease insulin delivery

C. Increase the carbohydrate ratio to decrease insulin delivery for meals

D. Increase the correction factor to decrease automated insulin delivery by the device

E. Increase the target of the algorithm during activity

Answer: E) Increase the target of the algorithm during activity

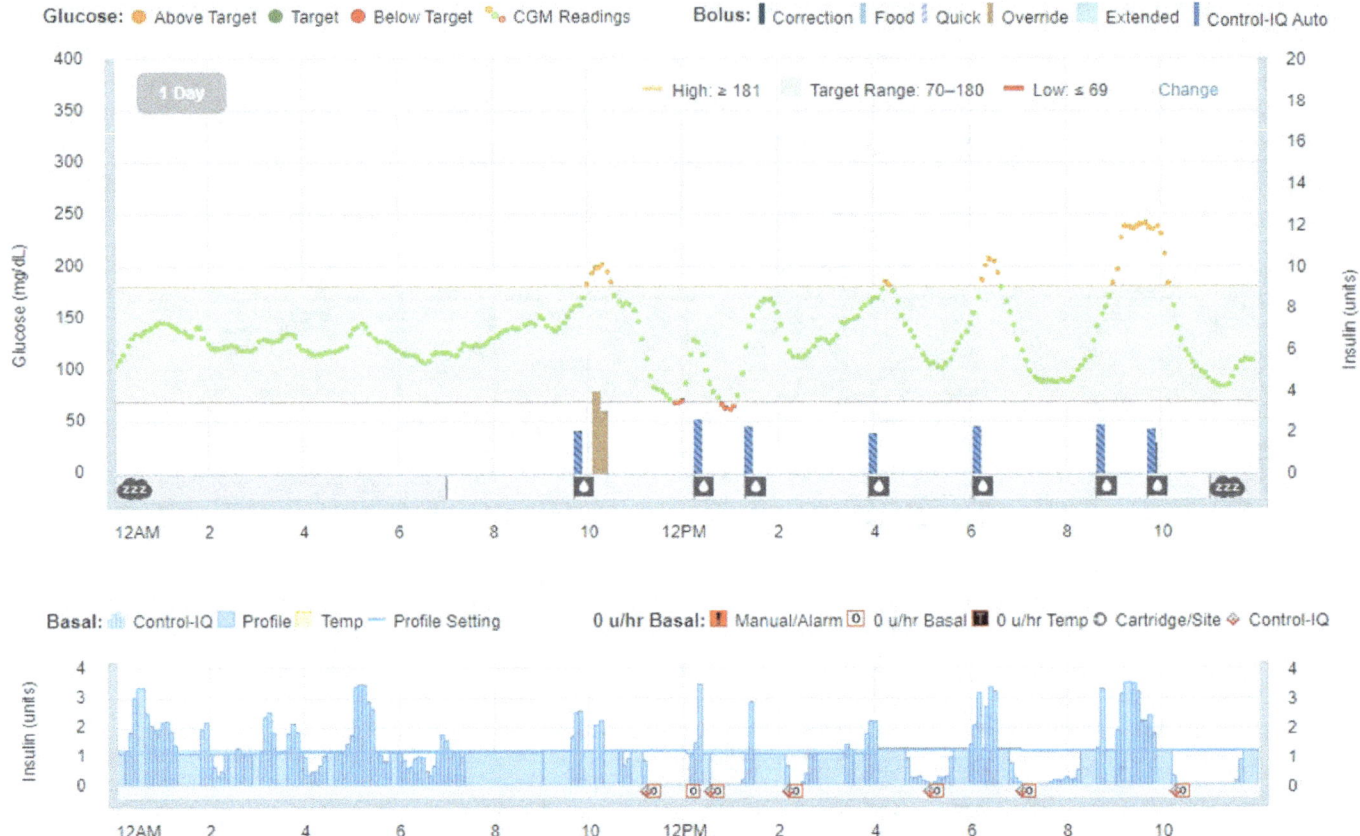

Decreasing the basal rate (Answer A), increasing the carbohydrate ratio (Answer C), increasing the correction factor (Answer D), and increasing the target of the algorithm during activity (Answer E) are all options that could be adjusted in this system and will affect insulin delivery.

Increasing the target of the algorithm (Answer E) is the preferred initial strategy, as he can activate the exercise activity option to temporarily increase the algorithm target to 140 to 160 mg/dL (7.8 to 8.9 mmol/L). He was not doing strenuous activity but rather sustained light activity that is likely to respond to this approach.

Increasing the correction factor (Answer D) would be the next best option, as this may directly lower the amount of the periodic automated correction boluses.

Decreasing the basal rate (Answer A) can affect insulin delivery, but it would have less of an intended effect, as the system can increase basal rates significantly if needed.

Increasing the carbohydrate ratio (Answer C) would not be as effective because there are not many user-requested boluses, and he has mostly automated correction boluses throughout the day.

Increasing insulin action time (Answer B), the duration of insulin action for the algorithm component, cannot be adjusted in this system.

Case 3

A 45-year-old woman has T1DM without complications and a recent hemogloblin A$_{1c}$ measurement of 7.6% (60 mmol/mol). She is currently using an insulin pump and CGM that are not connected and will be transitioning to an AID device (OP5). She does consistent meal bolusing during the day, and because of her concerns about hypoglycemia at night, she has a lower basal rate overnight. She notes she often wakes in the morning with higher glucose values.

What is the most effective parameter that could be adjusted to improve her glycemic outcomes once the OP5 AID device is initiated?

A. Decrease the carbohydrate ratio at dinner to increase insulin delivery for the meal

B. Decrease the correction factor to increase automated insulin delivery by the device

C. Decrease the duration of insulin action time

D. Increase the basal rate because that is the most direct way to affect automated insulin delivery by the device

E. Lower the target of the algorithm for postprandial dinner or overnight period

Answer: E) Lower the target of the algorithm for postprandial dinner or overnight period

Lowering the target of the algorithm for postprandial dinner or overnight period (Answer E) is the most effective method to adjust overall automated insulin delivery for this device. Therefore, it is reasonable to choose a lower target (eg, 110 or 120 mg/dL [6.1 or 6.7 mmol/L]).

Increasing the basal rate (Answer D) will not affect automated insulin delivery by the device after the very first pod has been changed and this is therefore not a long-term solution.

Decreasing the correction factor to increase automated insulin delivery by the device (Answer B) is not preferred solution as written because adjusting the correction factor with this system will only affect the user-directed boluses, not the automated insulin delivery for this device.

Decreasing the carbohydrate ratio at dinner (Answer A) and decreasing the duration of insulin action time (Answer C) are adjustable factors that will affect user-direct boluses and are reasonable to consider if more nuanced adjustments are needed once the algorithmic targets are set.

References

1. Bergenstal RM, Garg S, Weinzimer SA, et al. Safety of a hybrid closed-loop insulin delivery system in patients with type 1 diabetes. *JAMA*. 2016;316(13):1407-1408. PMID: 27629148

2. Garg SK, Weinzimer SA, Tamborlane WV, et al. Glucose outcomes with the in-home use of a hybrid closed-loop insulin delivery system in adolescents and adults with type 1 diabetes. *Diabetes Technol Ther*. 2017;19(3):155-163. PMID: 28134564

3. Brown SA, Kovatchev BP, Raghinaru D, et al; IDCL Trial Research Group. Six-month randomized, multicenter trial of closed-loop control in type 1 diabetes. *N Engl J Med*. 2019;381(18):1707-1717. PMID: 31618560

4. Brown SA, Forlenza GP, Bode BW, et al; Omnipod 5 Research Group. Multicenter trial of a tubeless, on-body automated insulin delivery system with customizable glycemic targets in pediatric and adult participants with type 1 diabetes. *Diabetes Care*. 2021;44(7):1630-1640. PMID: 34099518

5. Foster NC, Beck RW, Miller KM, et al. State of type 1 diabetes management and outcomes from the T1D exchange in 2016-2018. *Diabetes Technol Ther*. 2019;21(2):66-72. PMID: 30657336

6. Miller KM, Foster NC, Beck RW, et al; T1D Exchange Clinic Network. Current state of type 1 diabetes treatment in the U.S.: updated data from the T1D exchange clinic registry. *Diabetes Care*. 2015;38:971-978. PMID: 25998289

7. Messer LH, Forlenza GP, Sherr JL, et al. Optimizing hybrid closed-loop therapy in adolescents and emerging adults using the MiniMed 670G system. *Diabetes Care*. 2018;41(4):789-796. PMID: 29444895

8. O'Malley G, Messer LH, Levy CJ, et al; iDCL Trial Research Group. Clinical management and pump parameter adjustment of the control-IQ closed-loop control system: results from a 6-month, multicenter, randomized clinical trial. *Diabetes Technol Ther*. 2021;23(4):245-252. PMID: 33155824

9. Berget C, Sherr JL, DeSalvo DJ, et al. Clinical implementation of the Omnipod 5 automated insulin delivery system: key considerations for training and onboarding people with diabetes. *Clinical Diabetes*. 2022;40(2):168-184.

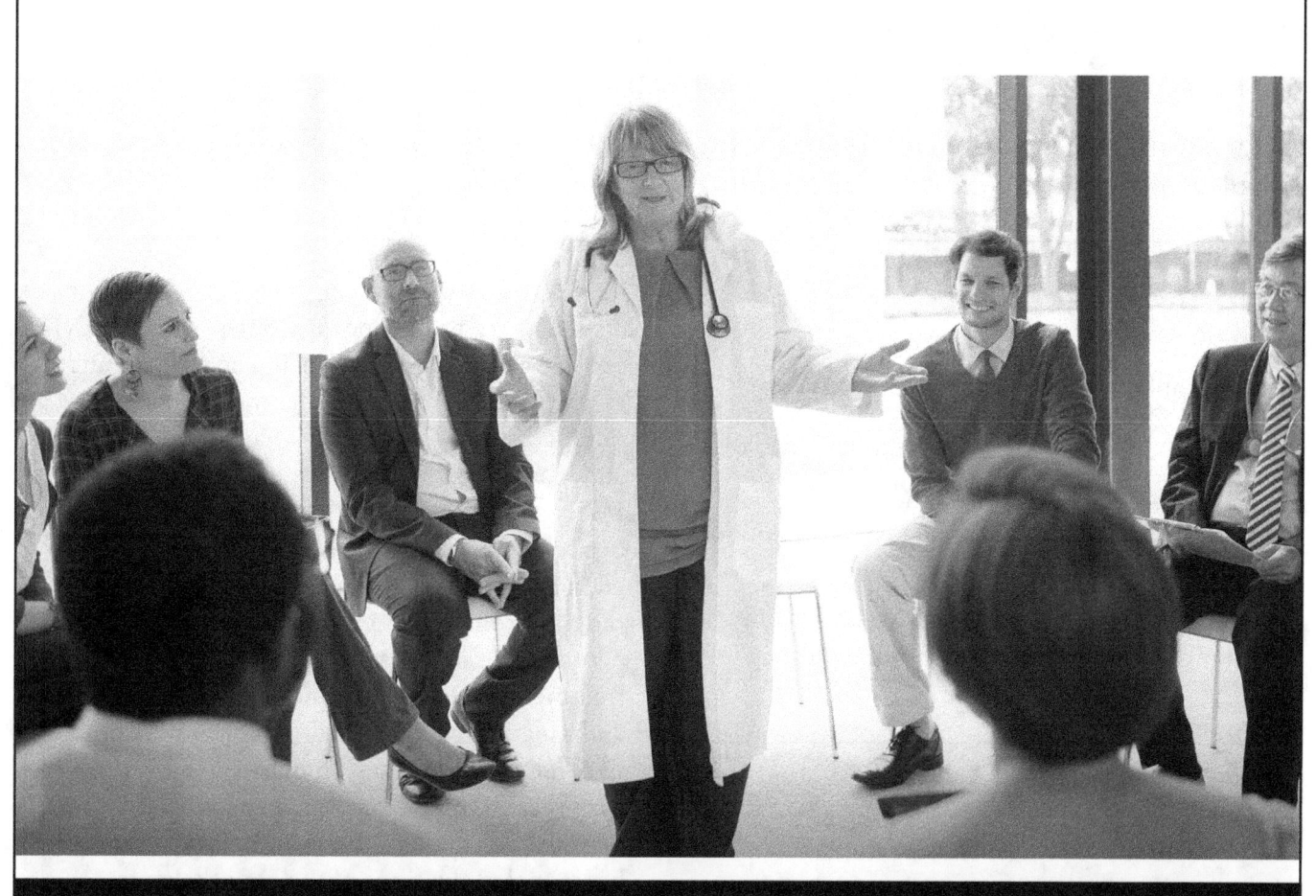

NEUROENDOCRINOLOGY AND PITUITARY

Perioperative Management of Pituitary Adenomas

Ismat Shafiq, MD. Division of Endocrinology and Metabolism, University of Rochester, NY; E-mail: Ismat_shafiq@urmc.rochester.edu

Learning Objectives

As a result of participating in this session, learners should be able to:

- Perform preoperative assessment and manage pituitary hormonal dysfunction.

- Explain the need for intraoperative stress-dose glucocorticoid treatment.

- Assess pituitary function postoperatively in functional and nonfunctional adenomas.

Main Conclusions

The perioperative management of pituitary adenomas requires an experienced multidisciplinary team that includes an endocrinologist, neuroophthalmologist, and neurosurgeon for optimal patient care. Appropriate preoperative assessment is crucial to guide perioperative and postoperative management decisions. All patients should have a thorough evaluation for hormonal overproduction and deficiencies. Close monitoring for adrenal insufficiency (AI), diabetes insipidus (DI), and syndrome of inappropriate antidiuretic hormone secretion (SIADH)/hyponatremia is necessary in the early postoperative period.

Significance of the Clinical Problem

Pituitary adenomas are benign intracranial neoplasms that are categorized based on functional status or size. Functional adenomas include cortisol-producing adenomas (Cushing disease), GH-producing adenomas (acromegaly), prolactinomas, TSH-producing adenomas, and rare FSH/LH-producing adenomas. Pituitary microadenomas are smaller than 10 mm, and macroadenomas are larger than 10 mm. Macroadenomas larger than 40 mm are giant tumors. Population-based studies have indicated an increase in the incidence of pituitary adenomas ranging from about 3.9 to 7.4 cases per 100,000 per year.[1] Transsphenoidal surgery is the primary treatment for large nonfunctioning adenomas and functioning adenomas except prolactinomas.[2] Crowder et al reported an increase in pituitary surgeries from 26.7 to 36.2 per million per year over the last decade.[3] Thorough preoperative hormonal evaluations of the hypothalamic-pituitary axis are imperative to guide management decisions during the perioperative and postoperative periods. The postoperative period requires close monitoring for AI, DI, and hyponatremia/SIADH to prevent mortality.

Barriers to Optimal Practice

- Limited and variable information to identify appropriate treatment strategies for pituitary adenomas in the perioperative period.

- Limited experience of endocrinologists and neurosurgeons managing pituitary adenomas in hospitals with a low volume of patients with these tumors.

Strategies for Diagnosis, Therapy, and/or Management

Preoperative Evaluation and Management

According to society guidelines and consensus statements, all patients with pituitary incidentalomas should undergo laboratory evaluation for hormone excess and deficiency.[2,4,5] The initial preoperative workup of pituitary adenomas should include evaluation for hormone excess and hormone deficiency.

Evaluation for Hormone Excess

Measuring serum prolactin is crucial to exclude a prolactinoma, as medical therapy with dopamine agonists is the first-line treatment for this type of tumor. Serum prolactin levels generally correspond to the tumor size. A serum prolactin concentration greater than 250 ng/mL (>10.9 nmol/L) suggests a macroprolactinoma. There may be a discrepancy between tumor size and prolactin level in the setting of cystic adenoma and assay artifact. If the prolactin concentration is between 20 and 200 ng/dL (0.9 and 8.7 nmol/L) in a patient with a macroadenoma, consider obtaining serum prolactin in serial dilution to assess for evaluation of a falsely low level due to the hook effect in the assay, especially in patients with giant tumors. Current prolactin immunoassays are sensitive, and falsely low prolactin levels are infrequently observed.[6]

IGF-1 should be measured for GH assessment. If the IGF-1 is equivocal, further confirmation tests can be performed in selected patients.

Glucocorticoid excess should be evaluated by measuring salivary cortisol on 2 consecutive nights or by 24-hour urine collection for free cortisol excretion or a 1-mg overnight dexamethasone-suppression test.

Evaluation for Hormone Deficiency

Current guidelines recommend evaluation for hypopituitarism in all patients with pituitary adenomas.

Measurement of basal serum cortisol at 8:00 AM is an easy and reliable way to assess the hypothalamic-pituitary-adrenal axis (HPA), and it should be done in all patients with pituitary adenomas. A morning serum cortisol concentration between 8 and 15 µg/dL (220 and 413 nmol/L) suggests an intact HPA axis. A morning serum cortisol concentration less than 3 µg/dL (<83 nmol/L) confirms AI. A serum cortisol concentration less than 8 µg/dL (<220 nmol/L) warrants further investigation with a cosyntropin-stimulation test (CST). A normal CST result is defined by an increase in cortisol greater than 18 µg/dL (>500 nmol/L) after injection of 250 mcg of an ACTH analogue. All patients with adrenal insufficiency should be started on glucocorticoid replacement preoperatively. The standard dosages for glucocorticoid replacement are prednisone, 5 to 7.5 mg daily, or hydrocortisone, 15 to 30 mg daily.[7-10] At our pituitary center, we use prednisone, 5 mg, or hydrocortisone, 15 mg, in divided doses preoperatively in patients diagnosed with AI.

Free T_4 should be measured in patients with pituitary adenomas. TSH measurement is not a reliable test in patients with pituitary disease, and the result can be low, normal, or minimally elevated. The Endocrine Society recommends treating all patients with central hypothyroidism preoperatively. Emerging data suggest treating patients based on the degree of hypothyroidism. The degree of hypothyroidism defines perioperative risk and mortality. Perioperative treatment with levothyroxine is recommended for patients with severe hypothyroidism (myxedema coma, severe symptoms of hypothyroidism, free T_4 <0.5 ng/dL [<6.4 pmol/L]) to avoid cardiac and respiratory compromise, postoperative ileus, and hyponatremia. Preoperative treatment may not be necessary for mild to moderate hypothyroidism since studies have not shown any difference in mortality or cardiovascular outcomes.[11-13] However, given the paucity of data, the decision to treat patients with central hypothyroidism should be individualized based on history, symptoms, and other comorbidities.

IGF-1 should be measured to assess for GH deficiency. GH deficiency does not warrant further preoperative testing or treatment.

Evaluation of gonadal function depends on the patient's sex and age. There is no need to measure gonadotropins in premenopausal women with regular periods. In premenopausal women with irregular menses, LH, FSH, and estradiol can be used to screen for hypogonadotropic hypogonadism. FSH measurement in postmenopausal women can be helpful, as low levels suggest hypopituitarism. Morning testosterone and gonadotropin levels should be measured in all men. Treatment of hypogonadism can be deferred until 3 months after surgery if it persists.

DI is rare in patients with pituitary adenomas. DI is common in craniopharyngiomas, hypophysitis, and metastatic disease. In patients with polyuria and polydipsia, a diagnosis can be established by measuring serum sodium and urine osmolality. DI should be suspected if the serum sodium concentration is at or greater than 145 mEq/L (≥145 mmol/L) with urine osmolality less than 100 mOsm/kg. Preoperative medical treatment with desmopressin can be considered to relieve symptoms in selected patients.

Intraoperative Management

Glucocorticoid management at the time of surgery varies among local practices. The main questions when considering glucocorticoid management are: (1) who should receive stress-dose steroids preoperatively and (2) what is the optimal glucocorticoid stress dose?

Historically, intraoperative empiric "stress-dose" glucocorticoids have been given to all patients undergoing pituitary surgery to prevent adrenal crisis. Several clinical studies have demonstrated that intraoperative stress-dose steroids are not necessary in patients with an intact HPA axis.[14-16] At our institution, we do not give stress-dose steroids preoperatively to patients with a preserved HPA axis. Intraoperative stress-dose glucocorticoids are advisable in patients with known or suspected adrenal insufficiency.

Glucocorticoid stress dosing varies among practices. Inder et al recommend using hydrocortisone, 50 mg every 8 hours, with rapid tapering to a physiologic dose within 48 hours. The use of dexamethasone, 4 mg, on the day of surgery followed by a quick taper has also been suggested.[16] Others have used hydrocortisone, 30 mg intravenously every 8 hours, on the day of surgery with a taper in the next 48 hours. At our center, all patients receive dexamethasone, 4 mg, as stress-dose glucocorticoids during anesthesia induction.

Postoperative Evaluation and Management

Postoperative follow-up includes assessment of the HPA axis, monitoring DI and/or hyponatremia, assessing the thyroid/gonadal axis, and evaluating functional adenoma.[13]

HPA Axis

The Pituitary Society Delphi panel recommends checking basal morning cortisol levels 1 to 5 days postoperatively to evaluate the HPA axis. Published studies have measured basal morning cortisol on the first postoperative day. The threshold for a normal morning serum cortisol value in this context varies among studies. A morning serum cortisol concentration of 8 to 15 μg/dL (220 to 413 nmol/L) generally suggests an intact HPA axis.

- In patients with an intact HPA axis preoperatively, we check morning cortisol on postoperative day 1. We currently use a cortisol cutoff of 10 μg/dL (275 nmol/L) to define intact HPA axis, in contrast to a cutoff of 14 μg/dL (386 nmol/L) in our previously published study.[17] We have not noticed any change in postoperative outcomes using the lower cortisol cutoff. If the morning cortisol concentration is greater than 10 μg/dL (>275 nmol/L), patients are not discharged on any glucocorticoids. If the morning cortisol concentration is less than 10 μg/dL (<275 nmol/L), patients are started on prednisone, 5 mg daily. Morning cortisol is checked on postoperative day 5 to reassess the HPA axis and to assess the need for glucocorticoid replacement.

- In patients with a preoperative cortisol concentration less than 10 µg/dL (<275 nmol/L)/AI, hydrocortisone, 20 mg twice daily, is given on postoperative day 1; the dosage is then decreased to 10 mg twice daily on postoperative day 2, followed by hydrocortisone 10 mg/5 mg. We measure morning cortisol 1 to 2 weeks later, after holding hydrocortisone for 24 hours. An attempt is made to decrease the hydrocortisone dosage or reassess soon if the morning cortisol concentration is greater than 10 µg/dL (>275 nmol/L). If the morning cortisol concentration remains less than 10 µg/dL (<275 nmol/L), glucocorticoid replacement is continued. Three months postoperatively, dynamic testing is performed to evaluate the HPA axis.

Diabetes Insipidus

The postsurgical triphasic response includes transient DI, followed by SIADH/hyponatremia, and then permanent DI.

- The initial DI phase is from surgical traction and disruption of the nerve terminal at the posterior pituitary leading to polyuria and polydipsia. The DI phase is most common and occurs in about 25% to 30% of patients. Most DI resolves spontaneously within 7 days. Close monitoring of patient symptoms, fluid intake, urine output, and serial plasma sodium with urine osmolarity is paramount for early diagnosis in the postoperative period. At our center, we monitor patient symptoms and perform laboratory assessment if urine output is greater than 200 cc/h for 3 hours. We routinely measure serum sodium and urine osmolality on postoperative day 1 in all patients after surgery. We instruct the patient to drink to thirst in the immediate postoperative period. Most patients do not need any medical treatment because they have intact thirst mechanisms. In selected patients with a serum sodium concentration greater than 145 mEq/L (>145 mmol/L), desmopressin, 0.10 mg (oral dose), is given to relieve symptoms at night. Alternatively, desmopressin, 1 to 2 mcg subcutaneously, can be used. Intranasal desmopressin is often avoided immediately after surgery due to nasal congestion. A continuous desmopressin dose is not favored, as DI is transient and may be followed by the second phase of SIADH.[13,18,19]

- SIADH may occur independently from DI. The hyponatremia associated with SIADH is due to the aberrant release of ADH, surgical manipulation of the gland, untreated adrenal insufficiency, and central hypothyroidism. SIADH generally occurs 5 to 7 days after surgery and lasts 14 days. The incidence varies from 1.8% to 25%. At our institution, we measure serum sodium on postoperative day 6. Most cases of SIADH-induced hyponatremia are mild and treated with fluid restriction. Severe hyponatremia is defined as a sodium level less than 125 mEq/L (<125 mmol/L). The management of severe hyponatremia requires hospital admission and treatment with fluid restriction, sodium tablets, and/or hypertonic saline.[13,18,19]

- The third phase is DI again, which can be permanent. Chronic DI is present in 2% of patients after pituitary surgery. The treatment aim is to reduce symptoms of polyuria and polydipsia. Desmopressin should be used at the lowest possible dosage with a goal serum sodium value greater than 140 mEq/L (>140 mmol/L). Oral tablets (dose ranges from 0.1 to 0.2 mg tablets) or nasal spray (10 mcg) can be used for long-term replacement in divided doses. We generally recommend patients hold off desmopressin 1 day a week to assess for spontaneous late recovery from DI.[18,19]

Postoperative Evaluation and Management of Thyroid and Gonadal Axis

- Thyroid axis: The consensus is to check thyroid function 6 to 8 weeks after pituitary surgery. At our institution, we assess thyroid function 2 weeks after surgery.

- Gonadal axis: The guidelines recommend checking the gonadal axis 6 to 12 weeks after surgery. At our institution, we evaluate patients 12 weeks postoperatively.

Postoperative Evaluation and Management in Patients With Functioning Adenomas

- Prolactinomas: Surgery is recommended for patients with prolactinomas for whom medical treatment fails. Dopamine agonists are usually held the day before surgery in patients with macroprolactinomas. The serum prolactin level may be checked on postoperative day 1 or 2 to evaluate for remission. A prolactin concentration less than 10 ng/mL (<0.43 nmol/L) is suggestive of cure, especially in the setting of a microadenoma.[6,20]

- Acromegaly: GH may be measured postoperatively for evaluation, although the cutoff to define remission is unclear. IGF-1 takes longer to normalize, so it should be measured 6 to 12 weeks postoperatively.

- Cushing disease: Serum morning cortisol is measured postoperatively to see if a patient is in remission. Disease remission is defined as a serum cortisol concentration less than 5 µg/dL (<138 nmol/L), preferably less than 2 µg/dL (<55 nmol/L) in the immediate postoperative period. Persistent disease should be suspected if the morning cortisol concentration is greater than 5 µg/dL (>138 nmol/L).[21] A small subset of patients may develop hypocortisolemia in the late postoperative period. The decision to start glucocorticoids varies from center to center. Most experts recommend starting glucocorticoid treatment if the cortisol concentration is less than 5 µg/dL

(<138 nmol/L). If the value is greater than 5 µg/dL (>138 nmol/L), close monitoring with serial serum cortisol measurements is recommended. Some pituitary centers start glucocorticoids regardless of the cortisol value to avoid the risk of AI. At our institution, we measure morning cortisol and ACTH on postoperative day 1. We generally treat with glucocorticoids if the morning value is less than 10 µg/dL (<275 nmol/L). Hydrocortisone, 30 mg in divided doses, is initially prescribed, followed by a drop of 5 mg every 2 weeks.

Clinical Case Vignettes
Case 1

A 66-year-old woman has peripheral vision loss on routine eye examination. Neuropathology examination confirms bitemporal visual field defects. MRI reveals a 3.2-cm pituitary adenoma with suprasellar extension and compression of the optic apparatus.

Laboratory test results:

> Prolactin = 57.8 ng/mL (4-30 ng/mL)
>   (SI: 2.51 nmol/L [0.17-1.30 nmol/L])
> Cortisol (8 AM) = 12.6 µg/dL (5.0-25 µg/dL)
>   (SI: 347.6 nmol/L [137.9-689.7 nmol/L])
> Free T$_4$ = 0.8 ng/dL (0.8-1.8 ng/dL)
>   (SI: 10.3 pmol/L [10.30-23.17 pmol/L])
> IGF-1 = 71 ng/mL (67-195 ng/mL)
>   (SI: 9.3 nmol/L [8.8-25.5 nmol/L])

Her gonadotropin levels are inappropriately low for menopause.

Medications include sertraline, 50 mg daily, and a multivitamin.

On physical examination, her blood pressure is 159/83 mm Hg, pulse rate is 63 beats/min, and BMI is 35.19 kg/m².

A nonfunctioning pituitary adenoma is diagnosed.

In preparation for surgery, the patient should be treated with which of the following?

A. Hydrocortisone

B. Hydrocortisone and levothyroxine

C. Levothyroxine

D. No changes

Answer: C) Levothyroxine

This patient has a nonfunctioning pituitary adenoma with evidence of multiple axis insufficiency in the form of inappropriately low sex hormones for menopause and mild central hypothyroidism. The morning cortisol concentration is greater than 10 μg/dL (>275 nmol/L) and there is no clinical evidence of AI. Thus, preoperative glucocorticoid treatment (Answers A and B) is not necessary. The Endocrine Society guidelines and the Pituitary Society Delphi panel recommend treating patients with central hypothyroidism (thus, Answer C is correct and Answer D is incorrect). However, some experts may decide to monitor patients with mild hypothyroidism because the risk of developing cardiac or respiratory problems is low in a patient with mild to moderate hypothyroidism.

Case 2

A 38-year-old woman has an incidental 1.5-cm pituitary macroadenoma found on imaging for evaluation of headaches.

Preoperative laboratory test results:

> Prolactin = 52.2 ng/mL (4-30 ng/mL)
>   (SI: 2.27 nmol/L [0.17-1.30 nmol/L])
> Free T_4, normal
> Cortisol (8 AM), normal

She has an intrauterine device for contraception. She underwent transsphenoidal surgery, with final pathology showing gonadotroph cell type adenoma.

Postoperative laboratory test results:

> Cortisol (8 AM) = 28 μg/dL (5.0-25 μg/dL)
>   (SI: 772.5 nmol/L [137.9-689.7 nmol/L])
> Sodium = 140 mEq/L (136-142 mEq/L)
>   (SI: 140 mmol/L [136-142 mmol/L])
> Urine osmolality = 187 mOsm/kg
>   (150-1150 mOsm/kg) (SI: 187 mmol/kg
>   [150-1150 mmol/kg]) (with symptoms of
>   polyuria)

She is not treated with desmopressin.

Which of the following is the best next step in this patient's care?

A. Advise fluid restriction

B. Follow-up in 2 weeks in the clinic

C. Measure serum sodium on postoperative day 5 to 7

D. Prescribe desmopressin at bedtime and advise to use if symptomatic

Answer: C) Measure serum sodium on postoperative day 5 to 7

SIADH-related hyponatremia is one of the reasons for hospital admission following pituitary surgery. Symptoms vary depending on the degree of hyponatremia. The common symptoms with mild to moderate hyponatremia are headaches, confusion, weakness, nausea, and decreased appetite. SIADH usually occurs 5 to 7 days after transsphenoidal surgery; thus, following up in 2 weeks (Answer B) is incorrect. According to society guidelines, serum sodium levels should be measured on postoperative day 5 to 7 (Answer C). DI is transient and is expected to resolve spontaneously; thus, medical therapy with desmopressin (Answer D) should be avoided to prevent hyponatremia. Fluid restriction alone (Answer A) would not be helpful in managing hyponatremia.

Case 3

A 36-year-old woman with a left 1.4-cm adrenal incidentaloma is found to have an elevated cortisol concentration of 9.1 μg/dL (251.0 nmol/L) after 1 mg of dexamethasone is administered at 11:00 PM.

Laboratory test results:

> Salivary cortisol measurements (11:00 PM-
> 12:00 AM) = 0.17, 0.16, 0.13 µg/dL)
> (<0.13 µg/dL) (SI: 4.7 nmol/L, 4.4 nmol/L,
> 3.6 nmol/L [<3.6 nmol/L])
> Urinary cortisol = 85 µg/24 h (4-50 µg/24 h)
> (SI: 234.6 nmol/d [11-138 nmol/d])
> ACTH = 123 pg/mL (10-60 pg/mL)
> (SI: 12.1 pmol/L [2.2-13.2 pmol/L])

She undergoes transsphenoidal surgery, and the final pathology describes a pituitary adenoma, with densely granulated corticotroph (ACTH) cells.

Postoperative laboratory test results:

> ACTH = 28 pg/mL (10-60 pg/mL)
> (SI: 6.2 pmol/L [2.2-13.2 pmol/L])
> Cortisol = 11.3 µg/dL (5.0-25 µg/dL)
> (SI: 311.7 nmol/L [137.9-689.7 nmol/L])

Which of the following is the best next step?

A. Initiation of glucocorticoid replacement

B. Radiation treatment

C. Repeated surgery

D. Serial serum morning cortisol measurement with instructions to call if symptoms of AI develop

Answer: D) Serial serum morning cortisol measurement with instructions to call if symptoms of AI develop

Delayed remission is described in patients with Cushing disease after surgery. Frequent monitoring of morning cortisol with detailed information on signs and symptoms of AI is recommended (Answer D). It is advised to discharge the patient with hydrocortisone or prednisone with instructions to start glucocorticoids if symptoms develop during a weekend or if she does not have access to the laboratory.

Glucocorticoid treatment is initated when the serum cortisol concentration is less than 5 µg/dL (<138 nmol/L) after pituitary surgery in patients with Cushing disease (thus, Answer A is incorrect).

Repeated surgery (Answer C) and radiation treatment (Answer B) are indicated in patients with persistent hypercortisolemia after initial surgery, which is too soon to assess immediately after surgery.

References

1. Daly AF, Beckers A. The epidemiology of pituitary adenomas. *Endocrinol Metab Clin North Am.* 2020;49(3):347-355. PMID: 32741475

2. Freda PU, Beckers AM, Katznelson L, et al; Endocrine Society. Pituitary incidentaloma: an Endocrine Society clinical practice guideline. *J Clin Endocrinol Metab.* 2011;96(4):894-904. PMID: 21474686

3. Crowther S, Rushworth RL, Rankin W, Falhammar H, Phillips LK, Torpy DJ. Trends in surgery, hospital admissions and imaging for pituitary adenomas in Australia. *Endocrine.* 2018;59(2):373-382. PMID: 29103185

4. Fleseriu M, Bodach ME, Tumialan LM, et al. Congress of Neurological Surgeons systematic review and evidence-based guideline for pretreatment endocrine evaluation of patients with nonfunctioning pituitary adenomas. *Neurosurgery.* 2016;79(4):E527-E529. PMID: 27635959

5. Tritos NA, Fazeli PK, McCormack A, et al; Pituitary Society Delphi Collavorative Group. Pituitary Society Delphi Survey: an international perspective on endocrine management of patients undergoing transsphenoidal surgery for pituitary adenomas. *Pituitary.* 2022;25(1):64-73. PMID: 34283370

6. Melmed S, Casanueva FF, Hoffman AR, et al; Endocrine Society. Diagnosis and treatment of hyperprolactinemia: an Endocrine Society clinical practice guideline. *J Clin Endocrinol Metab.* 2011;96(2):273-288. PMID: 21296991

7. Karaca Z, Tanriverdi F, Atmaca H, et al. Can basal cortisol measurement be an alternative to the insulin tolerance test in the assessment of the hypothalamic-pituitary-adrenal axis before and after pituitary surgery? *Eur J Endocrinol.* 2010;163(3):377-382. PMID: 20530552

8. Montes-Villarreal J, Perez-Arredondo LA, Rodriguez-Gutierrez R, et al. Serum morning cortisol as a screening test for adrenal insufficiency. *Endocr Pract.* 2020;26(1):30-35. PMID: 31461355

9. Gasco V, Bima C, Geranzani A, et al. Morning serum cortisol level predicts central adrenal insufficiency diagnosed by insulin tolerance test. *Neuroendocrinology.* 2021;111(12):1238-1248. PMID: 33406519

10. Kumar R, Carr P, Wassif W. Diagnostic performance of morning serum cortisol as an alternative to short synacthen test for the assessment of adrenal reserve; a retrospective study. *Postgrad Med J.* 2020;98(1156):113-118. PMID: 33122342

11. Himes CP, Ganesh R, Wight EC, Simha V, Liebow M. Perioperative evaluation and management of endocrine disorders. *Mayo Clin Proc.* 2020;95(12):2760-2774. PMID: 33168157

12. Kohl BA, Schwartz S. Surgery in the patient with endocrine dysfunction. *Med Clin North Am.* 2009;93(5):1031-1047. PMID: 19665618

13. Woodmansee WW, Carmichael J, Kelly D, Katznelson L; AACE Neuroendocrine and Pituitary Scientific Committee. American Association of Clinical Endocrinologists and American College of Endocrinology Disease State Clinical Review: postoperative management following pituitary surgery. *Endocr Pract.* 2015;21(7):832-838. PMID: 26172128

14. Tohti M, Junyang L, Zhou Y, Yuebing H, Zhuang Y, Chiyuan M. Is perioperative steroid replacement therapy necessary for the pituitary adenomas treated with surgery? A systematic review and meta-analysis. *PLoS One.* 2015;10(3):e0119621. PMID: 25775019

15. Garcia-Luna PP, Leal-Cerro A, Rocha JL, Trujillo F, Garcia-Pesquera F, Astorga R. Evaluation of the pituitary-adrenal axis before, during, and after pituitary adenomectomy. Is perioperative glucocorticoid therapy necessary? *Acta Endocrinol (Copenh)*. 1990;122(1):83-88. PMID: 2154904

16. Inder WJ, Hunt PJ. Glucocorticoid replacement in pituitary surgery: guidelines for perioperative assessment and management. *J Clin Endocrinol Metab*. 2002;87(6): 2745-2750. PMID: 12050244

17. Manuylova E, Calvi LM, Vates GE, Hastings C, Shafiq. Morning serum cortisol level after transsphenoidal surgery for pituitary adenoma predicts hypothalamic-pituitary-adrenal function despite intraoperative dexamethasone use. *Endocr Pract*. 2015;21(8):897-902. PMID: 26121454

18. Whitaker SJ, Meanock CI, Turner GF, et al. Fluid balance and secretion of antidiuretic hormone following transsphenoidal pituitary surgery. A preliminary series. *J Neurosurg*. 1985;63(3):404-412. PMID: 4020468

19. Burke WT, Cote DJ, Penn DL, et al. Diabetes insipidus after endoscopic transsphenoidal surgery. *Neurosurgery*. 2020;87(5):949-955. PMID: 32503055

20. Amar AP, Couldwell WT, Chen JCT, Weiss MH. Predictive value of serum prolactin levels measured immediately after transsphenoidal surgery. *J Neurosurg*. 2002;97(2):307-314. PMID: 12186458

21. Rutkowski MJ, Breshears JD, Kunwar S, Aghi MK, Blevins LS. Approach to the postoperative patient with Cushing's disease. *Pituitary*. 2015;18(2):232-237. PMID: 25702104

Shifting Fluids: Syndrome of Inappropriate Antidiuretic Hormone Secretion and Diabetes Insipidus

Julia Kharlip, MD. Penn Pituitary Center, University of Pennsylvania, Philadelphia, PA;
E-mail: julia.kharlip@pennmedicine.upenn.edu

Learning Objectives

- Describe approaches to monitor for and prevent delayed hyponatremia following pituitary surgery.

- Evaluate and manage hyponatremia in patients with permanent central diabetes insipidus (DI).

- Recognize the importance of education for patients with permanent DI.

Main Conclusions

- Fluid restriction as a part of structured follow-up program is a promising approach to delayed hyponatremia after pituitary surgery.

- Severe hyponatremia can lead to neurologic sequalae requiring expedient therapy; however, this must be balanced against a risk of osmotic demyelination syndrome (ODS) with rapid overcorrection. Patients with chronic DI treated with desmopressin are at high risk for this dual-risk scenario at a time of gastrointestinal illness, trauma, procedures, or surgeries.

- Accurate diagnosis of DI is essential to avoid iatrogenic hyponatremia related to inappropriate desmopressin therapy.

Significance of the Clinical Problem

Delayed hyponatremia due to syndrome of inappropriate antidiuretic hormone secretion (SIADH) is the most common cause of readmission for patients undergoing pituitary surgery. While mild in most, SIADH is symptomatic and severe in some patients. It can be flanked by 2 transitions of fluid volume status when preceded and followed by DI, presenting a significant treatment challenge due to the rapidity of transitions.

Gastrointestinal illness in a patient chronically treated for central DI can lead to severe hyponatremia as a result of continued desmopressin administration. Once hyponatremia sets in, its treatment presents its own challenge of avoiding overly rapid correction and ODS.

Hyponatremia is common in patients chronically treated for DI, but it should always prompt an investigation for causes and treatment adjustment to eliminate it. For example, central DI can resolve in some patients with pituitary lesions or history of surgery and clinicians should stay attuned to this possibility to be prepared to discontinue therapy that puts the patient at risk for hyponatremia.

Barriers to Optimal Practice

• Clinical states of salt-water abnormalities often present at transition or when multiple derangements are present at once, creating diagnostic dilemmas.

• The rapid nature of autodiuresis that follows hyponatremia presents a significant management challenge to avoid ODS even in the critical care setting. Accurate input/output monitoring is required, as well as exceedingly rapid access to laboratory data and significant investment of time and expertise. This challenge is magnified in patients with DI due to a potential for an even greater degree of sodium rise if DI is left untreated.

Strategies for Diagnosis, Therapy, and/or Management

Delayed Hyponatremia

Delayed hyponatremia due to SIADH is the most common cause of hospital readmission for patients undergoing pituitary surgery.[1-3] A recent meta-analysis of 27 studies found an incidence of overall and symptomatic delayed hyponatremia to be 10.5% (95% CI, 7.4%-14.7%) and 5.0% (95% CI, 3.6%-6.9%), respectively.[3]

Delayed hyponatremia is preceded by DI in 3% to 4% of patients ("biphasic response") and is preceded by and followed by permanent DI ("triphasic response") in 1.1% patients.[2] The shift from DI (the first phase) to SIADH (the second phase) commonly occurs rapidly over several hours on postoperative days 6 to 8,[1,4,5] so hyponatremia in this situation is always acute (<48 hours of duration). The treatment approach mirrors that of other causes of SIADH and depends on the presence of alterations in mental status as seen in patients with severe hyponatremia (serum sodium <125 mEq/L [<125 mmol/L]) or mild to moderate hyponatremia (mild: 130-134 mEq/L [130-134 mmol/L]; moderate: 125-129 mEq/L [125-129 mmol/L]). While hypertonic saline must be used for severe hyponatremia accompanied

by depressed mental status, mild to moderate hyponatremia is treated with volume restriction or vaptans.[1,4,5] In most patients, treatment is weaned within days when SIADH resolves, but one must stay vigilant for the possibility of the third phase of DI to ensure that alert patients have free access to water and that DDAVP is available to prevent a rapid sodium rise.

Gastrointestinal Illness in Patients With Chronic DI

A shift to and from hypovolemic hyponatremia accompanies several clinical situations that are likely to arise in the lifetime of a patient chronically treated for DI: gastrointestinal illness, blood loss, and need for hospitalization/anesthesia are among most common.

Patient education is critical, and "sick-day rules" can be used for patients with DI, similar to those used for patients with adrenal insufficiency (*Box 1*).

Box 1. Patient Instructions for Self-Care in Case of Diabetes Insipidus During a Diarrheal Illness

1. **Early contact:** If you develop a diarrheal illness, please notify us early in the illness by calling the on-call line and stay in touch for the duration of the illness if managing at home.

2. **Hydration by mouth:** Please try to hydrate as much as possible with an electrolyte-rich fluid (Pedialyte, broth, or WHO oral rehydration solution, which can be made at home: http://www.rehydrate.org/ors/ort.htm).

3. **Stay vigilant for signs of severe dehydration:** Please keep an eye on your hydration status: you should be able to see bubbles of saliva under the tongue. Dry lips, coated tongue, small amounts of dark urine, or feeling dizzy are signs of dehydration. If starting to feel week, lethargic, or lightheaded, please head to the emergency department and call us when on the way, so we can communicate with your emergency care team.

4. **Desmopressin:** During dehydrated state from diarrhea, the requirement for desmopressin/DDAVP temporarily goes away/decreases.

   ◦ Please take your next scheduled DDAVP only at the time of "breakthrough"/when symptoms of diabetes insipidus symptoms return: high output of light-colored urine and significant thirst.

   ◦ Once you have breakthrough symptoms, please resume taking desmopressin/DDAVP without delay.

   ◦ If going to the emergency department, please bring desmopressin/DDAVP with you.

5. **Vomiting or febrile diarrheal illness:** A reminder that a vomiting or a febrile diarrheal illness always requires care at a medical facility.

Patients with a vomiting illness must be cared for at a medical facility because vomiting makes oral rehydration impossible. Patients who are otherwise well with self-limited diarrhea can be treated at home, but with a low threshold for transition to hospital care.

Patients with DI requiring hospitalization need close endocrine care for the duration of their hospital stay. Providing the emergency care staff with a letter or procedure/hospitalization recommendations for patients can facilitate safe care (*Box 2*). Patients with DI and hyponatremia are at risk for ODS during autodiuresis unless desmopressin is resumed in a timely fashion and free water is actively replaced. Considerations for hospitalized patients are shown in Box 3.

Box 2. Sample Procedure Letter for Patients With Diabetes Insipidus Requiring Anesthesia*

As you know, Ms/Mr. @NAME@ (@DOB@) has diabetes insipidus. This should not preclude her/him from having surgical procedures. I understand she/he is scheduled to undergo an outpatient procedure with you under general anesthesia.

Diabetes insipidus makes the patient sensitive to fluid shifts.

1. The patient should continue to take the oral desmopressin as prescribed the day before and the day of the procedure.

2. As the patient will be NPO from midnight prior to the procedure, I recommend that she/he be scheduled first thing in the morning to avoid being deprived of free water for too long.

3. A STAT sodium measurement should be checked prior to induction of anesthesia. Depending on duration of the procedure, sodium should be checked every 3 to 4 hours.

4. If the patient is excessively thirsty before the procedure or if the procedure will take longer than an hour, please consider giving her/him D5W1/2NS intravenously at a maintenance rate during the procedure.

5. Please avoid administration of hypotonic fluids when the patient is in an antidiuresis state (desmopressin had been given and the urine output is <200 mL/h)

6. If the patient's mental status does change at any time, I recommend checking a stat serum sodium level. After the procedure, she/he should have access to free water to drink to thirst.

These recommendations have been discussed with @name@.

Please do not hesitate to call me with any further questions.

Sincerely,

* Developed with Dr. Lauren Fishbein.

Box 3. Considerations for Hospitalized Patients With Diabetes Insipidus

- Encourage patients to bring desmopressin to the emergency department or hospital and allow physician-directed administration to avoid delays related to procuring the medication

- In case of severe hyponatremia (serum sodium <125 mEq/L [<125 mmol/L]):
  - Transfer patient to higher level of care for close sodium monitoring every 4 to 6 hours and strict input/output monitoring
  - Identify treatment strategy based on severity of hyponatremia and the presence of mental status change
  - Determine sodium goal of correction based on risk of osmotic demyelination syndrome
  - Correct any potassium deficits accounting for the expected sodium increase as part of the overall sodium goal of correction
  - Provide free access to water in awake patients and identify water replacement plan in patients experiencing autodiuresis
  - Hold desmopressin for shortest period needed to confirm autodiuresis:
    - We use urine output ≥500 mL over any 2 hours and bedside specific gravity <1.010 to resume desmopressin as long as the sodium measured within the previous 6 hours was at the low limit or normal
    - We order STAT sodium and urine osmolality prior to desmopressin to use for the next round of clinical decision-making*

*Others have described an approach concurrent with measures for hyponatremia and preventive desmopressin administration.[6]

Accurate Diagnosis of Central DI

Accurate diagnosis of central DI can be challenging, but it is critical to avoiding iatrogenic hyponatremia. In a patient with polyuria (urine output >3 L daily) and urine osmolality less than 800 mOsm/kg, DI can be diagnosed by either using a traditional water-deprivation or copeptin-based algorithm (*Figure*).

Clinical Case Vignettes

Case 1

A 54-year-old woman with a pituitary adenoma traveled out of state for transsphenoidal resection. Postoperatively, her urine output was 6 L per day, and she was given desmopressin on postoperative days 1 and 2. After discharge, she was staying at

Figure. Algorithm for Diagnosing Diabetes Insipidus

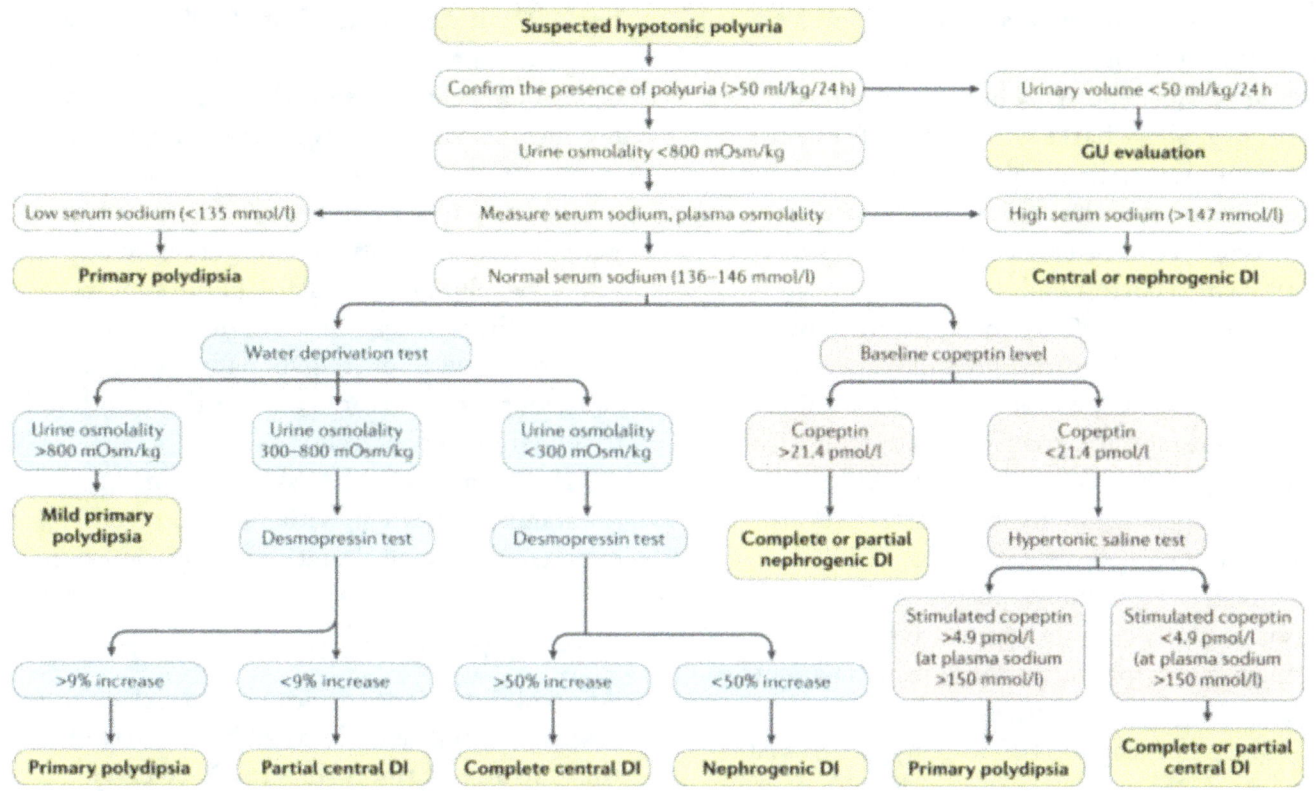

Reprinted with permission from Christ-Crain M et al. *Nat Rev Dis Primers*, 2019; 5(1) © Springer Nature Limited.

a local hotel in anticipation of her postoperative visit. She was drinking large amounts of water because her mouth was dry from mouth breathing due to nasal packing and the heat (the air conditioner at the hotel was broken). On postoperative day 7, she experiences headache, became rapidly obtunded, and is brought to the emergency department where her blood pressure is documented to be 148/76 mm Hg with a pulse rate of 72 beats/min. She appears euvolemic.

Laboratory test results:

> Serum sodium = 113 mEq/L (136-144 mEq/L)
> (SI: 113 mmol/L [136-144 mmol/L])
> Serum potassium = 4.1 mEq/L (3.6-5.1 mEq/L)
> (SI: 4.1 mmol/L [3.6-5.1 mmol/L])
> Rapid urine specific gravity by dipstick = 1.004
> (1.010-1.030)
> Cortisol, normal
> TSH, normal
> Free T$_4$, normal

In view of her recent history of postoperative DI, the report of marked thirst in recent days, and low specific gravity, the emergency department physician prescribes desmopressin.

Which of the following is the best next treatment step in addition to close monitoring of sodium and mental status in the intensive care unit setting?

A. Continue desmopressin

B. Stop desmopressin; initiate 3% saline until mental status improves

C. Stop desmopressin; initiate 800 mL fluid restriction

D. Stop desmopressin; initiate tolvaptan

E. B or D

Answer: B) Stop desmopressin; initiate 3% saline until mental status improves

This patient's hyponatremia on postoperative day 7 was not due to prior doses of desmopressin administered on postoperative days 1 and 2 given this medication's short half-life (12 to 24 hours). Her reportedly high water intake after hospital discharge was most likely due to dry mouth rather than polydipsia and had most likely exacerbated the degree of hyponatremia. Importantly, the observed specific gravity of 1.004 (which corresponds to a urine osmolality of approximately 190 mOsm/kg), while low, does not point to DI. A normal physiologic response to severe hyponatremia is production of maximally dilute urine (specific gravity, undetectable; urine osmolality <100 mOsm/kg). Thus, her low but detectible specific gravity in the face of severe hyponatremia is consistent with SIADH.

Given the timeline of postoperative day 7, this is most likely acute hyponatremia as part of a biphasic or triphasic response seen in patients undergoing pituitary surgery.[1-3]

Given her diagnosis of acute hyponatremia due to SIADH, continued treatment with desmopressin is contraindicated (thus, Answer A is incorrect). In patients with acute, severe hyponatremia (sodium <120 mEq/L [<120 mmol/L]) and depressed mental status, the primary goal of therapy is the expedient correction of sodium to restore consciousness.[8] The standard of care is administration of 3% saline as a bolus or continuous infusion with close sodium monitoring due to hypertonic saline's rapid efficacy and reliability. The initial goal of correction is a sodium level that restores consciousness (rather than to a specific increment or to a completely normal level). Otherwise well outpatients who recently underwent pituitary surgery are generally at low risk for ODS. While the exact degree of sodium correction needed to restore consciousness varies among patients, the range corresponds to 4 to 8 mEq/L (4 to 8 mmol/L) in the first 24 hours—the same conservative increment that is known to be safe for other patients who are not at very high risk for ODS. Once the SIADH phase resolves, these patients experience autodiuresis and even subsequent aquaresis if DI follows ("the third phase"), so it is important to ensure adequate access to water and desmopressin therapy (in the case of DI) if yet another shift of fluid status occurs.

Treating with fluid restriction only (Answer C) is not expeditious enough, as it is likely to produce a change of only several mEq/L (mmol/L) over days.

The role of vaptans (Answer D) in patients with SIADH after pituitary surgery is being actively explored, particularly in the context of using them instead of water deprivation for patients with severe hyponatremia once consciousness is restored and for those with mild to moderate hyponatremia.[5]

Hypertonic saline (Answer B) remains the standard of care in patients with severe hyponatremia with alteration of consciousness.

Case 1 (continued)

Appropriate steps to reduce the risk of readmission due to delayed hyponatremia include any of the following EXCEPT?

A. Daily phone contact with her treatment team during first postoperative week

B. Fluid restriction to 1 L during postoperative days 4 through 8

C. Laboratory measurement of serum sodium at a laboratory offering STAT processing on postoperative day 7

D. Patient education to (1) drink only to thirst once discharged and (2) to notify her treatment team immediately if symptoms of hyponatremia occur

E. Self-directed desmopressin administration by the patient at home

Answer: E) Self-directed desmopressin administration by the patient at home

Self-directed desmopressin administration by patients at home (Answer E) has not been studied as an approach to the management of postoperative diabetes insipidus and can potentially increase the risk of readmission due to delayed hyponatremia given a rapid transition from DI to the SIADH phase. The risk of delayed hyponatremia can be increased by inappropriate self-dosing by a patient as they enter the SIADH stage.[1,5,9] Timely discontinuation of desmopressin used during the first DI phase is important before the patient enters the SIADH stage, and it often requires daily contact with the patient recovering at home (as happens in patients treated on a fast-track discharge pathway, an approach used by some pituitary centers.[10]

Patient education regarding the risk of SIADH and its symptoms (Answer D), daily phone contact (Answer A), and routine sodium monitoring on postoperative days 7 or 8 (Answer C) have been described by several centers dedicated to pituitary surgery.[4,9-11] However, few factors have been consistently identified as risk factors for SIADH beyond patient age,[3] and given its precipitous onset, none of the described interventions have been able to reduce hospital readmission or prevent severe symptomatic hyponatremia.[9,11] A recently described approach of 1 L fluid restriction on postoperative days 4 to 8 (Answer B) for patients without preceding DI appears to reduce readmission rates[12] and will most likely become the prevailing strategy in managing these patients once there is a better understanding of the approach to the 5% to 6% of patients with preceding DI.[13] The fluid restriction approach does require close contact with patients during the first postoperative week, especially for those patients who are managed on a fast-track to discharge pathway.

Case 2

A 27-year-old woman with a history of childhood craniopharyngioma resection, hypopituitarism, and DI has just moved and seeks to establish endocrine care locally. She is on an appropriate regimen for hypopituitarism and takes desmopressin spray, 10 mcg each nostril twice daily. Review of her recent laboratory data shows appropriate free T_4 and IGF-1 levels and sodium concentrations ranging from 139 to 141 mEq/L (139 to 141 mmol/L).

She sends a portal message reporting a brief visit to a local emergency department (at the height of COVID-19 pandemic) for "adrenal insufficiency" in a setting of a diarrheal illness. She reports her blood pressure was in the 120s/80s mm Hg with a fast heart rate. She was given intravenous hydrocortisone for presumed adrenal insufficiency causing hyponatremia (sodium = 126 mEq/L [126 mmol/L]). Her potassium concentration was normal. She was subsequently discharged. Her COVID test result was negative, and no other cause of her diarrheal illness was identified. She is now at home, still feeling unwell, weak, and with continued diarrhea. She notes that her mouth feels very dry. She is pushing fluids (water) per emergency department recommendations.

In addition to increasing her oral hydrocortisone dosage (to account for rapid gastrointestinal transit) for the duration of her diarrheal illness, which of the following is the most appropriate step to address her condition?

A. Consider use of an antidiarrheal agent because a bacterial cause of diarrhea is not suspected

B. Hold desmopressin spray until there is a clear breakthrough with increased thirst and frequency and volume of light-colored urine

C. Hydrate with a solute-containing liquids (Pedialyte, WHO homemade rehydration solution) until mouth/lips are no longer dry and there are bubbles of saliva under the tongue

D. Maintain close contact, monitor orthostatic blood pressure and heart rate at home, reassess sodium and urine osmolality/specific gravity in 24 to 48 hours provided there is a trend for clinical improvement, but have a low threshold to return to emergency department, particularly if she has difficulty tolerating oral intake, worsening lethargy, lightheadedness, or a long duration of hyponatremia is suspected

E. All of the above

Answer: E) All of the above

Hypovolemic hyponatremia is a well-recognized clinical scenario in the general population and is caused by the loss of gastrointestinal secretions, which are hypotonic. However, the increased risk of hyponatremia due to continued use of desmopressin despite hypovolemia is a common but underrecognized clinical scenario for patients with chronic DI.

Excessive loss of hypotonic solute via the gastrointestinal tract with concurrent water and desmopressin administration leads to disproportionate water retention and likely hyponatremia. At the time of intravascular depletion (such as due to gastrointestinal illness, excessive sweating, or blood loss), there is an increase in proximal sodium and water reabsorption, which leads to reduced delivery of water to collecting tubules that are under AVP control. Consequently, DI temporarily remits, and continued administration of desmopressin further leads to hyponatremia. Hence, desmopressin should be held (Answer B). Once intravascular volume is restored, (which at home can be achieved with oral hydration with solute-containing fluids [Answer C] in patients who are able to drink and are otherwise hemodynamically stable) the aquaresis resumes, indicated by the usual DI breakthrough symptoms of increased thirst and urination, and it is safe to resume desmopressin.

Importantly, this outpatient management approach is not appropriate for most patients because of risk of ODS following autocorrection and resumption of aquaresis, especially if resumption of desmopressin therapy is delayed.[8,14] Risk of ODS is especially high in patients with a serum sodium concentration less than 125 mEq/L (<125 mmol/L), hypokalemia, alcohol abuse, malnutrition, liver disease, poor health literacy, and lack of social support. Patients who are otherwise well, hemodynamically stable, able to hydrate orally, have access to solute-containing oral rehydration solutions, and have a short duration of diarrheal illness might be cautiously managed at home with close supervision and instructions to resume desmopressin right at breakthrough (Answer D).

By the time this patient's portal message was received, she was back in the emergency department (brought in by her husband due to lethargy), and she had a sodium concentration of 117 mEq/L (117 mmol/L). She, in fact, continued to take her desmopressin spray over the weekend "to avoid excessive urination in addition to diarrhea." In the hospital, she was managed by holding desmopressin and repleting intravascular volume. Her urine output was followed closely. Her sodium normalized. Once urine output was greater than 500 mL over 2 hours with a low bedside specific gravity, desmopressin was appropriately resumed (48 hours after hospital admission).

At a subsequent clinic telehealth visit, she was reminded to call the office on-call line at the time of an illness. "Sick-day rules" were reviewed for both adrenal insufficiency and DI, and she took a picture of the strategies to keep on her phone. Both she and her husband programmed the on-call phone number into their cell phones. A conversation with the emergency department colleague caring for her during her first admission would have most likely prevented the chain of the events that led to her severe hyponatremia.

Case 3

A 44-year-old woman with Cushing disease undergoes pituitary surgery. She is not cured but has now developed DI that persists past the immediate postoperative period. Subsequently, she undergoes bilateral adrenalectomy. Her regimen now includes hydrocortisone, 10 mg on awakening and 10 mg at 3 PM; fludrocortisone, 0.1 mg daily; and desmopressin tablets, 0.1 mg at bedtime and 0.05 mg at 10 AM.

On physical examination, her blood pressure is 127/75 mm Hg, pulse rate is 72 beats/min, and body surface area is 1.52 m².

Laboratory test results:

ACTH = 130 pg/mL (10-60 pg/mL)
(SI: 28.6 pmol/L [2.2-13.2 pmol/L])
Sodium = 137 mEq/L (136-144 mEq/L)
(SI: 137 mmol/L [136-144 mmol/L])
Potassium = 4.2 mEq/L (3.6-5.1 mEq/L)
(SI: 4.2 mmol/L [3.6-5.1 mmol/L])
Plasma renin activity = 0.3 ng/mL per h
(0.6-4.3 ng/mL per h)

Three years after the initial pituitary surgery, she reports she has been feeling well and her cushingoid physical findings have mostly resolved. She describes daily breakthrough symptoms of increased thirst with frequent urination of straw-colored urine between 7 PM and bedtime. While she finds these symptoms tolerable, over the past 6 months she has had 3 episodes of headache and nausea that led to emergency department visits. Review of these records reveals stable vital signs on arrival and a pattern of hyponatremia with a serum sodium concentration that ranges from 128 to 131 mEq/L (128 to 131 mmol/L). One episode occurred while presenting at a high-stakes professional dinner meeting that was causing much psychological stress. She recalls taking an extra dose of 0.05 mg of desmopressin that evening to eliminate breakthrough during the meeting.

Which of the following are the most likely cause(s) of her emergency department visits and the best approaches to address them?

A. Her headaches and nausea with associated hyponatremia represent acute adrenal insufficiency and should be addressed with an increased daily hydrocortisone dosage

B. Her severe headaches cause symptoms of acute adrenal insufficiency, including nausea and hyponatremia; these should be addressed with early pain control and appropriate stress doses of hydrocortisone

C. Her headaches and nausea are caused by hyponatremia due to an inadequate fludrocortisone dosage, which should be increased

D. Her headaches and nausea are caused by hyponatremia; the hyponatremia is caused by periodic excessive water and/or desmopressin intake

E. B and D

Answer: E) B and D

While this patient's presentation during emergency department visits may represent acute adrenal insufficiency due to a mismatch between physiologic stress related to painful headache and her daily hydrocortisone dosage, increasing her

daily hydrocortisone dosage (Answer A) that is appropriate for her body surface area and allows her to feel well on most days is not the right approach and would likely lead to overtreatment.

It is also unlikely that her fludrocortisone dosage is insufficient given her appropriate vital signs, appropriate sodium and potassium concentrations outside of these episodes, and plasma renin activity suggesting a plentiful fludrocortisone dosage. Thus, increasing her fludrocortisone dosage (Answer C) is incorrect.

Both a change in the approach to managing her headaches to prevent acute adrenal insufficiency (Answer B), as well as eliminating excessive water retention causing hyponatremia (Answer D) are plausible approaches that should be further explored.

Case 3 (continued)

The patient is seen by a headache specialist who prescribes an effective abortive regimen, and she is given instructions to take an additional hydrocortisone dose with the onset of headache. She is instructed to eliminate as-needed desmopressin self-dosing and is reminded "to drink only to thirst." She follows the instructions meticulously, but she has another 2 episodes over the next 4 months.

Which of the following is the best next step to address this patient's periodic hyponatremia?

A. Monitor sodium at regular intervals to determine whether hyponatremia occurs outside of these episodes and occurs while she is asymptomatic

B. Reduce the desmopressin dosage

C. Monitor intake and output via patient-provided timed logs

D. Give guidance regarding safe intake parameters

E. All of the above

Answer: E) All of the above

Because concerns related to acute adrenal insufficiency have now been excluded, all of the listed strategies (Answer E) can be used to try to address periodic hyponatremia related to suspected mismatch between water intake and desmopressin dosing. Periodic hyponatremia is not uncommon in patients chronically treated for DI and has been reported in up to one-third of patients,[15] but it should always be investigated and addressed. Although daily breakthrough to allow for release of any retained water is not routinely required for chronic care of patients with DI,[7] it is particularly surprising that this patient continues to experience hyponatremia despite reporting daily breakthrough symptoms.

Case 3 (continued)

Over the next 2 months, the patient's desmopressin dosage is reduced, and routine weekly monitoring of sodium is arranged. The patient is asked to provide intake and output logs, which show that input and output are well matched. She reports more uncomfortable breakthrough symptoms, as would be expected given the desmopressin dosage reduction, and yet hyponatremia is still noted during routine monitoring. The patient undergoes water-deprivation testing (*see Table*).

Based on the results of the water-deprivation test, which of the following is the best next step?

A. Administer a saline-stimulated copeptin test

B. Continue desmopressin at a lower dosage and impose a strict daily fluid intake limit

C. Continue desmopressin but at a lower dosage

D. Stop desmopressin; she no longer has DI

Answer: D) Stop desmopressin she no longer has DI

After approximately 8 hours of fluid deprivation, the patient's urine osmolality had reached more than 700 mOsm/kg and had plateaued over 3 successive measurements, at which point the calculated serum osmolality was 302 mOsm/kg. At that time, 2 mcg of subcutaneous DDAVP was administered, but the urine osmolality failed to increase more than 9% (~5% increase). These data are consistent with a normal concentrating ability.

Of note, plasma antidiuretic hormone, although appropriately processed and sent to a reference laboratory, returned undetectable at the beginning and at the end of test—a common false-positive result best explained by the high preanalytical instability of AVP (arginine vasopressin) in samples.[7,16]

In summary, results of this patient's water-deprivation test support intact concentrating ability and resolution of DI. In fact, amelioration or resolution of DI within years of pituitary

Time	Sodium	Serum osmolality	Urine osmolality	Urine output	Antidiuretic hormone	Other
8:46	139 mEq/L (SI: 139 mmol/L)	292 mOsm/kg	238 mOsm/kg	500 mL	<0.5 pg/mL	Weight: 80.7 kg
10:36	141 mEq/L (SI: 141 mmol/L)	295 mOsm/kg	291 mOsm/kg	400 mL		...
13:39	143 mEq/L (SI: 143 mmol/L)	295 mOsm/kg	586 mOsm/kg	300 mL		...
14:55	142 mEq/L (SI: 142 mmol/L)	295 mOsm/kg	743 mOsm/kg	325 mL		...
17:00	143 mEq/L (SI: 143 mmol/L)	293 mOsm/kg	719 mOsm/kg	175 mL	<0.5 pg/mL	Weight: 80 kg (<1% decrease)
19:00	141 mEq/L (SI: 141 mmol/L)	302 mOsm/kg	772 mOsm/kg	100 mL		19:41 2 mcg subcutaneous DDAVP
20:20	143 mEq/L (SI: 143 mmol/L)	292 mOsm/kg	818 mOsm/kg	50 mL		Protocol stopped

Antidiuretic hormone reference range: 0-6.9 pg/mL.

surgery or neurohypophysitis has been previously described.[17,18] This patient has been feeling well off desmopressin therapy (Answer D).

Continuing a lower dosage of desmopressin with or without fluid restriction (Answers B and C) would lead to hyponatremia.

A saline-stimulated copeptin test (Answer A) could have been used in this clinical circumstance instead of a water-deprivation test, but this was not available at the time of this patient's evaluation. Given the clear evidence of resolved DI, a saline-stimulated copeptin test would not add value.

References

1. Loh JA, Verbalis JG. Disorders of water and salt metabolism associated with pituitary disease. *Endocrinol Metab Clin North Am*. 2008;37(1):213-234, x. PMID: 18226738

2. Hensen J, Henig A, Fahlbusch R, Meyer M, Boehnert M, Buchfelder M. Prevalence, predictors and patterns of postoperative polyuria and hyponatraemia in the immediate course after transsphenoidal surgery for pituitary adenomas. *Clin Endocrinol (Oxf)*. 1999;50(4):431-439. PMID: 10468901

3. Lee C-C, Wang Y-C, Liu YT, Huang Y-C, et al. Incidence and factors associated with postoperative delayed hyponatremia after transsphenoidal pituitary surgery: a meta-analysis and systematic review. *Int J Endocrinol*. 2021;2021:6659152. PMID: 33936198

4. Bohl MA, Ahmad S, Jahnke H, Shepherd D, Knecht L, White WL, Little AS. Delayed hyponatremia is the most common cause of 30-day unplanned readmission after transsphenoidal surgery for pituitary tumors. *Neurosurgery*. 2016;78(1):84-90. PMID: 26348011

5. Kleindienst A, Georgiev S, Schlaffer SM, Buchfelder M. Tolvaptan versus fluid restriction in the treatment of hyponatremia resulting from SIADH following pituitary surgery. *J Endocr Soc*. 2020;4(7):bvaa068. PMID: 32666012

6. MacMillan TE, Tang T, Cavalcanti RB. Desmopressin to prevent rapid sodium correction in severe hyponatremia: a systematic review. *Am J Med*. 2015;128(12):1362.e15-24. PMID: 26031887

7. Christ-Crain M, Bichet DG, Fenske WK, et al. Diabetes insipidus. *Nat Rev Dis Primers*. 2019;5(1):54. PMID: 31395885

8. Verbalis JG, Goldsmith SR, Greenberg A, et al. Diagnosis, evaluation, and treatment of hyponatremia: expert panel recommendations. *Am J Med*. 2013;126(10 Suppl 1):S1-S42. PMID: 24074529

9. Bohl MA, Ahmad S, White WL, Little AS. Implementation of a postoperative outpatient care pathway for eelayed hyponatremia following transsphenoidal surgery. *Neurosurgery*. 2018;82(1):110-117. PMID: 28449052

10. Lobatto DJ, Vliet Vlieland TPM, van den Hout WB, et al. Feasibility, safety, and outcomes of a stratified fast-track care trajectory in pituitary surgery. *Endocrine*. 2020;69(1):175-187. PMID: 32361869

11. Deaver KE, Catel CP, Lillehei KO, Wierman ME, Kerr JM. Strategies to reduce readmissions for hyponatremia after transsphenoidal surgery for pituitary adenomas. *Endocrine*. 2018;62(2):333-339. PMID: 29961198

12. Winograd D, Staggers KA, Sebastian S, Takashima M, Yoshor D, Samson SL. An effective and practical fluid restriction protocol to decrease the risk of hyponatremia and readmissions after transsphenoidal surgery. *Neurosurgery*. 2020;87(4):761-769. PMID: 31993647

13. Perez-Vega C, Tripathi S, Domingo RA, et al. Fluid restriction after transsphenoidal surgery for the prevention of delayed hyponatremia: a systematic review and meta-analysis. *Endocr Pract*. 2021;27(9):966-972. PMID: 34265453

14. Achinger SG, Arieff AI, Kalantar-Zadeh K, Ayus JC. Desmopressin acetate (DDAVP)-associated hyponatremia and brain damage: a case series. *Nephrol Dial Transplant*. 2014;29(12):2310-2315. PMID: 25107337

15. Behan LA, Sherlock M, Moyles P, et al. Abnormal plasma sodium concentrations in patients treated with desmopressin for cranial diabetes insipidus: results of a long-term retrospective study. *Eur J Endocrinol*. 2015;172(3):243-250. PMID: 25430399

16. Morgenthaler NG. Struck J, Alonso C, Bergmann A. Assay for the measurement of copeptin, a stable peptide derived from the precursor of vasopressin. *Clin Chem*. 2006;52(1):112-119. PMID: 16269513

17. Nishizawa S, Ohta S, Oki Y. Spontaneous resolution of diabetes insipidus after pituitary stalk sectioning during surgery for large craniopharyngioma. Endocrinological evaluation and clinical implications for surgical strategy. *Neurol Med Chir (Tokyo)*. 2006;46(3):126-134; discussion 134-135. PMID: 16565582

18. Glynn N, O'Brien D, Agha A. Late recovery of cranial diabetes insipidus following pituitary surgery. *Horm Res Paediatr*. 2013;80(3):217-220. PMID: 24051558

Multiple Endocrine Neoplasia Type 1 Across the Lifespan

Maria Luisa Brandi, MD, PhD. FIRMO Foundation, Florence, Italy; E-mail: marialuisa@ marialuisabrandi.it

Learning Objectives

As a result of participating in this session, learners should be able to:

- Diagnose multiple endocrine neoplasia type 1 (MEN 1) and perform periodic clinical monitoring in young patients.

- Recognize classic and nonclassic tumors of MEN 1, as the latter are increasingly relevant in the course of the disease.

Main Conclusions

MEN 1 is a rare autosomal dominant disorder caused by alterations in the *MEN1* gene located on chromosome 11q13.[1] Patients with MEN 1 classically develop tumors of the endocrine glands and also nonendocrine neoplasia, with potential involvement of more than 20 organs.[1] The most harmful MEN 1–related tumors are pancreatic and gastroduodenal neuroendocrine tumors, thymic carcinoids, and adrenocortical carcinomas. Patients with MEN 1 have a decreased life expectancy. The disease has a long course; however, the late course of the disease, including causes of death, are not fully understood.

MEN 1 is often viewed exclusively as a disorder that is only symptomatic during adulthood. As a result, children and adolescents with MEN 1 may receive inadequate care because their signs and symptoms are misdiagnosed as unrelated to MEN 1. Because adverse consequences of lack of care are potentially permanent and progressive, this delay is harmful to patients.

We have identified key steps to assist clinicians in providing comprehensive care when treating this disorder. Acquiring the knowledge and skills to make an early diagnosis can mitigate the burden of MEN 1 for patients and their families.

Genetic testing of patients with a clinical diagnosis of MEN 1 can confirm the diagnosis. Genetic testing can identify asymptomatic family members carrying the *MEN1* pathogenic variant, as well as determine which family members can be excluded from clinical monitoring if they do not carry the *MEN1* pathogenic variant. Genetic testing can also help to recognize potential phenocopies that occur in 5% to 10% of families with MEN 1. The risk of developing malignant tumors justifies early recognition of the disease and early pharmacological or surgical treatments. Early diagnosis allows for early screening, thus decreasing morbidity and increasing quality of life and life expectancy. Moreover, young adults with MEN 1 face difficult family-planning decisions, as MEN 1 is an inherited disorder with the potential to be passed on to children. Genetic counseling and the option of in vitro fertilization with preimplantation genetic diagnosis are substantial undertakings for these patients.

The MEN 1 phenotype encompasses varying combinations of more than 20 different endocrine and nonendocrine tumor types. These are characterized by loss of heterozygosity at 11q13 in the tumor tissue (*Figure*). Endocrine tumors are diagnosed either by hormone measurements or imaging techniques. The clinical diagnosis of MEN 1 requires the presence of 2 or more of the following neoplasms in the proband: parathyroid gland tumors, anterior pituitary tumors, and duodeno-pancreatic neuroendocrine tumors. Other tumors associated with MEN 1 include thymus and lung neuroendocrine tumors, type 2 gastric neuroendocrine tumors, adrenocortical tumors, pheochromocytomas, facial angiofibromas, hibernomas, meningiomas, ependymomas, leiomyomas, lipomas, and breast cancer (increased risk in female patients). While lung neuroendocrine tumors, breast cancer, parathyroid carcinoma, and adrenocortical carcinoma are rare in patients with MEN 1, they are potentially deadly neoplasias.[1]

Significance of the Clinical Problem

MEN 1 is often viewed exclusively as a disorder expressed in adulthood and, as a result, children with MEN 1 may receive inadequate care because their symptoms are overlooked. Recent studies support the need for comprehensive screening for endocrine neoplasms during childhood to enable early tumor recognition and intervention before the development of adverse sequelae. However, in general, screening for MEN 1 begins relatively late in childhood.

MEN 1 is a complex disorder. The array of tumors linked to MEN 1 is constantly increasing.

Figure. Neoplasms associated with MEN 1.

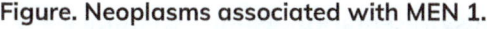

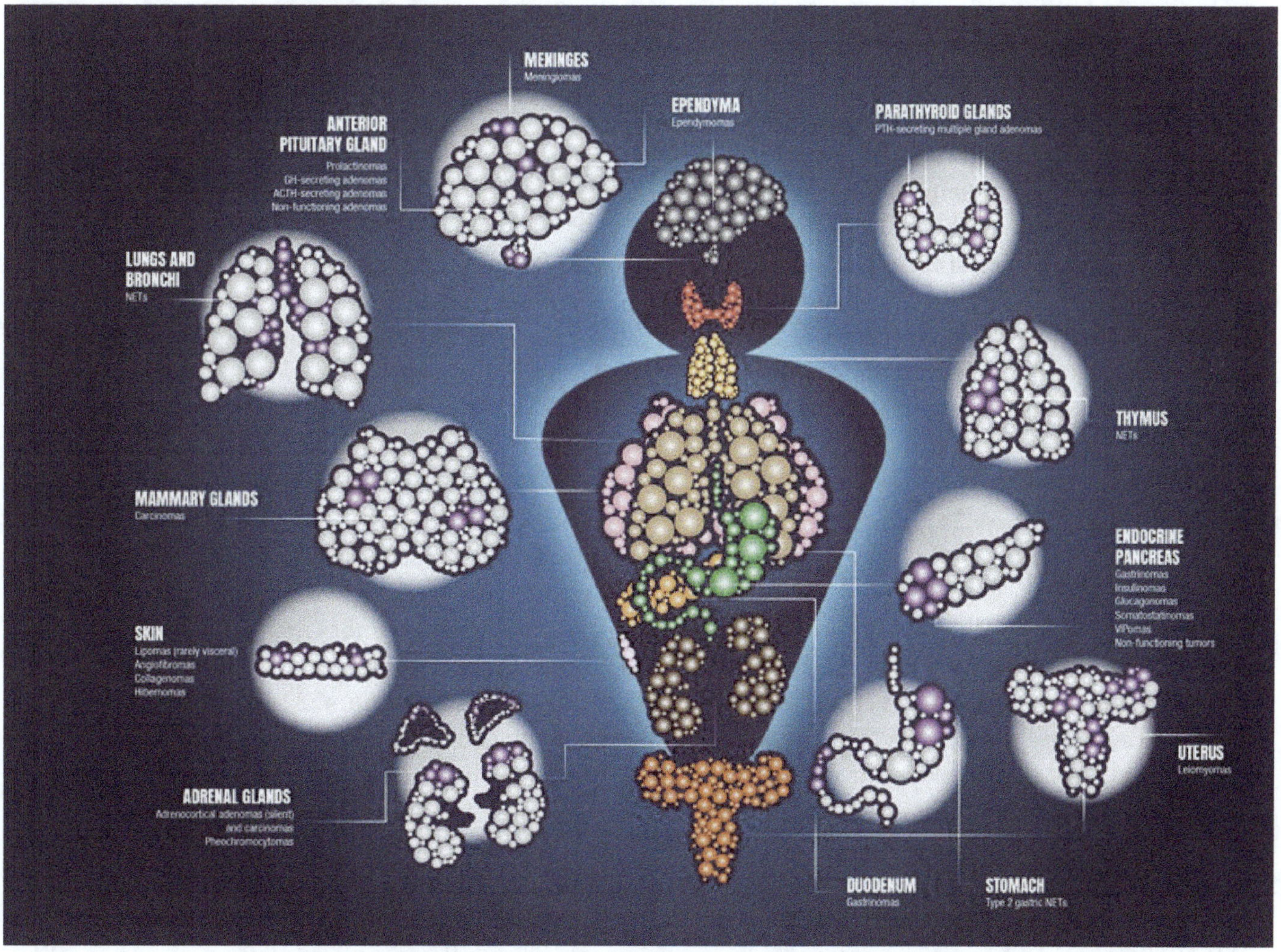

Adapted from Brandi M et al. Endocr Rev, 2021; 42(2) © Endocrine Society.

Physicians of different specialties must be educated to avoid missing the diagnosis. A practical MEN 1 chart should be developed and distributed to clinicians who may encounter patients with undiagnosed MEN 1. A basic understanding of MEN 1 as a condition affecting patients' whole bodies, lives, and families is the first step toward accomplishing improved patient care.

Barriers to Optimal Practice

The incidence of MEN 1 manifestations in childhood is not well characterized and may be underestimated. Moreover, there is lack of consensus regarding the optimal management of MEN 1–associated tumors in children. Finally, genetic testing should be performed at birth in children who have a parent with MEN 1, but this is not routinely done.

Constrained office visit time restricts clinicians from providing all-inclusive management of patients with MEN 1. Clinicians may feel pressured to focus on the most obvious MEN 1 manifestations, but they should be aware that patients are likely to experience additional ongoing MEN 1–related manifestations. Furthermore, given the complex nature of this disorder, not all manifestations of MEN 1 can be handled by the same specialist, risking disorganized communication among different departments. A checklist for testing for manifestations should be developed.

Strategies for Diagnosis, Therapy, and/or Management

The burden of MEN 1 influences the lives of patients' families, friends, and colleagues. Recognizing the disease at an early stage and evaluating the overall signs, symptoms, and complications with sustained attention to detail has the potential to reduce this disease burden. This requires continuous engagement from the informed patient.

In this Meet the Professor session dedicated to MEN 1 across the lifespan, clinicians will be educated on the importance of early disease recognition and on monitoring for various neoplasms during a patient's lifetime, as the disease is chronic and progressive. Patients require treatment regimens that prevent tumoral progression as early as possible. Early recognition of associated tumors can be achieved with well-designed follow-up that includes regular biochemical monitoring to assess endocrine status and radiological examinations to detect tumor development or growth. Understandably, not all endocrinologists are experts in every rare disease. Nonetheless, endocrinologists are likely to be the first health care provider to see patients with MEN 1, so their understanding of the nuances of this particular disorder can aid in its diagnosis and treatment. This includes awareness that MEN 1 also affects children and can have a highly heterogeneous presentation. Failure to unite a constellation of MEN 1 manifestations may result in delayed or incorrect diagnosis and inappropriate surgery or other treatments.

Disorders Linked to MEN1 Pathogenic Variants

MEN 1 is characterized by a large array of endocrine and nonendocrine tumors. Tumors attributed to the disorder are usually characterized by loss of heterozygosity at 11q13, the location of the *MEN1* gene, resulting in biallelic loss of *MEN1*. Tumors can be diagnosed by detection of hormonal oversecretion or by imaging.

Classic MEN 1–associated endocrinopathies include parathyroid tumors, pituitary tumors, and duodeno-pancreatic neuroendocrine tumors. Other endocrine tumors include thymus and lung neuroendocrine tumors, type 2 gastric neuroendocrine tumors, adrenocortical tumors, and pheochromocytomas. Nonendocrine tumors include collagenomas, hibernomas, facial angiofibromas, lipomas, meningiomas ependymomas, leiomyomas, and breast cancer. Screening should be conducted for all of these conditions as part of follow-up. Guidelines do not indicate the need for radiological or clinical examination by specialists (eg, dermatologists) with regard to nonendocrine tumors. Future guidance about management of MEN 1 will hopefully include this information.

Recently, the prevalence of hypercoagulability with increased risk of venous thromboembolism was shown to be higher in germline pathogenic variant–positive patients with MEN 1 relative to the general population.[2] Risk was similar to that found in patients with different types of cancer and Cushing syndrome. MEN 1–associated lifetime incidence rates are about 2-fold higher than the estimated incidence rate in the general population and are comparable to the known risk in the setting of various cancer types. Neuroendocrine tumors were present in 80% of the affected patient population, and 42% of patients experienced perioperative venous thromboembolism.[2]

Management of Children With MEN1 Pathogenic Variants

Parental MEN 1 was shown to be associated with high vulnerability of neonates, and this did not seem to correlate with antenatal maternal hypercalcemia.[1] Newborns whose parents have MEN 1 exhibit a number of complications, such as lower body weight, hypoglycemia, hypocalcemia, and increased postnatal mortality, mostly linked to infections. The excess risk was not fully explained by maternal MEN 1 or antenatal hypercalcemia.

The penetrance of MEN 1 manifestations is age-dependent, but this does not mean that children are never affected. Until recently, epidemiological and clinical information on MEN 1 in childhood was derived mainly from clinical case reports. Only in the last few years have there been publications that include screening data. While approximately 20% of affected patients are diagnosed with the disease in the first 2 decades of life, clinically relevant symptoms and signs are rare in children. In a recent retrospective analysis of 80 patients with MEN 1 who commenced tumor surveillance at 18 years or younger, 70% developed an endocrine tumor by age 18 years. These findings will affect counseling for young patients with MEN 1, underscoring the need to perform genetic testing and to start surveillance screening in early childhood.[3] The current guidelines, published in 2012, recommend phenotype screening in children by age 5 years, along with early genetic testing.[4] However, in a recent publication, a child was reported to be affected by primary hyperparathyroidism at age 4 years. Presymptomatic screening recommendations for patients with MEN 1 have been based on the youngest age at which disease manifestations have been described and this may not be the optimal timing, as disease signs in children can be overlooked.

Genetic testing in clinical practice has become widespread and is considered routine in tertiary medical centers. In a recent report, young patients with MEN 1 and an exon 2 pathogenic variant appear to have a 2-fold greater risk for developing both neuroendocrine tumor and distant metastasis.[5] However, genetic testing in the pediatric population is not without complexities and ethical challenges that must be considered. Early recognition of MEN 1 can prompt close monitoring for MEN 1–related neoplasms, hopefully resulting in decreased morbidity and mortality.

Primary hyperparathyroidism is often the first and most commonly observed endocrinopathy in young patients with MEN 1 (75%). Primary hyperparathyroidism in children with MEN 1 is usually asymptomatic, even if a higher incidence of rickets and osteomalacia is demonstrated in the pediatric population than in adults. Published data on parathyroidectomy in these patients are limited to adolescents. In any case, the parathyroidectomy should be subtotal to avoid secondary hypoparathyroidism. No data are available on the use of cinacalcet in children with MEN 1.

Pituitary tumors are the second most common tumor in young patients with MEN 1 (>30%), with the earliest documented manifestation at age 10 years. Prolactinomas are the most frequently diagnosed pituitary tumors in children with MEN 1. The possibility of progression to malignancy and resistance to dopamine therapy in some but not others represent important reasons to screen young patients with MEN 1.

Clinically relevant neuroendocrine tumors are rarely described in children with MEN 1, with the youngest patient diagnosed at age 8 years. However, the systematic use of endoscopic ultrasonography in patients with MEN 1 brought the occurrence of occult neuroendocrine tumors to 42% of pediatric cases. The aggressiveness of gastrinomas in children with MEN 1 and brain damage caused by hypoglycemia in the setting of insulinomas support the need for active surveillance for neuroendocrine tumors in children.

Children with MEN 1 who present with a single endocrine tumor should be evaluated through multiple imaging modalities for other potential endocrine tumors. Moreover, children who present with a tumor type described in MEN 1 (usually rare at young ages) should be tested for germline *MEN1* pathogenic variants.

In the last decade, several reports have indicated that morbidity is not uncommon in children and young adults affected by MEN 1. Early diagnosis in these patients could potentially contribute to lowering morbidity and even mortality in adulthood. Problems to be considered in the decision to activate active tumor surveillance are psychological and financial burden. Expert physicians who communicate well with parents and children are crucial in the construction of appropriate diagnostic and therapeutic paths for young patients with MEN 1. Following recommendations in the most recent guidance articles is certainly important, but we must bear in mind that their application in real life can be challenging.

Clinical Case Vignettes

Case 1

A 7-year-old boy is admitted to the emergency department due to loss of consciousness while biking. A history of headaches and visual disturbances is noted. He is neurologically intact upon arrival, except for recall deficit. Brain and pituitary MRI shows a 2.5 × 1.8 × 1.9-cm enhancing mass expanding the sella turcica (*Figure*). In the last year, he has had reduced growth velocity, and his height declined to the 11th percentile.

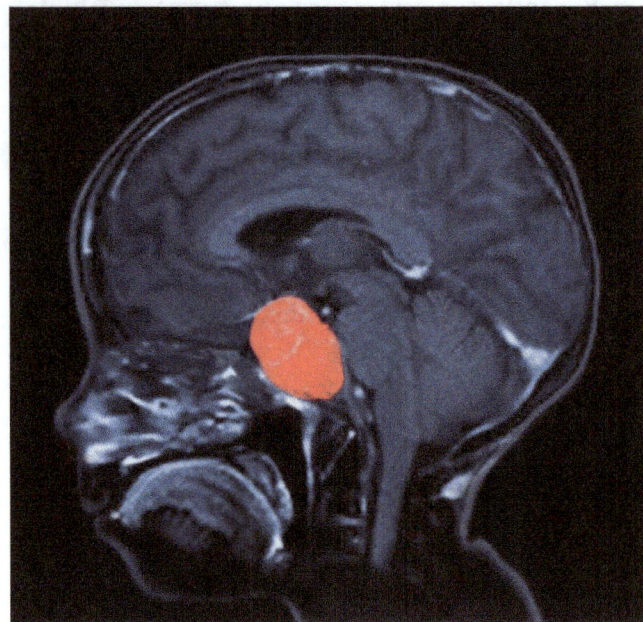

His prolactin concentration is 2776 ng/mL (121 nmol/L) in the emergency department, and GH levels are undetectable.

In a recent systematic review, macroprolactinomas were more common in girls than in boys in the younger-than-20 years age group, but the proportion of macroprolactinomas vs microprolactinoms was greater in males, particularly for large invasive tumors.[6] Recognition of pituitary disease and effective treatments for MEN 1 have made this a rare cause of morbidity and death in affected patients.

This patient had no maternal history of MEN 1. However, the father and paternal grandmother were affected by MEN 1, but this information had never been relayed to the divorced wife. Genetic testing confirmed that the patient had the same *MEN1* pathogenic variant as his father (in exon 2).

Medical therapy was initiated with cabergoline, 0.25 mg twice weekly. Long-term medical treatment in children and adolescents is safe and is effective in three-quarters of patients, with surgery or radiotherapy needed in some patients with resistant disease. In this patient, tumor shrinkage (>50% after 6 months) was achieved with a cabergoline dosage of 2.0 mg weekly. His prolactin concentration normalized and signs and symptoms resolved. The patient's growth rate improved while treated with cabergoline, and his serum GH concentration normalized as well. At 11 months of follow-up, his height was at the 19th percentile.

After 15 years follow-up, the patient was still being treated with cabergoline at a dosage of 0.25 mg twice weekly. His height was 72.8 in (185 cm), and sexual development was normal. The patient was monitored every 6 months for pituitary function, and MRI was performed annually. Once a year, the patient was evaluated for all potential MEN 1–associated tumors. He had hyperparathyroidism by age 11 years, and 2 cutaneous lipomas were evident at age 12 years. He had no signs or symptoms of excessive neuroendocrine function.

Genetic testing at birth would have been useful for this patient, so appropriate biochemical screening could have been undertaken and hyperprolactinemia could have been diagnosed before complications developed. Given the rarity of pediatric pituitary tumors, children presenting with a pituitary tumor should undergo genetic testing for pathogenic variants in genes known to cause pituitary tumors in children (*MEN1, AIP, PRKAR1A, CDKN2A, DICER1*, among others). A panel approach could be applied, or individual genes could be selected based on the phenotype.

References

1. Brandi ML, Agarwal SK, Perrier ND, Lines KE, Valk GD. Multiple endocrine neoplasia type 1: latest insights. *Endocr Rev.* 2021;42(2):133-170. PMID: 33249439

2. Lee ME, Ortega-Sustache YM, Agartala SK, et al. Patients with MEN1 are at increased risk for venous thromboembolism. *J Clin Endocrinol Metab.* 2021;106(2):e460-e468. PMID: 32756962

3. Shariq OA, Lines KE, English KA, et al. Multiple endocrine neoplasia type 1 in children and adolescents: clinical features and treatment outcomes. *Surgery.* 2021;171(1)77-87. PMID: 34183184

4. Thakker RV, Newey PJ, Walls GV, et al; Endocrine Society. Clinical practice guidelines for multiple endocrine neoplasia type 1 (MEN1). *J Clin Endocrinol Metab.* 2012;97(9):2990-3011. PMID: 22723327

5. Christakis I, Qiu W, Hyde SM, et al. Genotype-phenotype pancreatic neuroendocrine tumor relationship in multiple endocrine neoplasia type 1 patients: a 23-year experience at a single institution. *Surgery.* 2017;163(1):212-217. PMID: 29122330

6. Yang A, Cho SY, Park H, et al. Clinical, hormonal, and neuroradiological characteristics and therapeutic outcomes of prolactinomas in children and adolescents at a single center. *Front Endocrinol (Lausanne).* 2020;11:527. PMID: 32849307

Aggressive Pituitary Tumors

Nienke Biermasz, MD. Department of Internal Medicine, Division of Endocrinology, Leiden University Medical Center, Leiden, The Netherlands; E-mail: nrbiermasz@lumc.nl

Learning Objectives

As a result of participating in this session, learners should be able to:

- Distinguish aggressive tumors from benign-behaving pituitary adenomas and recognize tumors at risk for aggressive behavior.

- Use currently identified predictive factors for pituitary tumor aggressiveness in individualized follow-up planning in clinic.

- Discuss current state-of-the-art multidisciplinary management of aggressive pituitary tumors.

Main Conclusions

Aggressive pituitary tumors comprise a very small subset of pituitary lesions. Although ideally these rare tumors are treated in expert centers, awareness that regular pituitary tumors may develop into aggressive tumors after many years is important for all physicians providing surveillance for pituitary tumors.[1]

An aggressive tumor is best defined by a combination of aggressive behavior; invasiveness in surrounding tissues; multiple recurrences; rapid growth; and/or resistance to conventional treatments with endocrine drugs, surgery, and radiotherapy. Pituitary carcinoma may also metastasize. These features, when isolated, can also be observed in nonaggressive tumors, which makes identifying aggressive tumors very challenging.[2] Clinical predictive factors are invasion and growth, and pathological predictive factors are Ki-67 labeling index and mitotic count.

First-line multidisciplinary management is repeated surgery and radiotherapy, as well as drugs if the tumor is functioning. For patients with refractory disease, temozolomide is the formally recommended drug, although it is effective in only 30% to 40% of cases. Last-resort or emerging treatments are radionuclide treatment, immunotherapy, angiogenesis-directed therapies, and possibly rescue surgery and radiotherapy. These treatments do not yet have an established role in management and should be considered on a patient-by-patient basis.[3-5] Trials of new drugs are urgently needed.

Significance of the Clinical Problem

Aggressive pituitary tumors cause significant morbidity due to local invasion and uncontrolled hormone excess and increased mortality, especially in patients who do not respond to temozolomide. Early identification of an aggressive pituitary tumor is challenging because such tumors may initially seem unremarkable or because risk factors such as the Ki-67 labeling index and invasiveness are not perfectly discriminative. Emerging treatment options are needed for a small subset of patients, but investigational drug trials are not widely available, and optimal management should be determined with a multidisciplinary care team.

Barriers to Optimal Practice

Given the lack of reliable outcome data on specific treatment options, management of these tumors depends on real-world experience. Ideally, groups of experts could provide guidance regarding management. Recording cases in registries would be helpful to start collecting better outcomes data. Prevalence data are also lacking.

Collaboration among care team members could assist in flagging patients at risk for developing aggressive disease, and a more intensive surveillance protocol could be designed to detect aggressive behavior early, leaving more time for surgical and radiotherapeutic strategies. Centralized evaluation of pathology specimens would be an important step in better understanding the biological behavior of these tumors. Better descriptions of clinical behavior are also key in understanding the clinical course.

Guidance on how care of patients with aggressive pituitary tumors deviates from care of patients with nonaggressive pituitary adenomas has been difficult to provide because outcomes are heterogenous. Ongoing endocrine care for hormone excess and deficiency, in addition to the oncological trajectory, remains important.

Strategies for Diagnosis, Therapy, and/or Management

A small subset (<5%) of generally benign-behaving pituitary adenomas evolve into aggressive pituitary tumors. In contrast to patients with nonaggressive pituitary adenomas who are treated according to well-known algorithms with a combination of neurosurgery, endocrine drugs, and/or radiotherapy with no concern of tumor progression, aggressive pituitary tumors present with unpredictable, unusual growth patterns. These tumors can metastasize and are refractory to standard treatments. There is a clinical impression that the prevalence of aggressive pituitary tumors is rising, but epidemiological data are scarce.[6-9]

The European Society of Endocrinology recommends considering the presence of an aggressive pituitary tumor in patients with radiologically invasive tumors, unusually rapid tumor growth rate, or clinically relevant tumor growth despite optimal standard therapies. These features share considerable overlap with other adenomas; invasiveness alone is not a discriminating feature. In addition, the definition of growth is not straightforward.

There are several issues with the clinical components of the definition:

- An invasive tumor is not always an aggressive tumor, as this feature can also be seen in nonaggressive adenomas (eg, drug-sensitive tumors or tumors without a tendency to grow fast). However, once a tumor is determined to have radiological invasiveness, it is probably irresectable. Radiological invasiveness is described by the Knosp classification (cavernous sinus) or by the less-used HARDY classification. Invasiveness as observed during surgery may be different from expected based on preoperative imaging, and therefore surgical outcomes may differ among stages. There is also biological invasiveness; for example, invasiveness in the medical cavernous sinus wall or in the skull base. Giant adenomas may invade the skull base or grow intraventricularly. They are usually not aggressive, although they might be considered as such. The definition of invasiveness is not straightforward.

- Rapid tumor growth rate is not a straightforward clinical component. There is no consensus for defining a rapid growth rate because evidence-based data are not available and there is no consensus about the way such growth should be evaluated in clinical practice. Tumor volume measurements are the most precise assessment; however, a maximal diameter would probably suffice, even though tumors are noncircular and sometimes difficult to demarcate precisely. Maximal diameter can be measured in the outpatient setting. The RECIST guidelines align with oncology evaluation protocols. According to RECIST criteria, progressive disease is defined as a new lesion or a 20% or greater increase in longest diameter (or at least 5 mm). With pituitary disease, there is usually a single lesion and evaluation is done with MRI instead of CT. There is a practical definition proposed for clinically relevant tumor growth: new, worsening, or imminent signs and symptoms related to the complications caused by the tumor growth, independent of the relative or absolute increase in tumor size. Unusually rapid tumor growth by 20% or greater in the longest diameter or in the sum of the longest diameters (when multiloculated residual disease) in less than 6 to 12 months, independent of whether this constitutes clinically relevant tumor growth, constitutes rapid tumor growth. Even in patients who have tumors with unusual growth velocity, reviewing sequential MRI is important.

- Optimal standard therapy is currently left to an individual clinician's judgment. Many patients with tumors considered to be aggressive have a history of repeated surgery, radiotherapy, and drug treatment. Despite these treatment efforts, the tumors tend to recur. Some prolactinomas require higher than recommended dosages of cabergoline. Growth despite these strategies is suspicious for aggressiveness.

Several additional diagnostic tools can help distinguish aggressive from nonaggressive pituitary tumors. These tools are not evidence-based, but used in experienced hands, they can be used to help optimize treatment. The cornerstone of diagnostic imaging for pituitary tumors is dedicated pituitary MRI with 2- to 3-mm slices. In addition to standard series, axial coupes are helpful. The skull base is best evaluated with CT. Suitability of peptide radioreceptor therapy could be evaluated with somatostatin receptor PET-CT. Determining the best schedule for surveillance MRI is critical. Generally, we recommend every 3 to 6 months for tumors with suspected aggressiveness unless very stable. Clinicians must also be aware of the possibility of distant metastases. Endocrine workup is needed to evaluate for hormone excess and deficiency. There might be a discrepancy in radiological progression and endocrine progression, so laboratory evaluation and imaging are both needed. Ophthalmological function is critical to monitor in patients with pituitary tumors that may affect vision. For patients with aggressive tumors, there is ideally continuity of ophthalmological care (by one ophthalmologist). This parameter may guide treatment decisions, and there should be a low threshold to reevaluate if the patient has new-onset symptoms. Screening for metastasis should be considered if a patient has site-specific symptoms and discrepant hormone excess for the pituitary lesions. Most cases of metastasis are in the cranium or the spinal cord. Also, if a nonfunctioning tumor shifts to become a functioning tumor, this can be a sign of aggressiveness.

Histopathologic characteristics may indicate potential aggressiveness. As a first step, determining the Ki-67 labeling index is recommended. In patients with a Ki-67 labeling index greater than 3%, determining the mitotic index and p53 is advised. Tumors often develop aggressive behavior many years after initial diagnosis and pathologic evaluation. Ki-67 is related to aggressiveness; however, it may also be low in patients with aggressive disease. A higher Ki-67 index is a red flag for potential aggressiveness, and surveillance protocols for such patients should be more rigorous. The European Pituitary Pathology Club has proposed a practical 5-tiered classification: 1a noninvasive, nonproliferative; 1b proliferative, noninvasive; 2a invasive but nonproliferative; 2b proliferative and invasive; and 3 pituitary carcinoma. In this classification, proliferation is defined by the presence of 2 of 3 proliferation markers (p53, Ki-67, mitotic index).

Debulking surgery carefully planned with a multidisciplinary team may be a good option, although the anatomical relationships can be challenging. Many patients receive radiotherapy. When standard medical options fail, temozolomide, and possibly immunotherapy should be considered.

Several factors are involved in tumorigenesis, but their relationship to aggressiveness is not well studied (changes in tumor cells and microenvironment).

Temozolomide is the cornerstone for treating aggressive pituitary tumors, but this drug is not effective in a relevant subset. There are innovations with peptide receptor radionuclide therapy and immunotherapy. These approaches are highly individualized. Outcome data of drugs other than temozolomide have been mainly limited to case reports.

Clinical Case Vignettes

Case 1

A 52-year-old woman presents with a giant pituitary adenoma that has destroyed the skull base and the left orbit. There is suprasellar extension intracranially, encasement of the carotid artery, and compression of the temporal lobe. She has no pituitary hormone deficiencies, but she does have partial epilepsy related to the pituitary adenoma. There are increased ACTH values (262 pg/mL [57.6 pmol/L]) without clear signs of biochemical or clinical Cushing disease. She has severe visual field defects, and surgery is scheduled for debulking of tumor mass. The Ki-67 labeling index is less than 2%, and there is weak ACTH staining.

Which of the following is the most likely diagnosis?

A. Aggressive pituitary tumor

B. Giant adenoma

C. Silent corticotroph tumor

D. Both A and B

E. Either B or C

Answer: E) Either B or C

At this stage, it is difficult to judge whether this giant adenoma is also "aggressive." Findings on pathological evaluation are unremarkable. The tumor's growth pattern fits with being aggressive. There is ACTH secretion and ACTH-positive staining. However, there is not clear hypercortisolism. This is either a silent corticotroph tumor (Answer C) or simply a giant adenoma (Answer B). Thus, Answer E is correct. This patient requires close follow-up.

Case 1 (Continued)

Over the next 5 years, there is gradual tumor growth with increasing optic chiasmatic compression. Reoperation is required, and pathologic examination again shows a low Ki-67 labeling index. The patient's ACTH concentration is 300 pg/mL (66 pmol/L).

Is there any reason to change the above-mentioned diagnosis?

A. Yes

B. No

Answer: B) No

There are no additional arguments to revise the diagnosis (Answer B). Watchful waiting should be continued. Additional radiotherapy could be an option.

Case 2

A 49-year-old woman presents with Cushing syndrome. She has a Hardy grade IIA macroadenoma and undergoes endoscopic surgery. She is subsequently in remission and is temporarily hydrocortisone-dependent. Pathologic staining is positive for ACTH, there are no mitoses, and the Ki-67 labeling index is not available. Postoperative MRI shows no residual disease.

Three years later, she has a biochemical recurrence and now there is an 18-mm macroadenoma with invasion in the cavernous sinus, grade 3BE. Pathology documents a Ki-67 labeling index of 7%, p53 is negative, and there is minor cellular polymorphy.

Which of the following is the most likely diagnosis?

A. Aggressive tumor

B. Recurrence of Cushing disease

C. Either an aggressive tumor or recurrence of Cushing disease—difficult to discriminate

Answer: C) Either an aggressive tumor or recurrence of Cushing disease—difficult to discriminate

The pathology and clinical course in this vignette are consistent with the diagnosis of an aggressive tumor, as well as recurrence of Cushing disease. However, the patient had not yet received radiotherapy, so in theory, this tumor could have been stabilized with radiotherapy.

Case 2 (Continued)

Two years later, the patient experiences a new recurrence. Radical resection is not possible. The Ki-67 labeling index is again 7%. Postoperative radiotherapy is administered. Two years later, there is growth despite radiotherapy. She has some ophthalmoplegia. Temozolomide is started with good response 1.5 years later. The patient's condition and the tumor are stable; she is wondering about stopping temozolomide.

What is your suggestion? What is this patient's prognosis?

This is a highly individualized plan, with advantages and disadvantages. The standard advice is to evaluate after 3 months. If there is a positive response, temozolomide will be continued, as long as the patient tolerates it and continues responding. There are no evidence-based trials on best practices.

References

1. Raverot G, Ilie MD, Lasolle H, et al. Aggressive pituitary tumours and pituitary carcinomas. *Nat Rev Endocrinol.* 2021;17(11):671-684. PMID: 34493834

2. Raverot G, Burman P, McCormack A, et al; European Society of Endocrinology. European Society of Endocrinology Clinical Practice Guidelines for the management of aggressive pituitary tumours and carcinomas. *Eur J Endocrinol.* 2018;178(1):G1-G24. PMID: 29046323

3. McCormack A, Dekkers OM, Petersenn S, Popovic V, Trouillas J, Raverot G, Burman P; ESE survey collaborators. Treatment of aggressive pituitary tumours and carcinomas: results of a European Society of Endocrinology (ESE) survey 2016. *Eur J Endocrinol.* 2018;178(3):265-276. PMID: 29330228

4. Trouillas J, Burman P, McCormack A, Petersenn S, Popovic V, Dekkers O, Raverot G. Aggressive pituitary tumours and carcinomas: two sides of the same coin? *Eur J Endocrinol.* 2018;178(6):C7-C9. PMID: 29588294

5. Duhamel C, Ilie MD, Salle H, et al. Immunotherapy in corticotroph and lactotroph aggressive tumors and carcinomas: two case reports and a review of the literature. *J Pers Med.* 2020;10(3):88. PMID: 32823651

6. Ilie MD, Jouanneau E, Raverot G. Aggressive pituitary adenomas and carcinomas. *Endocrinol Metab Clin North Am.* 2020;49(3):505-515. PMID: 32741485

7. Trouillas J, Jaffrain-Rea M-L, Vasiljevic A, et al. Are aggressive pituitary tumors and carcinomas two sides of the same coin? Pathologists reply to clinician's questions. *Rev Endocr Metab Disord.* 2020;21(2):243-251. PMID: 32504268

8. Honegger J, Reincke M, Petersenn S, eds. *Pituitary Tumors: A Comprehensive and Interdisciplinary Approach.* Elsevier Press; 2021.

9. Trouillas J, Jaffrain-Rea M-L, Vasiljevic A, Raverot G, Roncaroli F, Villa C. How to classify the pituitary neuroendocrine tumors (PitNETs) in 2020. *Cancers (Basel).* 2020;12(2):514. PMID: 32098443

Controversies in the Field of Acromegaly

Elena V. Varlamov, MD. Departments of Medicine (Endocrinology, Diabetes, and Clinical Nutrition) and Neurological Surgery, and Pituitary Center, Oregon Health & Science University, Portland, OR; E-mail: varlamoe@ohsu.edu

Maria Fleseriu, MD. Departments of Medicine (Endocrinology, Diabetes, and Clinical Nutrition) and Neurological Surgery, and Pituitary Center, Oregon Health & Science University, Portland, OR; E-mail: fleseriu@ohsu.edu

Learning Objectives

As a result of participating in this session, learners should be able to:

- List possible limitations of IGF-1 and GH assays in the diagnosis of acromegaly.

- Describe indications for adjuvant medical therapy for patients with acromegaly after pituitary surgery.

- Explain the role of a personalized approach to medical management of patients with acromegaly.

- Select medical therapy for acromegaly based on tumor characteristics, IGF-1 and GH levels, comorbidities, and patient goals.

Main Conclusions

- The oral glucose tolerance test (OGTT) GH cutoff for diagnosis of acromegaly is 0.4 ng/mL (0.4 µg/L) using modern GH assays. Patients with mild acromegaly may have a GH concentration less than 0.4 ng/mL (<0.4 µg/L) assessed by OGTT.

- IGF-1 and GH levels are affected by various physiologic and pathologic states, as well as medications. Careful clinical evaluation, repeat testing, and pituitary MRI are necessary in patients for whom suspicion of acromegaly is reasonably high.

- Pituitary surgery is first-line treatment for most patients in the United States, unless contraindicated, not feasible, or declined by the patient. Use of primary medical therapy has increased over time.

- First-generation somatostatin receptor ligands (SRLs), lanreotide Autogel and octreotide (injectable and oral), are most commonly used for persistent biochemical/radiologic disease postoperatively, although pegvisomant could also be used as initial therapy in some patients. The SRL dosage should be escalated for biochemical control (normal IGF-1 and GH <1.0 ng/mL [<1.0 µg/L]) to the maximal dosage approved/tolerated. If a tumor has characteristics associated with resistance to SRLs (negative somatostatin receptor type 2 receptor, sparsely granulated type, T2-weighted MRI hyperintensity, pathogenic variant in the aryl hydrocarbon receptor-interacting protein gene [*AIP*], high Ki67 index), pasireotide LAR or a combination of an SRL and pegvisomant could be considered. Cabergoline can be useful in selected patients with mild acromegaly.

- Radiation therapy is third-line treatment for most patients, except those who have large, invasive, or enlarging residual tumors after surgery. Radiation therapy is associated with hypopituitarism and requires medical therapy for GH excess while awaiting effects.

- Quality of life and symptom improvement are important determinants of successful treatment outcomes; clinicians should evaluate symptoms in all patients even after biochemical control is achieved.

Significance of the Clinical Problem

Acromegaly is a rare condition resulting from chronic GH and IGF-1 excess.[1] Most cases are due to a GH-secreting pituitary adenoma; less than 1% are caused by an ectopic GHRH- or GH-producing neuroendocrine tumor.[2] Prevalence of acromegaly is 85 in 10 million,[3] which is higher than previously thought, probably due to increased awareness and improved diagnostic means.

Untreated or uncontrolled acromegaly is associated with multisystem complications resulting in a roughly 2-fold increased mortality rate, primarily driven by cardiovascular disease. Cerebrovascular disease (often attributed to pituitary radiation therapy), sleep apnea, and cancer likely also add to the increased mortality, although this has not been demonstrated consistently.[3,4] Normalization of GH and IGF-1, as well as identification and treatment of comorbidities, reduces mortality rates to that of the general population.[1,5-8] In addition to attaining biochemical control, treatment goals also include tumor removal/shrinkage, symptom control, and improved quality of life.

Transsphenoidal removal of a GH-producing adenoma is usually first-line treatment in the United States and should be performed by an experienced neurosurgeon. Despite technological advances, the long-term surgical cure rate is less than 65%,[9] most likely because many patients present with larger and invasive tumors, making complete tumor excision difficult.[5] Adjunctive medical therapy to normalize GH and/or IGF-1 levels, as well as to shrink the tumor, is

implemented in patients not cured by surgery. Radiotherapy is generally reserved for patients in whom medical therapy fails and those with invasive and aggressive tumors.[10]

Development of new medical therapies, discovery of predictive factors for success or failure of different treatments, increased awareness of possible treatment-related complications, as well as understanding the patient's personal goals have led to the new concept of personalized management of acromegaly. This approach takes into consideration tumor type, size, IGF-1 and GH levels, patient symptoms, comorbid conditions, and patient preferences.[11]

Although biochemical control typically results in significant improvement of a patient's symptoms, the "goal" target (normal age- and sex-adjusted IGF-1 concentration and GH concentration <1 ng/mL [<1.0 µg/L]) is sometimes still associated with persistent symptomatology (arthralgias, sweating, fatigue, soft-tissue swelling).[12] Clinicians should consider therapy adjustment in patients with ongoing symptoms.

Lastly, long-term follow-up and regular reassessment of biochemical and tumor control are important. Patients in clinical and biochemical remission should be periodically screened for recurrence.

Barriers to Optimal Practice

- GH and IGF-1 assays are heterogeneous. Discrepancies exist among laboratories, complicating diagnosis and monitoring if testing is performed in different laboratories.

- OGTT and IGF-1 measurement have limitations in the diagnosis of mild acromegaly.

- Histopathology reports do not always include information that can guide treatment choice or determine prognosis (eg, sparsely vs granulated GH-secreting tumors, presence of somatostatin receptor type 2).

- SRL monotherapy is effective in less than 50% of patients in unselected populations; thus, patients often require a switch to a different agent or combination therapy.

Strategies for Diagnosis, Therapy, and/or Management

Clinical Scenario

A 63-year-old woman with a history of hypertension, prediabetes, sleep apnea, benign thyroid nodules, breast cancer in remission, and meningioma resection 10 years ago presents with a 1.5 × 0.9-cm pituitary adenoma found on surveillance MRI. The adenoma does not touch the optic chiasm. She also has meningioma recurrence.

Laboratory test results:

> IGF-1 = 312 ng/mL (53-287 ng/mL) (SI: 40.9 nmol/L [6.9-37.6 nmol/L])
> Random GH = 0.9 ng/mL (≤4.9 ng/mL) (SI: 0.9 μg/L [≤4.9 μg/L])

The rest of her pituitary function is normal. OGTT shows GH suppression to 0.31 ng/mL (0.31 μg/L) with a concurrent glucose value of 242 mg/dL (13.4 nmol/L). This is regarded as normal at an outside institution and the patient is followed up conservatively for pituitary adenoma but undergoes another resection of meningioma. On follow-up, IGF-1 remains persistently mildly elevated. The patient has headaches but no changes in hand or foot size, sweating, or joint pain. On 3-year follow-up imaging, the pituitary adenoma has enlarged to 1.7 × 1.4 × 1.3 cm with optic chiasm compression. She is referred to your institution and undergoes transsphenoidal surgery. Pathologic examination reveals a sparsely granulated somatotroph adenoma. Her postoperative IGF-1 concentration is 98 ng/mL (49-279 ng/mL) (SI: 12.8 nmol/L [6.4-36.5 nmol/L]).

How should one interpret discrepant biochemical results when evaluating for acromegaly?

Difficulties in the Diagnosis of Acromegaly

Diagnosis of acromegaly is not always straightforward. Patients may lack "classic" clinical symptoms and signs, particularly in mild cases. Some present only with complications, such as sleep apnea, glucose intolerance or diabetes, osteoarthritis, carpal tunnel syndrome, or hypertension, which leads to suspicion of acromegaly. IGF-1 is the recommended screening test in all patients who present with classic symptoms and with a combination of comorbidities associated with acromegaly, as well as in patients with a pituitary mass.[5] OGTT with assessment of GH nadir is performed when IGF-1 levels are mildly elevated or equivocal. Both tests have limitations related to established cutoffs, assay performance, physiologic factors affecting the results as well as the clinical scenario—whether they are performed to establish a diagnosis or to assess for remission after surgery.

IGF-1 is a protein secreted in the liver under GH stimulation. Its half-life is 15 hours, and it is a surrogate marker for GH disorders, especially GH excess.[5] IGF-1 levels should be interpreted in the context of established age- and sex-adjusted reference ranges. Since these differ between various IGF-1 assays, borderline results can create difficulties in both diagnosis and decision making, particularly for monitoring patients during treatment. Various physiologic factors can influence IGF-1 levels (*Table 1*).[13,14] "Falsely" elevated IGF-1 may be related to inadequately established reference ranges in a reference population.[15]

GH has a pulsatile secretion pattern and is also subject to different physiologic influences (*Table 1*). In healthy individuals, glucose loading suppresses GH by inhibiting GHRH and/or potentiating somatostatin release. The cutoff of nadir GH less than 1.0 ng/mL (<1.0 μg/L) on 75-g OGTT was recommended,[5] but using new ultrasensitive assays, a GH value less than 0.4 ng/mL (<0.4 μg/L) has been proposed as a revised cutoff.[10] However, some patients with acromegaly suppress to less than 0.4 ng/mL (<0.4 μg/L).[16] One study found that 7 of 40 of patients had a GH value

Table 1. Factors That Affect IGF-1 and GH Levels

Factors that ↑ IGF-1	Factors that ↓ IGF-1	Factors that ↑ GH	Factors that ↓ GH
• Parenteral testosterone • Pregnancy • Late-stage adolescence • Inadequate limits of normality • Assay interference	• Oral estrogen, selective estrogen receptor modulators • Severe obesity • Prolonged fasting and malnutrition • Liver disease • Kidney disease • Uncontrolled diabetes • Acute illness	• Oral estrogen, midcycle • Significantly uncontrolled diabetes • Kidney failure • Prolonged fasting and malnutrition • Liver disease • Acute critical illness	• Age (postmenopausal) • High BMI

less than 0.4 ng/mL (<0.4 µg/L) on 100-g OGTT; these patients had baseline GH values less than 4.3 ng/mL (<4.3 µg/L) and most had microadenomas. However, nonsuppression of GH (GH >0.4 ng/mL [>0.4 µg/L]) has been demonstrated in healthy slim individuals and in women taking oral estrogen.[17] Additionally, patients with uncontrolled diabetes can have nonsuppressed GH levels. Therefore, these factors must be considered when interpreting OGTT results.

When the initial evaluation is equivocal and results are discrepant and/or do not fit with the clinical picture, retesting is recommended. MRI should be obtained if clinical suspicion for acromegaly is high, even if OGTT is normal. Repeated MRI is warranted if biochemical and clinical progression is evident when the patient is followed by observation.

Clinical Scenario

A 35-year-old woman presents with a 1.9-cm pituitary adenoma identified radiographically during amenorrhea workup. She also has headaches, hirsutism, increased sweating, increased shoe and ring size, puffiness under her eyes, and occasional snoring.

Laboratory test results:

> IGF-1 = 963 ng/mL (113-297 ng/mL)
>   (SI: 126.1 nmol/L [14.8-38.9 nmol/L])
> Prolactin = 148 ng/mL (4-23 ng/mL)
>   (SI: 6.44 nmol/L [0.17-1.00 nmol/L])

Pituitary surgery is performed, and pathologic examination shows a mammosomatotroph adenoma, somatostatin receptor type 2 receptor negative. Her 3-month postoperative IGF-1 concentration is 469 ng/mL (61.4 nmol/L) and her GH concentration is 10.2 ng/mL (10.2 µg/L), indicating persistent acromegaly. MRI shows interval resection of a pituitary mass and postsurgical changes.

How should one decide what adjuvant treatment option to choose in the era of personalized medicine?

Surgical Remission Criteria

Disease control after surgery or on medical therapy is defined as normal IGF-1 and a random GH concentration less than 1.0 ng/mL (<1.0 µg/L), the biochemical profile associated with normalization of mortality.[5] Patients with a GH value greater than 1.0 ng/mL (>1.0 µg/L) may benefit from OGTT for additional evaluation. Discrepant results, most commonly GH less than 1 ng/mL (<1.0 µg/L) and elevated IGF-1 levels, may occur postoperatively, and the current consensus statement recommends relying on IGF-1 with close follow-up. IGF-1 seems to correlate better with comorbidities than GH nadir levels; furthermore, IGF-1 is more predictive than nadir GH in assessing insulin sensitivity and clinical symptoms after surgery.[18]

Persistent Disease After Surgery

Persistent disease after surgery is treated with medical therapy for which there are a variety of options.

Somatostatin Receptor Ligands

SRLs remain the first-line medical treatment for many patients.[1,5,19] These agents bind to somatostatin receptors on somatotroph adenoma cells, suppressing both GH secretion and tumor cell proliferation. Octreotide long-acting release (LAR), and deep subcutaneous lanreotide depot/Autogel are equally effective injectable formulations of first-generation SRLs (*Table 2*). Approximately 30% to 60% of patients[19] achieve biochemical control; such variable response is thought to be related to preselection of patients for GH responsiveness in the studies, different definitions of remission, prior treatments, duration of follow-up, and other factors. Dosage escalation often leads to better biochemical control. More than 70% of patients achieve greater than 20% tumor volume reduction on SRL therapy.[20] Oral octreotide capsules are approved for patients whose disease is controlled on injectable SRLs. In a double-blind randomized controlled trial of 56 patients who previously responded to long-acting injectable SRLs, approximately 60% vs 20% in the placebo group maintained biochemical control.[21] Another phase 3 trial, assessing maintenance of response to oral octreotide capsules vs switching to injectable SRLs showed noninferiority of oral octreotide capsules (91% [CI: 80%-97%]) to injectable SRLs (100% [CI: 91%-100%]) at 36 weeks for patients who responded to both therapies.[22] Therefore, oral octreotide capsules may be considered as an alternative for patients whose disease is controlled on injectable SRLs and for whom injections present

Table 2. Summary of Medical Therapies for Acromegaly

Class	Agent	Notes	Possible adverse effects
First-generation SRL Affinity to somatostatin receptor type, arranged by order from the strongest to the weakest: 2 > 5, 3 > 1 > 4	Octreotide LAR, 10 to 40 mg every 4 weeks, intramuscularly	• Administered by a health care professional, as it requires reconstitution	Gastrointestinal distress cholelithiasis, liver function enzyme elevation, hyperglycemia or hypoglycemia, bradycardia Intolerance of 1 drug does not indicate cross-intolerance to other
	Lanreotide Autogel, 60 to 120 mg every 4 to 8 weeks, deep subcutaneously	• May be self-administered (prefilled syringes)	
	Octreotide, 50 to 100 mcg 3 times daily, subcutaneously	• Rarely used alone • Sometimes used for treatment of acromegaly related headaches	
	Octreotide capsules, 20 mg twice daily, up to 80 mg daily, orally	• Indicated for patients controlled on injectable SRL • Could improve several symptoms in selected patients • Must be taken on empty stomach or 2 hours after meal	
Newer-generation SRL Higher affinity to somatostatin receptor type 5	Pasireotide LAR, 40 to 60 mg every 4 weeks, intramuscularly	• Biochemical control in 20% of cases resistant to first-generation SRL	Hyperglycemia/diabetes mellitus (~60%), QT prolongation, liver function enzyme elevation
D2 receptor agonist	Cabergoline, 1 to 5 mg weekly, orally	• For mild IGF-1 elevation or in combination therapy	Nausea, dizziness, worsening mood disorders and impulse control disorders
GH receptor antagonist	Pegvisomant, 10 to 40 mg daily, subcutaneously 2 to 3 times per week regimens can be used	• Effective in >60% in real-life scenario • Could improve glycemic control • No antitumor effect • GH levels remain elevated and should not be monitored	Liver function enzyme elevation QT prolongation

a burden, as well as for those who experience breakthrough symptoms at the end of the injection cycle due to wear-off. Food reduces absorption of oral octreotide capsules; thus, lack of adherence to correct food-medication instructions can decrease efficacy.

Resistance to first-generation SRLs has been observed in patients with sparsely granulated somatotroph adenomas, somatostatin receptor type 2-negative adenomas, T2-MRI hyperintense adenomas, large and invasive tumors, *AIP* gene pathogenic variants, high Ki67 proliferation index, and younger age.[5,23,24] Pasireotide LAR is a newer-generation SRL with greater somatostatin receptor type 5 affinity and higher efficacy than octreotide LAR (31.3% vs 19.2%, P = .007)[25] or LAN[25-27]; tumor volume reduction is approximately 40%.[25] However, biochemical response may also be driven by action on somatostatin receptor type 2.[28] Efficacy in patients resistant to first-generation SRLs is approximately 20%. The adverse effect profile is similar, except for higher rates of hyperglycemia/diabetes (~60%). Therefore, close monitoring and the addition of metformin, a GLP-1 receptor agonist, and a DPP-4 inhibitor has been recommended.[29] Hyperglycemia is less likely to occur in younger patients, those with normal glucose tolerance, and those without hypertension or dyslipidemia history. Hyperglycemia is reversible with pasireotide LAR discontinuation.[30]

Pegvisomant, a GH receptor antagonist, blocks IGF-1 production in the liver. It reduces IGF-1 in a dose-dependent manner, achieving IGF-1 control in greater than 90% of patients at dosages of up to 40 mg daily. Real-life observation data show a lower control rate, 53% at year 1 and 75% at year 10, attributed to lower dosages (mean = 14.0 mg daily at year 1 and 18.2 mg daily at year 10) and slower titration rates outside of clinical trials.[31] Tumor volume increase is 3% to 7%.[31] Pegvisomant improves fasting and postprandial glycemia and could be beneficial for patients with diabetes. Additionally, a long half-life (60 to 138 hours) allows reduced frequency of injections (2 to 3 times weekly), thus lessening the injection burden.

Dopamine agonists effectively achieve biochemical control in some patients, with variable degree of tumor volume reduction. Because of limited efficacy, cabergoline is considered mainly in patients with very mild disease or in those treated with combination therapy.[32]

Combination medical therapy is used when monotherapy fails to achieve control or when lower dosages are desired to minimize adverse effects of individual medications.[24] A combination of a first-generation SRL and pegvisomant provides 80% to 97% IGF-1 normalization, allowing lower or less frequent pegvisomant dosages (once or twice weekly), with lower cost and improved tolerability.[33,34] The combination of pasireotide LAR and pegvisomant allows for reduction in the pegvisomant dosage by as much as 66% compared with the combination of a first-generation SRL and PEG. However, the frequency of diabetes doubles.[35] As both types of drugs are associated with liver function enzyme elevation, close monitoring is needed. The combination of an SRL and cabergoline is also relatively well-tolerated and may be considered for patients with mild IGF-1 elevations. The combination of pegvisomant and cabergoline is reasonable if a patient with mild disease is intolerant to SRLs or when combination of an SRL and pegvisomant is cost prohibitive. Long-term efficacy and safety of various combination therapies need further study.[5,24]

Emerging medical therapies for acromegaly include a nonpeptide selective somatostatin receptor type 2 agonist paltusotine, antisense oligonucleotides (cimdelirsen), long-acting subcutaneous octreotide, and another SRL, somatoprim. Temozolomide is used off-label in combination with other medical therapies for patients with aggressive GH-secreting tumors.[6,24]

Primary medical therapy in lieu of surgery may be considered for patients with smaller adenomas without optic chiasm compromise, those who are not surgical candidates or decline surgery, and those with empty sella due to "burnt-out" adenoma. SRLs are most commonly used for this purpose as they reduce tumor volume and control GH hypersecretion; pegvisomant is also an option in these patients, as risk of tumor progression is low. Data on preoperative use of medial therapy in order to improve postsurgery biochemical outcomes are conflicting; therefore, this strategy is not used routinely. In rare clinical scenarios, such as a patient with severe pharyngeal thickness and severe sleep apnea syndrome, preoperative therapy may be considered to possibly reduce perioperative morbidity. Further study is needed to assess utility of presurgical medical treatment in patients with acromegaly.[5,36]

Radiation (conventional and stereotactic) is mostly third-line treatment in those for whom surgery and medical therapy fail, but it is recommended postoperatively in patients with aggressive somatotroph adenomas. Due to slow effect onset, bridge medical therapy is required until the radiation "kicks in," which occurs in 40% to 60% of patients at 5 years.[37] Hypopituitarism occurs in 25% to 50% at 5 years.[10] Radiation-induced cerebrovascular disease, secondary tumors, and cranial nerve palsy may be less frequent with modern focused stereotactic techniques.[10]

Reoperation is considered for patients with identifiable resectable tumor for whom postoperative medical therapy failed after initial surgery or with tumor regrowth. New developing nuclear medicine techniques (eg, 11C-Met PET-CT) may help localize residual somatotroph adenomas if no visible tumor is seen on MRI.[38]

The Figure summarizes the algorithm for medical management of acromegaly.

Figure. Suggested Algorithm for Medical Management of Acromegaly[1,5-8,9,10,32]

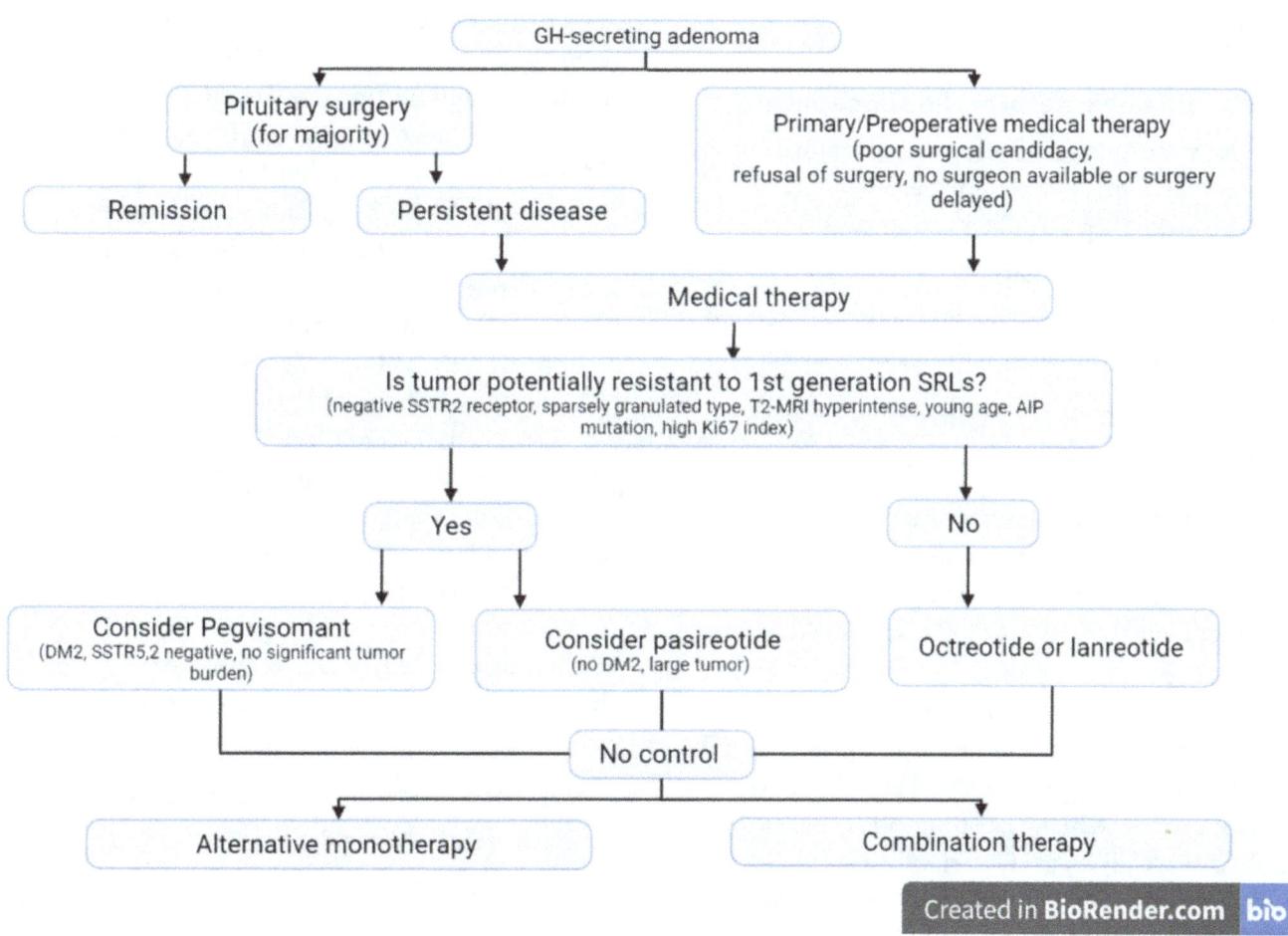

Adapted from Ting Lim DS & Fleseriu M. Endocr Pract, 2022; 28(3) © AACE. Published by Elsevier Inc. All rights reserved.

Clinical Case Vignettes

Case 1

A 59-year-old woman presents with a 6 × 6 × 9-mm pituitary adenoma discovered incidentally during workup for dizziness and ataxia. She has diabetes mellitus controlled on metformin and neuropathy. She has no obvious acromegalic features, no hand enlargement, excessive sweating, joint pain, or headache. IGF-1 measurement is mildly elevated at 276 ng/mL (40-217 ng/mL) (SI: 36.2 nmol/L [5.3-28.4 nmol/L]). A repeated IGF-1 measurement in a different laboratory is 266 ng/mL (53-287 ng/mL) (SI: 34.8 nmol/L [6.9-37.6 nmol/L]). GH levels on OGTT are 1.3 ng/mL (1.3 µg/L), 1.4 ng/mL (1.4 µg/L), 2.0 ng/mL (2.0 µg/L), and 1.6 ng/mL (1.6 µg/L) with glucose values of 195 mg/dL (10.8 mmol/L), 119 mg/dL (6.6 mmol/L), 83 mg/dL (4.6 mmol/L), and 70 mg/dL (3.9 mmol/L). Other pituitary function is normal.

How should one interpret the above results?

A. Patient's results are discrepant; therefore, a diagnosis cannot be established

B. Patient's OGTT results are abnormal, confirming acromegaly

C. Patient's first IGF-1 value is falsely high, second IGF-1 value is normal; acromegaly is excluded

Answer: B) Patient's OGTT results are abnormal, confirming acromegaly

This patient presented with an incidental microadenoma, and management depends on the presence or absence of mass effect and hormonal hypersecretion. There is no mass effect and seemingly no symptoms, but she has some comorbidities potentially related to acromegaly, namely type 2 diabetes and neuropathy. Her initial IGF-1 measurement was elevated and the second one was normal, which is a common scenario in mild disease given assay variability, as well as intra-patient IGF-1 variability. One should consider factors that can reduce IGF-1 levels such as oral estrogen, uncontrolled diabetes, and liver or kidney disease (*Table 1*) (thus, Answers A and C are incorrect). This patient lacked any confounders.

In the setting of equivocal results, OGTT could help make the diagnosis; here it clearly demonstrated GH nonsuppression after documented hyperglycemia, confirming the diagnosis of mild acromegaly (Answer B). The patient underwent pituitary surgery, and pathologic examination confirmed a GH-positive pituitary adenoma with biochemical remission. Her postoperative IGF-1 concentration was 152 ng/mL (37-208 ng/mL) (SI: 19.9 nmol/L [4.8-27.2 nmol/L]) and GH concentration was 0.16 ng/mL (0.16 µg/L).

Case 2

A 66-year-old woman has acromegaly due to a 1.5-cm pituitary macroadenoma. She has a history of osteopenia, colonic polyps, sleep apnea, controlled type 2 diabetes mellitus, and hypertension. Her IGF-1 value is 652 ng/mL (75-263 ng/mL) (SI: 85.4 nmol/L [9.8-34.4 nmol/L]), and her GH value is 20.3 ng/mL (SI: 20.3 µg/L). She undergoes pituitary surgery, and pathologic examination shows mammosomatotroph adenoma. Postoperatively at 3 months, her IGF-1 value is 262 ng/mL (32-238 ng/mL) (SI: 34.3 nmol/L [4.2-31.2 nmol/L]), and her GH value is 0.4 ng/mL (SI: 0.4 µg/L). IGF-1 continues to be high 6 months after surgery. MRI shows postoperative changes and a possible small residual adenoma. Many of her acromegaly symptoms have improved or resolved.

Which of the following is the best therapeutic choice for this patient?

A. Lanreotide, 60 mg every 6 weeks

B. Oral octreotide capsules, 20 mg twice daily

C. Pasireotide, 40 mg daily

D. Pegvisomant, 10 mg daily

E. No therapy

Answer: A) Lanreotide, 60 mg every 6 weeks

This patient presents with mildly elevated IGF-1 and nonsuppressed GH 3 to 6 months postoperatively, which indicates persistent disease. If results of a laboratory workup at 3 months are borderline, a repeated biochemical evaluation is warranted, and medical therapy should be started for persistently elevated IGF-1, as in this scenario. Thus, recommending no therapy (Answer E) is incorrect.

Long-acting first-generation SRLs such as lanreotide or octreotide are the first choice for persistent, biochemically active acromegaly, particularly in patients with a low likelihood for resistance. Lanreotide, 60 mg every 6 weeks (Answer A), is correct. Although the typical lanreotide regimen is every 4 weeks, it is FDA approved with extended interval between doses, which also maintains control in mild disease and reduces the injection burden.

Pegvisomant (Answer D), although effective, is rarely first-line therapy in patients with mild disease, except in selected patients.

Among SRLs, pasireotide LAR (Answer C) is also second-line therapy and is mostly considered for resistant cases. It also carries a risk of worsening diabetes in this patient.

Oral octreotide capsules (Answer B) could be effective if her acromegaly is controlled on a long-acting SRL; this maybe a good option if she demonstrates control on lanreotide but has end-cycle breakthrough symptoms or dislike of injections.

Cabergoline (not given as a choice here) is not FDA approved but can potentially control GH and IGF-1 in patients with mild acromegaly and as part of combination therapy. Dosages required are higher than what is prescribed to treat prolactinoma; if the dosage exceeds 2 to 3 mg weekly, echocardiography should be performed at baseline and after treatment is initiated as needed, depending on the clinical picture and national guidelines.

Case 3

A 40-year-old woman with acromegaly presents to discuss treatment. She has a history of a 2.7-cm mixed GH- and prolactin-secreting pituitary macroadenoma (somatostatin receptor type 2 staining not available), with an initial IGF-1 concentration of 513 ng/mL (106-368 ng/mL) (SI: 67.2 nmol/L [13.9-48.2 nmol/L]) and prolactin concentration of 73 ng/mL (3-20 ng/mL) (SI: 3.17 nmol/L [0.13-0.87 nmol/L]). Postoperatively, her IGF-1 value is 375 ng/mL (106-368 ng/mL) (SI: 49.1 nmol/L [13.9-48.2 nmol/L]) and GH value is 2.62 ng/mL (2.62 µg/L). Notably, she is on a combined oral contraceptive. MRI shows a 1.6. × 1.1-cm residual pituitary adenoma with bilateral extension into the cavernous sinuses, but she declines reoperation and is started on octreotide LAR, 30 mg every 4 weeks. IGF-1 normalizes within 4 months, but GH remains greater than 1.0 ng/mL (>1.0 µg/L). The residual tumor shrinks to 1.1 × 0.7 cm on follow-up MRI at 1 year. Additionally, cabergoline, 0.25 mg twice weekly, is prescribed for hyperprolactinemia and persistent galactorrhea.

Laboratory test results after 3 years of treatment:

> IGF-1 = 320 ng/mL (79-276 ng/mL) (SI: 41.9 nmol/L [10.3-36.2 nmol/L])
> GH = 3.4 ng/mL (SI: 3.4 µg/L)

Tumor size is stable. She is no longer on an oral contraceptive pill and notes mild headaches and increased sweating.

How should this patient's therapy be adjusted to control her disease?

A. Add pegvisomant

B. Administer radiation therapy

C. Increase the octreotide LAR dosage to 40 mg every 4 weeks

D. Perform reoperation

E. Switch to different first-generation SRL, such as lanreotide

Answer: C) Increase the octreotide LAR dosage to 40 mg every 4 weeks

This patient showed both biochemical and clinical response to octreotide LAR plus cabergoline. However, it was an incomplete response, evident after stopping the oral contraceptive pill. Estrogen in the oral contraceptive pill was most likely decreasing IGF-1 liver production, while GH production remained abnormal. Since she has not yet tried a maximum dosage of octreotide, one should attempt to maximize the dosage (Answer C).

Switching to lanreotide (Answer E) is not expected to improve biochemical control, as it is not more effective than octreotide; switching could play a role if there are issues with octreotide LAR injections administration per se.

Adding pegvisomant (Answer A) would be a reasonable next step if the patient does not achieve biochemical control with the maximum octreotide dosage or she does not tolerate it. Of note, when adding pegvisomant, it would be reasonable to simultaneously reduce the octreotide dosage. Radiation is usually third-line treatment if medical therapy fails.

Reoperation (Answer D) may be offered to some patients; however, this patient previously declined another surgery.

Case 4

A 56-year-old woman is diagnosed with acromegaly due to a 2-cm pituitary adenoma, which is T2-isointense with areas of hyperintensity. The adenoma does not touch the optic chiasm.

Laboratory test results:

> IGF-1 = 781 ng/mL (53-287 ng/mL)
> (SI: 102.3 nmol/L [6.9-37.6 nmol/L])
> GH = 20.6 ng/mL (0.01-3.61 ng/mL)
> (SI: 20.6 μg/L [0.01-3.61 μg/L])
> Prolactin = 7 ng/mL (4-30 ng/mL)
> (SI: 0.30 nmol/L [0.17-1.30 nmol/L])
> Hemoglobin A_{1c} = 5.6% (4.0%-5.6%) (38 mmol/mol
> [20-38 mmol/mol])

She has vocal cord paralysis related to previous surgery for compressive goiter and has a difficult airway for intubation noted by otolaryngology. She would like to avoid surgery, and her treatment team also prefers a nonoperative approach at this time, but surgery will be considered if her laryngeal edema improves with treatment.

Which of the following therapies should this patient start?

A. Combination therapy with lanreotide and pegvisomant

B. Octreotide LAR, 20 mg every 4 weeks

C. Pasireotide, 60 mg every 4 weeks

D. Pegvisomant, 40 mg daily

Answer: C) Pasireotide, 60 mg every 4 weeks

This patient needs therapy that will effectively lower her IGF-1 and reduce tumor size. Tumor size reduction is an important therapeutic goal. Since her tumor is T2-isointense with areas of hyperintensity, it may potentially be resistant to first-generation SRLs. This patient does not have diabetes mellitus. Therefore, pasireotide (Answer C) is a good choice for this patient, but close monitoring for hyperglycemia will still be required.

Octreotide LAR may also be used; however, the dosage of 20 mg every 4 weeks (Answer B) is unlikely to achieve biochemical control, especially given risk factors for resistance.

Pegvisomant (Answer D) will likely effectively lower her IGF-1, although it will not reduce tumor size (and she has a large tumor).

Combination therapy with lanreotide and pegvisomant (Answer A) may also be effective, but rarely are 2 medications started simultaneously. The goal in this case is to shrink the tumor and achieve faster biochemical control.

References

1. Melmed S. Acromegaly pathogenesis and treatment. *J Clin Invest.* 2009;119(11):3189-3202. PMID: 19884662

2. Ghazi AA, Amirbaigloo A, Dezfooli AA, et al. Ectopic acromegaly due to growth hormone releasing hormone. *Endocrine.* 2013;43(2):293-302. PMID: 22983831

3. Dal J, Feldt-Rasmussen U, Andersen M, et al. Acromegaly incidence, prevalence, complications and long-term prognosis: a nationwide cohort study. *Eur J Endocrinol.* 2016;175(3):181-190. PMID: 27280374

4. Gadelha MR, Kasuki L, Lim DST, Fleseriu M. Systemic complications of acromegaly and the impact of the current treatment landscape: an update. *Endocr Rev.* 2019;40(1):268-332. PMID: 30184064

5. Katznelson L, Laws ER Jr, Melmed S, et al; Endocrine Society. Acromegaly: an Endocrine Society clinical practice guideline. *J Clin Endocrinol Metab.* 2014;99(11):3933-3951. PMID: 25356808

6. Melmed S. New therapeutic agents for acromegaly. *Nat Rev Endocrinol.* 2016;12(2):90-98. PMID: 26610414

7. Giustina A, Barkan A, Beckers A, et al. A consensus on the diagnosis and treatment of acromegaly comorbidities: an update. *J Clin Endocrinol Metab.* 2020;105(4):dgz096. PMID: 31606735

8. Fleseriu M, Biller BMK, Freda PU, et al. A Pituitary Society update to acromegaly management guidelines. *Pituitary.* 2021;24(1):1-13. PMID: 33079318

9. Melmed S, Bronstein MD, Chanson P, et al. A consensus statement on acromegaly therapeutic outcomes. *Nat Rev Endocrinol.* 2018;14(9):552-561. PMID: 30050156

10. Giustina A, Barkhoudarian G, Beckers A, et al. Multidisciplinary management of acromegaly: a consensus. *Rev Endocr Metab Disord.* 2020;21(4):667-678. PMID: 32914330

11. Fleseriu M, Barkan A, Del Pilar Schneider M, et al. Prevalence of comorbidities and concomitant medication use in acromegaly: analysis of real-world data from the United States. *Pituitary.* 2022 [online ahead of print] PMID: 34973139

12. Broersen LHA, Zamanipoor Najafabadi AH, Pereira AM, Dekkers OM, van Furth WR, Biermasz NR. Improvement in symptoms and health-related quality of life in acromegaly patients: a systematic review and meta-analysis. *J Clin Endocrinol Metab.* 2021;106(2):577-587. PMID: 33245343

13. Akirov A, Masri-Iraqi H, Dotan I, Shimon I. The biochemical diagnosis of acromegaly. *J Clin Med.* 2021;10(5):1147. PMID: 33803429

14. Schilbach K, Strasburger CJ, Bidlingmaier M. Biochemical investigations in diagnosis and follow up of acromegaly. *Pituitary.* 2017;20(1):33-45. PMID: 28168377

15. Bancos I, Algeciras-Schimnich A, Grebe SK, Donato LJ, Nippoldt TB, Erickson D. Evaluation of variables influencing the measurement of insulin-like growth factor-1. *Endocr Pract.* 2014;20(5):421-426. PMID: 24326002

16. Ribeiro-Oliveira A Jr, Faje AT, Barkan AL. Limited utility of oral glucose tolerance test in biochemically active acromegaly. *Eur J Endocrinol.* 2011;164(1):17-22. PMID: 20926592

17. Schilbach K, Gar C, Lechner A, et al. Determinants of the growth hormone nadir during oral glucose tolerance test in adults. *Eur J Endocrinol.* 2019;181(1):55-67. PMID: 31096183

18. Bidlingmaier M, Friedrich N, Emeny RT, et al. Reference intervals for insulin-like growth factor-1 (igf-i) from birth to senescence: results from a multicenter study using a new automated chemiluminescence IGF-I immunoassay conforming to recent international recommendations. *J Clin Endocrinol Metab.* 2014;99(5):1712-1721. PMID: 24606072

19. Carmichael JD, Bonert VS, Nuno M, Ly D, Melmed S. Acromegaly clinical trial methodology impact on reported biochemical efficacy rates of somatostatin receptor ligand treatments: a meta-analysis. *J Clin Endocrinol Metab.* 2014;99(5):1825-1833. PMID: 24606084

20. Caron PJ, Bevan JS, Petersenn S, et al; PRIMARYS Investigators. Tumor shrinkage with lanreotide Autogel 120 mg as primary therapy in acromegaly: results of a prospective multicenter clinical trial. *J Clin Endocrinol Metab.* 2014;99(4):1282-1290. PMID: 24423301

21. Samson SL, Nachtigall LB, Fleseriu M, et al. Maintenance of acromegaly control in patients switching from injectable somatostatin receptor ligands to oral octreotide. *J Clin Endocrinol Metab.* 2020;105(10):e3785-e3797. PMID: 32882036

22. Fleseriu M, Dreval A, Bondar I, et al. Maintenance of response to oral octreotide compared with injectable somatostatin receptor ligands in patients with acromegaly: a phase 3, multicentre, randomised controlled trial. *Lancet Diabetes Endocrinol.* 2022;10(2):102-111. PMID: 34953531

23. Cuevas-Ramos D, Fleseriu M. Somatostatin receptor ligands and resistance to treatment in pituitary adenomas. *J Mol Endocrinol.* 2014;52(3):R223-R240. PMID: 24647046

24. Lim DS, Fleseriu M. The role of combination medical therapy in the treatment of acromegaly. *Pituitary.* 2017;20(1):136-148. PMID: 27522663

25. Colao A, Bronstein MD, Freda P, et al; Pasireotide C2305 Study Group. Pasireotide versus octreotide in acromegaly: a head-to-head superiority study. *J Clin Endocrinol Metab.* 2014;99(3):791-799. PMID: 24423324

26. Bronstein MD, Fleseriu M, Neggers S, et al; Pasireotide C2305 Study Group. Switching patients with acromegaly from octreotide to pasireotide improves biochemical control: crossover extension to a randomized, double-blind, phase III study. *BMC Endocr Disord.* 2016;16:16. PMID: 27039081

27. Gadelha MR, Bronstein MD, Brue T, et al; Pasireotide C2402 Study Group. Pasireotide versus continued treatment with octreotide or lanreotide in patients with inadequately controlled acromegaly (PAOLA): a randomised, phase 3 trial. *Lancet Diabetes Endocrinol.* 2014;2(11):875-884. PMID: 25260838

28. Muhammad A, Coopmans EC, Gatto F, et al. Pasireotide responsiveness in acromegaly is mainly driven by somatostatin receptor subtype 2 expression. *J Clin Endocrinol Metab.* 2019;104(3):915-924. PMID: 30346538

29. Samson SL. Management of hyperglycemia in patients with acromegaly treated with pasireotide LAR. *Drugs.* 2016;76(13):1235-1243. PMID: 27473537

30. Gadelha MR, Gu F, Bronstein MD, et al. Risk factors and management of pasireotide-associated hyperglycemia in acromegaly. *Endocr Connect.* 2020;9(12):1178-1190. PMID: 33434154

31. Fleseriu M, Fuhrer-Sakel D, van der Lely AJ, et al. More than a decade of real-world experience of pegvisomant for acromegaly: ACROSTUDY. *Eur J Endocrinol.* 2021;185(4):525-538. PMID: 34342594

32. Lim DST, Fleseriu M. Personalized medical treatment of patients with acromegaly: a review. *Endocr Pract.* 2022 [Online ahead of print] PMID: 35032649

33. Neggers SJ, Franck SE, de Rooij FW, et al. Long-term efficacy and safety of pegvisomant in combination with long-acting somatostatin analogs in acromegaly. *J Clin Endocrinol Metab.* 2014;99(10):3644-3652. PMID: 24937542

34. Bonert V, Mirocha J, Carmichael J, Yuen KCJ, Araki T, Melmed S. Cost-effectiveness and efficacy of a novel combination regimen in acromegaly: a prospective, randomized trial. *J Clin Endocrinol Metab.* 2020;105(9):dgaa444. PMID: 32754748

35. Muhammad A, Coopmans EC, Delhanty PJD, et al. Efficacy and safety of switching to pasireotide in acromegaly patients controlled with pegvisomant and somatostatin analogues: PAPE extension study. *Eur J Endocrinol.* 2018;179(5):269-277. PMID: 30076159

36. Fleseriu M, Hoffman AR, Katznelson L; AACE Neuroendocrine and Pituitary Scientific Committee. American Association of Clinical Endocrinologists and American College of Endocrinology Disease State Clinical Review: management of acromegaly patients: what is the role of pre-operative medical therapy? *Endocr Pract.* 2015;21(6):668-673. PMID: 26135961

37. Gheorghiu ML. Updates in outcomes of stereotactic radiation therapy in acromegaly. *Pituitary.* 2017;20(1):154-168. PMID: 28210908

38. Koulouri O, Kandasamy N, Hoole AC, et al. Successful treatment of residual pituitary adenoma in persistent acromegaly following localisation by 11C-methionine PET co-registered with MRI. *Eur J Endocrinol.* 2016;175(5):485-498. PMID: 27562400

Management of Nonsecretory Pituitary Tumors When Surgery Fails

Mark Gurnell, MD, PhD. Wellcome–MRC Institute of Metabolic Science, University of Cambridge and Addenbrooke's Hospital, Cambridge, United Kingdom; E-mail: mg299@medschl.cam.ac.uk

Learning Objectives

As a result of participating in this session, learners should be able to:

- Adopt a systematic approach to the assessment of patients with nonfunctioning pituitary adenomas (NFPAs) who have undergone primary surgery.

- Explain the limitations of standard MRI techniques in discriminating residual disease from posttreatment remodeling and in predicting future aggressive vs indolent behavior.

- Determine which patients with NFPAs require additional therapy following surgery and which patients can be managed through surveillance.

- Advise when radiotherapy should be considered or when alternative medical therapies may be indicated.

Main Conclusions

Surgery remains the primary treatment for most patients with NFPAs in whom there are clinical grounds for intervention (eg, compression of the visual pathways). However, in a significant proportion of patients, persistent or recurrent disease is suspected or confirmed. In this context, multidisciplinary expertise (provided through a pituitary tumor center of excellence) is required to guide further management and should be informed by:

- High-quality postsurgical imaging of the sella and parasellar regions.

- Detailed pathological characterization of the resected tumor, including cell lineage markers.

- Assessment of the patient's endocrine status (extent of hypopituitarism).

- Assessment of the patient's nonendocrine status (eg, visual function, presence or absence of comorbidities, pregnancy, childhood).

- Local expertise, including neurosurgery/otolaryngology, neurooncology, clinical trials.

Management options include:

- Surveillance (clinical, ophthalmic, radiological).

- Repeated surgery and/or radiotherapy.

- Trial of existing pituitary-directed medical therapy (eg, dopamine agonist).

- Systemic chemotherapy (eg, temozolomide) in aggressive tumors/pituitary carcinoma.

- Trial of novel therapies (ideally in the context of a clinical trial).

Significance of the Clinical Problem

Pituitary adenomas affect 1 in 1200 persons. A significant proportion (25%-50%) are nonsecretory (NFPA) and come to attention when they have enlarged sufficiently to compress adjacent neurological structures (eg, optic chiasm) and/or cause pituitary hormone insufficiency (hypopituitarism). Another subgroup is diagnosed incidentally during imaging of the brain performed for an unrelated indication. When required, transsphenoidal surgery is the preferred primary treatment and permits rapid and effective decompression of the visual pathways. However, complete surgical resection is not possible in all patients, with the attendant risk of tumor regrowth.[1]

Current clinical, laboratory, pathological, and radiological parameters do not reliably distinguish tumors that are likely to recur and/or behave more aggressively from those that will follow a more indolent course (*Figures 1 and 2*). Accordingly, most centers initially recommend a standard "one-size-fits-all" approach to postoperative surveillance, combining periodic MRI, ophthalmic assessment, and evaluation of endocrine status.[1,2] Traditionally, radiotherapy has been favored when there is a significant remnant in the anticipation of mitigating tumor regrowth, although it carries a risk of additional impairment of pituitary function.[1,2] There is also increasing recognition that apparent residual disease is not universally associated with regrowth/expansion (*Figure 2*). However, if a conservative approach is pursued, this is often resource intensive and may be associated with increased patient anxiety.

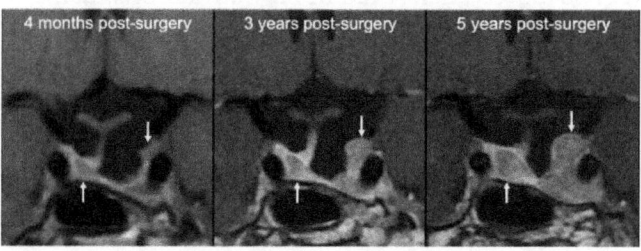

Figure 1. Progressive pituitary tumor regrowth following primary surgery.

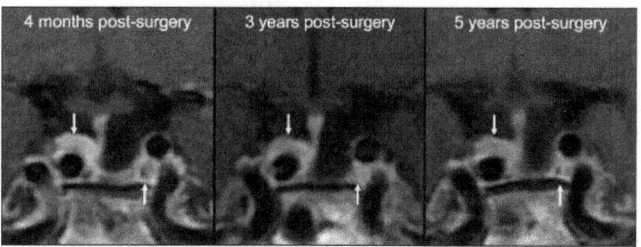

Figure 2. Suspected residual pituitary tumor following primary surgery, but with stable appearance over time.

Barriers to Optimal Practice

- Current disease biomarkers (clinical, laboratory, pathological) have limited ability to distinguish tumors that are likely to regrow and/or behave aggressively from those with more indolent behavior.

- Standard clinical MRI sequences do not always reliably discriminate postoperative remodeling from residual tumor or identify remnants that are likely to enlarge.

- High rates of additional pituitary hormone deficits have been reported in patients undergoing repeat surgery and/or radiotherapy (30%-60%).

- Prospective multicenter studies examining the efficacy and tolerability of existing pituitary-directed medical treatments (eg, dopamine agonists, somatostatin receptor ligands) and novel therapies in mitigating NFPA tumor (re)growth are lacking.

Strategies for Diagnosis, Therapy, and/or Management

NFPA is a diagnosis of exclusion. It is appropriate, therefore, to consider all available information (clinical features, previous endocrine investigations, histopathology) before deciding on the next step in the management of NFPA after primary surgery. Low-grade hormonal hypersecretion (eg, GH or ACTH) is sometimes overlooked and may require dynamic testing for exclusion. This is particularly relevant if immunohistochemistry reveals PIT-1 or T-PIT transcription factor expression. Similarly, comprehensive screening for hypopituitarism should be undertaken to help inform the discussion regarding the potential risks of further treatment. Genetic screening (eg, for familial isolated pituitary adenoma) should also be considered in young patients and in those with a suggestive personal or family history.

What constitutes surgical failure?

To fail

> *verb:* to be unsuccessful in achieving one's goal

In the absence of pathological hormone secretion, the main goals of pituitary surgery for NFPAs are:

- Protection, stabilization, and rescue of vision.

- Preservation and recovery of pituitary function.

These goals may be achieved without complete resection of the tumor, and indeed more "aggressive surgery" can result in less favorable outcomes, including injury to key neurovascular structures within the cavernous sinus or damage to the remaining normal gland with more widespread pituitary dysfunction (including cranial diabetes insipidus). The demonstration of possible, or even likely, residual tumor on early postoperative imaging should not therefore be considered an immediate indication for adjuvant therapy, especially if the visual pathways have been adequately decompressed. Surveillance is a reasonable option, especially in the early phase following surgery when histology has not identified any concerning features.

In addition, it is important to recognize the potential limitations of standard clinical MRI in the discrimination of residual tumor from postoperative remodeling—not all apparent remnants will turn out to be tumor (*Figure 3*).

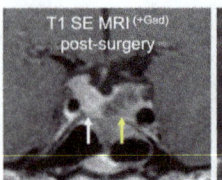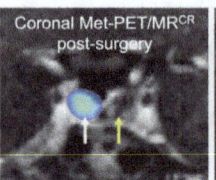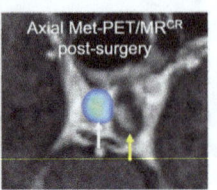

Figure 3. Standard clinical imaging (T1 spin echo MRI with gadolinium [T1 SE MRI [+Gad]]) demonstrating suspected residual tumor (*yellow arrow*) following primary surgery, with normal pituitary tissue displaced to the right of the sella (*white arrow*). However, molecular imaging (^{11}C-methionine PET/CT coregistered with volumetric MRI (Met-PET/MR[CR]) shows tracer uptake only within the normal gland, consistent with postoperative remodeling in the left hemi-sella rather than residual adenoma.

Treatment Options Following Primary Pituitary Surgery[1-3]

Further Surgery

The decision to proceed with adjuvant therapy following primary surgery for NFPA should ideally be guided by a multidisciplinary specialist team in a pituitary tumor center of excellence. This allows a full and careful evaluation of whether a repeated surgery by a highly skilled pituitary surgeon could provide added benefit without significantly increasing risk (eg, more extensive debulking to facilitate radiotherapy without causing additional pituitary deficits).

Pituitary Radiotherapy

As already highlighted, the routine use of radiotherapy postoperatively to mitigate regrowth of NFPA is no longer supported. However, in patients with significant tumor remnants that are enlarging and not amenable to further surgery, radiotherapy may arrest growth or induce tumor shrinkage. Conventional fractionated radiotherapy (eg, 45-55 Gy, delivered in 25-30 fractions, using image-guided, intensity-modulated techniques) achieves high control rates at 10 and 20 years (75%-90%), but carries a risk of hypopituitarism (~50% at 10 years) and second tumors (~1%-2%), and may predispose to premature cerebrovascular disease, although the latter is debated. Stereotactic radiosurgery has been reported to achieve control rates of up to 95% at 5 years; however, larger tumors, suprasellar extension, and lower radiation doses have all been linked with suboptimal control, while hypopituitarism, visual disturbance, and cranial neuropathies may complicate treatment. Case selection bias may also at least partially explain why outcomes from conventional fractionated radiotherapy can appear less impressive.

Medical Therapy

Dopamine Agonists

Several retrospective studies have reported tumor stabilization or even shrinkage in patients with residual or recurrent NFPAs treated with dopamine agonists (most commonly cabergoline) following primary surgery. Timing of treatment initiation (early [preventative—ie, when residual tumor suspected on postoperative MRI] vs delayed [remedial—ie, upon detection of regrowth during follow-up]) may influence effectiveness. However, routine adoption of such an approach must be balanced against the potential risks of long-term dopamine agonist therapy, and further prospective multicenter studies will be required to establish the effectiveness and safety of this approach.

Somatostatin Receptor Ligands

Evidence for the routine use of first-generation somatostatin receptor ligands (octreotide, lanreotide) in the management of residual or recurrent NFPAs is currently lacking. Although tumor stabilization has been reported in some small-scale studies, there is little evidence of tumor shrinkage. Similarly, there is a paucity of data to support combined treatment with dopamine agonists and somatostatin receptor ligands or with second-generation somatostatin receptor ligand therapy (eg, pasireotide).

Temozolomide

Temozolomide, an oral alkylating agent, is normally reserved for the treatment of aggressive pituitary adenomas and pituitary carcinomas.[3] Findings in patients with NFPAs indicate 20% to 25% response with a further 50% of patients achieving stable disease.

Novel Therapeutic Approaches

Several novel treatment targets have been identified in NFPAs, which may permit targeting with small-molecule modulators, although clinical trials are awaited. These include the folate receptor and the PI3K/AKT/mTOR pathway. Peptide receptor radionuclide therapy, which is dependent on tumoral somatostatin receptor expression, has also been tried, but with limited success.

Clinical Case Vignettes
Case 1

A 59-year-old man is seen in the endocrinology clinic. He underwent transsphenoidal pituitary surgery 3 years ago for an NFPA (immunohistochemistry of the resected tumor demonstrated SF-1 positivity, with Ki-67 labeling index of 1.6%). Twelve months ago, he received adjunctive conventional fractionated radiotherapy (45 Gy in 25 fractions) for an enlarging right cavernous sinus remnant.

On physical examination, there are no stigmata of endocrine dysfunction. Visual fields are normal. There is no cranial neuropathy.

Laboratory test results:

Prolactin = 39 ng/mL (4-23 ng/mL) (SI: 1.70 nmol/L [0.17-1.00 nmol/L])
TSH = 1.22 mIU/L (0.5-5.0 mIU/L)
Free T$_4$ = 1.10 ng/dL (0.8-1.8 ng/dL) (SI: 14.2 pmol/L [10.30-23.17 pmol/L])
Cortisol (8 AM) = 15.5 µg/dL (5-25 µg/dL) (SI: 427.6 nmol/L [137.9-689.7 nmol/L])
IGF-1 = 179 ng/mL (78-220 ng/mL) (SI: 23.4 nmol/L [10.2-28.8 nmol/L])
FSH = 3.5 mIU/mL (1.0-13.0 mIU/mL) (SI: 3.5 IU/L [1.0-13.0 IU/L])
LH = 2.7 mIU/mL (1.0-9.0 mIU/mL) (SI: 2.7 IU/L [1.0-9.0 IU/L])
Total testosterone = 237 ng/dL (300-900 ng/dL) (SI: 8.2 nmol/L [10.4-31.2 nmol/L])

Pituitary MRI is shown (*see Images*).

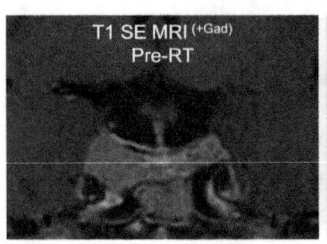

T1 SE MRI (+Gad)
Pre-RT

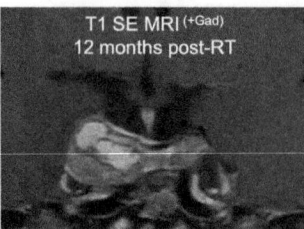

T1 SE MRI (+Gad)
12 months post-RT

Which of the following is the most appropriate next step in this patient's management?

A. Arrange another transsphenoidal surgery

B. Arrange for surveillance MRI in 6 to 12 months

C. Commence dopamine agonist therapy

D. Commence somatostatin receptor ligand therapy

E. Commence temozolomide chemotherapy

Answer: B) Arrange for surveillance MRI in 6 to 12 months

The patient is clinically well, with no neuroophthalmic complications and well-preserved pituitary function. The radiological appearances on the latest scan are consistent with postradiotherapy changes. No further intervention is required at this stage. Surveillance (Answer B) is therefore the most appropriate approach.

Case 2

A 53-year-old man is seen in the pituitary multidisciplinary clinic. He has undergone transsphenoidal pituitary surgery on 2 previous occasions for an NFPA. Following the second operation, immunohistochemistry demonstrated T-PIT positivity, weak positive staining for ACTH, and a Ki-67 labeling index of 8%. He then underwent conventional fractionated radiotherapy (50 Gy in 30 fractions), which was completed 18 months ago.

On physical examination, there are no stigmata of Cushing syndrome. He is otherwise eupituitary. Visual fields are normal. There is no cranial neuropathy.

Laboratory test results:

Prolactin = 17 ng/mL (4-23 ng/mL) (SI: 0.74 nmol/L [0.17-1.00 nmol/L])

TSH = 2.68 mIU/L (0.5-5.0 mIU/L)

Free T_4 = 1.13 ng/dL (0.8-1.8 ng/dL) (SI: 14.5 pmol/L [10.30-23.17 pmol/L])

Cortisol (8 AM) = 17.0 µg/dL (5-25 µg/dL) (SI: 469.0 nmol/L [137.9-689.7 nmol/L])

ACTH = 52 pg/mL (10-60 pg/mL) (SI: 11.4 pmol/L [2.2-13.2 pmol/L])

IGF-1 = 179 ng/mL (84-223 ng/mL) (SI: 23.4 nmol/L [11.0-30.5 nmol/L])

FSH = 5.5 mIU/mL (1.0-13.0 mIU/mL) (SI: 5.5 IU/L [1.0-13.0 IU/L])

LH = 2.2 mIU/mL (1.0-9.0 mIU/mL) (SI: 2.2 IU/L [1.0-9.0 IU/L])

Total testosterone = 265 ng/dL (300-900 ng/dL) (SI: 9.2 nmol/L [10.4-31.2 nmol/L])

Pituitary MRI is shown (*see Images*).

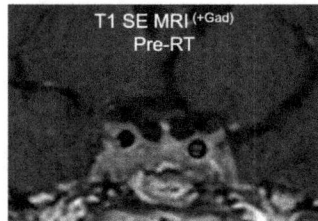

T1 SE MRI (+Gad)
Pre-RT

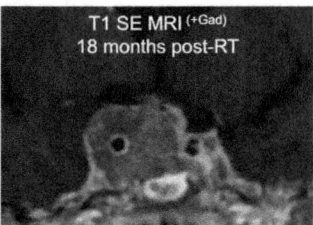

T1 SE MRI (+Gad)
18 months post-RT

Which of the following is the most appropriate next treatment?

A. Dopamine agonist therapy

B. Somatostatin receptor ligand therapy

C. Stereotactic radiosurgery

D. Temozolomide chemotherapy

E. Transcranial pituitary surgery

Answer: D) Temozolomide chemotherapy

This patient has an aggressive pituitary tumor, exhibiting radiological invasiveness with significant tumor growth despite optimal standard treatments. Conventional pituitary-directed medical therapies typically have limited efficacy in this context, whereas temozolomide (Answer D) yields a clear survival benefit.

References

1. Yavropoulou MP, Tsoli M, Barkas K, Kaltsas G, Grossman A. The natural history and treatment of non-functioning pituitary adenomas (non-functioning PitNETs). *Endocr Relat Cancer*. 2020;27(10):R375-R390. PMID: 32674070

2. Esposito D, Olsson DS, Ragnarsson O, Buchfelder M, Skoglund T, Johannsson G. Non-functioning pituitary adenomas: indications for pituitary surgery and post-surgical management. *Pituitary*. 2019;22(4):422-434. PMID: 31011999

3. Raverot G, Burman P, McCormack A, et al; European Society of Endocrinology. European Society of Endocrinology Clinical Practice Guidelines for the management of aggressive pituitary tumours and carcinomas. *Eur J Endocrinol*. 2018;178(1):G1-G24. PMID: 29046323

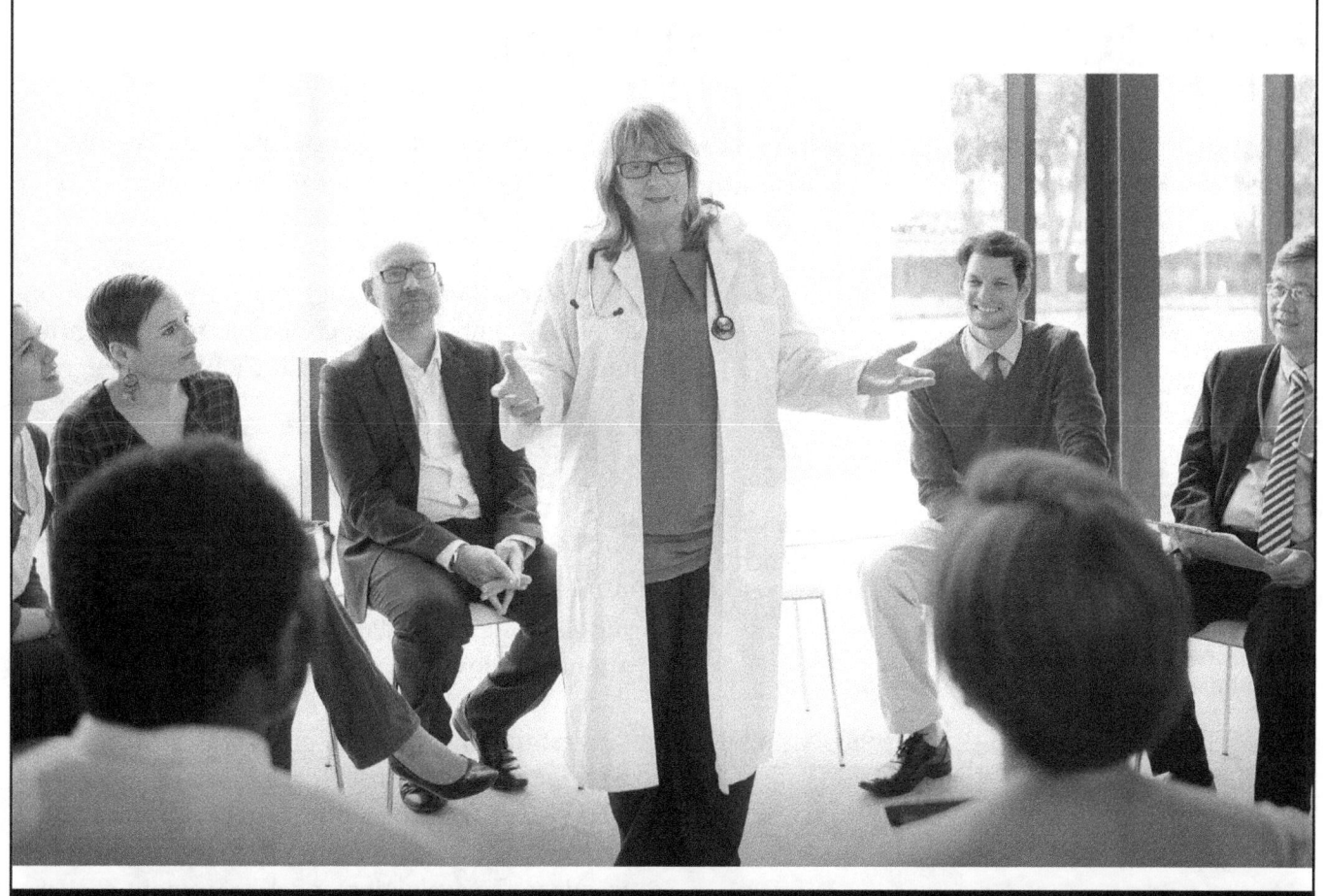

PEDIATRIC
ENDOCRINOLOGY

Precocious Puberty: Evidence-Based Management

Maria G. Vogiatzi, MD. Department of Pediatrics, Division of Endocrinology and Diabetes, Children's Hospital of Philadelphia, Philadelphia, PA; E-mail: vogiatzim@chop.edu

Learning Objectives

As a result of participating in this session, learners should be able to:

- Describe secular trends for onset of thelarche and menarche and associations with body weight, and explain their clinical relevance when evaluating a child with signs of sexual precocity.

- Develop an approach to the evaluation and management of a child with central precocious puberty (CPP).

- List various forms of GnRH analogues, explain monitoring of therapeutic effectiveness, and describe short- and long-term treatment outcomes.

Main Conclusions

A decrease in the age of onset of thelarche that is linked to obesity has been reported over the past several years. However, the tempo of pubertal progression is slower in many girls older than 7 years, and adult height may not be adversely affected. For this group of patients, clinicians must distinguish between rapidly advancing puberty and slowly progressing puberty. A period of careful monitoring has been suggested as an approach in the decision-making process for starting GnRH analogue therapy. In addition, the number of longer-acting GnRH analogue options has increased. Monitoring the effectiveness of GnRH analogue treatment is primarily clinical rather than hormonal based. Height outcomes in treated girls older than 7 years remain unclear.

Long-term therapeutic outcomes are reassuring. Advancements in genetics have started to identify monogenic causes of idiopathic CPP.

Significance of the Clinical Problem

A decrease in the age of thelarche brings a growing number of girls aged 6 to 8 years to medical attention. However, the age of menarche has decreased minimally, and longitudinal studies suggest that the tempo of puberty is slower among those with earlier breast development.[1] CNS pathology is rare at this age. Pediatric endocrinologists must consider these secular trends in the evaluation and management of such girls.

Clinical care using GnRH analogue therapy has changed over the last several years. New longer-acting GnRH analogue formulations have entered the market.[1] Widespread use of ultrasensitive LH assays has decreased the need for stimulation testing for diagnostic purposes and treatment monitoring. Regardless, there is paucity of well-designed, controlled studies to guide evidence-based care for children with CPP, and more research is needed to compare the efficacy and long-term outcomes of the most recent depot preparations. Long-term outcomes of GnRH analogue administration regarding obesity, cardiovascular risk factors, fertility, and bone mass are reassuring.[1] The effect of GnRH analogue therapy on the psychosocial adjustment in children with CPP is uncertain.

Barriers to Optimal Practice

- Clinical studies in CPP are hampered by the lack of well-designed controlled studies, small sample size, and heterogeneous design. Management decisions are frequently not supported by clear practice guidelines.

- Data regarding boys with CPP, associations of gonadarche with obesity, response to GnRH analogue therapy, and long-term outcomes are limited.

Strategies for Diagnosis, Therapy, and/or Management

Diagnosis

Secular Trends on Gonadarche and How They May Influence Decisions About Initiation of GnRH Analogue Therapy

In recent years, many studies have reported a decrease in the age of onset of thelarche. The Breast Cancer and Environment Research Program, a large prospective longitudinal study in the United States, observed the median ages for onset of Tanner stage 2 breast development at 8.8, 9.3, 9.7, and 9.7 years for Black, Hispanic, White, and Asian girls, respectively. Girls with high BMI tend to achieve stage 2 breast development at younger ages. Similar trends have been observed in Europe and Asia.[2] This has led some investigators to propose a younger age than 8 years as a cutoff for definition of sexual precocity in girls. Despite this pronounced decrease in the age of thelarche, however, the age of menarche has decreased minimally. Longitudinal studies suggest that the tempo of pubertal progression is slower among those with earlier breast development.[1,2] In addition, population-based gonadotropin levels among girls who experience earlier breast development does not support activation of the hypothalamic-pituitary-gonadal axis, suggesting that many cases of breast development around age 6 to 8 years represent benign thelarche. Data are less consistent in boys, although the preponderance of studies also support an earlier onset of puberty in association with increased BMI. Based on the above secular trends, clinical observation for 4 to 6 months has been proposed for girls who experience onset of breast development between age 7 and 8 years to assess the tempo of pubertal progression and before considering suppression of puberty.[1] Evidence of rapid pubertal progression increases the risk for short adult height and supports starting a GnRH analogue.

Laboratory Assessment

With the introduction of ultrasensitive LH assays, random LH measurements have become the most valuable laboratory tool in the diagnosis of CPP. The use of GnRH or GnRH analogue–stimulation tests is typically reserved for patients in whom there is a strong clinical suspicion for CPP and a prepubertal random LH value.[1] Pelvic ultrasonography is not always useful for the diagnosis of CPP. Brain MRI is recommended in all boys with CPP given their greater risk for pathology. The risk of CNS pathology in girls between age 6 and 8 years is small. In this age range, the incidence of tumors that would require intervention is 1.6% according to a recent meta-analysis that included approximately 1800 girls.[1] Based on these results, it has been suggested that girls with CPP should have brain MRI performed routinely if they are younger than 6 years or have symptoms suggestive of CNS pathology.

Genetics of CPP

Approximately 90% of girls and 25% to 60% of boys have idiopathic CPP, with no identifiable causes explaining the sexual precocity. The onset of puberty is regulated by a functionally connected and well-organized neuronal network that can send signals that either stimulate or inhibit the generation of GnRH pulses.[3] Environmental factors, such as nutritional status or adoption, can influence the age of gonadarche via interactions with this GnRH neuronal network. Genes, such as kisspeptin (*KISS1*), kisspeptin receptor (*KISS1R*), makorin ring finger 41 protein 3 (*MKRN3*), and delta-like homolog 1 (*DLK1*), have a key role in

GnRH pulse regulation. Pathogenic variants in these genes are associated with idiopathic CPP. Of these genes, loss-of-function pathogenic variants in *MKRN3* have been identified so far as the most frequent monogenic cause of idiopathic CPP.[3]

Management

GnRH Analogue Formulations and Monitoring of Therapy

The number of available long-acting GnRH analogue formulations has increased over the years in the United States with the use of the histrelin implant in 2007 and the most recent introduction of leuprolide acetate intramuscular 3-month depot at doses of 11.25 mg and 30 mg; intramuscular triptorelin 6-month depot; and subcutaneous leuprolide acetate 6-month depot. Clinical suppression and growth rate appear similar with all formulations. Data on adult height and long-term outcomes with the 6-month triprorelin and 6-month subcutaneous leuprolide are still unavailable. Decisions about what formulations to use are based on family and patient preference and cost rather than specific guidelines.[1] While the prescription of a GnRH analogue is not weight-based in the United States, the GnRH analogue dosages used in different countries, such as Europe, China, or Japan, are much smaller and in the range of 10 to 350 mcg/kg.

Monitoring during therapy has been shifted to clinical evidence of suppression rather than strict hormonal monitoring. During therapy with longer-acting formulations, values of random LH with ultrasensitive assays are frequently above the established prepubertal range despite clinical evidence of pubertal suppression.[1]

Effect of GnRH Analogue Therapy on Height

In older published reports, untreated CPP leads to a height loss in adults of about 20 cm in men and 12 cm in women compared with height in the average population.[4] Height loss in CPP is inversely correlated with the age at puberty onset. GnRH analogue therapy leads to improved adult height compared with predicted adult height at the start of therapy. Height outcomes are less clear for girls with onset of puberty at age 7 years or older. A systematic review of 6 controlled studies (2 randomized) of GnRH analogues vs no treatment in 332 girls with onset of puberty older than 7 years found no evidence that GnRH analogue therapy improves adult height, while untreated girls reached an adult height similar to midparental height.[1,4]

GnRH analogue therapy may lead to a decrease in height velocity. To improve growth rate in children with CPP and persistently low adult height prediction, the use of a GnRH analogue combined either with low-dosage estrogen or oxandrolone was examined in a limited number of studies. Although the results were promising, there have not been further studies to support this practice.[4] Adding GH to GnRH analogue therapy to the regimen of patients with CPP was examined in several studies. The results show modest improvement in adult height of approximately 3 cm in those who received GH, according to a recent meta-analysis.[4]

Psychosocial Adjustment in CPP and Effect of GnRH Analogue Therapy

Previous studies of patients with CPP have described high rates of depression, suicidal thoughts, and behavior problems. These findings have been inconsistent. More recently, the National Longitudinal Study of Adolescent and Adult Health has linked early age of menarche with higher rates of depression and antisocial behavior in adult life.[5] These associations may be partially explained by postpubertal stressful life events, such as increased likelihood of teenage pregnancy and childbearing, as well as sexual and physical assault, that perpetuate long-term vulnerabilities. Whether GnRH analogue therapy has any effect on these parameters is unknown. Smaller studies of children treated with GnRH analogues provide inconsistent results about rates of psychologic concerns and how they are influenced by GnRH analogue therapy.

GnRH Analogue Adverse Effects and Long-Term Outcomes

Adverse effects of GnRH analogue therapy are rare and include local reactions, sterile abscess formation after depot injections, hot flushes, withdrawal bleeding in girls with advanced puberty, and sporadic case reports of convulsions. Hypertension with use of triptorelin has rarely been reported. Pituitary apoplexy and prolonged QT interval in association with GnRH analogue therapy have been reported in men with prostate cancer but not in pediatric patients. Screening electrocardiography is recommended in children with cardiac disease or those who are treated with medications that increase the QT interval.

Long-term outcome data focus primarily on girls, while data in boys are limited. Although children with CPP have increased body weight compared with their peers at diagnosis, GnRH analogue therapy does not appear to lead to obesity in adulthood. In a study by Lazar et al, women with a history of CPP (treated or untreated) had the same BMI and cardiovascular risk as matched healthy control participants. In this cohort, education, marital status, and pregnancy rates were the same as those of control participants and not affected by GnRH analogue therapy. Data are conflicting about the development polycystic ovary syndrome in women with a history of CPP, while a small number of studies indicate that GnRH analogue therapy does not increase the risk for polycystic ovary syndrome. Changes in bone mass with GnRH analogue therapy are addressed in a few studies that do not provide long-term follow up. Results indicate a decrease in bone mineral density during GnRH analogue therapy and a resumption of bone accrual after GnRH analogue discontinuation. Bone mineral density has been reported in the normal range in late adolescence.

Clinical Case Vignettes

Case 1

A 7-and-3/12-year-old girl presents with a 6-month history of breast development. She has a history of rapid weight gain with a BMI greater than the 99th percentile since her toddler years and body odor and pubic hair development since age 5 years. Examination findings are significant for Tanner 2 breast development with additional adipomastia. Pubic hair is Tanner stage 3. She has generalized obesity with acanthosis on the neck and in the axillae. Her family history is negative for precocity, and review of her growth shows stable linear growth at the 75th percentile with no recent acceleration.

Laboratory test results:

> Baseline ultrasensitive LH =
> 0.1 mIU/mL (0.02-0.30 mIU/mL)
> (SI: 0.1 IU/L [0.02-0.30 IU/L])
> FSH = 2.3 mIU/mL (0.26-3.0 mIU/mL)
> (SI: 2.3 IU/L [0.26-3.0 IU/L])
> 17-Hydroxyprogesterone (8 AM) = 75 ng/dL
> (0-90 ng/dL) (SI: 2.27 nmol/L [0-2.72 nmol/L])
> DHEA-S = 85 μg/dL (16-96 μg/dL) (SI: 2.3 μmol/L
> [0.43-2.60 μmol/L])

Her bone age is 8 years and 10 months. Adult height prediction is 61 in (155 cm) according to Bailey-Pinneau (average maturation table) compared with midparental height of 63 in (160 cm).

Which of the following is the best next step in this patient's management?

A. Observation

B. Order pelvic ultrasonography

C. Perform a GnRH-stimulation test

D. Both B and C

Answer: A) Observation

The girl in this vignette has Tanner stage 2 breast development and a random LH measurement by ultrasensitive assay in the prepubertal range. Her bone age is advanced, but the advancement may be related to obesity. A LH random measurement may miss the diagnosis of CPP in approximately 25% of children, and a GnRH-stimulation test (Answer C) should be performed if CPP is clinically suspected and the provider wants to consider GnRH analogue therapy.[1] However, the onset of thelarche in girls with obesity is increasingly common above age of 7 years in many instances, and pubertal progression in such girls tends to be slow and adult height is not affected.[1,2] It has been suggested, therefore, to observe these girls (Answer A) for 4 to 6 months to assess the tempo of puberty before starting GnRH analogue therapy.[1,2] Findings from pelvic ultrasonography (Answer B) are not a diagnostic criterion for CPP.

Case 1 (continued)

The child returns 6 months later at age 7 and 9/12 years. Her mother reports some increase in both breast and pubic hair development. Review of systems is otherwise unremarkable. Her growth chart indicates an increase in growth rate, while her BMI percentile is unchanged at greater than the 99th. Her repeated LH measurement is 0.4 mIU/mL and repeated bone age is interpreted to be 10 years. The family is interested in GnRH analogue treatment.

How would you counsel the family about GnRH analogue therapy for this girl?

A. GnRH analogue therapy is unlikely to improve adult height

B. GnRH analogue therapy is likely to worsen adult BMI

C. MRI of the brain should be performed before therapy initiation

D. Both A and C

Answer: A) GnRH analogue therapy is unlikely to improve adult height

There is no clear evidence that GnRH analogue therapy improves final height in girls with CPP who are older than 7 years (Answer A).[1,4] Long-term outcomes in women with a history of CPP show similar BMI and cardiovascular risk factors regardless of GnRH analogue therapy (thus, Answer B is incorrect).[1] The risk of CNS pathology in girls aged 6 to 8 years appears small, and MRI of the brain has been suggested in this age group if they have relevant symptoms. The girl in this vignette has no headaches or other symptoms suggestive of a CNS process, thus MRI of the brain (Answer C) is incorrect.[1]

Case 1 (continued)

The child is treated with a histrelin implant. She returns a year after implant at age 9 years. There is no progression in breast development (Tanner stage 2) and minimal advancement in pubic hair growth. Her growth rate is stable, as it was pretreatment. BMI percentiles remain in the same range and greater than the 99th. Repeated bone age is interpreted as having advanced from 10 years to between 10 and 11 years over the course of the past year. A random LH measurement (by ultrasensitive assay) is 0.6 mIU/mL 10 months after implantation.

Which of the following is the best next step in this patient's management?

A. Order pelvic ultrasonography

B. Perform a GnRH-stimulation test

C. Provide reassurance about the treatment course

D. Replace the histrelin implant

Answer: C) Provide reassurance about the treatment course

Random ultrasensitive LH values above the established prepubertal range have been described with histrelin despite clinical suppression of puberty. No additional workup such as pelvic ultrasonography (Answer A) or a GnRH-stimulation test (Answer B) is suggested unless there is clinical evidence that puberty is not suppressed.[1] Thus, the patient should be reassured about the treatment course (Answer C). Current evidence indicates that histrelin can effectively suppress puberty for longer than 12 months; thus, replacement (Answer D) is not necessary now.

Case 1 (continued)

The family has questions about length of GnRH analogue therapy and resumption of puberty.

What should this family be told about GnRH analogue therapy?

A. Age of menarche after stopping GnRH analogue therapy is variable

B. The decision to discontinue GnRH analogues should consider the psychological readiness of the child

C. Treatment beyond the bone age of 12.5 years is unlikely to significantly improve adult height

D. All the above

Answer: D) All the above

There are no clear guidelines for therapy discontinuation.[1] The decision is individualized based on the child's readiness to progress in puberty and growth assessment (Answer B). In terms of growth, it appears that height gains decrease beyond the bone age of 12.5 years in girls and 14 in boys (Answer C),[1,4] although more recent data support further therapy in select patients. Resumption of menses after stopping GnRH analogue therapy varies from several months to more than 2 years (Answer A).[1]

Case 2

An 8-and-10/12-year-old girl experienced menarche 4 months ago. Breast development was first appreciated at age 7-and-6/12 years. She is otherwise healthy and is doing well in school. Menses have been regular.

On physical examination, her height is 57 in (145 cm), and BMI is at the 75th percentile, Breast and pubic hair are Tanner stage 4. Her bone age is interpreted to be 13.5 years. Her midparental height is 64 in (163 cm). Her mother reports initial difficulties handling menses, but "things are getting better."

What should this family be told about depression and psychosocial distress in this patient group?

A. Girls with early menarche are at greater risk for depression as adolescents and adults

B. GnRH analogue therapy significantly ameliorates psychosocial distress

C. Neither A nor B

D. Both A and B

Answer: A) Girls with early menarche are at greater risk for depression as adolescents and adults

According to a large recent epidemiological study, earlier age at menarche is associated with higher rates of depressive symptoms in adolescence and adulthood (Answer A).[6] Whether GnRH analogue therapy ameliorates these symptoms (Answer B) is unclear.[1]

Case 2 (continued)

The patient's mother requests evaluation of the younger sister. She is 6 and 6/12 years old and has had recent onset of breast development.

On physical examination, breast development is Tanner stage 2. A random ultrasensitive LH measurement is 1.2 mIU/mL and bone age is interpreted to be 8 years.

Genetic analysis is considered.

Which of the following is true about genetic analysis in this patient's case?

A. Genetic analysis is likely to yield negative results

B. Genetic analysis is likely to reveal an activating pathogenic variant in *MKRN3*

C. Genetic analysis is likely to reveal an activating pathogenic variant in *KISS1*

D. Kisspeptin and MKRN3 levels can serve as biomarkers for genetic causes of CPP

Answer: A) Genetic analysis is likely to yield negative results

The overall estimated prevalence of *MKRN3* variants in persons with CPP is 9.0%. The prevalence of pathogenic variants in familial cases of CPP is variable among different studies, but according to a recent meta-analysis, the estimated pooled prevalence is 19.0% (95% CI, 0.05-0.36).[5] Thus, genetic analysis is unlikely to reveal an etiology (Answer A).

MKRN3 has an inhibitory role in pubertal onset, and loss-of-function pathogenic variants (not activating variants [Answer B]) in the *MKRN3* gene are the most frequent monogenic cause of CPP.[6]

Activating pathogenic variants in the *KISS1* gene have been identified in persons with CPP, but they are rare (thus, Answer C is incorrect).[6]

Serum concentrations of kisspeptin increase with puberty, while MKRN3 concentrations decrease. Serum concentrations of kisspeptin and MKRN3 are being considered as biomarkers of puberty. However, neither serves as a biomarker for genetic causes of CPP (thus, Answer D is incorrect).

References

1. Bangalore Krishna K, Fuqua JS, Rogol AD, et al. Use of gonadotropin-releasing hormone analogs in children: update by an international consortium. *Horm Res Paediatr.* 2019;91(6):357-372. PMID: 31319416

2. Tenedero CB, Oei K, Palmert MR. An approach to the evaluation and management of the obese child with early puberty. *J Endocr Soc.* 2021;6(1):bvab173. PMID: 34909516

3. Schneider Aguirre R, Eugster EA. Central precocious puberty: from genetics to treatment. *Best Pract Res Clin Endocrinol Metab.* 2018;32(4):343-354. PMID: 30086862

4. Wit JM. Should skeletal maturation be manipulated for extra height gain? *Front Endocrinol (Lausanne).* 2021;12:812196. PMID: 34975773

5. Valadares LP, Meireles CG, De Toledo IP, et al. MKRN3 mutations in central precocious puberty: a systematic review and meta-analysis. *J Endocr Soc.* 2019;3(5):979-995. PMID: 31041429

6. Mendle J, Ryan RM, McKone KMP. Early menarche and internalizing and externalizing in adulthood: explaining the persistence of effects. *J Adolesc Health.* 2019;65(5):599-606. PMID: 31500947

Dilemmas in Diabetes Mellitus in Youth

Philip S. Zeitler, MD, PhD. Department of Pediatrics, Section of Endocrinology, University of Colorado School of Medicine, Anschutz Medical Campus, Aurora, CO; E-mail: Philip.Zeitler@ childrenscolorado.org

Learning Objectives

As a result of participating in this session, learners should be able to:

- Describe the challenges related to evaluation and management of prediabetes in youth.

- Guide the evaluation and management of adolescents with obesity who have new-onset diabetes mellitus.

Main Conclusions

The pediatric diabetologist is faced with limitations in the evaluation and management of diabetes in adolescents, including unique features of pathophysiology, the effect of childhood obesity and puberty, the substantial clinical overlap between type 1 and type 2 diabetes mellitus (T1DM and T2DM), and limited information on the earliest periods of disease. Emerging information suggests that mild glycemic elevations are normal during puberty and that there is very substantial reversion to normoglycemia in youth. Thus, the current criteria used for identification of youth with "prediabetes" are suspect. These realities have made it difficult to design studies of optimal treatment of "prediabetes" in youth and for pediatric clinicians to be confident in managing mild dysglycemia. Although the incidence of T2DM diabetes has increased dramatically in youth over the last 3 decades, T1DM diabetes remains as, or more, common than T2DM, even among high-risk youth based on their ethnic heritage and/or family history. Furthermore, the prevalence of obesity in the entire western population is rising, but this does not protect against T1DM. In the United States, approximately 30% of youth with T1DM diabetes have obesity. Because of this overlap, clinical features are insufficient for determination of diabetes type, and the clinician is often faced with a patient with T1DM who also has features of insulin resistance (eg, dyslipidemia, hypertension, fatty liver, polycystic ovary syndrome, etc). This requires changes to the historical management of T1DM. Taken together, the changing nature of pediatric diabetes necessitates informed physiology-based approaches to evaluation and management, including familiarity with changing guidelines for management of glycemic and nonglycemic outcomes.

Significance of the Clinical Problem

The incidence and prevalence of diabetes in youth, both T1DM and T2DM, are increasing in the United States and in many other regions of the globe.[1] At the same time, the prevalence of obesity is increasing in the general population, and this is mirrored in the rate of obesity among youth with diabetes. This makes the distinction between T1DM and T2DM more complex than in the past. Furthermore, the distinction of diabetes type in children is even more challenging than in adults with new-onset diabetes. While the pathophysiology of T1DM has been well described and includes a steady loss of β-cell function until the typical metabolic decompensation that characterizes onset of clinical disease, the course of youth-onset T2DM is only beginning to be understood. Studies indicate that youth-onset T2DM has several unique aspects. For example, there is an important association of T2DM with pubertal development, most likely related to the transient reduction in insulin sensitivity that occurs in children as they enter puberty[2] and the need for compensation in insulin secretion, which may lead to hyperglycemia in youth with limited β-cell capacity. Furthermore, dysglycemia occurring during puberty, including both "prediabetes" and clinically overt diabetes, may be reversible in some youth due to the dynamic nature of the underlying insulin resistance. Yet, it is critical to understand that while decline in β-cell function also occurs in adults with T2DM, when there is progressive β-cell failure leading to overt diabetes in youth, it is more rapid, resulting in more frequent presentation with metabolic decompensation and greater challenges in achieving and maintaining glycemic targets after initiation of therapy.[3-8] Finally, there is evidence of microvascular complications and risk markers for macrovascular complications at the time of diagnosis, along with rapid progression of complications in youth with T2DM.[9-11] Importantly, many of the microvascular and macrovascular complications seen in youth-onset T2DM are associated with visceral adiposity and insulin resistance, suggesting similar risk in individuals with T1DM complicated by obesity and obesity-related comorbidities.[12]

Taken together, the changing epidemiology of diabetes in youth, the unique features of T2DM in youth, and the increasing prevalence of obesity in the population create challenges for the clinician evaluating and managing adolescents with obesity and evidence of dysglycemia, metabolic dysfunction, and/or new-onset diabetes. This evolution requires reconsideration of historical approaches to managing and monitoring of youth with diabetes and a deeper familiarity with approaches to mitigate cardiorenal risk.

Barriers to Optimal Practice

- There is no well-established, physiologically valid definition of prediabetes in youth, and most youth found to have prediabetes by current definitions (based on adult American Diabetes Association criteria) will revert to normoglycemia without intervention. This creates challenges for both study design in this population, as well as selection of optimal treatment approaches.

- Lifestyle change, the backbone of obesity treatment and mitigating risk for diabetes, is difficult to achieve in youth with obesity, who often come from challenged backgrounds and family environments. There is currently limited evidence to support pharmacologic approaches for youth at risk for diabetes.

- Despite rising incidence of T2DM, T1DM remains prevalent, even among high-risk youth. Furthermore, rising rates of obesity and minority representation in the general population are mirrored in the pediatric T1DM population, such that presenting clinical features are not reliable for determination of diabetes type.

- The rising rates of obesity in individuals with T1DM, as well as the increased percentage of individuals with T1DM who come from ethnic and cultural backgrounds at increased risk for obesity-related cardiovascular disease, mean that the pediatric diabetologist is increasingly called on to manage cardiovascular risk factors, which have not historically been a focus of T1DM care.

Strategies for Diagnosis, Therapy, and/or Management

With the rise of childhood obesity and youth-onset T2DM, greater attention has been paid to the trajectory of disease development, whereas historically the focus has been dominated by T1DM. Pediatric clinician knowledge of the concept and treatment of prediabetes in adults has resulted in interest in identifying prediabetes in youth and potentially initiating treatment to prevent disease progression. Yet, the meaning of glycemic measures in youth are not fully understood, as all youth experience metabolic changes during puberty, including transient insulin resistance, and little is known about the effect of these metabolic changes on the distribution of glycemia. However, despite this lack of knowledge, the American Diabetes Association adult criteria for the diagnosis of diabetes and prediabetes have been extrapolated to youth. In 2010, the American Diabetes Association added criteria for use of hemoglobin A_{1c} for screening and diagnosis of diabetes (ie, >6.5% [>48 mmol/mol]) and prediabetes (ie, >5.7%-6.4% [39-46 mmol/mol]).[13] Indeed, hemoglobin A_{1c} measurement has some advantages over the traditional diagnostic tests (fasting or 2-hour glucose), including no need for fasting and less influence of acute circumstances of the testing day. The decision to add hemoglobin A_{1c} to the criteria was based on improvements in assay standardization, correlation with 2-hour glucose values, and population studies demonstrating increased prevalence of retinopathy in adults at high risk for T2DM.[14,15] In adults, a prediabetes hemoglobin A_{1c} value has been shown to predict progression to diabetes, as well as risk for retinopathy. However, studies validating the use of a prediabetes hemoglobin A_{1c} value to predict risk for progression to diabetes or diabetes complications in youth are lacking. We and others have shown correlation of hemoglobin A_{1c} with other measures of glycemia (eg, oral glucose tolerance testing [OGTT] and continuous glucose monitoring) in the context of screening for T2DM in youth with obesity.[16,17] In the absence of a full understanding of physiologic changes in glycemia during puberty, the meaning of any of these measures of glycemia remains unclear. In a large cohort of racially and ethnically diverse midpubertal youth, 1 of 50 healthy-weight youth had a hemoglobin A_{1c} measurement in the "prediabetes" range.[18] These elevated hemoglobin A_{1c} values are highly unlikely to represent

evolving diabetes based on previously published epidemiologic data showing a much lower prevalence of diabetes in this group of normal-weight youth.[19,20] In adults, hemoglobin A_{1c} values in the prediabetes range have been shown to correlate with impaired glucose tolerance (IGT) and impaired fasting glucose (IFG) by OGTT.[21] No similar study has been performed to date in youth.

OGTT is often considered the gold standard test for diagnosing diabetes. While there is evidence that adults with a 2-hour glucose value in the prediabetes range are at high risk for progression to diabetes,[15] the evidence for this association in youth is lacking. In fact, in a study of 117 adolescents with obesity, 45.5% of 33 youth with IGT reverted to normal glucose tolerance after a mean of 20.4 months of follow-up.[22] The substantial variability in OGTT seen over time may be, in part, related to variability in the physiologic changes in glucose metabolism occurring during the well-described transient insulin resistance of puberty.[23,24] This transient insulin resistance of puberty may also alter glucose metabolism in normal-weight youth and lead to transient increases in glycemia, similar to changes seen with lipids during puberty.[25-27] Therefore, there is not a full understanding of whether elevations into the adult prediabetes range with any measure of glycemia are meaningful in youth. While the mean hemoglobin A_{1c} value was slightly higher in youth who were overweight or obese, the distribution of hemoglobin A_{1c} in the overweight/obese cohort was very similar to the distribution in the normal-weight cohort. Thus, a proportion of youth with obesity have a hemoglobin A_{1c} value in the adult "prediabetes" range, but these same hemoglobin A_{1c} values are within the distribution for normal-weight youth, raising questions about how meaningful the adult-based cutoffs are for defining prediabetes in youth. In fact, analysis of the HEALTHY cohort reported that of those with a prediabetes hemoglobin A_{1c} level at baseline (6th grade, n = 128), only 1 progressed to diabetes, while 53% had a normal hemoglobin A_{1c} value, and the rest continued to have a hemoglobin A_{1c} value in the prediabetes range at follow-up (8th grade).[28] While large, prospective, longitudinal cohort studies exploring whether hemoglobin A_{1c}, or any other measure of glycemia, can predict progression to diabetes in youth have not been done, a large retrospective study of more than 11,000 youth with obesity has reported that progression to diabetes among youth with a hemoglobin A_{1c} value less than 6.0% (<42 mmol/mol) occurs in less than 6% and even for those with a hemoglobin A_{1c} value between 6.0% and 6.5% (42 and 48 mmol/mol), progression is only around 18%.[29] Therefore, clinicians caring for youth with obesity and dysglycemia should be cautious when undertaking interventions beyond lifestyle change until efficacy has been directly demonstrated in the pediatric population.

When a child or adolescent with obesity presents with apparent diabetes-range hyperglycemia, definitive diagnosis and typing of diabetes requires 2 steps: (1) confirmation of the presence of diabetes followed by (2) determination of diabetes type. This is rarely a problem in T1DM because of the characteristic symptomatic presentation with metabolic decompensation, but on occasion, youth are identified with mild to moderate dysglycemia without the other hallmark features of T1DM, and the confirmation of diabetes may need to be considered more carefully. The criteria and classification of diabetes are provided in the American Diabetes Association annual guidelines and the International Society for Pediatric and Adolescent Diabetes clinical practice consensus guidelines.[30,31] While the American Diabetes Association has added hemoglobin A_{1c} as a diagnostic criterion based on prediction of retinopathy risk, this assumes use of a laboratory-measured, DCCT-aligned assay—not point-of-care testing. In the absence of symptoms, hyperglycemia detected incidentally or under conditions of acute physiologic stress may be transitory and should not be regarded as diagnostic of diabetes. Therefore, in the absence of unambiguous chronic symptoms of hyperglycemia, a second test on a different day is required.

After the diagnosis of diabetes is established, careful consideration should be given to determining diabetes type. There are features of presentation and phenotype that may be useful in developing a presumption of T1DM or T2DM, although there is substantial overlap between characteristics of T2DM and T1DM in adolescents with obesity, making these features of limited value. The degree of pubertal development may be the most useful, although in a negative fashion: youth with T2DM are almost always in puberty, with a mean age of diagnosis of 13 to 14 years and Tanner stage 4 to 5. They are rarely prepubertal.[32,33] Most importantly, diabetes autoantibody testing should be done in all youth with the clinical diagnosis of T2DM because of the high frequency of islet-cell autoimmunity in patients with otherwise "typical" T2DM[34]; the presence of antibodies predicts rapid development of insulin requirement, as well as risk for development of other autoimmune disorders. Diabetes autoantibody testing also should also be considered in overweight/obese pubertal children with a clinical picture of T1DM (weight loss, ketosis/ketoacidosis), some of whom may have T2DM and be able to be weaned off insulin for extended periods.[35,36] Finally, monogenic forms of diabetes, such as maturity-onset diabetes of the young should be considered in individuals who have a presentation and course that are not characteristic of either T1DM or T2DM.

Initial treatment of the adolescent with obesity and diabetes must consider that diabetes type is often not certain in the first few weeks of treatment, that 10% to 15% of adolescents with new-onset diabetes and obesity have T1DM, and that a substantial percentage of adolescents with T2DM present with clinically significant ketoacidosis.[37,38] Therefore, initial treatment should be based on the clinical presentation, while maintaining an open mind regarding both the diabetes type and eventual therapy.

Adolescents presenting with acidosis require initiation of intravenous insulin, no matter the diabetes type. However, once acidosis is resolved, subsequent therapy depends on the provisional clinical diagnosis. In those patients for whom the provisional diagnosis is T1DM, the diabetes care team should proceed with the usual education and insulin therapy. In those patients for whom the clinical impression is T2DM or antibodies have been shown to be negative, basal insulin at a dose of 0.2 to 0.4 units/kg once daily is started and titrated based on fingerstick glucose measurements. Insulin is administered at whatever time of day is the most likely to promote good engagement with therapy. At the same time, metformin is initiated at 500 mg once daily and is titrated weekly to a maximally tolerated dosage, with a target of 2000 mg daily. Insulin can generally be discontinued within a few weeks once antibody negativity has been confirmed. Asymptomatic patients with an initial hemoglobin A_{1c} value greater than 9.0% or 10.0% (75 or 86 mmol/mol) may also require initiation of once-daily basal insulin therapy to allow sufficient recovery of β-cell function for successful monotherapy with oral medication. However, results from the TODAY study suggest that initiation of metformin and basic dietary intervention results in a hemoglobin A_{1c} value in the nondiabetic range, with or without insulin.[35,36] Asymptomatic adolescents with obesity who present with less decompensation can be started on metformin alone, with a high likelihood of initial success.

Lifestyle change is critical to treatment of obesity, whether the patient has T1DM or T2DM, and clinicians should initiate a lifestyle modification program, including nutrition and physical activity, for children and adolescents at the time of T2DM diagnosis.[38] Interventions include promoting a healthy lifestyle through behavior change, including nutrition, exercise training, weight management, and cigarette smoking cessation. However, the challenges in implementing lifestyle modifications in adolescents are greater than in adults because adolescents with obesity typically come from families where overeating and sedentary lifestyle are the norm. Thus, many adolescents with T2DM do not maintain the recommended lifestyle changes and remain overweight with suboptimal diabetes control. The role of weight-loss medications for adolescents with diabetes and obesity remains unclear and poorly studied. Although the GLP-1 receptor agonist liraglutide has been approved for use in adolescents with T2DM, weight loss in the pivotal study was not as impressive as seen in adults. While potentially more effective GLP-1 receptor agonists such as dulaglutide and semaglutide are being actively studied in youth, no data are yet available. Similarly, although SGLT-2 inhibitors have been shown to improve hyperglycemia, as well as lead to substantial weight loss (and reduction in cardiorenal risk) in adults, data are not yet available in youth. Similarly, the role for antihyperglycemia agents, such as metformin, GLP-1 receptor agonists, and SGLT-2 inhibitors, as adjunct agents in youth with obesity and T1DM is intriguing, as they offer potential reduction in weight, insulin resistance, and cardiorenal risk, but studies are only now being undertaken, and use of these agents is optimally done in the setting of a research study.

There are currently distinctions between recommendations for monitoring comorbidities and complications in youth with T1DM and T2DM, with earlier and more aggressive monitoring in T2DM because of the evidence for earlier and more rapid onset of microvascular and macrovascular abnormalities.[39] However, the presence of insulin resistance in youth with T1DM and obesity and the association of kidney, retinal, nerve, vascular, and heart disease with insulin resistance, as well as glycemia, suggest that it may be appropriate to undertake an approach to monitoring in these individuals that is more like the recommendations for T2DM. Studies addressing this question are needed but may be difficult to undertake because of the need to prevent acute and chronic negative outcomes in individual patients.

Clinical Case Vignettes
Case 1

A 10-year-old African American girl sees a new primary care provider who notes that she has had longstanding elevation in BMI (>98th percentile) and has moderate acanthosis nigricans on examination. She has Tanner stage 3 breast and pubic hair development and has not had menarche. Family history is notable for T2DM in her mother, who had diabetes during pregnancy, as well as in her maternal grandmother. A point-of-care hemoglobin A_{1c} measurement is 5.9% (41 mmol/mol). The primary care provider tells the family that the patient has prediabetes and refers her to the diabetes center.

Which of the following is the most important next step in this patient's management?

A. Measure liver transaminases

B. Order lipid panel

C. Refer for multidisciplinary lifestyle intervention

D. Repeat the hemoglobin A_{1c} measurement to confirm prediabetes

E. Start metformin, 500 mg daily

Answer: C) Refer for multidisciplinary lifestyle intervention

Although the patient has a mildly elevated hemoglobin A_{1c} value in the adult prediabetes range on point-of-care hemoglobin A_{1c} testing, the implication of a hemoglobin A_{1c} value in this range in youth is unclear. Evidence suggests that such elevations are likely to be nonprogressive and often transient. Therefore, there is no compelling argument supporting initiation of pharmacologic therapy (Answer E) in adolescents with mild degrees of glycemia. Since there is little value in diagnosing "prediabetes" in youth, there is no value in repeating the test (Answer D).

Although abnormal lipids (Answer B) and elevated liver transaminases (Answer A) suggesting fatty liver are often seen in youth with obesity, the patient is African American, making fatty liver and elevated triglycerides (the only lipid abnormality that may be of clinical relevance at this age) less likely.

Referral of this patient to a structured multidisciplinary program (Answer C) is warranted given her longstanding obesity and family history of diabetes risk.

Case 2

A 16-year-old Latina girl was diagnosed with diabetes 3 years ago by her primary care physician. At that time, diabetes type was determined based on presentation and family history of T2DM. She was started on metformin, 2000 mg daily, but she reports that she took this for only a few months. Since that time, she has been off all medications and reports no symptoms of diabetes, including no polyuria, polydipsia, or weight loss. One month ago, she was admitted to the hospital following a suicide attempt. During that admission, she was noted to have a glucose value of 550 ng/dL (30.5 mmol/L) and glucosuria, with small ketones and normal pH. Her hemoglobin A_{1c} value was 12.5% (113 mmol/mol). She was treated by the inpatient team with subcutaneous basal-bolus insulin and restarted on metformin. She is referred to the diabetes center for further evaluation. At that visit, her BMI is 28 kg/m² and blood pressure is 125/72 mm Hg.

Given the length of time since her initial diagnosis, obtaining which of the following is the most important next step in this patient's evaluation?

A. Fasting and stimulated C-peptide measurements

B. Fasting lipid panel

C. Home glucose measurements

D. Liver transaminase measurements

E. Pancreatic autoantibody assessment

Answer: E) Pancreatic autoantibody assessment

Even though this patient has had diabetes for 3 years without severe metabolic decompensation off treatment, there is no clinical characteristic with 100% sensitivity in excluding T1DM. Since T1DM remains more common than T2DM at all ages and in most ethnicities, the a priori risk for T1DM is higher than T2DM, despite "typical" characteristics. Furthermore, even among those racial/ethnic groups where T2DM is more common in adolescents (African American, American Indian), T1DM still occurs. Furthermore, a substantial percentage of adolescents with T1DM in the United States have obesity and obesity does not protect from autoimmunity. Therefore, even in this setting, the most important step in the evaluation of an adolescent with diabetes is rigorous determination of diabetes type (Answer E). The presence of positive antibodies, no matter the phenotype, is associated with more rapid progression to insulin requirement, and patients with positive antibodies should be treated with insulin irrespective of how they are doing on oral therapy.

Measurement of fasting C-peptide (Answer A) may be helpful in determining degree of insulin resistance, and stimulated C-peptide may be a reasonable measure of insulin secretory capacity, potentially contributing to the distinction of T2DM from T1DM. However, this is only true in the setting of stable metabolic status. During acute decompensation, insulin and C-peptide secretion are transiently decreased. Measurement of C-peptide may be more useful in asymptomatic patients, in patients who have recovered from decompensation, or in patients with presumed T2DM who have a persistent insulin requirement.

The remaining options would be important to obtain at diagnosis in individuals with obesity and diabetes, regardless of diabetes type but would be unlikely to make an immediate difference in therapeutic decisions. However, the specific screening done would depend on whether the individual has positive antibodies (TSH, celiac antibodies, lipids [Answer B]) or negative antibodies (lipids, AST/ALT [Answer D], urine albumin, creatinine clearance).

Case 3

A 15-year-old Latina girl has been recently diagnosed with diabetes after presenting with mild diabetic ketoacidosis. Metformin was initiated by her primary care provider based on clinical features suggesting T2DM, and she was referred to the diabetes center. She was previously healthy and took no medications. Findings on review of systems are normal.

On physical examination, her BMI is 35 kg/m^2 and blood pressure is 145/82 mm Hg. Her hemoglobin A_{1c} measurement is 7.8% (62 mmol/mol).

Laboratory test results:

> Glutamic acid decarboxylase antibodies, positive
> Islet antigen 2 antibodies, positive
> Zinc transporter 8 antibodies, positive
> ALT = 87 U/L (10-40 U/L) (SI: 1.45 μkat/L [0.17-0.67 μkat/L])
> LDL cholesterol = 160 mg/dL (SI: 4.14 mmol/L)
> HDL cholesterol = 24 mg/dL (SI: 0.62 mmol/L)
> Triglycerides = 545 mg/dL (SI: 6.16 mmol/L)
> Urine albumin-to-creatinine ratio = 45 mg/g creat (<30 mg/g creat)

Multiple daily insulin injections are started. At a follow-up visit 6 months later, her blood pressure is 148/84 mm Hg, and the following laboratory test results are documented:

> Hemoglobin A_{1c} = 7.1% (54 mmol/mol)
> ALT = 55 U/L (SI: 0.92 μkat/L)
> LDL cholesterol = 145 mg/dL (SI: 3.76 mmol/L)
> HDL cholesterol = 28 mg/dL (SI: 0.73 mmol/L)
> Triglycerides = 254 mg/dL (SI: 2.87 mmol/L)
> Urine albumin-to-creatinine = 22 mg/g creat

Which of the following is the best next step in this patient's management?

A. Start atorvastatin, 10 mg daily

B. Start canagliflozin, 100 mg daily

C. Start fenofibrate, 67 mg daily

D. Start lisinopril, 10 mg daily

E. Start vitamin E, 600 IU daily

Answer: D) Start lisinopril, 10 mg daily

Although guidelines suggest that treatment of both hypertension and elevated LDL cholesterol is indicated, evidence for clinical benefit of treating elevated blood pressure in adolescence is stronger. While an argument could be made for starting atorvastatin (Answer A), the increased risk in a reproductive-aged female patient relative to the risk of lisinopril would favor addressing hypertension first (thus, Answer D is correct).

Obesity in individuals of Latino heritage is often associated with insulin resistance abnormalities, including lipid abnormalities, endothelial and cardiac dysfunction, increased procoagulant and inflammatory markers, increased hepatic and muscle lipid deposition, mitochondrial dysfunction, increased plasma uric acid, ovarian hyperandrogenism, and sleep disorders, all of which increase cardiovascular risk. Given the increased prevalence of comorbidities in individuals with obesity and T1DM at the time of diagnosis, evaluation should occur either at the time of initial diagnosis or upon reestablishment of metabolic stability.

Blood pressure should be measured at every clinic visit and normalized for sex, height, and age. Initial treatment of blood pressure above the 95th percentile consists of weight loss, limitation of dietary salt, and increased physical activity. After 6 months, if blood pressure is still above the 95th percentile, an ACE inhibitor is started to achieve blood pressure values that are less than the 90th percentile. If the ACE inhibitor is not tolerated due to adverse effects (mainly cough), an angiotensin receptor blocker may be use. Combination therapy may be required if blood pressure does not normalize on single-agent therapy. Workup of hypertension not responsive to initial medication should also include kidney ultrasonography and echocardiography.

Urinary albumin excretion should be assessed at diagnosis and annually. Moderately increased albumin excretion is defined as an albumin-to-creatinine ratio of 30 to 299 mg/g creat in a spot urine sample and severely increased albumin excretion defined as greater than 300 mg/g. Because an elevated value can be secondary to exercise, cigarette smoking, menstruation, and orthostasis, the diagnosis of persistent abnormal albumin excretion requires documentation of 2 of 3 consecutive abnormal values obtained on different days, preferably on rising, as benign orthostatic proteinuria is common in adolescents. ACE inhibitors are the agents of choice due to proven kidney protection, even if blood pressure is normal. Albumin excretion should be repeated at 3- to 6-month intervals, and therapy should be titrated to achieve a normal albumin-to-creatinine ratio. Non–diabetes-related causes of kidney disease should be excluded, and consultation should be considered if an albumin-to-creatinine ratio greater than 300 mg/g is present. In adults, the use of SGLT-2 inhibitors (Answer B) has been shown to reduce progression of kidney disease and may become standard in prevention of diabetic kidney disease for all ages over time, but it is not yet approved for this use in youth with T1DM.

Testing for dyslipidemia should be performed soon after diagnosis when blood glucose control has been achieved and annually thereafter. Lipid goals are as follows:

> LDL cholesterol = <100 mg/dL (SI: <2.59 mmol/L)
> Triglycerides = <150 mg/dL (SI: <1.70 mmol/L)
> HDL cholesterol = >40 mg/dL (SI: >1.04 mmol/L)

If LDL cholesterol is above goal, blood glucose control should be maximized and dietary counseling should be provided (dietary cholesterol <200 mg daily, saturated fat <7% of total calories, and fat <30% of total calories). If LDL cholesterol remains higher than 130 mg/dL (>3.37 mmol/L) after 6 months, statin therapy should be started with a target of less than 100 mg/dL (<2.59 mmol/L). The use of statins in sexually active adolescent girls must be carefully considered and the risks explicitly discussed. Elevated triglycerides are not treated for cardiovascular disease prevention. However, if fasting triglycerides are greater than 500 mg/dL (>5.65 mmol/L), a fibric acid (Answer C) should be considered due to significantly increased risk for acute pancreatitis, with a treatment goal of less than 150 mg/dL (<1.70 mmol/L).

Hepatic steatosis is present in 25% to 50% of adolescents with obesity, particularly in individuals of Latino or Asian heritage, and more advanced forms of fatty liver disease are increasingly common and associated with progression to cirrhosis, portal hypertension, and liver failure. Fatty liver is now the most frequent cause of chronic liver disorders among youth with obesity and is the most common reason for liver transplant in adults in the United States. Although pharmacologic treatment with metformin and vitamin E (Answer E) has been studied, this has not been proven beneficial in adolescents with fatty liver. Therapies that improve insulin resistance appear to improve fatty liver.

However, due to the potential for progression to steatohepatitis, fibrosis, and cirrhosis, ongoing monitoring of liver enzymes is recommended, with referral for biopsy if enzymes remain markedly elevated.

In addition, the clinician should explore the possibility of polycystic ovary syndrome, depression, eating disorders, and sleep disturbance and address these as appropriate.

References

1. Dabelea D, Mayer-Davis EJ, Saydah S, et al. Prevalence of type 1 and type 2 diabetes among children and adolescents from 2001 to 2009. *JAMA*. 2014;311(17):1778-1786. PMID: 24794371

2. Hannon TS, Janosky J, Arslanian SA. Longitudinal study of physiologic insulin resistance and metabolic changes of puberty. *Pediatr Res*. 2006;60(6):759-763. PMID: 17065576

3. Rascati K, Richards K, Lopez D, Cheng L-I, Wilson J. Progression to insulin for patients with diabetes mellitus on dual oral antidiabetic therapy using the US Department of Defense Database. *Diabetes Obes Metab*. 2013;15(10):901-905. PMID: 23531154

4. Kahn SE. Clinical review 135: the importance of β-cell failure in the development and progression of type 2 diabetes. *J Clin Endocrinol Metab*. 2001;86(9):4047-4058. PMID: 11549624

5. Kahn SE, Lachin JM, Zinman B, et al; ADOPT Study Group. Effects of rosiglitazone, glyburide, and metformin on β-cell function and insulin sensitivity in ADOPT. *Diabetes*. 2011;60(5):1552-1560. PMID: 21415383

6. TODAY Study Group. Effects of metformin, metformin plus rosiglitazone, and metformin plus lifestyle on insulin sensitivity and β-cell function in TODAY. *Diabetes Care*. 2013;36(6):1749-1757. PMID: 23704674

7. Zeitler P, Hirst K, Copeland KC, et al; TODAY Study Group. HbA1c after a short period of monotherapy with metformin identifies durable glycemic control among adolescents with type 2 diabetes. *Diabetes Care*. 2015;38(12):2285-2292. PMID: 26537182

8. Copeland KC, Zeitler P, Geffner M, et al; TODAY Study Group. Characteristics of adolescents and youth with recent-onset type 2 diabetes: the TODAY cohort at baseline. *J Clin Endocrinol Metab*. 2011;96(1):159-167. PMID: 20962021

9. Sellers EAC, Yung G, Dean HJ. Dyslipidemia and other cardiovascular risk factors in a Canadian First Nation pediatric population with type 2 diabetes mellitus. *Pediatr Diabetes*. 2007;8(6):384-390. PMID: 18036065

10. Hannon TS, Arslanian SA. The changing face of diabetes in youth: lessons learned from studies of type 2 diabetes. *Ann N Y Acad Sci*. 2015;1353:113-137. PMID: 26448515

11. Dart AB, Martens PJ, Rigatto C, Brownell MD, Dean HJ, Sellers EA. Earlier onset of complications in youth with type 2 diabetes. *Diabetes Care*. 2014;37(2):436-443. PMID: 24130346

12. Today Study Group, Bjornstad P, Drews KL, Caprio S, et al. Long-term complications in youth-onset type 2 diabetes. *N Engl J Med*. 2021;385(5):416-426. PMID: 34320286

13. American Diabetes Association. 2. Classification and diagnosis of diabetes: standards of medical care in diabetes-2019. *Diabetes Care*. 2019;42(Suppl 1):S13-S28. PMID: 30559228

14. Report of the Expert Committee on the Diagnosis and Classification of Diabetes Mellitus. *Diabetes Care*. 1997;20(7):1183-1197. PMID: 9203460

15. International Expert Committee. International Expert Committee report on the role of the A1C assay in the diagnosis of diabetes. *Diabetes Care*. 2009;32(7):1327-1334. PMID: 19502545

16. Nowicka P, Santoro N, Liu H, et al. Utility of hemoglobin A(1c) for diagnosing prediabetes and diabetes in obese children and adolescents. *Diabetes Care*. 2011;34(6):1306-1311. PMID: 21515842

17. Chan CL, Pyle L, Newnes L, Nadeau KJ, Zeitler PS, Kelsey MM. Continuous glucose monitoring and its relationship to hemoglobin A1c and oral glucose tolerance testing in obese and prediabetic youth. *J Clin Endocrinol Metab*. 2015;100(3):902-910. PMID: 25532041

18. Kelsey MM, Severn C, Hilkin AM, Pyle L, Nadeau KJ, Zeitler PS. Puberty is associated with a rising hemoglobin A1c, even in youth with normal weight. *J Pediatr*. 2021;230:244-247. PMID: 33300876

19. Demmer RT, Zuk AM, Rosenbaum M, Desvarieux M. Prevalence of diagnosed and undiagnosed type 2 diabetes mellitus among US adolescents: results from the continuous NHANES, 1999-2010. *Am J Epidemiol*. 2013;178(7):1106-1113. PMID: 23887044

20. SEARCH for Diabetes in Youth Study Group, Liese AD, D'Agostino RB Jr, et al. The burden of diabetes mellitus among US youth: prevalence estimates from the SEARCH for Diabetes in Youth Study. *Pediatrics*. 2006;118(4):1510-1518. PMID: 17015542

21. American Diabetes Association. Diagnosis and classification of diabetes mellitus. *Diabetes Care*. 2010;33(Suppl 1):S62-S69. PMID: 20042775

22. Weiss R, Taksali SE, Tamborlane WV, Burgert TS, Savoye M, Caprio S. Predictors of changes in glucose tolerance status in obese youth. *Diabetes Care*. 2005;28:902-909. PMID: 15793193

23. Amiel SA, Sherwin RS, Simonson DC, Lauritano AA, Tamborlane WV. Impaired insulin action in puberty. A contributing factor to poor glycemic control in adolescents with diabetes. *N Engl J Med*. 1986;315(4):215-219. PMID: 3523245

24. Moran A, Jacobs DR Jr, Steinberger J, et al. Association between the insulin resistance of puberty and the insulin-like growth factor-I/growth hormone axis. *J Clin Endocrinol Metab*. 2002;87(10):4817-4820. PMID: 1234479

25. Morrison JA, Laskarzewski PM, Rauh JL, et al. Lipids, lipoproteins, and sexual maturation during adolescence: the Princeton maturation study. *Metabolism*. 1979;28(6):641-649. PMID: 449703

26. Tell GS, Mittelmark MB, Vellar OD. Cholesterol, high density lipoprotein cholesterol and triglycerides during puberty: the Oslo Youth Study. *Am J Epidemiol*. 1985;122(5):750-761. PMID: 4050768

27. Porkka KV, Viikari JS, Ronnemaa T, Marniemi J, Akerblom HK. Age and gender specific serum lipid and apolipoprotein fractiles of Finnish children and young adults. The Cardiovascular Risk in Young Finns Study. *Acta Paediatr*. 1994;83(8):838-848. PMID: 7981561

28. Buse JB, Kaufman FR, Linder B, et al; HEALTHY Study Group. Diabetes screening with hemoglobin A(1c) versus fasting plasma glucose in a

multiethnic middle-school cohort. *Diabetes Care.* 2013;36(2):429-435. PMID: 23193207

29. Love-Osborne KA, Sheeder JL, Nadeau KJ, Zeitler P. Longitudinal follow up of dysglycemia in overweight and obese pediatric patients. *Pediatr Diabetes.* 2018;19(2):199-204. PMID: 28856775

30. Zeitler P, Fu J, Tandon N, et al; International Society for Pediatric and Adolescent Diabetes. ISPAD clinical practice consensus guidelines 2014. Type 2 diabetes in the child and adolescent. *Pediatr Diabetes.* 2014;15(Suppl 20):26-46. PMID: 25182306

31. American Diabetes Association. 2. Classification and diagnosis of diabetes: standards of medical care in diabetes. *Diabetes Care.* 2021;44(Suppl 1):S15-S33. PMID: 33298413

32. Fagot-Campagna A, Pettitt DJ, Engelgau MM, et al. Type 2 diabetes among North American children and adolescents: an epidemiological review and public health perspective. *J Pediatr.* 2000;136(5):664-672. PMID: 10802501

33. Copeland KC, Zeitler P, Geffner M, et al; TODAY Study Group. Characteristics of adolescents and youth with recent-onset type 2 diabetes: the TODAY cohort at baseline. *J Clin Endocrinol Metab.* 2011;96(1):159-167. PMID: 20962021

34. Klingensmith GJ, Laffel L, Pyle L, et al; TODAY Study Group. The presence of GAD and IA-2 antibodies in youth with a type 2 diabetes phenotype. *Diabetes Care.* 2010;33(9):1970-1975. PMID: 20519658

35. Laffel L, Chang N, Grey M, et al; TODAY Study Group. Metformin monotherapy in youth with recent onset type 2 diabetes: experience from the prerandomization run-in phase of the TODAY study. *Pediatric Diabetes.* 2012;13(5):369-375. PMID: 22369102

36. Kelsey MM, Geffner ME, Guandalini C, et al; Treatment Options for Type 2 Diabetes in Adolescents and Youth Study Group. Presentation and effectiveness of early treatment of type 2 diabetes in youth: lessons from the TODAY study. *Pediatr Diabetes.* 2016;17(3):212-221. PMID: 25690268

37. Pinhas-Hamiel O, Dolan LM, Zeitler PS. Diabetic ketoacidosis among obese African-American adolescents with NIDDM. *Diabetes Care.* 1997;20(4):484-486. PMID: 9096965

38. Copeland KC, Silverstein J, Moore KR, et al; American Academy of Pediatrics. Management of newly diagnosed type 2 diabetes mellitus (T2DM) in children and adolescents. *Pediatrics.* 2013;131:e648-e664. PMID: 23359574

39. Arslanian S, Bacha F, Grey M, Marcus MD, White NH, Zeitler P. Evaluation and management of youth-onset type 2 diabetes: a position statement by the American Diabetes Association. *Diabetes Care.* 2018;41(12):2648-2668. PMID: 30425094

Novel Therapies in the Treatment of Congenital Hyperinsulinism

Diva D. De Leon-Crutchlow, MD, MSCE. Department of Pediatrics, Children's Hospital of Philadelphia and the Perelman School of Medicine at the University of Pennsylvania, Philadelphia, PA; E-mail: deleon@chop.edu

Learning Objectives

As a result of participating in this session, learners should be able to:

- Describe the clinical manifestations, genetics, and natural history of congenital hyperinsulinism (HI).

- Discuss the therapeutic approach to children with HI.

Main Conclusions

Hyperinsulinism is the most common cause of persistent hypoglycemia in neonates, infants, and children. Hyperinsulinism can be acquired secondary to perinatal factors, such as birth asphyxia, or it can be genetic. There are multiple genetic forms of hyperinsulinism, but the most common and severe form is due to inactivating pathogenic variants in the genes encoding the β-cell K_{ATP} channels. This form of hyperinsulinism can be diffuse or focal. Focal hyperinsulinism can be cured by surgical removal of the lesion. The diagnosis of hyperinsulinism is established by the demonstration that insulin secretion/actions are not appropriately turned off during hypoglycemia. However, one must be aware that during evaluation and diagnosis, plasma insulin concentrations are not always elevated in hyperinsulinism.

First-line therapy for hyperinsulinism is diazoxide, a K_{ATP} channel opener. Lack of responsiveness to diazoxide suggests that the hyperinsulinism is due to a K_{ATP} channel pathogenic variant and, therefore, the possibility of focal hyperinsulinism should be considered and genetic testing should be promptly ordered. The finding of a recessive paternally inherited variant in either 1 of the 2 genes encoding the K_{ATP} channel has a sensitivity of 97% for focal hyperinsulinism. When focal hyperinsulinism is suspected, specialized imaging with ^{18}F-DOPA PET for lesion localization and surgical resection is indicated. For patients with diazoxide-unresponsive, diffuse HI, somatostatin analogues are second-line therapy; when this fails, pancreatectomy may be required. Children with HI require ongoing monitoring of glycemic control, treatment-associated adverse effects, and growth and development. Several novel therapies are in development and are in clinical trials.

Significance of the Clinical Problem

HI is the most common cause of persistent hypoglycemia in neonates, infants, and children. HI is a rare condition with an estimated incidence in the United States and Europe of 1 in 20,000 live births. Despite advances in the understanding of the molecular genetics and pathophysiology of HI, affected children continue to have high rates of neurodevelopmental and neurobehavioral problems, which affect up to 50% of patients. Prompt diagnosis and establishment of effective therapy are critical for optimizing neurological outcomes. However, new therapies are needed for children who are unresponsive to currently available treatment.

Barriers to Optimal Practice

- Failure to identify neonates with persistent hypoglycemia due to HI before discharge from the newborn nursery.

- Lack of access to specific, accurate, and fast genetic testing with appropriate interpretation, which is critical to identifying children with the focal form of HI.

- Lack of access to specialized imaging and expertise for identifying, localizing, and surgically removing focal lesions.

- Lack of recognition and prevention of adverse effects associated with HI therapies.

- Limited therapeutic treatment options for children with diazoxide-unresponsive diffuse HI.

Strategies for Diagnosis, Therapy, and/or Management
Introduction

In the normal newborn, the plasma glucose concentration decreases after birth, reaching a nadir of about 55 to 60 mg/dL (3.0 to 3.3 mmol/L) at approximately 2 hours of life and staying lower than the normal range for older children and adults for 3 to 5 days. This phenomenon of physiological adaptation is known as transitional hypoglycemia. During this period of physiological transitional hypoglycemia, the plasma glucose concentration remains relatively stable and then increases steadily, reaching the normal range 3 to 5 days after birth. More severe hypoglycemia, symptomatic hypoglycemia, or hypoglycemia

that persists beyond this period should be further investigated.[1]

Hyperinsulinism due to dysregulation of insulin secretion is the most common cause of persistent hypoglycemia in neonates, infants, and children. Hyperinsulinism can be secondary to perinatal factors, such as perinatal asphyxia and maternal preeclampsia, or it can be caused by genetic defects in the pathway that regulates insulin secretion. HI may also be associated with syndromes in which HI is only one of the manifestations of the condition. The most common syndromes associated with HI are Beckwith-Wiedemann syndrome and Kabuki syndrome. The mechanisms by which perinatal stress causes hyperinsulinism is not yet elucidated, but this form of transient hyperinsulinism can be as severe as the genetic forms, and it is also associated with poor neurodevelopmental outcomes,[2] thus, at-risk neonates should be screened after birth for hypoglycemia and undergo an appropriate diagnostic evaluation.[1]

Genetic Forms of Hyperinsulinism

HI due to genetic defects in the insulin regulatory pathway is a genetically and phenotypically heterogenous condition.[3] More than 10 loci have been associated with HI, but the most common and severe form of HI is caused by inactivating pathogenic variants in *ABCC8* and *KCNJ11*, the genes encoding the β-cell ATP-sensitive potassium (K_{ATP}) channels, known as K_{ATP}-HI.[4] Histologically, K_{ATP}-HI can be diffuse or focal. Diffuse K_{ATP}-HI is caused by recessive biallelic variants or dominant monoallelic variants in *ABCC8* or *KCNJ11*. In focal K_{ATP}-HI, affected β cells are limited to a very small part of the pancreas, and it is caused by the combination of a paternally inherited recessive *ABCC8* variant or *KCNJ11* variant together with paternal isodisomy of the 11p15 chromosomal region confined to the pancreatic lesion. Focal HI can be cured if the lesion is surgically removed. The second most common HI subtype is hyperinsulinism hyperammonemia syndrome, which is caused by activating monoallelic variants in *GLUD1*, the gene encoding glutamate dehydrogenase. The phenotype of GLUD1-associated HI is characterized by fasting and protein-induced hypoglycemia, hyperammonemia, and neurological manifestations such as absence seizures and learning problems. A less common form of HI is caused by monoallelic activating variants in the *GCK* gene (encoding glucokinase) that sets the threshold for glucose-stimulated insulin secretion in the β cell. Activating variants in the *GCK* gene result in a lower threshold for glucose-stimulated insulin secretion and hyperinsulinism. Dominant inactivating variants in *HNF1A* and *HNF4A* cause a biphasic phenotype with transient hyperinsulinism early in infancy and childhood followed by diabetes later in life. Other less frequent genetic causes of HI include biallelic inactivating variants in the *HADH* gene, which encodes short-chain 3-hydroxyacyl-CoA (SCHAD), and monoallelic inactivating variants in the *UCP2* gene, which encodes uncoupling protein-2. Pathogenic variants in the promoter region of the *SCL16A1* gene, which encodes monocarboxylate transporter 1 (MCT1), result in the aberrant expression of this β-cell disallowed gene and cause a form of hyperinsulinism characterized by exercise-induced hypoglycemia. More recently, pathogenic variants in noncoding regions of the *HK1* gene (encoding hexokinase 1), another β-cell disallowed gene, have been recognize as a cause of HI.[5]

Diagnosis

The diagnosis of HI is established by demonstrating that insulin secretion/actions are not appropriately turned off in the presence of hypoglycemia (plasma glucose <50 mg/dL [<2.8 mmol/L]).[6] The typical laboratory findings include detectable insulin (sensitivity 82%; specificity 100%), low plasma free fatty acids (<1.7 mmol/L; sensitivity 87%; specificity 100%), low plasma β-hydroxybutyrate (<1.8 mmol/L; sensitivity 100%; specificity 100%), and a glycemic response to a pharmacologic dose of glucagon (>30 mg/dL (>1.7 mmol/L); sensitivity 89%;

specificity 100%).[6] A common misconception is that the plasma insulin concentration is always high in HI; however, it is not uncommon for plasma insulin to be "low" and even undetectable. Additional laboratory evaluation may help establish the diagnosis of the specific HI subtype. For example, plasma ammonia is elevated in HI due to activating pathogenic variants in *GLUD1*, and plasma C4-OH acylcarnitine and urine 3-hydroxyglutaric acid levels are elevated in HI due to inactivating pathogenic variants in *HADH*. Genetic testing is important for determining the specific genetic form of HI and for family counseling, but it is particularly essential for identifying children with focal HI. The finding of a paternally inherited recessive variant in *ABCC8* and *KCNJ11* predicts focal HI with a sensitivity of 97%.[4]

Treatment

Once the diagnosis of HI is established, specific treatment should be initiated. Diazoxide, a K_{ATP} channel opener, is the only drug with regulatory approval for the treatment of HI and is first-line therapy for this condition.[7] The dosage range of diazoxide is 5 to 15 mg/kg per day divided into 2 daily doses. To prevent complications from diazoxide-induced fluid retention, diuretic therapy should be initiated concomitantly with diazoxide. Dosage selection and dosage escalation should be carefully considered, weighing the response and potential for adverse effects. Because of its long half-life, it may take up to 5 days to achieve a full therapeutic effect. An important next step is to assess the responsiveness to diazoxide, which has important diagnostic and therapeutic implications. Responsiveness to diazoxide is defined by the demonstration that the cardinal feature of HI, hypoketotic hypoglycemia, is corrected by treatment. This is best assessed by a fasting test demonstrating that the child can fast for 12 to 18 hours with plasma glucose values of 70 mg/dL or higher (≥3.9 mmol/L) or that plasma β-hydroxybutyrate increases to greater than 1.8 mmol/L before plasma glucose decreases below 50 to 60 mg/dL (2.8 to 3.3 mmol/L) during fasting. Lack of responsiveness to diazoxide suggests the possibility that HI is due to inactivating variant(s) in the K_{ATP} channel genes, which account for up to 90% of cases of diazoxide-unresponsive HI. For these patients, rapid genetic testing for variants in *ABCC8* and *KCNJ11* is critical to determine the likelihood of focal HI.[4]

Surgery is the treatment of choice for focal HI, but before surgery, it is important to localize the lesion. These lesions are not visible using conventional imaging techniques such as ultrasonography, CT, and MRI; however, specialized imaging using ^{18}F-DOPA PET is almost 100% accurate in localizing focal lesions.[8] Expert assessment of the pancreatic histology during surgery using frozen biopsies and surgical expertise are key for surgical success. Therefore, these children should be referred to an HI center of excellence for management by a multidisciplinary team of experts. The reported cure rate for focal HI is 97%.[9]

For diazoxide-unresponsive patients with nonfocal HI, treatment options are limited. Off-label use of the somatostatin analogue octreotide has been the longstanding second-line treatment for HI,[10] but its effectiveness is limited by the development of tachyphylaxis. Because of its association with potentially fatal necrotizing enterocolitis, octreotide is not recommended for infants younger than 8 weeks. The recommended octreotide dosage range is 5 to 20 mcg/kg per day. Long-acting somatostatin analogues, octreotide LAR and lanreotide, are convenient options for children older than 1 year. An alternative treatment approach for diazoxide-unresponsive patients who are either not eligible or are unresponsive to octreotide is the use of a continuous infusion of dextrose through a gastrostomy tube.[11] Typically, dextrose 20% is used and because of tolerance, the maximal glucose infusion rate administrated through this route is 10 mg/kg per min. Continuous intragastric dextrose is also used in combination with octreotide, an approach that allows for less frequent dosing of octreotide and avoidance of

tachyphylaxis. In our HI program, we start with a continuous intragastric infusion of dextrose 20% given around the clock until the child is old enough to introduce octreotide. Typically, we introduce octreotide at 4 to 6 months of age and dose it twice daily, with a small dose of 2 to 3 mcg/kg given in the morning and a slightly higher dose of 4 to 5 mcg/kg given 6 hours later with continuous intragastric dextrose 20% for 12 hours overnight. At about 1 year of age, we transition from octreotide to lanreotide, 60 mg monthly. In some patients, the introduction of lanreotide allows for discontinuation of overnight dextrose.

Near-total pancreatectomy is indicated when medical therapy fails. Because hypoglycemia persists in up to 50% of children with diffuse HI after pancreatectomy, a gastrostomy tube is placed at the time of surgery to facilitate management of residual hypoglycemia using continuous intragastric dextrose.

The successful management of children with hyperinsulinism requires a stepwise approach with continuous assessment and adjustment of the treatment according to the response. Ongoing monitoring to assess for glycemic control, therapy-associated adverse effects, and growth and development is recommended. In addition to at-home monitoring of glycemic control, a yearly assessment of fasting tolerance in the hospital setting is important to guide treatment adjustments. Children who have undergone 50% or greater pancreatectomy should be monitored for diabetes and pancreatic insufficiency. Ninety-one percent of children who undergo near-total pancreatectomy require insulin by age 14 years. The frequency of neurodevelopmental and neurobehavioral problems in children with hyperinsulinism is 40% to 50%; therefore, neurodevelopmental assessments should be performed throughout childhood.

Multiple new therapies for HI are in development and promise to make possible a personalized approach to treatment of children with HI in an effort to improve their long-term outcomes. Therapies currently in clinical trials include a peptide antagonist of the GLP-1 receptor, a short-acting soluble glucagon analogue, a long-acting glucagon analogue, a selective nonpeptide somatostatin receptor 5 agonist, and an allosteric inhibitor of the insulin receptor. For up-to-date information about clinical trials in HI, visit www.clinicaltrials.gov.

Clinical Case Vignettes

Case 1

A 10-day-old male newborn has persistent hypoglycemia requiring a glucose infusion rate of 18 mg/kg per min. At 37 weeks' gestation, the infant was born by emergency cesarean delivery performed for fetal distress associated with maternal preeclampsia. Birth weight was 5 lb 4 oz (2373 g) (small for gestational age). His initial plasma glucose concentration was 16 mg/dL (0.89 mmol/L).

A critical sample was obtained during a spontaneous episode of hypoglycemia (plasma glucose = 50 mg/dL [2.8 mmol/L]):

Plasma insulin = 3 µIU/mL (should be undetectable during hypoglycemia) (SI: 20.8 pmol/L)
Plasma β-hydroxybutyrate = <0.3 mmol/L (≥1.8 mmol/L during hypoglycemia)
Plasma free fatty acids = 13.8 mg/dL (≥47.9 mg/dL during hypoglycemia) (SI: 0.49 mmol/L [≥1.7 mmol/L])
Cortisol = 3 µg/dL (≥10 ug/dL during hypoglycemia) (SI: 82.8 nmol/L [≥275.9 nmol/L])
GH = 10.0 ng/mL (≥10.0 ng/mL during hypoglycemia) (SI: 10.0 µg/L [≥10.0 µg/L])

In response to glucagon (1 mg), plasma glucose increases to 94 mg/dL (5.2 mmol/L).

Which of the following is the best next step in this patient's management?

A. Avoid diazoxide as it is contraindicated because of the high likelihood of adverse effects

B. Initiate diazoxide and chlorothiazide at the same time

C. Initiate hydrocortisone replacement therapy for adrenal insufficiency

D. Order rapid genetic testing for *ABCC8* and *KCNJ11* to assess the likelihood of diazoxide responsiveness

Answer: B) Initiate diazoxide and chlorothiazide at the same time

The clear history of perinatal stress suggests a diagnosis of perinatal stress-induced hyperinsulinism. Therefore, genetic testing (Answer D) is unlikely to be useful. Perinatal stress-induced hyperinsulinism may affect up to 50% of neonates at risk. The clinical course is heterogenous; some cases are mild and resolve within days, while others may be severe and persist for several weeks to months. This form of hyperinsulinism is responsive to therapy with diazoxide, but these infants may be more susceptible to developing diazoxide adverse effects, particularly edema.[12] Therefore, it is recommended that diuretic therapy be initiated concomitantly with diazoxide (Answer B). Although the likelihood of developing adverse events may be higher in this population of infants, this does not represent a contraindication of diazoxide treatment (Answer A), particularly because of the high risk of neurodevelopmental sequelae if hypoglycemia is not prevented.

A singe low GH or cortisol value at the time of fasting hypoglycemia has poor specificity for the respective diagnoses of GH deficiency and adrenal insufficiency.[13] Thus, hydrocortisone (Answer C) is not indicated now. If GH or cortisol deficiency is suspected, stimulation testing should be performed.

Case 2

A 5-month-old female infant presents to the emergency department after a witnessed seizure episode at home. Her parents report previous episodes of irritability and "eye deviation" that resolved after feedings. Birth history is remarkable for large-for-gestational birth weight (9 lb 9 oz [4335 g] at 38 weeks' gestation) and "transient" hypoglycemia that required intravenous dextrose for 5 days after birth.

At the time of presentation with seizures, a critical sample was obtained during a spontaneous episode of hypoglycemia:

Plasma glucose = 47 mg/dL (70-100 mg/dL) (SI: 2.6 mmol/L [3.9-5.6 mmol/L])

Plasma insulin = 12 μIU/mL (should be undetectable during hypoglycemia) (SI: 83.3 pmol/L)

Plasma β-hydroxybutyrate = <0.4 mmol/L (≥1.8 mmol/L during hypoglycemia)

Plasma free fatty acids = 8.5 mg/dL (≥47.9 mg/dL during hypoglycemia) (SI: 0.3 mmol/L [≥1.7 mmol/L])

In response to glucagon (1 mg), plasma glucose increases to 118 mg/dL (6.5 mmol/L). After 5 days of therapy with diazoxide, 15 mg/kg per day, and with feeds every 3 hours, prefeed plasma glucose values are in the range of 60 to 80 mg/dL (3.3 to 4.4 mmol/L).

Which of the following is the best next step in this patient's management?

A. Continue diazoxide; place a gastrostomy tube for initiation of overnight continuous feedings

B. Discontinue diazoxide; initiate octreotide in combination with continuous feedings overnight

C. Measure ammonia and treat for hyperammonemia to prevent further seizure episodes

D. Perform a fasting test to guide the next steps in addition to ordering genetic testing

Answer: D) Perform a fasting test to guide the next steps in addition to ordering genetic testing

Children with focal disease are more likely to present at an older age and have seizures at presentation compared with children with diffuse HI.[14] However, the history of "transient" hypoglycemia in the newborn period suggests late recognition of the HI diagnosis, rather than late presentation. Hyperinsulinism hyperammonemia syndrome is caused by an activating pathogenic variant in the *GLUD1* gene. It is the second most common genetic form of HI and may present later in infancy. The phenotype of this form of hyperinsulinism is characterized by hypoglycemia, hyperammonemia, and neurological manifestations with seizures in up to 60% of patients. Hyperinsulinism hyperammonemia syndrome is responsive to diazoxide and is associated with elevated ammonia. Genetic testing help establish the diagnosis. However, measuring ammonia and treating for hyperammonemia to prevent further seizure episodes (Answer C) is incorrect because treatment of hyperammonemia is not indicated.

Persistence of plasma glucose values lower than 70 mg/dL (<3.9 mmol/L), even with frequent feedings, suggests that the hyperinsulinism is not responsive to diazoxide. Ninety percent of diazoxide-unresponsive cases are due to inactivating pathogenic variants in the K_{ATP} channel genes, and up to 50% of these are focal. Thus, the appropriate next step is to assess diazoxide responsiveness by performing a fasting test in addition to obtaining genetic testing (Answer D).

The use of continuous feedings to treat hyperinsulinism (Answer A) should be avoided because it can result in feeding aversion.

Rather than committing to therapy with octreotide (Answer B), every effort should be made to evaluate for the possibility of focal disease, which is curable. If focal HI is ruled out, octreotide can then be considered for diazoxide-unresponsive patients.

Case 3

A 4-month-old female infant has persistent hypoglycemia and congenital hypothyroidism. The infant was born by vaginal delivery at 38 weeks' gestation with a birth weight of 7 lb 6 oz (3345 g). The neonatal period was complicated by respiratory distress, transient hypoglycemia, and feeding issues. Newborn screening was remarkable for an elevated TSH value of 80 mIU/L. Thyroid hormone replacement was initiated. She was also found to have a ventricular septal defect on echocardiography. The infant presented at 2 months of age with lethargy and was found to have hypoglycemia.

Results from a critical sample at the end of a diagnostic fast:

Plasma glucose = 48 mg/dL (70-100 mg/dL) (SI: 2.7 mmol/L [3.9-5.6 mmol/L])

Plasma insulin = <2 μIU/mL (should be undetectable during hypoglycemia) (SI: 13.9 pmol/L)

Plasma β-hydroxybutyrate = 1.3 mmol/L (≥1.8 mmol/L during hypoglycemia)

Plasma free fatty acids = 21.4 mg/dL (≥47.9 mg/dL during hypoglycemia) (SI:0.76 mmol/L [≥1.7 mmol/L during hypoglycemia])

In response to glucagon (1 mg), plasma glucose increases to 131 mg/dL (7.3 mmol/L). Physical examination findings are remarkable for microcephaly (head circumference <5th percentile), elongated eyelids, and persistent fetal finger pads.

Which of the following statements is true regarding this patient's evaluation and management?

A. A syndromic cause of hyperinsulinism should be considered and appropriate genetic testing should be ordered

B. Diazoxide is contraindicated because of the history of ventricular septal defect

C. Octreotide is contraindicated because of the history of hypothyroidism

D. The patient should be referred to a center of excellence for ^{18}F-DOPA PET

Answer: A) A syndromic cause of hyperinsulinism should be considered and appropriate genetic testing should be ordered

This infant's critical sample is consistent with the diagnosis of hyperinsulinism. Although plasma insulin was undetectable, it is not detectable in about 18% of patients with HI. There are a few explanations for this. Most commonly, the falsely low insulin concentration is due to hemolysis of the sample, which can happen when the critical sample is obtained from an indwelling catheter and results in degradation of insulin. The low plasma β-hydroxybutyrate and free fatty acids, as well as the robust glycemic response to glucagon, confirm the diagnosis of HI. The physical characteristics of the infant suggest the diagnosis of Kabuki syndrome; thus, genetic testing (Answer A) should include, in addition to HI-specific genes, testing for Kabuki syndrome, which is part of most HI genetic panels.

Before considering imaging with ^{18}F-DOPA PET (Answer D), diazoxide responsiveness should be assessed and genetic testing should be ordered. If the child is diazoxide-responsive and/or genetic testing confirms the diagnosis of Kabuki syndrome, ^{18}F-DOPA PET would not be indicated.

A ventricular septal defect is not necessarily a contraindication for the use of diazoxide (Answer B); a comprehensive assessment of the risk vs benefits should be performed for each case.

Hypothyroidism is not a contraindication for using octreotide (Answer C), but thyroid function should be followed in children receiving therapy with somatostatin analogues. If the child is unresponsive to diazoxide, octreotide should be considered as second-line therapy if focal HI is not suspected.

References

1. Thornton PS, Stanley CA, De Leon DD, et al; Pediatric Endocrine Society. Recommendations from the Pediatric Endocrine Society for evaluation and management of persistent hypoglycemia in neonates, infants, and children. *J Pediatr.* 2015;167(2):238-245. PMID: 25957977

2. Avatapalle HB, Banerjee I, Shah S, et al. Abnormal neurodevelopmental outcomes are common in children with transient congenital hyperinsulinism. *Front Endocrinol (Lausanne).* 2013;4:60. PMID: 23730298

3. Rosenfeld E, Ganguly A, De Leon DD. Congenital hyperinsulinism disorders: genetic and clinical characteristics. *Am J Med Genet C Semin Med Genet.* 2019;181(4):682-692. PMID: 31414570

4. Snider KE, Becker S, Boyajian L, et al. Genotype and phenotype correlations in 417 children with congenital hyperinsulinism. *J Clin Endocrinol Metab.* 2013;98(2):E355-E363. PMID: 23275527

5. Wakeling MN, Owens NDL, Hopkinson JR, et al. A novel disease mechanism leading to the expression of a disallowed gene in the pancreatic beta-cell identified by non-coding, regulatory mutations controlling HK1. *medRxiv.* 2022;doi: https://doi.org/10.1101/2021.12.03.21267240.

6. Ferrara C, Patel P, Becker S, Stanley CA, Kelly A. Biomarkers of insulin for the diagnosis of hyperinsulinemic hypoglycemia in infants and children. *J Pediatr.* 2016;168:212-219. PMID: 26490124

7. Brar PC, Heksch R, Cossen K, et al. Management and appropriate use of diazoxide in infants and children with hyperinsulinism. *J Clin Endocrinol Metab.* 2020;105(12):dgaa543.

8. States LJ, Saade-Lemus S, De Leon DD. 18-F-L 3,4-Dihydroxyphenylalanine PET/computed tomography in the management of congenital hyperinsulinism. *PET Clin.* 2020;15(3):349-359. PMID: 32498990

9. Adzick NS, De Leon DD, States LJ, et al. Surgical treatment of congenital hyperinsulinism: Results from 500 pancreatectomies in neonates and children. *J Pediatr Surg.* 2019;54(1):27-32. PMID: 30343978

10. Welters A, Lerch C, Kummer S, et al. Long-term medical treatment in congenital hyperinsulinism: a descriptive analysis in a large cohort of patients from different clinical centers. *Orphanet J Rare Dis.* 2015;10:150. PMID: 26608306

11. Vajravelu ME, Congdon M, Mitteer L, et al. Continuous intragastric dextrose: a therapeutic option for refractory hypoglycemia in congenital hyperinsulinism. *Horm Res Paediatr.* 2019;91(1):62-68. PMID: 30086540

12. Thornton P, Truong L, Reynolds C, Hamby T, Nedrelow J. Rate of serious adverse events associated with diazoxide treatment of patients with Hyperinsulinism. *Horm Res Paediatr.* 2019;91(1):25-32.

13. Kelly A, Tang R, Becker S, Stanley CA. Poor specificity of low growth hormone and cortisol levels during fasting hypoglycemia for the diagnoses of growth hormone deficiency and adrenal insufficiency. *Pediatrics.* 2008;122(3):e522-e528. PMID: 18694902

14. Lord K, Dzata E, Snider KE, Gallagher PR, De Leon DD. Clinical presentation and management of children with diffuse and focal hyperinsulinism: a review of 223 cases. *J Clin Endocrinol Metab.* 2013;98(11):E1786-E1789. PMID: 24057290

Approach to Pediatric Lipid Disorders

Ambika P. Ashraf, MD. Division of Pediatric Endocrinology & Diabetes, University of Alabama at Birmingham, Birmingham, AL; E-mail: aashraf@uabmc.edu

Learning Objectives

As a result of participating in this session, learners should be able to:

- Describe the initial evaluation and management of pediatric patients with lipid disorders.

- Provide an overview of dyslipidemia phenotypes: isolated elevation of LDL cholesterol (LDL-C), hypertriglyceridemia, and combined dyslipidemia with elevated triglycerides, low HDL cholesterol (HDL-C), and varying levels of LDL-C.

- Develop a practical management approach, including dietary and lifestyle recommendations and pharmacologic agents by dyslipidemia phenotype.

Main Conclusions

Dyslipidemias are highly prevalent in youth and can be due to genetic (monogenic or polygenic) causes or most commonly acquired due to secondary causes such as insulin resistance, obesity, and metabolic syndrome. Elevations of LDL-C, mild-to-moderate hypertriglyceridemia, and combined dyslipidemia are associated with risk for premature atherosclerotic cardiovascular disease (ASCVD) later in life, whereas severe hypertriglyceridemia is associated with acute pancreatitis risk. It is essential to rule out secondary factors and manage underlying risk factors.

Nonpharmacologic approaches involve therapeutic lifestyle changes, including appropriate dietary interventions, daily moderate-to-vigorous physical activity, maintenance of healthy weight, and avoidance of cigarette smoking.

Statins remains the initial lipid-lowering medication for children 10 years and older who have a persistently elevated LDL-C concentration of 190 mg/dL or higher (≥4.92 mmol/L) or for those who have LDL-C concentrations between 130 and 189 mg/dL (3.37 and 4.90 mmol/L), based on the presence of additional risk factor(s)/risk condition(s).

In patients with combined dyslipidemia, statin therapy is indicated for non–HDL-C concentrations greater than 145 mg/dL (>3.76 mmol/L) to reduce the ASCVD risk. Fibrates or omega-3 fatty acids can be used judiciously in patients with triglyceride concentrations greater than 400 mg/dL (>4.52 mmol/L) to prevent acute pancreatitis.

Currently, intense dietary fat restriction is the recommended treatment of severe hypertriglyceridemia, even though several novel therapeutic agents are in development.

Significance of the Clinical Problem

The field of pediatric lipidology is an emerging discipline in the United States and internationally. Premature cardiovascular diseases account for 30% of mortality in the United States. Children with dyslipidemia have an increased risk of becoming adults with dyslipidemia who are at risk for premature ASCVD and strokes. Early identification of the risk factors and early treatment may prevent future morbidity and mortality from ASCVD.

Both genetic and nongenetic dyslipidemias are widely prevalent[1] and are manifested at younger ages as a consequence of obesity and the diabetes epidemic. Factors implicated in the development of dyslipidemias include insulin resistance, metabolic syndrome, obesity, prediabetes, and diabetes. Children with familial hypercholesterolemia (FH) (prevalence = 1 in 300)[2] and familial combined hyperlipidemia (FCHL) (prevalence = 1 in 100)[3] experience lifelong cumulative exposure to elevated LDL-C concentrations and a projected 20% increase in risk for premature cardiovascular disease. Pediatric lipidologists increasingly confront an issue of epidemic proportions of dyslipidemia as the initial presentation of metabolic dysregulation associated with obesity.

Barriers to Optimal Practice

The absence of physical characteristics of FH (eg, xanthoma) in childhood makes it difficult to identify this at-risk population without universal screening. Use of family history can be inaccurate since family history may only be positive in a small proportion of patients due to a variety of factors such as incomplete or unknown family history, young age of parents, or unrecognized hyperlipidemia in family members. With the increasing incidence of obesity, insulin resistance, metabolic syndrome, prediabetes and type 2 diabetes, nongenetic causes of dyslipidemia are manifested at younger ages and dyslipidemia severity is exacerbated. Hence, all children and adolescents aged 2 years or older who have potential risk factors/conditions for premature cardiovascular disease should undergo selective screening. Moreover, FH may coexist with obesity or insulin resistance, and the dyslipidemia phenotype may be complex. The care of children with lipid disorders is currently spread among several subspecialists, including both pediatric and adult providers. These providers may lack the necessary

training and resources to administer high-quality care to this unique pediatric patient population.

Strategies for Diagnosis, Therapy, and/or Management
Screening

In 1992, the National Cholesterol Education Program presented the first guidelines for pediatric lipidology, focusing primarily on management of LDL-C. Today, the most comprehensive recommendations for screening and management come from the 2011 National Heart Lung and Blood Institute pediatric guidelines[4] and the 2019 American Heart Association updated guidelines.[5]

The National Heart Lung and Blood Institute guidelines recommend "universal screening" with a nonfasting lipid profile for children between ages 9 and 11 years and repeated measurements obtained between 17 and 21 years. This accounts for the fact that the total cholesterol concentration peaks at 9 to 11 years of age and decreases by 10% to 20% during puberty. In the case of an abnormal lipid profile, repeating a fasting lipid profile within 2 to 12 weeks of the initial lipid screening is recommended.

The National Heart Lung and Blood Institute pediatric guidelines were the first to emphasize screening for dyslipidemia in the presence of risk factors and conditions. Selective screening is recommended in all children 2 years or older who have potential risk factors for early cardiovascular disease (*Table*). Initial screening can be done with a nonfasting lipid profile to measure non–HDL-C; if abnormal, a fasting lipid profile can be obtained within 2 to 12 weeks. For borderline abnormal values (ie, between the 75th and 95th percentiles), repeated screening is suggested every 1 to 2 years. Decisions regarding medication therapy should be made on an individual basis.

Diagnosis

The dyslipidemia phenotype is often helpful in determining the mostly likely cause. It is also important to recognize that one etiology does not

Table. Cardiovascular Risk Factors and Risk Conditions

Risk-enhancing factors	Risk-enhancing conditions
• Obesity (BMI ≥95th to <99th percentile) • Insulin resistance–related comorbidities (eg, nonalcoholic fatty liver disease, polycystic ovary syndrome) • Current cigarette smoker or significant exposure to secondhand smoke • White-coat hypertension • HDL-C <40 mg/dL (<1.04 mmol/L) • Elevated lipoprotein (a) • Elevated apolipoprotein B	• Chronic inflammatory disease (eg, systemic lupus erythematosus, systemic juvenile idiopathic arthritis) • HIV infection • Childhood cancer survivor with cardiotoxic chemotherapy only • Adolescent depressive and bipolar disorders • Congenital heart disease involving (1) obstructive lesions of the left ventricle and aorta; (2) cyanotic congenital heart defects leading to Eisenmenger syndrome; and (3) congenital coronary artery anomalies in isolation or in association with other congenital defects
Moderate-risk factors	**Moderate-risk medical conditions**
• Confirmed hypertension (blood pressure >95th percentile or ≥130/80 mm Hg on 3 separate occasions) • Severe obesity (BMI ≥99th percentile or ≥35 kg/m²) • Multiple risk factors (≥3 risk enhancers)	• Kawasaki disease with regressed coronary aneurysms • Heterozygous familial hypercholesterolemia • Chronic inflammatory disease • Nephrotic syndrome • Childhood cancer survivor with exposure to chest irradiation • Chronic kidney disease
High-risk factors	**High-risk medical conditions**
• Current cigarette smoker • Multiple comorbidities—any moderate-risk condition plus ≥2 additional risk enhancers	• Diabetes mellitus, type 1 and type 2 • End-stage kidney disease/postkidney transplant • Postorthotopic heart transplant • Kawasaki disease with current aneurysms • Homozygous familial hypercholesterolemia
Positive family history: First-degree relatives (biological parents and siblings) or second-degree relatives (biological grandparents, aunts, and uncles) with any of the following before age 55 years in a male or 65 years in a female: myocardial infarction, stroke, angina, coronary artery bypass, stent, angioplasty, sudden cardiac death, or parent with total cholesterol >240 mg/dL (>6.22 mmol/L).	

From Expert panel on integrated guidelines for cardiovascular health and risk reduction in children and adolescents: summary report. *Pediatrics*, 128(Suppl 5), S213; De Ferranti et al. *Circulation*, 2019; 139(13); Ashraf AP et al. *J Clin Endocrinol Metab*, 2021; 106(12).

preclude another; namely, an underlying genetic etiology can be exacerbated by a secondary cause of dyslipidemia, such as diabetes. A substantial number of children with endocrinologic disorders have "mixed type" dyslipidemia with variable elevations of LDL-C and triglycerides.[6]

Therapy

Both LDL-C and non–HDL-C are used as targets to evaluate the cardiovascular disease–related risks associated with dyslipidemia. Recommendations for medical therapy, particularly for LDL-C elevation, are based on the number and severity of risk factors in addition to the actual LDL-C concentration. In the case

of combined dyslipidemia, it is important to calculate non–HDL-C. Non–HDL-C is calculated as the difference between total cholesterol and HDL-C. The management of elevated triglycerides is dependent on the etiology, concomitant symptoms, and degree of elevation.

Clinical Case Vignettes

Case 1

A 10-year-old girl with normal BMI and blood pressure has hypercholesterolemia. Her father has hypercholesterolemia and type 2 diabetes and had a myocardial infarction at age 42 years. He takes rosuvastatin, 40 mg daily.

The patient's lipid profile:

> Total cholesterol = 322 mg/dL (SI: 8.34 mmol/L)
> Triglycerides = 188 mg/dL (SI: 2.12 mmol/L)
> HDL-C = 47 mg/dL (SI: 1.22 mmol/L)
> LDL-C = 237 mg/dL (SI: 6.14 mmol/L)
> Thyroid function, normal
> Hemoglobin A_{1c}, normal
> Albumin, normal

She takes no medications. A repeated lipid profile obtained 6 months after implementing dietary and lifestyle changes has similar values.

Which of the following is the most likely diagnosis?

A. FCHL

B. FH

C. Metabolic syndrome

D. Polygenic hypercholesterolemia

Answer: B) FH

The dyslipidemia phenotype in this otherwise healthy, normal-weight child who has family history of premature cardiovascular disease is consistent with isolated LDL-C elevation. Notably, she does not have any secondary causes of hypercholesterolemia. Elevated LDL-C could be due to acquired causes, genetic predisposition, or both. It is important to rule out conditions such as hypothyroidism; nephrotic syndrome; diabetes; and drugs such as isotretinoin, atypical antipsychotic agents, or oral contraceptives.

The clinical picture in this patient is consistent with a diagnosis of FH (Answer B) based on the persistently elevated LDL-C concentration greater than 190 mg/dL (>4.92 mmol/L), a family history of premature cardiovascular disease in her father, and absence of secondary causes for elevated cholesterol. Children with an LDL-C level of 190 mg/dL or greater (≥4.92 mmol/L) without any secondary causes have a high likelihood of FH and almost certainly require pharmacotherapy.

Another differential diagnosis to consider is polygenic hypercholesterolemia (Answer D), which can be due to environmental factors, diet, or monogenic or polygenic factors affecting secretion and catabolism of apolipoprotein B–containing lipoproteins. However, given her positive family history, normal BMI, and absence of other contributing factors, polygenic hypercholesterolemia is not the correct choice.

FCHL (Answer A) and metabolic syndrome (Answer C) present with combined dyslipidemia in youth with obesity or insulin resistance-related conditions, in contrast to this patient who has isolated LDL-C elevation and normal BMI.

When should one consider a diagnosis of FH?
FH presents with isolated LDL-C elevations, usually greater than 160 mg/dL (>4.14 mmol/L), often with a family history of premature ASCVD-related events, such as angina, myocardial infarction, and stroke. FH can occur in the form of heterozygous hypercholesterolemia (HeFH) or the more severe homozygous disease (HoFH) where the LDL-C levels are greater than 400 mg/dL (>10.36 mmol/L). FH is due to impaired cholesterol metabolism from monogenic pathogenic variants that cause dysfunction of the LDL receptor (ie, variants in the gene encoding the LDL receptor, LDL receptor ligand, apolipoprotein B, LDL receptor regulating enzyme PCSK9, or LDL receptor adaptor protein-1 [LDLRAP1]).

What is the nonpharmacologic management of hypercholesterolemia?
Management of elevated LDL-C includes therapeutic lifestyle changes plus lipid-lowering medications, especially statins. Lifestyle modifications with the "cardiovascular health integrated lifestyle diet" (CHILD diet) and daily moderate to vigorous physical activity remain the cornerstone for management of pediatric hypercholesterolemia.[4] Sources of saturated fat include high-fat animal foods such as ground beef and processed meats, cheese, high-fat milk and ice cream, and tropical oils such as coconut and palm oils. Dietary cholesterol is only derived from animal foods, which also tend to be higher in saturated fat. Thus, decreasing saturated fat consumption is associated with reduction in

dietary cholesterol. Diet and exercise modifications can only reduce the LDL-C by 10% to 20%. After 3 to 6 months of lifestyle modification, statins can be used for the treatment of persistently elevated LDL-C concentrations of 160 mg/dL or higher (≥4.14 mmol/L).

What is the pharmacologic management of hypercholesterolemia?

Treatment of children with elevated LDL-C is based on assessment of lipid levels and associated risk factors or risk conditions. Statin therapy should be considered after a 6-month trial of lifestyle management with the CHILD-2 LDL diet in children 10 years or older: (1) if LDL-C is 190 mg/dL or greater (≥4.92 mmol/L), (2) if LDL-C is 160 mg/dL or greater (≥4.14 mmol/L) plus a positive family history *or* there is 1 high-risk factor/condition *or* 2 moderate risk factors/conditions, (3) if LDL-C is 130 mg/dL or greater (≥3.37 mmol/L) plus 2 high-risk factors/conditions *or* there is 1 high-risk factor/condition and 2 moderate-risk factors/conditions *or* clinical cardiovascular disease (*Table*).[7] Drug therapy can be considered for children as young as 8 years if LDL-C remains 190 mg/dL or greater (≥4.92 mmol/L) after a trial of lifestyle management and when there is a clinical suspicion or genetic diagnosis of FH, the presence of at least 1 high-risk factor or risk condition, or the presence of at least 2 moderate-risk factors or risk conditions.

All commercially available statins are FDA approved, with pravastatin, rosuvastatin, and pitavastatin starting at age 8 years and all others at age 10 years, for treatment of persistently elevated LDL-C of 160 mg/dL or greater (≥4.14 mmol/L) after 3 to 6 months of lifestyle modification in patients with clinical findings consistent with FH. Statins are well tolerated in children and have an excellent safety profile. The most commonly reported adverse effects are muscle-related symptoms, while hepatic transaminase elevations occur relatively infrequently. Pubertal girls should be advised about concerns of teratogenicity with statin use in pregnancy and counseled on the importance of concomitant contraceptive use. The goal of LDL-C lowering is to achieve an LDL-C level of 130 mg/dL or less (≤3.37 mmol/L). A lower LDL-C treatment goal may be considered if the child has diabetes or if there is a strong family history of premature cardiovascular disease.

Evolocumab is a PCSK9 inhibitor. A dose of 420 mg once monthly administered as a subcutaneous injection is approved for children 10 years and older with HeFH and HoFH if they have not achieved therapeutic goals on statin therapy.

In patients with HoFH, the management approach may include a maximally tolerated high-intensity statin along with ezetimibe and bile acid resins. Regular plasmapheresis is also recommended in the management of HoFH. Drugs acting through the LDL receptor such as PCSK9 inhibitors (eg, evolocumab for those older than 10 years and alirocumab for patients older than 18 years) are approved for use in HoFH. Drugs that act independently of LDL receptor such as ANGPTL3 inhibition (eg, evinacumab from age 12 years and lomitapide from age 18 years) are also treatment options.[8]

Is there any role for cardiac imaging?

Cardiovascular imaging is not required for children with HeFH. Cardiovascular imaging at diagnosis is indicated in children with HoFH (ie, electrocardiography, echocardiography, age-appropriate stress testing, and coronary artery imaging, including angiography).

Case 2

A 13-year-old boy with a BMI greater than the 99th percentile has the following lipid profile:

> Total cholesterol = 234 mg/dL (SI: 6.06 mmol/L)
> Triglycerides = 494 mg/dL (SI: 5.58 mmol/L)
> LDL-C = 126 mg/dL (SI: 2.59 mmol/L)
> Non–HDL-C = 201 mg/dL (SI: 5.21 mmol/L)
> HDL-C = 33 mg/dL (SI: 0.85 mmol/L)

His family history is notable for obesity, hypertriglyceridemia, hypercholesterolemia, and premature ASCVD in multiple relatives. After the implementation of therapeutic lifestyle changes, he loses 5 lb (2.3 kg).

A repeated fasting lipid profile obtained 12 weeks after the initial laboratory tests documents the following values:

> Total cholesterol = 286 mg/dL (SI: 7.41 mmol/L)
> Triglycerides = 173 mg/dL (SI: 1.95 mmol/L)
> LDL-C = 121 mg/dL (SI: 3.13 mmol/L)
> Non–HDL-C = 248 mg/dL (SI: 6.42 mmol/L)
> HDL-C = 38 mg/dL (SI: 0.98 mmol/L)

Which of the following is this patient's most likely diagnosis?

A. Familial hypertriglyceridemia

B. FCHL

C. Metabolic syndrome

D. Polygenic hypercholesterolemia

Answer: B) FCHL

This patient has combined dyslipidemia and obesity most likely due to FCHL (Answer B), given the variable elevations in LDL-C, persistently elevated non–HDL-C, positive family history of premature ASCVD, and marked variability in lipid profiles in patients and relatives.

Combined dyslipidemia (mixed dyslipidemia) manifests as elevated triglycerides and low HDL-C with variable LDL-C. Combined dyslipidemia is the most common lipid abnormality in childhood and adolescence. Usually, triglyceride levels are between 150 and 400 mg/dL (1.70 and 4.52 mmol/L) and HDL-C levels are less than 40 mg/dL (<1.04 mmol/L). The main differential diagnosis of combined dyslipidemia includes obesity-induced dyslipidemia (ie, dyslipidemia of metabolic syndrome due to visceral adiposity and insulin resistance) (Answer C) and FCHL (Answer B). Even though obesity-associated dyslipidemia overlaps phenotypically with FCHL, LDL-C concentrations are rarely greater than 160 mg/dL (>4.14 mmol/L) in patients with dyslipidemia due to obesity/metabolic syndrome. In the case of obesity-induced dyslipidemia, lipid abnormalities generally improve (ie,

triglycerides and non–HDL-C concentrations) with dietary modification or reduction in body weight. In contrast, patients with FCHL appear to have elevated non–HDL-C as does this patient (an indicator of excessive apolipoprotein B production).

Familial hypertriglyceridemia (Answer A) generally presents with hypertriglyceridemia. In the presence of secondary causes, such as type 2 diabetes, hypothyroidism, and certain medications, etc, combined dyslipidemia may be expressed in patients with associated minor variants in the genes controlling triglyceride metabolism. These patients have a higher ASCVD risk related to the degree of LDL-C and triglyceride elevation. Polygenic hypercholesterolemia (Answer D) is unlikely in this patient with combined dyslipidemia since polygenic hypercholesterolemia is predominantly characterized by elevated LDL-C concentrations, similar to FH.

What is the role of non–HDL-C?
Calculation of non–HDL-C is important in the management of these patients. Non–HDL-C encompasses all atherogenic molecules with an apolipoprotein B–containing particle. Non–HDL-C is elevated in this patient and hence he most likely has FCHL, which is associated with increased risk of premature ASCVD. Although triglyceride levels are typically between 200 and 500 mg/dL (2.26 and 5.65 mmol/L) in this setting, many gene-environment interactions (high-carbohydrate diet, obesity, sedentary lifestyle, estrogen, glucocorticoids, etc) can raise fasting serum triglyceride concentrations to greater than 500 mg/dL (>5.65 mmol/L) and postprandial triglycerides to greater than 1000 mg/dL (>11.30 mmol/L). For all patients with combined dyslipidemia, secondary factors must be ruled out.

What is the nonpharmacologic management of hypercholesterolemia?
The crucial step in treatment is intensive dietary and lifestyle changes and removal of offending drugs. In almost all cases, dyslipidemia of obesity responds well to lifestyle intervention, including

weight loss, changes in dietary composition, and increased physical activity. A decrease in weight/BMI will lead to significant improvement in triglycerides and HDL-C. Changes in dietary quality and composition (even without weight loss) are also effective in the management of high triglycerides and combined dyslipidemia. Such dietary modifications could include avoiding added sugars, limiting simple carbohydrates and replacing them with complex carbohydrates and/or low-glycemic load diets, increasing fiber intake, and reducing calorie intake. Each of these changes is an effective management strategy for combined dyslipidemia. Children and adolescents aged 5 to 17 years are recommended to have at least 60 minutes of moderate to vigorous intensity physical activity every day.

What is the pharmacologic management of hypercholesterolemia?

Judicious use of pharmaceutical agents such as statins, fibrates, or omega-3 fatty acids can be considered. Pharmacologic management is geared towards reduction of ASCVD risk later in life. The primary treatment target is LDL-C. If LDL-C is greater than 160 mg/dL (>4.14 mmol/L), statin treatment is recommended. The secondary treatment target is non–HDL-C. For triglyceride concentrations between 150 and 400 mg/dL (1.70 and 4.52 mmol/L) and non–HDL-C concentrations greater than 145 mg/dL (>3.76 mmol/L) despite 6 months of therapeutic lifestyle changes in children 10 years and older, statins are first-line therapy. In the case of a triglyceride concentration greater than 400 mg/dL (>4.52 mmol/L), fibrates are used along with therapeutic lifestyle changes. The role of omega-3 fatty acids in pediatric hypertriglyceridemia is debated. While over-the-counter omega-3 supplements are not beneficial, icosapent ethyl, 4 g daily, may be used in older children with hypertriglyceridemia. Treatment goals are triglyceride levels less than 150 mg/dL (<1.70 mmol/L) and non–HDL-C levels less than 145 mg/dL (<3.76 mmol/L).

Case 3

A 2-month-old girl presents with failure to thrive. Her serum is lipemic, and the following values are documented:

> Total cholesterol = 1295 mg/dL (SI: 33.54 mmol/L)
> Triglycerides = 26,000 mg/dL (SI: 293.8 mmol/L)
> HDL-C = 8 mg/dL (SI: 0.21 mmol/L)

Amylase and lipase levels are normal for age.

What is the most likely cause of severe hypertriglyceridemia in this patient?

A. Dysbetalipoproteinemia
B. Familial chylomicronemia syndrome
C. FCHL
D. Multifactorial chylomicronemia syndrome

Answer: B) Familial chylomicronemia syndrome

This patient has had hyperchylomicronemia from early infancy, indicating she has familial chylomicronemia syndrome (FCS) (Answer B), most likely secondary to autosomal recessive lipoprotein lipase deficiency. FCS is an autosomal recessive disorder due to homozygous or compound heterozygous pathogenic variants in the *LPL* gene, which encodes lipoprotein lipase (~80% of cases), or in genes regulating the lipoprotein lipase complex: *APOC2*, *APOA5*, *LMF1*, or *GPIHBP1*.

Mild-to-moderate triglyceride elevations typically reflect high VLDL and high numbers of remnant lipoprotein particles, while severe hypertriglyceridemia is due to excess accumulation of chylomicrons. Chylomicrons are produced in the intestine in response to dietary fat, and VLDL is produced in the liver. Lipoprotein lipase is the key enzyme involved in the hydrolysis of triglycerides in the circulating chylomicrons and VLDL. Lipoprotein lipase deficiency leads to impaired clearance of triglyceride-containing lipoproteins (ie, chylomicrons and VLDL) from the circulation. These severe triglyceride elevations could be due to monogenic causes such pathogenic variants in the lipoprotein lipase complex, known as FCS, or the multifactorial chylomicronemia syndrome.

Multifactorial chylomicronemia syndrome (Answer D) is due to coexistence of minor genetic variants (ie, rare heterozygous variants in the 5 FCS-related genes and/or accumulated common variants in many other loci associated with small increases in triglyceride levels identified in genome-wide association studies) and secondary factors. Such patients may present with baseline normal to moderate triglyceride levels, which may change to severe hypertriglyceridemia secondary to a metabolic insult. In this infant, the early onset of severe hypertriglyceridemia and lack of secondary factors make multifactorial chylomicronemia syndrome an unlikely diagnosis in this infant.

Familial dysbetalipoproteinemia (Answer A) is unlikely in this patient because it is characterized by equal elevations of total cholesterol and triglycerides (usually >300 mg/dL) due to the combination of homozygous apolipoprotein *E2* genotype or a rare binding-defective dominant variant in the *APOE* gene in the presence of a secondary metabolic insult.

FCHL (Answer C) can be excluded, as it is suggested by combined dyslipidemia of later onset, not isolated severe triglyceride elevations of early onset, as in this patient.

What is the management of severe hypertriglyceridemia?
Triglyceride concentrations greater than 1000 mg/dL (>11.30 mmol/L) are associated with a significant risk of acute pancreatitis. Proper dietary management of severe hypertriglyceridemia is crucial to prevent pancreatitis.[9] The treatment mainstay for FCS is restricting fat intake to less than 10% to 15% of dietary calories. Medium-chain triglycerides in the diet are absorbed directly into the portal circulation without the need for incorporation into chylomicron packaging and, hence, do not require lipoprotein lipase for absorption. Thus, part of the dietary fat could be consumed as medium-chain triglycerides. Over-the-counter medium-chain triglyceride oil and coconut oil are not recommended. In a child requiring a daily caloric intake of 1800 calories, medium-chain triglyceride oil should be limited to less than 1 to 2 tablespoons daily (eg, 2 tablespoons of medium-chain triglyceride oil have 28 g of fat and 252 calories). The primary objective is to prevent pancreatitis by maintaining triglyceride concentrations below 1000 mg/dL (<11.30 mmol/L). Medications are ineffective in the management of FCS.

In patients with multifactorial chylomicronemia syndrome, who almost always have a combination of genetic and secondary causes for triglyceride elevation, adding a fibrate is helpful to reduce the risk of acute pancreatitis. Currently, there are no FDA-approved medications to treat severe hypertriglyceridemia; hence, it is crucial to follow a strict low-fat diet. For patients older than 18 years, lomitapide and volanesorsen are clinical options in Europe.

Initial management of acute pancreatitis secondary to severe hypertriglyceridemia is administration of intravenous fluids and withholding oral intake. Insulin infusion can be tried in patients with diabetes or insulin deficiency to rapidly lower triglycerides. Withholding oral intake rapidly decreases chylomicron synthesis and reduces saturation of lipoprotein lipase sites with triglyceride-rich lipoproteins, leading to a rapid decrease in the serum triglyceride concentration. Once oral intake is resumed, a diet very low in fat (<15% of total calories) can be initiated. After the patient's condition is stable, dietary management for multifactorial chylomicronemia syndrome includes avoiding simple carbohydrates and following a low-fat diet, which can be slowly titrated to dietary fat content limited to less than 30% of total daily caloric intake to maintain triglycerides at a lower level. Strict glycemic control in patients with diabetes is also recommended. Weight loss is essential in patients who are overweight or obese.

Case 4

A 14-year-old boy with a BMI of 38 kg/m^2 presents for follow-up of type 2 diabetes.

Laboratory test results (sample drawn while fasting):

Hemoglobin A$_{1c}$ = 8.0% (4.0%-5.6%) (64 mmol/mol [20-38 mmol/mol])
Total cholesterol = 245 mg/dL (SI: 6.35 mmol/L)
Triglycerides = 380 mg/dL (SI: 4.29 mmol/L)
HDL-C = 36 mg/dL (SI: 0.93 mmol/L)
LDL-C = 133 mg/dL (SI: 3.44 mmol/L)
Amylase, normal
Lipase, normal

Which of the following is the best management option?

A. Fenofibrate

B. Omega-3 fatty acids

C. Statin

D. Stringent fat restriction to <15% of total dietary fat

Answer: C) Statin

How should dyslipidemia be managed in patients with type 2 diabetes?

Patients with type 2 diabetes require careful management. Dyslipidemia in these patients consists of elevated triglycerides, decreased HDL-C, and occasionally, elevated LDL-C. These patients also have elevated small, dense LDL particles, elevated VLDL-C, non–HDL-C, and apolipoprotein B increasing their high risk for future ASCVD. The American Diabetes Association and International Society for Pediatric and Adolescent Diabetes guidelines recommend lipid screening in patients with new-onset type 2 diabetes once glycemic control has been achieved or 3 months after diagnosis, with annual screening conducted thereafter.

- If LDL-C is above goal, glycemic control should be optimized, the American Heart Association Step 2 diet should be implemented (<30% of calories as total fat, <7% saturated fat, and <200 mg cholesterol daily), and testing should be repeated in 6 months. Hence, stringent fat restriction to less than 15% of total dietary fat (Answer D) is incorrect. If the fasting triglyceride concentration is greater than 1000 mg/dL (>11.30 mmol/L), this would be required.

- If repeated LDL-C is greater than 130 mg/dL (>3.37 mmol/L), statin treatment is recommended to achieve a goal value less than 130 mg/dL (<3.37 mmol/L) and ideally less than 100 mg/dL (<2.59 mmol/L). Therefore, statin treatment (Answer C) is correct.

- If triglycerides are greater than 400 mg/dL (>4.52 mmol/L) fasting or greater than 1000 mg/dL (>11.30 mmol/L) nonfasting, fibrates are recommended to reduce the risk for pancreatitis. Since this patient's triglycerides are less than 400 mg/dL (<4.52 mmol/L), fenofibrate (Answer A) and omega-3 fatty acids (Answer B) are incorrect.

- Strict glycemic control is recommended in patients with diabetes.

- Weight reduction, decreasing simple carbohydrates, and increasing dietary omega-3 fatty acids are also recommended.

- Lipid goals are: LDL-C <100 mg/dL (<2.59 mmol/L); HDL-C >35 mg/dL (>0.91 mmol/L); and triglycerides <150 mg/dL (<1.70 mmol/L).

How should dyslipidemia be managed in patients with type 1 diabetes?

According to the American Diabetes Association guidelines,[10] lipid testing should be performed in patients with type 1 diabetes when initial glycemic control has been achieved and the patient is 2 years or older. If LDL-C is 100 mg/dL or less (≤2.59 mmol/L), subsequent testing should be performed at age 9 to 11 years; if this is normal, the lipid profile should be repeated every 3 years.

- If LDL-C is abnormal, a lipid profile should be repeated in 6 months.

- After age 10 years, addition of a statin is suggested for patients who, despite medical nutrition therapy and lifestyle changes, continue to have LDL-C concentrations greater than 160 mg/dL (>4.14 mmol/L) or greater than 130 mg/dL (>3.37 mmol/L) plus 1 or more cardiovascular disease risk factor.

- In contrast, the International Society for Pediatric and Adolescent Diabetes guidelines[11] specify to consider treating at an LDL-C concentration greater than 130 mg/dL (>3.37 mmol/L) down to the same goal as above. Similarly, the American Heart Association classifies both type 1 diabetes and type 2 diabetes as high-risk conditions for which statin treatment is indicated when the LDL-C concentration is greater than 130 mg/dL (>3.37 mmol/L).[5,12]

- There are no recommendations regarding measurement of apolipoprotein B or screening lipoprotein (a).

- The goal LDL-C concentration is less than 100 mg/dL (<2.59 mmol/L).

References

1. Gidding SS, Leibel RL, Daniels S, Rosenbaum M, Van Horn L, Marx GR. Understanding obesity in youth. A statement for healthcare professionals from the Committee on Atherosclerosis and Hypertension in the Young of the Council on Cardiovascular Disease in the Young and the Nutrition Committee, American Heart Association. Writing Group. *Circulation.* 1996;94(12):3383-3387. PMID: 8989156

2. Sjouke B, Kusters DM, Kindt I, et al. Homozygous autosomal dominant hypercholesterolaemia in the Netherlands: prevalence, genotype-phenotype relationship, and clinical outcome. *Eur Heart J.* 2015;36(9):560-565. PMID: 24585268

3. Goldstein JL, Schrott HG, Hazzard WR, Bierman EL, Motulsky AG. Hyperlipidemia in coronary heart disease. II. Genetic analysis of lipid levels in 176 families and delineation of a new inherited disorder, combined hyperlipidemia. *J Clin Invest.* 1973;52(7):1544-1568. PMID: 4718953

4. Expert Panel on Integrated Guidelines for Cardiovascular Health and Risk Reduction in Children and Adolescents; National Heart, Lung, and Blood Institute. Expert panel on integrated guidelines for cardiovascular health and risk reduction in children and adolescents: summary report. *Pediatrics.* 2011;128(Suppl 5):S213-S256. PMID: 22084329

5. De Ferranti SD, Steinberger J, Ameduri R, et al. Cardiovascular risk reduction in high-risk pediatric patients: a scientific statement from the American Heart Association. *Circulation.* 2019;139(13):e603-e634. PMID: 30798614

6. Wilson DP, McNeal C, Blackett P. Pediatric dyslipidemia: recommendations for clinical management. *South Med J.* 2015;108(1):7-14. PMID: 25580750

7. Ashraf AP, Sunil B, Bamba V, et al. Case studies in pediatric lipid disorders and their management. *J Clin Endocrinol Metab.* 2021;106(12):3605-3620. PMID: 34363474

8. Sunil B, Foster C, Wilson DP, Ashraf AP. Novel therapeutic targets and agents for pediatric dyslipidemia. *Ther Adv Endocrinol Metab.* 2021;12:20420188211058323. PMID: 34868544

9. Valaiyapathi B, Sunil B, Ashraf AP. Approach to hypertriglyceridemia in the pediatric population. *Pediatr Rev.* 2017;38(9):424-434. PMID: 28864733

10. American Diabetes Association Professional Practice Committee; American Diabetes Association Professional Practice Committee; Draznin B, et al. 14. Children and adolescents: standards of medical care in diabetes–2021. *Diabetes Care.* 2021;44(Suppl 1):180-199. PMID: 34964865

11. Donaghue KC, Marcovecchio ML, Wadwa RP, et al. ISPAD clinical practice consensus guidelines 2018: microvascular and macrovascular complications in children and adolescents. *Pediatr Diabetes.* 2018;19(Suppl 27):262-274. PMID: 30079595

12. Sunil B, Ashraf AP. Dyslipidemia in pediatric type 2 diabetes mellitus. *Curr Diab Rep.* 2020;20(10):53. PMID: 32909078

Approach to Fractures in Children

Rachel I. Gafni, MD. Skeletal Disorders and Mineral Homeostasis Section, National Institute of Dental and Craniofacial Research, NIH, Bethesda, MD; E-mail: gafnir@nih.gov

Learning Objectives

As a result of participating in this session, learners should be able to:

- Recognize the most common causes of recurrent fractures in children and develop a plan of evaluation for these patients.

- List current indications for obtaining a dual-energy x-ray absorptiometry (DXA) scan and understand its interpretation and limitations in children.

- Develop a treatment and monitoring plan, keeping in mind the potential comorbidities that may be associated with the underlying disease and/or its therapy.

Main Conclusions

- Fractures are common in children and adolescents, particularly during times of peak growth.

- Low bone mineral density (BMD) and fragility fractures in children and adolescents may be caused by a variety of genetic, medical, or nutritional conditions.

- DXA is a useful screening tool for low BMD; however, correlation with fracture risk in sick populations has not been well established.

- Identifying the cause of low BMD and reversing the underlying disease may lead to partial or complete skeletal recovery.

- Off-label use of bisphosphonates may be considered in some patients, with appropriate monitoring.

Significance of the Clinical Problem

Fractures are frequent in children and adolescents due to the geometry of the growing skeleton and high levels of physical activity. Affected children may experience pain, skeletal deformity, and missed school days; with severe fractures, surgical intervention may be required. Thus, when fractures are recurrent, it is important to determine whether there are underlying pathologic factors contributing to bone fragility. The differential diagnosis for recurrent fractures is extensive, ranging from rare genetic disorders to common nutritional deficiencies, and thus an in-depth evaluation is required. While DXA is the standard screening tool, interpretation in the pediatric population differs from that in adults and is frequently misunderstood. Therefore, proper evaluation for children with recurrent fractures is critical for making the diagnosis and initiating the correct therapy.

Barriers to Optimal Practice

- Fractures are common in children, leading to delay in evaluation for underlying pathology.

- DXA is most commonly done in adults, particularly in postmenopausal women. Therefore, it is often difficult for practitioners to find a local densitometry center skilled in the performance and interpretation of DXA in children.

- There are no FDA-approved therapies for definitive treatment of osteoporosis in children.

Strategies for Diagnosis, Therapy, and/or Management

Fractures in Childhood

Fractures are common in children, occurring in approximately 50% of boys and 33% of girls. The fracture rate peaks between ages 11 and 15 years, with girls peaking earlier, consistent with the earlier pubertal growth spurt. The most common site for fracture is the forearm (about 25%-30% of fractures).[1] Risk factors for fractures include intrinsic factors such as bone density, size, and geometry, as well as extrinsic factors such as activity and impact. High participation in youth sports may be contributing to an increase in childhood fractures, including overuse insufficiency fractures.

When evaluating a child with fractures for underlying pathology, one should consider the site and mechanism of fracture, as well as any known medical conditions in the child. For example, a finger fracture sustained while playing basketball in an otherwise healthy child is generally not of concern, while a femur or a vertebral fracture after falling from a standing height would be unexpected. There is no set-in-stone rule for when a child with fractures should undergo DXA. In general, DXA is considered for children with a "clinically significant fracture history," defined as[2]:

1. A vertebral compression fracture or

2. 2 or more long bone fractures before age 10 years or

3. 3 or more long bone fractures before age 19 years

In addition, DXA should be considered for children with medical conditions or for children who are receiving treatments known to affect bone density, even in the absence of fractures.[3]

Evaluating the Child With Recurrent Fractures

History and Physical Examination

Given the long list of possible causes of skeletal fragility (*Box*), a systematic evaluation is crucial.[4,5] A careful history and physical examination with special attention to family history, comorbidities, kidney stones, dental issues, birthmarks/bruising, hyperextensibility, back/joint pain, rachitic deformities, and identification of dysmorphic features are important. Dietary habits should be reviewed to identify relevant nutritional or caloric insufficiencies. A detailed fracture history should include patient age, number of fractures, site, severity, and mechanism, as well as the adequacy of fracture healing. A history concerning for nonaccidental trauma should be addressed promptly. Minor finger and toe fractures occurring with an appropriate trauma are usually excluded from the definition of significant fracture history, unless excessive.

Laboratory Investigation

In a patient with a clinically significant fracture history, laboratory studies assessing bone and mineral metabolism should be completed. These include measurement of albumin-corrected calcium, phosphate, magnesium, creatinine, 25-hydroxyvitamin D, and intact PTH. Measurement of 1,25-dihydroxyvitamin D and FGF23 should be considered if the history suggests calcipenic or phosphopenic rickets. Additional screening laboratory tests such as complete chemistry panels, complete blood cell count, erythrocyte sedimentation rate, tissue transglutaminase antibodies, and thyroid function tests may be considered, driven by the history and physical examination, to identify systemic undiagnosed conditions. Age-appropriate normal ranges should be used for interpretation of laboratory results, especially blood phosphate, which is significantly higher in neonates and gradually decreases during childhood and adolescence until finally reaching the adult normal range. Urinary creatinine and calcium excretion should be measured; 24-hour collections are ideal. Again, age-specific urinary calcium and creatinine normal references should be applied and 24-hour collections should be corrected for body weight (normal calcium excretion: <4 mg/kg per 24 h or <0.1 mmol/kg per day). Genetic testing is commercially available for many of the causes of skeletal fragility.

Dual-Energy X-ray Absorptiometry

When ordering screening DXA in children, consensus guidelines recommend assessing the postero-anterior lumbar spine and the total body-less head.[2-4] The head is excluded because it is disproportionally large compared with the rest of the skeleton in children and may confound interpretation of low BMD. These 2 sites are the most reproducible with the greatest availability of normal reference databases. Reference databases used should be specific to the brand of densitometer. Using these databases, one can calculate the Z-score, which is the standard deviation score compared with age-, sex-, and race-matched healthy controls. T-scores, which calculate the standard deviation scores compared with young adults at peak bone mass, should never be used in children. Alternative sites such as the proximal femur and distal radius are more affected by changes in skeletal growth but may be informative in older adolescents. DXA acquisition requires careful positioning of the patient to ensure that the data generated can be interpreted compared with normal databases. In children with scoliosis, contractures, or skeletal deformity, appropriate positioning may be difficult or impossible. In such patients, lateral distal femur DXA may be performed and interpreted using published normative databases.[6]

Results from DXA include bone mineral content measured in grams, area in cm^2, and BMD reported in g/cm^2. As DXA is a 2-dimensional image of a 3-dimensional structure, this measurement output is better described as "areal BMD" (aBMD), as it does not represent true density, which is calculated as mass per volume. Therefore, aBMD is highly affected by bone size such that patients with short stature for age may have artifactually low aBMD. Conversely, aBMD

may be falsely elevated in patients with tall stature. Mathematical models have been developed to correct for variations in bone size; one method is to use the height Z-score to adjust the BMD Z-score. One online calculator specific to Hologic densitometers can be found here: https://zscore. research.chop.edu/calcpedbonedens.php.[7] Other factors that may confound DXA interpretation include altered pubertal timing, surgical hardware, and compression fractures (which decrease bone area and artifactually increase BMD).

A BMD Z-score between −2 and +2 SD is considered to be within the normal range. However, the correlation between BMD and fracture risk in children is not well-established, particularly in children with chronic diseases. Thus, the diagnosis of osteoporosis not based on DXA alone; rather, it is a clinical diagnosis.[2] For example, a child with an atraumatic vertebral compression fracture is considered to have osteoporosis, even when DXA results are within the normal range. Of note, BMD may be markedly elevated in sclerosing bone disorders such as osteopetrosis. Finally, DXA cannot distinguish between osteoporosis and osteomalacia (impaired mineralization).

Additional Testing

Guided by the history and physical examination, radiographs may be useful for identifying rickets, brachydactyly, fibrous dysplasia, or other skeletal abnormalities seen with several disorders associated with bone fragility. In patients at high risk for osteoporosis due to known underlying conditions or treatments (eg, leukemia, muscular dystrophy, chronic glucocorticoid use), lateral spine films may uncover asymptomatic vertebral fractures, particularly in the thoracic region.[8]

In cases of hypercalciuria, kidney ultrasonography is recommended to evaluate for nephrocalcinosis.

Collaboration with other specialists, including orthopedics, nephrology, hematology, neurology, rheumatology, genetics, and gastroenterology, is often essential in arriving at the correct diagnosis.

Box. Selected Causes of Skeletal Fragility in Children[4]

Primary bone disorders

- Osteogenesis imperfecta
- Osteoporosis pseudoglioma syndrome
- Ehlers-Danlos syndrome
- Marfan syndrome
- Homocystinuria
- Hajdu-Cheney syndrome
- Fibrous dysplasia
- Hypophosphatasia
- Pycnodysostosis
- Osteopetrosis
- Idiopathic juvenile osteoporosis

Secondary bone disorders

- Chronic inflammatory conditions
  - Rheumatologic disease
  - Inflammatory bowel disease
- Nephrology
  - Nephrotic syndrome
  - Renal insufficiency
  - Tubulopathies/acidosis
  - Hypercalciuria
- Neurology/reduced mobility
  - Cerebral palsy
  - Muscular dystrophies
  - Posttraumatic/spinal cord injury
- Hematology/oncology
  - Leukemia/malignancy
  - Thalassemia
  - Sickle cell anemia
  - Mastocytosis
- Endocrinology
  - Hypogonadism
  - Growth hormone deficiency
  - Cushing syndrome
  - Hyperthyroidism
  - Diabetes mellitus
  - Rickets (calcipenic and phosphopenic)

- Nutritional/malabsorptive
  - Vitamin D deficiency
  - Celiac disease
  - Anorexia nervosa
  - Relative energy deficiency in sport (RED-S)
  - Biliary atresia
  - Cystic fibrosis
- Iatrogenic
  - Glucocorticoids
  - Anticonvulsants
  - Methotrexate
  - Radiation therapy

Adapted from Boyce AM & Gafni RI. *J Clin Endocrinol Metab*, 2011; 96(7) © Endocrine Society.

Management

Once acute fractures are managed by the orthopedist, the primary goal is the prevention of future fractures. Optimization of nutrition and ensuring adequate calcium and vitamin D intake is appropriate for all patients. Weight-bearing exercise and/or physical therapy should be encouraged and tailored to the capacity of the individual, keeping in mind that patients with recurrent fractures due to anorexia nervosa or relative energy deficiency in sport (RED-S) will need to reduce or alter their exercise routine.[9] In otherwise healthy children with normal BMD and an explainable mechanism of injury, observation is often the best course. In children for whom a clear bone-impairing disease is identified, treating the underlying disorder is the first step, as the growing skeleton has tremendous capacity for remodeling and restoring bone density.[8] For example, vitamin D deficiency rickets in a toddler responds entirely over time with appropriate supplementation. However, many conditions are incompletely reversible, ongoing, or progressive, warranting pharmaceutical intervention.

Currently approved therapies for osteoporosis in adults include antiresorptive drugs (bisphosphonates, selective estrogen receptor modulators, RANK-ligand analogues) and anabolic drugs (teriparatide, PTHrP analogues, sclerostin antibody). To date, none of these medications have been approved for use in children. The greatest experience in pediatrics has been off-label use of bisphosphonates over the last 25 years.[10] Bisphosphates are analogues of pyrophosphates that are not degraded by skeletal pyrophosphatases. They are incorporated into newly forming bone where they can remain for decades. When released, bisphosphonates inhibit osteoclast function resulting in suppressed bone resorption. The most commonly used bisphosphonates in children are pamidronate and zoledronate, given intravenously every 3 months and every 6 to 12 months, respectively. The treatment regimen varies among institutions, but, in general, the initial dose is reduced to prevent the acute-phase reaction that is frequently seen with the first infusion.

The most common adverse effects seen with bisphosphonates are acute-phase reactions, hypocalcemia, hypophosphatemia, and bone pain. These transient adverse effects are usually easily managed with calcium, calcitriol, nonsteroidal antiinflammatory drugs and, occasionally, short bursts of glucocorticoids. Calcium and vitamin D intake should also be optimized prior to initiating bisphosphonate therapy. Oral nitrogen-containing bisphosphonates have not been well-studied in children and can cause irritant esophagitis; therefore, they are used less frequently in pediatric patients and should be avoided in those with reflux and cognitive impairment. Bisphosphonate-associated osteonecrosis of the jaw has been reported in adults but has not been seen in children. Regardless, a thorough dental evaluation with necessary extractions performed is recommended prior to the first bisphosphonate dose. Prolonged and excessive use of bisphosphonate can lead to bisphosphonate-induced osteopetrosis, characterized by defects in skeletal modeling. Thus, periodic DXA scans (every 6 to 12 months) and wrist or knee x-rays (every 1 to 3 years) are recommended to avoid overtreatment. The timing for bisphosphonate interruption (drug holidays) or discontinuation is not well established. In general, these strategies can be considered when the BMD Z-score is greater than –2 and/or the child is no longer having fractures.

Clinical Case Vignettes

Case 1

A 12-and-11/12-year-old girl presents with a history of 5 fractures: 3 supracondylar fractures at ages 3, 5, and 9 years; an L3 compression fracture at age 10 years while skiing; and an L1 compression fracture at age 12 years while sledding. She seems otherwise healthy with normal puberty, and height percentile was 85% to 90% before the vertebral fractures. DXA of the lumbar spine at age 10 years showed a Z-score –0.94; DXA was repeated at age 12 years with a Z-score of –1.4.

Which of the following is the most important thing to do next?

A. Counsel her on increasing dietary calcium and vitamin D intake

B. Perform genetic testing for type 1 osteogenesis imperfecta

C. Reassure her that these fractures are consistent with high-impact sports (sledding and skiing) and counsel her to be more careful

D. Recalculate her BMD Z-scores adjusted for height Z-score

Answer: D) Recalculate her BMD Z-scores adjusted for height Z-score

This patient has tall stature, which can artifactually increase aBMD measurement. In this case, the patient's height SD is approximately +1.5, while her uncorrected aBMD Z-scores are negative and decreasing. When the aBMD Z-scores were corrected for her tall stature (Answer D), the Z-score was –1.4 at age 10 years and –1.94 at age 12 years. Given that her fractures were in the lumbar vertebrae, which can reduce the DXA area measurement, the true aBMD may have been even lower than that.

Vertebral fractures are uncommon in children, even with vigorous activity (thus, Answer C is incorrect).

While patients with type 1 osteogenesis imperfecta often have normal stature, correct analysis of DXA and assessment of other laboratory tests should be done before genetic testing (Answer B).

Increasing calcium and vitamin D intake (Answer A) may be an important therapeutic option for this patient; however, it is important to appropriately interpret the results of testing prior to developing a treatment plan.

This patient was ultimately diagnosed with celiac disease, and her BMD improved on a gluten-free diet.

Case 2

A 15-year-old girl has sustained several stress fractures in her tibias that have healed very slowly. On questioning, you learn that she is a competitive runner and is hoping to get a scholarship to a division 1 college. Between school and practices, her eating is erratic, and she grabs quick meals and snacks whenever she can. She is very thin, and her last menses was 9 months ago. On DXA, her total body-less head Z-score is –2.2.

Which of the following should be recommended?

A. Leg brace to stabilize her tibia

B. Nutritional counseling and decreased running with cross-training and pool exercises

C. Oral contraceptive to restore her menses

D. Zoledronate infusion with reassessment of DXA in 6 months

Answer: B) Nutritional counseling and decreased running with cross-training and pool exercises

This patient has relative energy deficiency in sport (RED-S), formerly known as the "female athlete triad." RED-S is characterized by disordered eating, oligomenorrhea or amenorrhea, and decreased bone health. Affected patients can be difficult to treat because they are often very competitive and goal oriented. Treatment is centered on normalizing eating, increasing body fat, and reducing the repetitiveness of impact loading (Answer B). Over time, these efforts lead to return of menses and improved bone health.

While an oral contraceptive (Answer C) may be indicated in this patient to prevent pregnancy, this has not been shown to improve bone density in patients with RED-S. Studies in patients with anorexia nervosa indicate that when supplemental estrogen is needed, the transdermal route is more effective.

A leg brace (Answer A) may be useful in the acute management of a stress fracture but will not address the underlying pathology or prevent future fracture.

Bisphosphonate therapy (Answer D) would not be indicated before implementing these other measures and in the absence of a true fragility fracture.

Acknowledgment

Work in the author's laboratory is supported by the Intramural Research Program of the National Institutes of Health, National Institute of Dental and Craniofacial Research.

References

1. Hedström EM, Svensson O, Bergström U, Michno P. Epidemiology of fractures in children and adolescents. *Acta Orthop.* 2010;81(1):148-153. PMID: 20175744

2. Gordon CM, Leonard MB, Zemel BS; International Society for Clinical Densitometry. 2013 Pediatric Position Development Conference: executive summary and reflections [published correction appears in *J Clin Densitom.* 2014;17(4):517]. *J Clin Densitom.* 2014;17(2):219-224. PMID: 24657108

3. Guss CE, McAllister A, Gordon CM. DXA in children and adolescents. *J Clin Densitom.* 2021;24(1):28-35. PMID: 32111573

4. Boyce AM, Gafni RI. Approach to the child with fractures. *J Clin Endocrinol Metab.* 2011;96(7):1943-1952. PMID: 21734001

5. Weber DR. Bone health in childhood chronic disease. *Endocrinol Metab Clin North Am.* 2020;49(4):637-650. PMID: 33153671

6. Weber DR, Boyce A, Gordon C, et al. The utility of DXA assessment at the forearm, proximal femur, and lateral distal femur, and vertebral fracture assessment in the pediatric population: 2019 ISCD official position. *J Clin Densitom.* 2019;22(4):567-589. PMID: 31421951

7. Zemel BS, Kalkwarf HJ, Gilsanz V, et al. Revised reference curves for bone mineral content and areal bone mineral density according to age and sex for black and non-black children: results of the bone mineral density in childhood study [published correction appears in *J Clin Endocrinol Metab.* 2013;98(1):420]. *J Clin Endocrinol Metab.* 2011;96(10):3160-3169. PMID: 21917867

8. Ward LM, Ma J, Lang B, et al; Steroid-Associated Osteoporosis in the Pediatric Population (STOPP) Consortium. Bone morbidity and recovery in children with acute lymphoblastic leukemia: results of a six-year prospective cohort study. *J Bone Miner Res.* 2018;33(8):1435-1443. PMID: 29786884

9. Joy E, De Souza MJ, Nattiv A, et al. 2014 female athlete triad coalition consensus statement on treatment and return to play of the female athlete triad. *Curr Sports Med Rep.* 2014;13(4):219-232. PMID: 25014387

10. Ward LM. Part 2: when should bisphosphonates be used in children with chronic illness osteoporosis? *Curr Osteoporos Rep.* 2021;19(3):289-297. PMID: 34146247

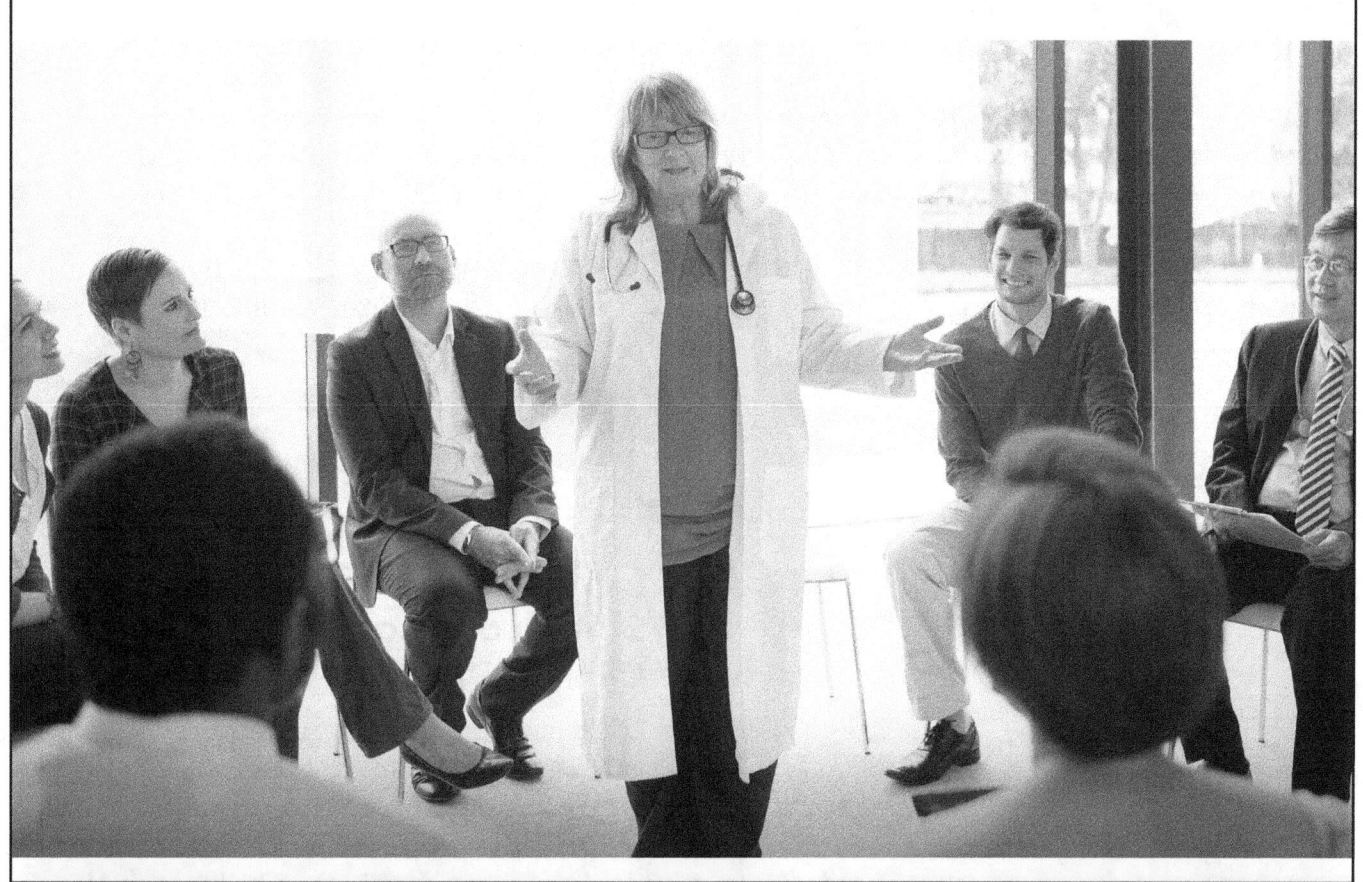

REPRODUCTIVE ENDOCRINOLOGY

Polycystic Ovary Syndrome Across the Lifespan

Melanie Cree Green, MD, PhD. Department of Pediatrics, Endocrine Section, University of Colorado Anschutz Campus and Children's Hospital Colorado, Aurora, CO; E-mail melanie.green@childrenscolorado.org

Kathleen M. Hoeger, MD, MPH. Department of Obstetrics and Gynecology, Division of Reproductive Endocrinology, University of Rochester, Rochester, NY; E-mail kathy_hoeger@urmc.rochester.edu

Learning Objectives

As a result of participating in this session, learners should be able to:

- Accurately diagnose polycystic ovary syndrome (PCOS) in patients of any age.

- Determine how and when to screen for and treat related metabolic disease.

- Explain management options for obesity-related PCOS concerns.

- Describe the best initial fertility options for patients with PCOS.

- Identify additional PCOS-related conditions to screen for and treat and determine when to refer to other specialists.

Main Conclusions

PCOS is a very common disorder in women and affects females from childhood through menopause. PCOS evaluation must be complete, but it should not include ovary ultrasonography in adolescents. PCOS can affect metabolic and psychologic health, and once it is diagnosed, affected patients should be screened for the full spectrum of associated conditions. Treatment plans should be developed with the patient to meet their unique needs and identified treatment goals.

Connection with peer-support networks should be encouraged.

Significance of the Clinical Problem

PCOS is a common menstrual disorder in women, estimated to affect 10% to 15% of all reproductive-aged women, and it can affect females across the lifespan.[1] The prevalence of PCOS in women who also have obesity may be even higher, up to 1 in 5 women. The underlying pathology of PCOS is not well understood, but it may be related to increased LH secretion, increased ovary sensitivity to LH and insulin, and excess insulin concentrations.[1] Some women have a genetic predisposition for PCOS.[2,3] Hormone differences can be detected in childhood in girls whose mothers have PCOS.[4] A history of early adrenarche (<8 years) and menarche (<10 years) is associated with a higher risk of developing PCOS.[5] PCOS can first be diagnosed in adolescence, with the presentation of irregular menses, although many women do not present until adulthood when they experience difficulty with conception.[6-9] Approximately 60% of women with PCOS become overweight; persistent weight gain and difficulty with weight loss are common presenting concerns.[1] PCOS symptoms can continue through menopause, when hormonal alterations resolve, but metabolic complications can continue, although potentially at the same rates as those of women without PCOS.[10,11]

A key component of PCOS is menstrual dysfunction, with many reproductive system consequences. Due to ovulatory dysfunction, PCOS is a leading cause of female infertility.[1] Ovulation induction is a primary therapy for infertility in patients with PCOS. Women with PCOS undergoing ovulation induction have increased risk of multiple gestation and ovarian hyperstimulation, so careful assessment is required and oral agents are preferred as the starting treatment. Additionally, long periods of amenorrhea increase the risk for endometrial hyperplasia. The rates of endometrial cancer are higher in women with PCOS and are thought to be related to extended periods without endometrial shedding.[12] There does not appear to be an increased risk for breast or ovarian cancer when controlled for obesity.[12]

PCOS is associated with many long-term detrimental metabolic consequences, including hypertension, central adiposity, dyslipidemia, hyperglycemia, type 2 diabetes, nonalcoholic fatty liver disease, and obstructive sleep apnea.[1,13-17] These metabolic risks are in excess in women with PCOS and are not just a consequence of related obesity. The relative risk of developing type 2 diabetes is almost 4 times higher in women with PCOS compared with risk in control patients after adjustment for age and is 2.4 times higher after further adjustment for BMI.[18] The risk for diabetes in adolescent girls is even higher.[16] Lipid abnormalities are common, in up to 70% of affected women, with low HDL cholesterol being the most common abnormality.[19] Epidemiological studies have not yet defined a clear increase in long-term cardiovascular events, but the risk factors for cardiovascular disease, early atherosclerosis deposition, and endothelial dysfunction are present in women with PCOS.[20] Rates of nonalcoholic fatty liver disease are 2- to 3-fold higher in women with PCOS, as are rates of obstructive sleep apnea.[21-24] The risks for metabolic disease seem to vary depending on a patient's race

and ethnicity, similar to risks for metabolic disease in women without PCOS.[25]

In addition to hormonal and metabolic consequences, PCOS affects many other aspects of health. Women with PCOS have higher rates of mood disruption and disordered eating.[26,27] Increased rates of depressive symptoms have been noted in adolescents with PCOS.[28] Sleep duration and circadian rhythms may also be altered in some women with PCOS, which can further contribute to metabolic disease.[17,29] Beyond the typical clinical manifestations of hyperandrogenism, including hirsutism, acne, and alopecia, PCOS is associated with hidradenitis suppurativa.[30] Acanthosis is also common, particularly in adolescents.[31]

Barriers to Optimal Practice

- Diagnosis of PCOS can be challenging, especially in adolescents.

- PCOS affects many systems, and patient care therefore requires longer appointment times and multidisciplinary care.

Strategies for Diagnosis, Therapy, and/or Management

Diagnosis

On average, it takes up to 4 physician visits and more than 2 years for patients to be diagnosed with PCOS. Efforts should be made to expedite an accurate diagnosis.[32] PCOS should be considered in any woman with irregular menses, especially if the patient also manifests signs of clinical hyperandrogenism. The diagnostic criteria were updated in the 2018 international guidelines, in particular for adolescents, and have been further clarified (*Table 1*).[1,31] History should be comprehensive, including age at menarche, timing of menses, signs or symptoms of hyperandrogenism, dermatologic history, sleep, obesity history if relevant, fertility plans, prior treatments, family history of PCOS, type 2 diabetes, and early cardiovascular death. Mood

Table 1. Diagnostic Characteristics of PCOS in Adolescents

1. Menstrual abnormalities	Primary amenorrhea	>15 years of age
		>3 years after thelarche
	Oligomenorrhea	Irregular menses are normal during the first gynecologic year
		>1 year postmenarche, >90 days for any cycle
		>1 to <3 years postmenarche cycle length <21 or >45 days
		>3 years postmenarche to perimenopause: <21 or >35 days or <8 cycles per year
2. Clinical or biochemical evidence of hyperandrogenism	Clinical hyperandrogenism	Acne: severe or cystic acne unresponsive to topical treatment
		Hirsutism: use Ferriman-Gallwey score, score of >4 to 8 is abnormal depending on race and ethnicity
		Androgenic alopecia: Ludwig alopecia scale (score of 0-4)
	Biochemical hyperandrogenism	Ideally liquid chromatography–tandem mass spectrometry should be used for most accurate measurement of total testosterone
		Calculated free testosterone concentration, free androgen index, or calculated bioavailable testosterone should be used, as those with obesity can have low SHBG and "normal" total testosterone
		A morning sample during menses will yield the highest concentrations
		Because of estrogen's effects on SHBG and altered gonadotropin-dependent androgen production, androgen concentrations cannot be interpreted if an individual is taking estrogen-containing medications
		When determination of androgen concentrations is essential for women on hormonal contraception, they must have ≥3 months of withdrawal with provision of alternative forms of contraception
Other diagnostic considerations	Ovarian imaging	<8 years postmenarche ovarian ultrasonography should not be used to diagnose polycystic ovary morphology due to the high prevalence of multifollicular ovary morphology
		>8 years postmenarche demonstrating ≥20 antral follicles per ovary or ≤10 cm volume in a single ovary is diagnostic
	PCOS is a diagnosis of exclusion	Exclude other causes of amenorrhea/oligomenorrhea: • Pregnancy: β-hCG • Thyroid abnormalities: TSH • Prolactinoma: prolactin • Primary gonadal failure: FSH • Hypothalamic amenorrhea: FSH, history • Absence of uterus, outflow obstruction: pelvic ultrasonography
		Exclude other causes of hyperandrogenism: • Congenital adrenal hyperplasia due to 21-hydroxylase deficiency: 17-hydroxyprogesterone • Other disorders of steroidogenesis • Tumor: consider imaging if testosterone or DHEA-S is greatly elevated • Cushing syndrome can be considered, but testing is not routine
	Other laboratory tests	Antimullerian hormone should not be used routinely to diagnose PCOS due to lack of assay standardization or validated cutoffs
	Additional considerations	Insulin resistance and hyperinsulinemia are not diagnostic criteria for PCOS
		Obesity is not a diagnostic criterion for PCOS

should be screened in all women with PCOS at the time of diagnosis. The physical examination should be comprehensive and assess for severity of acne, hirsutism as scored by the modified Ferriman-Gallwey scale,[33] androgenic alopecia,[34] acanthosis nigricans, skin tags, hidradenitis suppurativa, thyroid size, airway and tonsil size, liver size, peripheral edema, and striae size and color.

Management

Treatment Modalities

PCOS care should be delivered in an empathetic manner and be patient-centered. Goals should be set collaboratively, as there are currently high rates of treatment dissatisfaction.[1,32,36] Screening and treatment of conditions related to PCOS are described in Tables 2 and 3. All patients should be counseled on developing or maintaining a healthy lifestyle, including food, activity, and stress management components. Women may benefit from being connected with peer-support groups.[36]

Hormonal therapies are primarily to address endometrial health, and those with estrogen can reduce symptoms of hyperandrogenism.[1] Metformin (goal dosage 2000 mg daily) is prescribed to moderately decrease testosterone and hyperandrogenic symptoms and prevent diabetes in adults. Metformin can contribute to weight loss in patients of all ages. Metformin is thought to be more effective if a patient already has evidence of dysglycemia.[1] In women with obesity, early data suggest that GLP-1 receptor agonists are a promising option for PCOS, and bariatric surgery is highly effective.[37-41]

Clinical Case Vignettes

Case 1

A 14-year-old girl presents with irregular menses. She had menarche 15 months ago and has had 1 additional menses since then (5 months ago). She has acne on her face, chest, and back. She is not bothered by excess hair growth. She has struggled with weight since she started puberty. She stopped

Table 2. Screening for Conditions Related to PCOS

Condition	Testing modality	Frequency
Skin conditions	Physical exam, referral to dermatology if needed	Every visit
Infertility	Assessment of other factors contributing to fertility, ovulation induction; referral to fertility clinic if needed	When desired by the patient; should be discussed at regular visits to inform and advise
Hyperlipidemia	Fasting lipid panel	At diagnosis; frequency of repeated measurement depends on presence of hyperlipidemia and cardiovascular disease risk
Hypertension	Resting blood pressure 24-hour ambulatory blood pressure	Every visit
Dysglycemia	2-hour 75-g oral glucose tolerance test or hemoglobin A_{1c} measurement	At diagnosis, then every 1 to 3 years (every 3 to 6 months in adolescents with prediabetes)
Nonalcoholic fatty liver disease	Alanine aminotransferase, if elevated referral to hepatology for transient elastography or biopsy	At diagnosis, then every 1 to 3 years
Obstructive sleep apnea	Screening question on snoring, daytime sleepiness, morning headaches, restless sleep Referral to sleep/pulmonary for polysomnography if needed	At diagnosis, then every 1 to 3 years
Quality of life/sexual dysfunction	PCOS quality of life survey,[35] referral to psychology/psychiatry if needed	At diagnosis and at every visit if needed
Mood disorder	Mood screening survey, referral to psychology/psychiatry if needed	At diagnosis and at every visit if needed
Disordered eating	Eating history, referral to psychology/psychiatry if needed	At diagnosis and at every visit if needed

Table 3. Approaches to Treating Conditions Associated With PCOS

Endometrial health/contraception	Obesity or weight gain
• Combined hormonal contraceptive pills, patch, or ring • Cyclic progesterone every 3 months*† • Daily progesterone*† • Long-acting contraception; implantable 3-year progesterone or progesterone intrauterine device[42]* • Metformin†	• Nutritional modification • Activity/exercise plans ◦ No type of exercise is superior • Metformin • Weight-loss medication • Avoid weight gain–causing medications • Bariatric surgery
Fertility	**Dermatologic**
• Lifestyle modification with weight loss if patient has obesity • Metformin • Letrozole • Clomiphene citrate • In vitro fertilization Optimize metabolic control, especially glucose if patient has diabetes	• Hirsutism: combined hormonal contraceptive, spironolactone, topical eflornithine, laser hair reduction, electrolysis • Acne: combined hormonal contraceptives, spironolactone, benzoyl peroxide, salicylic acid, topical antibiotic, topical retinoid, oral retinoid • Hidradenitis: chlorhexidine gluconate, oral minocycline/doxycycline • Acanthosis: lactic acid lotion, metformin
Other metabolic conditions such as diabetes, nonalcoholic fatty liver disease, obstructive sleep apnea, hypertension, hyperlipidemia, depression, or anxiety should be treated in standard-of-care fashion for each condition	

* Will not decrease testosterone or dermatologic manifestations of PCOS.

† Not effective contraception.

playing sports partly because she felt like it was exacerbating the boils on her groin and under her bra. She is now home schooled as she was having problems with friends and having trouble getting up in the morning. Her family history is notable for type 2 diabetes in her mother and PCOS in a paternal aunt.

On physical examination, she is overweight (BMI = 92nd percentile) and is not hypertensive. She has moderate acne. Her Ferriman-Gallwey score is 12, including scores of 3 on the upper lip and chin. She also has active hidradenitis under the breasts and on the groin and grade 4 acanthosis on the neck.

Does this patient meet international guideline criteria for PCOS?

A. No, she is only 15 months postmenarche

B. Yes, she had menarche 4 years after breast development, so technically had delayed menses

C. Yes, she has gone >90 days between menses in the second menarcheal year

D. No, we do not know her serum testosterone concentration

E. Yes, this is a classic presentation for PCOS

Answer: C) Yes, she has gone >90 days between menses in the second menarcheal year

For adolescents, oligomenorrhea in the second menarcheal year is considered abnormal if there are more than 90 days between menses (Answer C). Primary amenorrhea 3 years after thelarche is also considered abnormal, but the age of thelarche was not noted in the vignette—a reminder to be comprehensive in obtaining pubertal history. The diagnosis of PCOS can be made based on oligomenorrhea and clinical signs of hyperandrogenism after all other causes of each have been ruled out.

Additional questions: What would be the benefits of combined oral contraceptives for her? What would you recommend regarding her hirsutism? What can you suggest for the hidradenitis and acanthosis? What other conditions would you like to get more information about?

Elevated testosterone can contribute to acne, hirsutism, and hidradenitis, and all may be improved with treatment of combined hormonal contraception. A combined hormonal contraceptive could decrease her risk for endometrial cancer and cause regular (or suppressed) menses, if desired. Note that the patient states that she is not bothered by hirsutism despite a clinically significant Ferriman-Gallwey score. This is a reminder that treatments should be patient-led. She is describing symptoms of hidradenitis, which can be managed with topical chlorhexidine gluconate and referral to dermatology. Hidradenitis is noted as a barrier to implementing an exercise program and treating this may be necessary before the patient is willing to increase activity. Other barriers to implementing lifestyle changes could be explored. Her history of being home-schooled and having trouble with friends is concerning for possible struggles with mood. Her difficulty getting up in the morning could be related to obstructive sleep apnea or a circadian rhythm shift and may require referral to sleep medicine for a full evaluation. Metabolic screening should be performed and, because of her weight, family history of diabetes, and presence of acanthosis, she may be at higher risk for dysglycemia. If she has evidence of dysglycemia, she would be a good candidate for metformin. Because she is overweight but not obese, neither appetite suppressants nor bariatric surgery would be recommended. However, if she had obesity, those treatments would be considerations, in conjunction with an intensive lifestyle program.

Case 2

A 35-year-old G1P1001 woman with PCOS and obesity (BMI = 55 kg/m²) presents with concerns about weight gain and metabolic risks. Her weight has fluctuated over time, and she has been unsuccessful sustaining weight loss (*see Figure*).

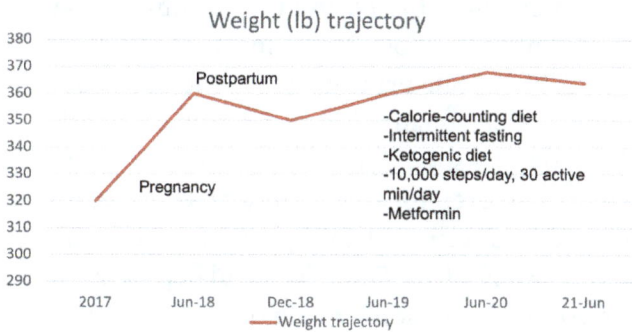

She is interested in options for losing weight and controlling her metabolic risks. She has a levonorgestrel intrauterine device in place and is experiencing amenorrhea with this treatment. She has not had significant hair growth changes since delivery.

Recommended testing includes an oral glucose tolerance test, lipid panel, and TSH measurement. She currently takes metformin. While this has not been effective in achieving her weight-loss goals, she has lost 3% to 4% of her peak weight. Her hemoglobin A_{1c} measurement is 5.9% (41 mmol/mol).

Which of the following treatment options would you NOT discuss for metabolic health and weight loss?

A. Meeting with a dietician to see if she is properly following a ketogenic diet

B. Encouraging her to increase her active minutes per day from 30 to 60

C. Starting a weight-loss medication

D. Doubling her dosage of metformin

E. Inquiring about sleep habits and ordering a sleep study if suspicious for obstructive sleep apnea

Answer: D) Doubling her dosage of metformin

The metformin dosage could be increased to 2000 mg daily, but exceeding this dosage is not advised (Answer D). This patient is at very high risk for metabolic disease, and this risk is increased by having PCOS. The risk for nonalcoholic fatty liver disease is 2-fold higher in women with PCOS, rates of type 2 diabetes are 8-fold higher in women with obesity, and rates of obstructive sleep apnea are 2-fold higher in patients with PCOS.[18,22,23,43] She presents with concerns about obesity. A personalized conversation around this chief concern should include reinforcement of dietary and exercise education with consideration of a dietician visit and discussion of options to sustain weight loss. Poor sleep and depression can contribute to weight gain or failure to lose weight and may need to be addressed first. Options include FDA-approved medications for weight loss (*Table 4*).

Overall, there are limited data on GLP-1 receptor agonists in patients with PCOS from randomized controlled trials but a meta-analysis of trials comparing GLP-1 receptor agonists with metformin suggests improved weight reduction with GLP-1 receptor agonists.[12]

Bariatric surgery in patients with PCOS promotes significant weight loss within 1 year, which is associated with amelioration of insulin resistance, hyperandrogenism, menstrual irregularity, and ovulatory dysfunction. Compared with metformin, bariatric surgery is associated with improved menstrual control. While data suggest improved odds of conception with bariatric surgery compared with metformin, current data are insufficient to use it as a primary fertility intervention.

Case 3

A 32-year-old G0 woman would like to conceive. She has used combined oral contraceptive pills for the past 10 years with no adverse effects. She has had routine gynecologic examinations with no significant medical problems. She was married 2 years ago and stopped using combined oral contraceptive pills 6 months ago. As her menses did not resume spontaneously, her gynecologist ordered bloodwork and ultrasonography. PCOS was subsequently diagnosed. In her medical records, her blood pressure is 126/74 mm Hg, BMI is 42.4 kg/m^2, TSH and prolactin concentrations are normal, and total testosterone concentration is 63 ng/dL (2.2 nmol/L). Both ovaries have a volume greater than 10 mL.

Table 4. FDA-Approved Medications for Weight Loss

FDA-approved antiobesity medications	Mechanism of action	Placebo-subtracted weight loss	Contraindications
Orlistat	Lipase inhibitor, fat malabsorption	-2.6 kg	Pregnancy, malabsorption syndromes, cholestasis
Lorcaserin	Selective 5HT receptor antagonist, promotes satiety	-3.2 kg	Pregnancy
Phentermine-toprimate	Norepinephrine-releasing agent/GABA receptor modulator, reduces appetite	-8.8 kg	Pregnancy, hyperthyroidism, glaucoma, MAOIs
Naltrexone-buproprion	Opioid antagonist/dopamine and norepinephrine reuptake inhibitor, reduces food intake	-5.0 kg	Pregnancy, uncontrolled hypertension, seizure disorder, anorexia, bulimia, drug or alcohol withdrawal, long-term opioid use, MAOIs
Liraglutide	GLP-1 agonist, delays gastric emptying	-5.3 kg	Pregnancy, personal or family history of medullary thyroid cancer or multiple endocrine neoplasia type 2
Semaglutide (2021)	GLP-1 analogue, reduces appetite	-12.7 kg	Pregnancy, personal or family history of medullary thyroid cancer or multiple endocrine neoplasia type 2

Courtesy W. Vitek.

Which of the following is the best next step in this patient's management?

A. Review the use of letrozole as a first-line agent for ovulation induction

B. Screen for diabetes, dyslipidemia, and depression and then initiate letrozole

C. Recommend a nutrition consult and return to the office after 3 months of lifestyle modification

Answer: B) Screen for diabetes, dyslipidemia, and depression and then initiate letrozole

In this setting, the preconception counseling should include metabolic assessment (Answer B) to determine whether there is glucose intolerance before attempting pregnancy. Additional assessments should include male partner evaluation and evaluation of the uterus and fallopian tubes. Ovulation induction (Answer A) is the next line of intervention as she has anovulation. The international guidelines for the management of infertility in PCOS note that letrozole should be considered first-line pharmacological treatment to improve ovulation, pregnancy, and live birth rates in women with PCOS with anovulatory infertility and no other infertility factors.[1]

Data regarding weight reduction prior to fertility attempts (Answer C) in the setting of normal glycemia are mixed for PCOS. However, a randomized controlled trial evaluating 6 months of weight reduction prior to fertility attempts improved ovulation rates in response to medical ovulation induction.[44]

References

1. Teede HJ, Misso ML, Costello MF, et al; International PCOS Network. Recommendations from the international evidence-based guideline for the assessment and management of polycystic ovary syndrome. *Fertil Steril.* 2018;110(3):364-379. PMID: 30033227

2. Dapas M, Lin FTJ, Nadkarni GN, et al. Distinct subtypes of polycystic ovary syndrome with novel genetic associations: An unsupervised, phenotypic clustering analysis. *PLoS Med.* 2020;17(6):e1003132. PMID: 32574161

3. Lerchbaum E, Schwetz V, Giuliani A, Obermayer-Pietsch B. Influence of a positive family history of both type 2 diabetes and PCOS on metabolic and endocrine parameters in a large cohort of PCOS women. *Eur J Endocrinol.* 2014;170(5):727-739. PMID: 24591551

4. Torchen LC, Legro RS, Dunaif A. Distinctive reproductive phenotypes in peripubertal girls at risk for polycystic ovary syndrome. *J Clin Endocrinol Metab.* 2019;104(8):3355-3361. PMID: 30844044

5. Ibanez L, Potau N, Zampolli M, Prat N, Virdis R, Vicens-Calvet E, Carrascosa A. Hyperinsulinemia in postpubertal girls with a history of premature pubarche and functional ovarian hyperandrogenism. *J Clin Endocrinol Metab.* 1996;81(3):1237-1243. PMID: 8772605

6. Legro RS, Arslanian SA, Ehrmann DA, et al; Endocrine Society. Diagnosis and treatment of polycystic ovary syndrome: an Endocrine Society clinical practice guideline. *J Clin Endocrinol and Metab.* 2013;98(12):4565-4592. PMID: 24151290

7. Martin KA, Anderson RR, Chang RJ, et al. Evaluation and treatment of hirsutism in premenopausal women: an Endocrine Society clinical practice guideline. *J Clin Endocrinol Metab.* 2018;103(4):1233-1257. PMID: 29522147

8. Goodman NF, Cobin RH, Futterweit W, et al; American Association of Clinical Endocrinologists (AACE); American College of Endocrinology (ACE); Androgen Excess and PCOS Society. American Association of Clinical Endocrinologists, American College of Endocrinology, and Androgen Excess and PCOS Society disease state clinical review: guide to the best practices in the evaluation and treatment of polycystic ovary syndrome - Part 2. *Endocr Pract.* 2015;21(12):1415-1426. PMID: 26642102

9. Goodman NF, Cobin RH, Futterweit W, et al; American Association of Clinical Endocrinologists (AACE), American College of Endocrinology (ACE); Androgen Excess and PCOS Society (AES). American Association of Clinical Endocrinologists, American College of Endocrinology, and Androgen Excess and PCOS Society disease state clinical review: guide to the best practices in the evaluation and treatment of polycystic ovary syndrome--Part 1. *Endocr Pract.* 2015;21(11):1291-1300. PMID: 26509855

10. Robeva R, Mladenovic D, Veskovic M, et al. The interplay between metabolic dysregulations and non-alcoholic fatty liver disease in women after menopause. *Maturitas.* 2021;151:22-30. PMID: 34446275

11. Helvaci N, Yildiz BO. The impact of ageing and menopause in women with polycystic ovary syndrome. *Clin Endocrinol (Oxf).* 2021 [Online ahead of print]

12. Barry JA, Azizia MM, Hardiman PJ. Risk of endometrial, ovarian and breast cancer in women with polycystic ovary syndrome: a systematic review and meta-analysis. *Hum Reprod Update.* 2014;20(5):748-758. PMID: 24688118

13. Mo L, Mansfield DR, Joham A, et al. Sleep disturbances in women with and without polycystic ovary syndrome in an Australian National Cohort. *Clin Endocrinol (Oxf).* 2019;90(4):570-578. PMID: 30585648

14. Lim SS, Kakoly NS, Tan JWJ, et al. Metabolic syndrome in polycystic ovary syndrome: a systematic review, meta-analysis and meta-regression. *Obes Rev.* 2019;20(2):339-352. PMID: 30339316

15. Sarkar M, Terrault N, Chan W, et al. Polycystic ovary syndrome (PCOS) is associated with NASH severity and advanced fibrosis. *Liver Int.* 2019;40:355-359. PMID: 31627243

16. Hudnut-Beumler J, Kaar JL, Taylor A, Kelsey MM, Nadeau KJ, Zeitler P, et al. Development of type 2 diabetes in adolescent girls with polycystic ovary syndrome and obesity. *Pediatr Diabetes.* 2021;22(5):699-706. PMID: 33870630

17. Simon S, Rahat H, Carreau A-M, et al. Poor sleep is related to metabolic syndrome severity in adolescents with PCOS and obesity. *J Clin Endocrinol Metab.* 2020;105(4):e1827-e1834. PMID: 31901092

18. Kakoly NS, Earnest A, Teede HJ, Moran LJ, Joham AE. The impact of obesity on the incidence of type 2 diabetes among women with polycystic ovary syndrome. *Diabetes Care.* 2019;42(4):560-567. PMID: 30705063

19. Wild RA, Rizzo M, Clifton S, Carmina E. Lipid levels in polycystic ovary syndrome: systematic review and meta-analysis. *Fertil Steril.* 2011;95(3):1073-1079 e1-e11. PMID: 21247558

20. Wild RA, Carmina E, Diamanti-Kandarakis E, et al. Assessment of cardiovascular risk and prevention of cardiovascular disease in women with the polycystic ovary syndrome: a consensus statement by the Androgen Excess and Polycystic Ovary Syndrome (AE-PCOS) Society. *J Clin Endocrinol Metab.* 2010;95(5):2038-2049. PMID: 20375205

21. Cree-Green M, Bergman BC, Coe GV, et al. Hepatic steatosis is common in adolescents with obesity and PCOS and relates to de novo lipogenesis but not insulin resistance. *Obesity (Silver Spring).* 2016;24(11):2399-2406. PMID: 27804265

22. Kumarendran B, Sumilo D, O'Reilly MW, et al. Increased risk of obstructive sleep apnoea in women with polycystic ovary syndrome: a population-based cohort study. *Eur J Endocrinol.* 2019;180(4):265-272. PMID: 30763274

23. Fernandez RC, Moore VM, Van Ryswyk EM, et al. Sleep disturbances in women with polycystic ovary syndrome: prevalence, pathophysiology, impact and management strategies. *Nat Sci Sleep.* 2018;10:45-64. PMID: 29440941

24. Gutierrez-Grobe Y, Ponciano-Rodriguez G, Ramos MH, Uribe M, Mendez-Sanchez N. Prevalence of non alcoholic fatty liver disease in premenopausal, posmenopausal and polycystic ovary syndrome women. The role of estrogens. *Ann Hepatol.* 2010;9(4):402-409. PMID: 21057159

25. Andrisse S, Garcia-Reyes Y, Pyle L, Kelsey MM, Nadeau KJ, Cree-Green M. Racial and ethnic differences in metabolic disease in adolescents with obesity and polycystic ovary syndrome. *J Endocr Soc.* 2021;5(4):bvab008. PMID: 33644620

26. Cooney LG, Dokras A. Depression and anxiety in polycystic ovary syndrome: etiology and treatment. *Curr Psychiatry Rep.* 2017;19(11):83. PMID: 28929349

27. Cooney LG, Lee I, Sammel MD, Dokras A. High prevalence of moderate and severe depressive and anxiety symptoms in polycystic ovary syndrome: a systematic review and meta-analysis. *Hum Reprod.* 2017;32(5):1075-1091. PMID: 28333286

28. Benson J, Severn C, Hudnut-Beumler J, et al. Depression in girls with obesity and polycystic ovary syndrome and/or type 2 diabetes. *Can J Diabetes.* 2020;44(6):507-513. PMID: 32792104

29. Wang F, Xie N, Wu Y, et al. Association between circadian rhythm disruption and polycystic ovary syndrome. *Fertil Steril.* 2021;115(3):771-781. PMID: 33358334

30. Garg A, Neuren E, Strunk A. Hidradenitis suppurativa is associated with polycystic ovary syndrome: a population-based analysis in the United States. *J Invest Dermatol.* 2018;138(6):1288-1292. PMID: 29378201

31. Pena AS, Witchel SF, Hoeger KM, et al. Adolescent polycystic ovary syndrome according to the international evidence-based guideline. *BMC Med.* 2020;18(1):72. PMID: 32204714

32. Gibson-Helm M, Teede H, Dunaif A, Dokras A. Delayed diagnosis and a lack of information associated with dissatisfaction in women with polycystic ovary syndrome. *J Clin Endocrinol Metab.* 2017;102(2):604-612. PMID: 27906550

33. Yildiz BO, Bolour S, Woods K, Moore A, Azziz R. Visually scoring hirsutism. *Hum Reprod Update.* 2010;16(1):51-64. PMID: 19567450

34. Ludwig E. Classification of the types of androgenetic alopecia (common baldness) occurring in the female sex. *Br J Dermatol.* 1977;97(3):247-254. PMID: 921894

35. Williams S, Sheffield D, Knibb RC. The polycystic ovary syndrome quality of life scale (PCOSQOL): development and preliminary validation. *Health Psychol Open.* 2018;5(2):2055102918788195. PMID: 30038788

36. Cree-Green M. Worldwide dissatisfaction with the diagnostic process and initial treatment of PCOS. *J Clin Endocrinol Metab.* 2017;102(2):375-378. PMID: 28359108

37. Lee R, Joy Mathew C, Jose MT, Elshaikh AO, Shah L, Cancarevic I. A review of the impact of bariatric surgery in women with polycystic ovary syndrome. *Cureus.* 2020;12(10):e10811. PMID: 33042653

38. Frossing S, Nylander M, Chabanova E, et al. Effect of liraglutide on ectopic fat in polycystic ovary syndrome: a randomized clinical trial. *Diabetes Obes Metab.* 2018;20(1):215-218. PMID: 28681988

39. Jensterle M, Goricar K, Janez A. Metformin as an initial adjunct to low-dose liraglutide enhances the weight-decreasing potential of liraglutide in obese polycystic ovary syndrome: randomized control study. *Exp Ther Med.* 2016;11(4):1194-1200. PMID: 27073422

40. Jensterle M, Kravos NA, Goricar K, Janez A. Short-term effectiveness of low dose liraglutide in combination with metformin versus high dose liraglutide alone in treatment of obese PCOS: randomized trial. *BMC Endocr Disord.* 2017;17(1):5. PMID: 28143456

41. Nylander M, Frossing S, Clausen HV, Kistorp C, Faber J, Skouby SO. Effects of liraglutide on ovarian dysfunction in polycystic ovary syndrome: a randomized clinical trial. *Reprod Biomed Online.* 2017;35(1):121-127. PMID: 28479118

42. Buyers E, Sass AE, Severn CD, Pyle L, Cree-Green M. Twelve-month continuation of the etonogestrel implant in adolescents with polycystic ovary syndrome. *J Pediatr Adolesc Gynecol.* 2021;34(1):33-39. PMID: 32919086

43. Kumarendran B, O'Reilly MW, Manolopoulos KN, et al. Polycystic ovary syndrome, androgen excess, and the risk of nonalcoholic fatty liver disease in women: a longitudinal study based on a United Kingdom primary care database. *PLoS Med.* 2018;15(3):e1002542. PMID: 29590099

44. Legro RS, Dodson WC, Kris-Etherton PM, et al. Randomized controlled trial of preconception interventions in infertile women with polycystic ovary syndrome. *J Clin Endocrinol Metab.* 2015;100(11):4048-4058. PMID: 26401593

Beginner's Guide to Gender-Affirming Hormone Therapy for Transgender and Gender-Diverse Adults

Caroline J. Davidge-Pitts, MB, BCh. Division of Endocrinology, Diabetes, Metabolism, and Nutrition, Mayo Clinic, Rochester, MN; E-mail: davidge-pitts.caroline@mayo.edu

Sean J. Iwamoto, MD. Division of Endocrinology, Metabolism, and Diabetes, Department of Medicine, University of Colorado School of Medicine, Anschutz Medical Campus; Endocrinology Service, Medicine Service, Rocky Mountain Regional Veterans Affairs Medical Center; and UCHealth Integrated Transgender Program, Aurora, CO; E-mail: sean.iwamoto@cuanschutz.edu

Learning Objectives

As a result of participating in this session, learners should be able to:

- Recognize that gender-affirming hormone therapy (GAHT) can be provided to transgender and gender-diverse (TGD) patients in safe and effective ways.

- Describe GAHT regimens and monitoring recommendations.

- Interpret laboratory test results of patients taking GAHT.

- Review screening recommendations and special considerations in older TGD individuals.

Main Conclusions

TGD patients continue to face challenges related to health care access and health disparities. There is growing interest among clinicians to provide safe and effective gender-affirming care (including GAHT) and among researchers to investigate ways to mitigate and prevent potential GAHT-related risks. Feminizing GAHT typically relies on exogenous estrogen and antiandrogen therapies, while the mainstay of masculinizing GAHT is exogenous testosterone. Feminization or masculinization with these regimens improves mental health and quality of life for TGD individuals. Endocrine Society guidelines recommend evaluating patients every 3 months during the first year and then 1 to 2 times per year to measure hormone levels and monitor for appropriate signs of physical changes or adverse effects.[1] More data are being published on how GAHT affects laboratory values in TGD patients, with most analyte concentrations moving into physiologic reference ranges that align with patients' gender identity (eg, feminizing GAHT is associated with decreases in serum creatinine and hematocrit). It is also recommended to screen for conditions in TGD patients if organs or tissues are present for which screening guidelines exist for cisgender adults. More research is needed to inform future guidelines on TGD-specific screening, especially related to cardiovascular disease risk.

Significance of the Clinical Problem

TGD individuals have gender identities that differ from their sex recorded at birth. This gender incongruence can lead to clinically significant distress or impaired ability to function in social, occupational, or other important areas.[2] Insurance coverage for TGD-related services has improved over recent years, with subsequent increased demand for providers with competence in TGD health care; however, barriers to obtaining gender-affirming care remain.[3] The health care profession continues to face challenges in providing optimal care for the TGD population, and there is a significant paucity of TGD-related education in medical school and postgraduate training programs.[4] Considering the central role of endocrinologists in medical management of gender dysphoria/incongruence, particularly with GAHT, it is essential that endocrinologists receive the necessary education to optimize gender-affirming care for TGD patients.

Barriers to Optimal Practice

TGD individuals can be marginalized by negative social stigma, internalized transphobia, and prejudices, and they face multiple obstacles in seeking and maintaining health care compared with the general population.[5,6] Epidemiologic studies have repeatedly shown high rates of adverse health outcomes in the setting of minority stress.

Although, in general, access to care has greatly improved in the last decade due to increased social awareness and improved insurance coverage, several barriers to receiving optimal care remain for TGD individuals. Access to gender-affirming providers continues to be limited. This is in part due to limited education in TGD health. Many specialties, including endocrinology, report lack of training in this area,[7] thereby leading to a downstream lack of confidence and competence in providing care to TGD patients. Despite improvements in insurance coverage overall, there continues to be inequity among insurance plans on what services are covered.[8]

Although the COVID-19 pandemic has led to significant strains on the health care system, access to telemedicine has allowed marginalized communities, particularly in rural areas, to obtain care. However, it is important to also recognize that telehealth visits could exacerbate voice dysphoria and appearance anxiety for TGD patients. Many patients might have concerns about safety and privacy, and internet access might not always be reliable.[9] Nonetheless, for TGD patients with a preference for telemedicine, virtual health can be an important tool to close some of the gaps in gender-affirming care access.

Strategies for Diagnosis, Therapy, and/or Management

The goal of GAHT is to induce physical changes that align with an individual's gender identity, thereby alleviating the distress associated with gender dysphoria/gender incongruence. Several organizations (eg, Endocrine Society,[1] World Professional Association for Transgender Health,[10] and the University of California, San Francisco[11]) provide guidelines to aid clinicians who care for TGD individuals. Studies have demonstrated that gender-affirming medical and surgical interventions help to alleviate gender dysphoria and improve well-being.[12,13] The Table includes terminology often used in this space.

Criteria for Initiating GAHT in Adults

Per the most recent Endocrine Society (2017) and World Professional Association for Transgender Health (version 7) guidelines, the criteria for initiating GAHT in adults include: (1) persistent, well-documented gender dysphoria/gender incongruence, (2) the capacity to make a fully informed decision and to consent to treatment, (3) the age of majority in a given country, and (4) mental health concerns, if present, must be reasonably well-controlled.

Table. Selected Terminology in the Care of TGD Individuals

Term	Definition
Terms representing independent aspects of one's identity (ie, not the same things)	
Gender identity	The innate and internal sense of gender that is not visible to other people
Sex recorded at birth	Also hear "sex assigned at birth," "assigned female at birth," "assigned male at birth"
Gender expression	The external manifestations of a person's gender; may or may not conform to the socially defined behaviors and external characteristics that are historically referred to as masculine or feminine (eg, clothing, haircut, jewelry, social interactions, speech patterns)
Sexual orientation	Term that characterizes pattern of romantic or sexual attraction to other people, independent of gender identity
Terms used when discussing gender identity	
Gender incongruence	When a person's gender identity or gender expression differs from that person's sex recorded at birth or what is typically associated with the designated sex recorded at birth; not everyone with gender incongruence has gender dysphoria or seeks treatment
Gender dysphoria	The distress and unease associated with gender incongruence; the phrase "gender identity disorder" is no longer used, particularly after the 2013 American Psychiatric Association's DSM-5 replaced it with "gender dysphoria"
Transgender	An adjective that encompasses people whose gender identity or gender expression differs from their sex recorded at birth; independent of the decision whether to use GAHT or undergo gender-affirming surgery, and inclusive of gender nonbinary people; the terms "transgendered" and "transgenders" should not be used
	Examples:
	A person who was assigned female at birth but whose gender identity or gender expression is (more) male/masculine may identify as a transgender man, transgender male, transmasculine, or something else
	A person who was assigned male at birth but whose gender identity or gender expression is (more) female/feminine may identify as a transgender woman, a transgender female, transfeminine, or something else
Gender nonbinary	May represent people who identify and present themselves as both or alternatively male and female, as neither male nor female, or with a gender identity outside the male/female binary; may include genderqueer, gender-fluid, pan-gender, polygender
Cisgender	An adjective for people whose gender identity and gender expression align with their sex recorded at birth (ie, not transgender)

Adapted from Iwamoto SJ et al. *Ther Adv Endocrinol Metab*, 2019;10 © SAGE Publications.

We acknowledge that most current GAHT guidelines are binary in their recommendations for hormone dosages, meaning that hormone dosages and goal hormone levels are extrapolated from physiologic cisgender female and male reference ranges. The University of California San Francisco provides useful "initial-low" dosing recommendations for patients who may desire lower dosages of GAHT or slower titration (eg, some gender nonbinary patients) or need less GAHT due to medical history. For our growing number of nonbinary and gender-diverse patients who identify outside the transgender female-male binary, it is equally as important to guide GAHT initiation and management with their goals and expectations in mind, but also acknowledge the need for more outcomes research related to these alternative dosages or regimens to guide evidence-based GAHT recommendations. For this GAHT chapter, we will focus on current binary GAHT recommendations.

Feminizing Gender-Affirming Hormone Therapy

Endocrine Society guidelines, most recently updated in 2017,[1] recommend evaluation of medical conditions that could be exacerbated by feminizing GAHT (fGAHT). Baseline laboratory workup, which can vary depending on patient risk profile and age, could assess metabolic status, complete blood cell count, liver enzymes, electrolytes, and sex steroid hormones (if relevant). We also recommend assessment of immunization status, evaluation for substance use, and testing for HIV and other sexually transmitted infections. All patients initiating fGAHT should be informed about fertility effects and counseled regarding options for fertility preservation prior to initiation.

The approach to fGAHT depends on several factors including patient preference, differences in the regional availability of medications, and cost considerations. fGAHT aims to lower and/or block testosterone along with estrogen to inhibit testosterone secretion and provide feminizing physical changes.

Estrogen lowers testosterone secretion from the gonads by inhibiting the hypothalamic-pituitary-gonadal (HPG) axis. 17β-Estradiol is recommended over other estrogen preparations such as ethinyl estradiol and conjugated equine estrogens due to a more favorable risk profile.[1] In addition, 17β-estradiol can be measured and monitored with commercial estradiol assays. Transdermal and parenteral preparations are potentially less thrombogenic by avoiding the first-pass effect, as opposed to oral estrogens.[1,15]

Antiandrogens block androgen action and can have an inhibitory effect on testosterone secretion. Spironolactone is a mineralocorticoid receptor antagonist that blocks the androgen receptor at higher dosages. Spironolactone also inhibits the secretion of testosterone from the gonads, possibly due to progestin and estrogenlike effects. It is generally safe and well-tolerated, although it can induce hyperkalemia, hypotension, and increased urination. Cyproterone acetate is a progestin with androgen-blocking properties. Adverse effects include hepatotoxicity, mood disturbances, and multifocal meningiomas. Although cyproterone acetate is widely used in Europe, it is not available in the United States. 5α-Reductase inhibitors (eg, finasteride) block conversion of testosterone to dihydrotestosterone, potentially increasing the testosterone level. 5α-Reductase inhibitors have been associated with adverse mood alterations and are therefore not recommended as first-line agents. Nonsteroidal androgen receptor antagonists (eg, bicalutamide) do not reduce

testosterone levels and are not recommended as first-line therapy because of potentially serious hepatotoxic effects.

Gonadotropin-releasing hormone (GnRH) analogues reduce the secretion of gonadotropins, which in turn decreases stimulation of gonadal testosterone production. GnRH analogues can be considered in TGD individuals who cannot tolerate other antiandrogens, in situations where adequate testosterone suppression cannot be achieved with standard antiandrogen therapy, or in patients who require a lower estrogen dosage (eg, older patients and those at risk of venous thromboembolism or vascular disease).[16] In practice, the use of GnRH analogues is limited in many countries because of cost.

The role of progestins in fGAHT remains unclear, although they are often requested to enhance breast development and improve mood.[17] Currently, progestins are not recommended by Endocrine Society guidelines as part of standard fGAHT but can be considered as part of an individualized approach.

On initiation of fGAHT, sex steroid hormones should be maintained in the physiologic range for cisgender women: estradiol, 100-200 pg/mL (367-734 pmol/L) and testosterone, <50 ng/dL (<1.7 nmol/L). Although precise onset and timing of feminizing physical changes in response to medical interventions are not well-defined, most physical changes begin within a few months and continue to progress over 2 to 3 years.

fGAHT is generally considered safe when prescribed and monitored by an experienced medical provider. Nevertheless, it is important to acknowledge risks, so that precipitating factors can be addressed. In a recent large electronic medical record–based study of transgender women in the United States who were mostly on oral estradiol, the incidence rate for venous thromboembolism was higher than both cisgender male and cisgender female control groups, and the difference was more pronounced with increased follow-up over time.[18] Evidence on the risks of fGAHT in transgender women older than 50 years is lacking. Outcomes data are limited by hormone regimens, type, and route, and cardiovascular risk profiles and are difficult to match. The goal of fGAHT in aging transgender women is to promote feminizing hormone effects and limit venous thrombosis, cardiovascular, and breast cancer risks. It is important to discuss potentially tapering the estradiol dosage and/or switching from oral to transdermal/injectable estradiol to minimize risks. However, estradiol dosages that are decreased too much could risk increased masculinization in individuals without gonadectomy. There continues to be a paucity of data with respect to cardiovascular risk in older transgender women. However, a recent Dutch mortality study revealed more observed deaths due to cardiovascular disease compared with the number of deaths of the same cause in the general population over 5 decades.[19] Risk of ischemic stroke is also higher with use of oral estrogens as opposed to transdermal preparations. In a systematic review, 8 cases of stroke were reported in a pooled population of 859 individuals on estrogen therapy.[20] The recent transfeminine cohort study showed that the incidence rate of ischemic stroke was 4.8 per 1000 person-years as opposed to 1.2 in reference men and 1.9 in reference women, with a particular increase in incidence after 6 years of treatment.[18] While it is important to consider cardiovascular risk and risk factors in fGAHT management due to increases in relative risk in some studies, absolute risks remain low. These potential long-term risks due to fGAHT must be balanced (and better studied) with the well-documented short-term mental health risks related to withholding fGAHT.

Masculinizing Gender-Affirming Hormone Therapy

Unlike fGAHT, masculinizing GAHT (mGAHT) typically relies on administering a single hormone, testosterone, to initiate and maintain masculinization. Testosterone alone is usually enough to suppress the HPG axis and, therefore, endogenous estradiol production. Patient preferences, regional availability of medications, and cost should also be considered when selecting route of testosterone administration.

Testosterone is available in parenteral and transdermal formulations. Testosterone esters (cypionate or enanthate) drawn from a vial into a syringe can be administered weekly or every other week, subcutaneously or intramuscularly, with both routes producing similar testosterone levels. Subcutaneous injections are preferred by many patients.[21] A new autoinjector with testosterone enanthate provides subcutaneous testosterone; however, it is only available in 3 doses and insurance coverage can be limited. Testosterone undecanoate is much longer-acting, requiring an injection every 3 months (in the clinic setting, with rare risks of pulmonary oil microembolism and anaphylaxis). It is more common outside the United States, but it is available through a Risk Evaluation and Mitigation Strategy program. Transdermal testosterone comes in the form of gels (of varying percentages depending on preparation) and patches. Gels and patches are applied to clean and dry skin daily. Currently, Endocrine Society guidelines and others acknowledge the lack of data on the safety and efficacy of masculinization with other routes of testosterone administration, including buccal, implants/pellets, compounded preparations, and the recently FDA-approved oral testosterone.

Parenteral or transdermal testosterone can be used to achieve total testosterone levels within the physiologic range for cisgender men. Target concentrations of total testosterone are 400 to 700 ng/dL (13.9-24.3 nmol/L), with caveats based on route and timing of administration. Testosterone ester injections (cypionate or enanthate) can result in peak (1 to 2 days after injecting) and trough (1 to 2 days prior to next injection) levels, depending on the timing of the laboratory test and the most recent injection. If drawn midway between injections, the above target range can be the goal. If patients are unable to have a mid-dose blood draw, measuring a peak or trough level to ensure the serum total testosterone concentration remains within the laboratory's reference range for cisgender men may be more appropriate. Testosterone undecanoate can result in steady testosterone levels over several months, with levels drawn just prior to the next injection. Transdermal preparations also provide stable levels of serum testosterone over time. The testosterone concentration can be measured after 1 week of daily application, at least 2 hours after that day's application. We do not currently have recommendations for the goal concentration for free testosterone while on mGAHT; however, accurate assays to measure free testosterone remain unavailable for most.

mGAHT is also considered safe when prescribed and monitored by a gender-affirming clinician. After starting testosterone, masculinizing physical changes typically begin within a few months and continue to progress for 1 to 2 years but may take up to 5 years. During discussions about effects, we mention that some mGAHT-related physical effects may be permanent if testosterone is discontinued, including facial hair, androgenic alopecia, deeper voice, and clitoromegaly.

In most TGD patients, testosterone use results in menstrual suppression within the first year, more often with parenteral testosterone than with transdermal testosterone.[22] When bleeding persists and other medications are desired (ie, not surgery), norethindrone acetate and other progestins (eg, oral, parenteral, intrauterine device) or a GnRH analogue (if available and affordable) can be prescribed.

An increase in hematocrit leading to erythrocytosis (hematocrit >50%) is well-documented in TGD persons taking mGAHT.[23,24] If testosterone levels are elevated above goal, the testosterone dosage can be decreased in this setting. Other causes of secondary erythrocytosis should also be evaluated, including tobacco smoking and obstructive sleep apnea. The concerns about secondary erythrocytosis increasing the risk for cardiovascular disease in this population have not borne out in recent studies. In the previous systematic review, venous thromboembolism was reported in 1 of 771

individuals, while there were 0 cases of stroke in 340 participants. The recent transmasculine cohort study showed no significant increase in incidence of venous thromboembolism, ischemic stroke, or myocardial infarction compared with rates in either cisgender men or women.[18] However, a Dutch cohort recently documented a higher rate of myocardial infarction among transgender men than in reference cisgender women but not in reference cisgender men.[25] More research is needed regarding long-term cardiovascular disease risk in patients taking mGAHT, with particular focus on duration of mGAHT and age at initiation.

Clinical Case Vignettes
Case 1

A 19-year-old transgender woman is referred for initiation of fGAHT. The patient's sex recorded at birth was male, but she experienced a persistent desire to be female since age 7 years. She has followed with her local therapist since age 16 years who confirms persistent gender dysphoria/incongruence. She has a history of depression, which is stable. There are no other medical concerns, and she does not smoke cigarettes. Physical examination findings are unremarkable.

You initiate fGAHT with estradiol and spironolactone.

Which of the following laboratory changes is expected with this medical therapy?

A. Decrease in HDL cholesterol

B. Decrease in hemoglobin and hematocrit

C. Decrease in potassium

D. Increase in serum creatinine

Answer: B) Decrease in hemoglobin and hematocrit

It is important for clinicians to understand how GAHT will affect laboratory testing, although this is an evolving area in transgender health.

With the decrease in endogenous testosterone levels, hemoglobin and hematocrit are expected to decrease into the female range due to reduced erythropoiesis (thus, Answer B is correct).[23]

Regarding the renal system, androgen deprivation is one factor that reduces creatinine (thus, Answer D is incorrect). There is also likely a direct effect of the estradiol on the kidney.[26]

With respect to lipid panel changes, estradiol can have a neutral effect on HDL cholesterol, or increase its value (thus, Answer A is incorrect).[20]

Considering this patient is taking spironolactone, one would not expect a decrease in potassium, as this is a potassium-sparing diuretic (thus, Answer C is incorrect).

Case 2

A 60-year-old transgender woman presents for her annual visit. She has been on fGAHT for 6 years. She has not undergone gender-affirming surgeries. She has no acute concerns. Her only medication is lisinopril for hypertension. Family history is pertinent for prostate cancer in her father. Blood pressure is normal at the visit.

Which of the following general screenings should be recommended?

A. Mammography

B. Bone density assessment

C. Prostate-specific antigen measurement

D. A and C

E. No screening advised

Answer: D) A and C

Preventive care for patients on GAHT includes standard recommendations for sex recorded at birth and age, with few TGD-specific screening recommendations from the Endocrine Society and other organizations.[27] Advising no screening for this patient (Answer E) is incorrect.

Baseline bone mineral density testing is indicated for TGD patients who have any of the following[28]:

- History of gonadectomy or therapy that lowers endogenous gonadal steroid levels before initiation of hormone therapy

- Hypogonadism with no plan to take hormone therapy

- Presence of risk factors for bone loss and/or fracture (eg, glucocorticoid use, hyperparathyroidism)

- Follow-up bone mineral density testing is indicated when the results are likely to influence treatment decisions. Examples include:

  ○ Baseline low bone density

  ○ Use of GnRH analogues without hormone therapy

  ○ Nonadherence to or inadequate doses of hormone therapy

  ○ Plan to discontinue hormone therapy

  ○ Presence of risk factors for bone loss and/or fracture (eg, glucocorticoid use, hyperparathyroidism)

Bone mineral density testing intervals are based on the clinical scenario—typically every 1 to 2 years until bone mineral density is stable or improved, followed by longer intervals thereafter. Calcium and vitamin D supplementation is also recommended (following age-appropriate recommendations for cisgender women). Bone mineral density screening (Answer B) is not indicated in this patient because she has not undergone gonadectomy, she has been on stable hormone therapy with estradiol, and she has no other risk factors for bone loss.

Clinicians should follow age-appropriate breast cancer screening recommendations after 5 years of estrogen therapy plus monthly self-examination or follow individualized recommendations if the patient has a family history of breast or ovarian cancer. Clinicians should also follow age-appropriate prostate cancer screening recommendations for cisgender men. Expect prostate-specific antigen levels to decrease by approximately 50% (even in the presence of prostate cancer). Normal laboratory reference ranges may not apply. Thus, the best answer is both mammography (Answer A) and prostate-specific antigen measurement (Answer C).

Case 3

A 49-year-old transgender man presents to endocrine clinic for follow-up after starting testosterone 1 year ago. He is happy with masculinizing effects and is excited about his upcoming gender-affirming chest surgery. He has noticed a 10-lb (4.5-kg) weight gain despite exercising 5 days per week. He has a family history of cardiovascular disease, and he is anxious about his risk. His BMI is 24.5 kg/m², up from 22.8 kg/m² 1 year ago.

Which of the following is also likely to be increased now compared with baseline?

A. Systolic blood pressure

B. LDL cholesterol

C. HDL cholesterol

D. Triglycerides

E. A and B

Answer: E) A and B

Per Endocrine Society guidelines, weight, blood pressure, and lipids should be measured at regular intervals while a patient is on mGAHT. Testosterone can lead to weight gain, thought to be associated with increases in muscle/lean mass and abdominal fat.[29] However, some patients may lose weight, which can be due to increased physical activity, self-esteem, and energy associated with taking mGAHT.

Testosterone is also associated with consistent increases in systolic blood pressure (Answer A) and less consistent increases in diastolic blood pressure.[30]

At 1 year, LDL cholesterol is increased from baseline (Answer B), and HDL cholesterol is decreased (not increased [Answer C]). Changes in total cholesterol and triglycerides are less consistent (thus, Answer D is incorrect).[20]

Cardiovascular disease risk in TGD adults is an important area in need of more research. We lack data on how to best calculate cardiovascular disease risk in this population. Factors include age at initiation of GAHT and length of GAHT exposure. As such, clinicians may choose to calculate risk based on sex recorded at birth, affirmed gender, or average the two.[27]

References

1. Hembree WC, Cohen-Kettenis PT, Gooren L, et al. Endocrine treatment of gender-dysphoric/gender-incongruent persons: an Endocrine Society clinical practice guideline. *J Clin Endocrinol Metab.* 2017;102(11):3869-3903. PMID: 28945902

2. Valentine SE, Shipherd JC. A systematic review of social stress and mental health among transgender and gender non-conforming people in the United States. *Clin Psychol Rev.* 2018;66:24-38. PMID: 29627104

3. Warner DM 2nd, Mehta AH. Identifying and addressing barriers to transgender healthcare: where we are and what we need to do about it. *J Gen Intern Med.* 2021;36(11):3559-3561. PMID: 34254221

4. Fraser L, Knudson G. Education needs of providers of transgender population. *Endocrinol Metab Clin North Am.* 2019;48(2):465-477. PMID: 31027553

5. Feldman JL, Luhur WE, Herman JL, Poteat T, Meyer IH. Health and health care access in the US transgender population health (TransPop) survey. *Andrology.* 2021;9(6):1707-1718. PMID: 34080788

6. Pellicane MJ, Ciesla JA. Associations between minority stress, depression, and suicidal ideation and attempts in transgender and gender diverse (TGD) individuals: systematic review and meta-analysis. *Clin Psychol Rev.* 2022;91:102113. PMID: 34973649

7. Davidge-Pitts C, Nippoldt TB, Danoff A, Radziejewski L, Natt N. Transgender health in endocrinology: current status of endocrinology fellowship programs and practicing clinicians. *J Clin Endocrinol Metab.* 2017;102(4):1286-1290. PMID: 28324050

8. Bakko M, Kattari SK. Transgender-related insurance denials as barriers to transgender healthcare: differences in experience by insurance type. *J Gen Intern Med.* 2020;35(6):1693-1700. PMID: 32128693

9. Pankey TL, Heredia D Jr, Vencill JA, Gonzalez CA. Gender-affirming telepsychology during and after the COVID-19 pandemic: recommendations for adult transgender and gender diverse populations. *J Health Serv Psychol.* 2021;47(4):181-189. PMID: 34693297.

10. Coleman E, Bockting W, Botzer M, Cohen-Kettenis PT, De Cuypere G, Feldman J, Fraser L, Green J, Knudson G, Meyer W, Monstrey S. Standards of care for the health of transsexual, transgender, and gender-nonconforming people, version 7. *Int J Transgenderism.* 2012;13:165-232.

11. UCSF Transgender Care, Department of Family and Community Medicine, University of California San Francisco. Guidelines for the primary and gender-affirming care of transgender and gender nonbinary people. 2nd ed. Deutsch MB, ed. June 2016. Available at transcare.ucsf.edu/guidelines. Access May 2022.

12. Nguyen HB, Chavez AM, Lipner E, et al. Gender-affirming hormone use in transgender individuals: impact on behavioral health and cognition. *Curr Psychiatry Rep.* 2018;20(12):110. PMID: 30306351

13. Wernick JA, Busa S, Matouk K, Nicholson J, Janssen A. A systematic review of the psychological benefits of gender-affirming surgery. *Urol Clin North Am.* 2019;46(4):475-486. PMID: 31582022

14. Iwamoto SJ, Defreyne J, Rothman MS, et al. Health considerations for transgender women and remaining unknowns: a narrative review. *Ther Adv Endocrinol Metab.* 2019;10:2042018819871166. PMID: 31516689

15. Zucker R, Reisman T, Safer JD. Minimizing venous thromboembolism in feminizing hormone therapy: applying lessons from cisgender women and previous data. *Endocr Pract.* 2021;27(6):621-625. PMID: 33819637

16. Maheshwari A, Nippoldt T, Davidge-Pitts C. An approach to nonsuppressed testosterone in transgender women receiving gender-affirming feminizing hormonal therapy. *J Endocr Soc.* 2021;5(9):bvab068. PMID: 34278180

17. Iwamoto SJ, T'Sjoen G, Safer JD, et al. Letter to the editor: "Progesterone is important for transgender women's therapy-applying evidence for the benefits of progesterone in ciswomen". *J Clin Endocrinol Metab.* 2019;104(8):3127-3128. PMID: 30860591

18. Getahun D, Nash R, Flanders WD, et al. Cross-sex hormones and acute cardiovascular events in transgender persons: a cohort study. *Ann Intern Med.* 2018;169(4):205-213. PMID: 29987313

19. de Blok CJ, Wiepjes CM, van Velzen DM, et al. Mortality trends over five decades in adult transgender people receiving hormone treatment: a report from the Amsterdam cohort of gender dysphoria. *Lancet Diabetes Endocrinol.* 2021;9(10):663-670. PMID: 34481559

20. Maraka S, Singh Ospina N, Rodriguez-Gutierrez R, et al. Sex steroids and cardiovascular outcomes in transgender individuals: a systematic review and meta-analysis. *J Clin Endocrinol Metab.* 2017;102(11):3914-3923. PMID: 28945852

21. Figueiredo MG, Gagliano-Juca T, Basaria S. Testosterone therapy with subcutaneous injections: a safe, practical, and reasonable option. *J Clin Endocrinol Metab.* 2022;107(3)614-626. PMID: 34698352

22. Defreyne J, Vanwonterghem Y, Collet S, et al. Vaginal bleeding and spotting in transgender men after initiation of testosterone therapy: a prospective cohort study (ENIGI). *Int J Transgend Health.* 2020;21(2):163-175. PMID: 32935087

23. Madsen MC, van Dijk D, Wiepjes CM, Conemans EB, Thijs A, den Heijer M. Erythrocytosis in a large cohort of trans men using testosterone: a long-term follow-up study on prevalence, determinants, and exposure years. *J Clin Endocrinol Metab.* 2021;106(6):1710-1717. PMID: 33599731

24. Oakes M, Arastu A, Kato C, et al. Erythrocytosis and thromboembolic events in transgender individuals receiving gender-affirming testosterone. *Thromb Res.* 2021;207:96-98. PMID: 34592628

25. Nota NM, Wiepjes CM, de Blok CJM, Gooren LJG, Kreukels BPC, den Heijer M. Occurrence of acute cardiovascular events in transgender individuals receiving hormone therapy. *Circulation.* 2019;139(11):1461-1462. PMID: 30776252

26. Maheshwari A, Dines V, Saul D, Nippoldt T, Kattah A, Davidge-Pitts C. The effect of gender-affirming hormone therapy on serum creatinine in transgender individuals. *Endocr Pract.* 2022;28(1):52-57. PMID: 34474185

27. Iwamoto SJ, Grimstad F, Irwig MS, Rothman MS. Routine screening for transgender and gender diverse adults taking gender-affirming hormone therapy: a narrative review. *J Gen Intern Med.* 2021;36(5):1380-1389. PMID: 33547576

28. Rosen HN, Hamnvik O-PR, Jaisamrarn U, et al. Bone densitometry in transgender and gender non-conforming (TGNC) individuals: 2019 ISCD official position. *J Clin Densitom.* 2019;22(4):544-553. PMID: 31327665

29. Irwig MS. Testosterone therapy for transgender men. *Lancet Diabetes Endocrinol.* 2017;5(4):301-311. PMID: 27084565

30. Irwig MS. Cardiovascular health in transgender people. *Rev Endocr Metab Disord.* 2018;19(3):243-251. PMID: 30073551

Diagnosis and Treatment of Male Hypogonadism

Channa N. Jayasena, PhD. Department of Endocrinology, Imperial College London, Hammersmith Hospital, London, United Kingdom; E-mail: c.jayasena@imperial.ac.uk

Learning Objectives

As a result of participating in this session, learners should be able to:

- Confidently diagnose hypogonadism.
- Guide the approach to treatment of hypogonadism, including judgment of risk-benefit of testosterone therapy.

Main Conclusions

Primary hypogonadism is a straightforward diagnosis identified by elevated serum gonadotropin and low serum testosterone concentrations. Furthermore, men with serum morning fasted total testosterone concentrations less than 230 ng/dL (<8 nmol/L) are likely to be hypogonadal. When testosterone levels are borderline (230-350 ng/dL [8-12 nmol/L]), it is important to consider the strength of clinical features together with other biological markers, including hematocrit. Calculated free testosterone may be considered when SHBG levels are abnormal, but its utility is entirely dependent on total testosterone and SHBG assay performance. Testosterone treatment is commonly administered using transdermal gels, long-acting testosterone injections, and short-acting testosterone injections, but other methods are available. Patient needs and preferences should be taken into account when selecting the appropriate treatment regimen for hypogonadism. "Peak and trough" symptoms and erythrocytosis may be problematic when using testosterone injections, in which case changing to transdermal gels may be preferable. Testosterone does not cause prostate cancer, but it might unmask an incidental prostate tumor. The Endocrine Society recommends prostate surveillance using digital rectal examination and serum PSA measurement in men older than 40 years. Testosterone may increase thrombosis risk, but the absolute risk is very small. There is uncertainty about the cardiovascular safety of testosterone, and this should be discussed with hypogonadal men who have established cardiac disease.

Significance of the Clinical Problem

Hypogonadism is a common endocrine condition that is becoming more challenging to manage. An increasing proportion of evaluated men have manifestations of "functional" hypogonadism such as aging and comorbidities including obesity. Furthermore, there is no binary biochemical threshold of testosterone that can reliably distinguish hypogonadal from eugonadal men. Unless biochemical features are compelling, they need to be framed within the likely etiology and clinical context to make a secure diagnosis.

This session will provide a pragmatic, evidence-based discussion to optimize the diagnosis and management of hypogonadism. Focus will be given to borderline cases that are most challenging in real-world clinical practice.

Barriers to Optimal Practice

- Diagnosis requires interpretation of biochemistry within the clinical context; inconsistency between assays and "cut-points" creates variation among clinicians in defining which patients have male hypogonadism.

- Some nonhypogonadal men display testosterone-seeking behavior due to the perception that testosterone treatment may improve many nonspecific symptoms.

- Concerns remain over the cardiovascular safety of testosterone treatment, particularly in older men with hypogonadism, which may modify prescribing habits.

Strategies for Diagnosis, Therapy, and/or Management

Diagnosis

The diagnosis of male hypogonadism requires both convincing clinical features and indicative biochemistry.[1]

History

Look for specific clinical features of male hypogonadism, which may be sexual (reduced libido/sexual activity, erectile dysfunction, and reduced spontaneous erections), developmental (delayed puberty, cryptorchidism, known Klinefelter syndrome), or hematological (anemia); drugs (androgenic steroids, strong opioids); bone fractures or osteoporosis; vasomotor flushes; prior cancer treatment; and anemia.[1,2] However, the following clinical features are nonspecific, not helpful diagnostically, and are less likely to improve with testosterone treatment: disturbances of mood or sleep and reduced concentration (sometimes termed "brain fog").

Examination

Check if the voice pitch is postpubertal. Look for male-pattern hair growth, gynecomastia, testicular volume, and evidence of cryptorchidism or orchidopexy (groin scars, affected testis is often reduced in size).[1,2]

Laboratory Investigations

Obvious biochemical features of hypogonadism include the following: serum LH >10.0 mIU/mL (>10.0 IU/L) (ie, primary hypogonadism); serum LH far below the reference range (ie, hypogonadotropic hypogonadism); serum morning fasted total testosterone <230 ng/dL (<8 nmol/L) (requires 2 measurements).[3]

Serum Morning Fasted Total Testosterone Concentration 230-350 ng/dL (8-12 nmol/L)
Patients with values in this range may be normal or hypogonadal, so consideration of other evidence is important. In the United States, 300 ng/dL (10.4 nmol/L) is commonly quoted as a "threshold" for diagnosing hypogonadism.[1] However, assays and hormonal levels may result in variation. The 2.5th and 97.5th percentiles for serum total testosterone were reported as 265 ng/dL (9.2 nmol/L) and 916 ng/dL (31.8 nmol/L), respectively, in more than 9000 healthy nonobese young men from Europe and North America using the Centers for Disease Control and Prevention reference method.[4,5] Furthermore, the European Male Ageing Study observed that in approximately 3400 men aged 40 to 79 years, the odds of experiencing sexual symptoms increased with either a total testosterone concentration less than 230 ng/dL (<8 nmol/L) (regardless of calculated free testosterone) or total testosterone concentration less than 317 ng/dL (<11 nmol/L) (with calculated free testosterone <6.3 ng/dL [<220 pmol/L]).[6] When serum testosterone results are borderline, the strength of clinical features together with diagnostic features such as anemia and low bone mineral density can help decide on the diagnosis if results are equivocal.

Testosterone Concentration >350 ng/dL (>12 nmol/L)
There is very little published evidence from interventional trials that testosterone treatment improves symptoms better than placebo in men with hypogonadism and a testosterone concentration greater than 345 ng/dL (>12 nmol/L).[2]

Role of Free Testosterone in Diagnosis

Free testosterone estimation may add value if total testosterone levels are borderline *and* SHBG levels are abnormally high or low. Someone with a serum testosterone concentration of 300 ng/dL (10.4 nmol/L) and SHBG concentration of 1.12 µg/mL (10 nmol/L) will have a higher free testosterone than if the SHBG concentration is 11.24 µg/mL (100 nmol/L). Free testosterone is difficult to measure reliably within laboratories (using equilibrium dialysis), and results may be inaccurate.[1] Calculated free testosterone using the Vermeulen formula is a broadly accepted surrogate of free testosterone measurement, which has shown clinical validity in many studies.[7] The original Vermeulen equation was validated using assays for testosterone and SHBG that are no longer available but has recently been revalidated using current state-of-the-art methods.[8] Controversy remains about the level of importance that should be placed on calculated free testosterone in the diagnosis of male hypogonadism.[9] Furthermore, its performance is entirely dependent on assay performance of serum total testosterone and SHBG. Clinicians should liaise closely with clinical biochemistry colleagues in their own clinic to be informed regarding the limitations of current assays. In summary, calculated free testosterone is a second-line test when SHBG is abnormal or when total testosterone is in the borderline range for patients with clinical features suggestive of androgen deficiency.

Testosterone Therapy

Currently available testosterone formulations, dosages, administration, and their benefits and disadvantages are presented in the Table.[2,10,11] The clinician should support the patient to identify a suitable testosterone formulation through a structured needs assessment and by providing the patient with a rationale of benefits and disadvantages of each testosterone formulation.

Monitoring Testosterone Treatment

Treatment Efficacy and Satisfaction

The most important aspect of monitoring is to ensure that the patient tolerates treatment and feels symptom relief from the testosterone therapy chosen. Inadequate symptom control may indicate subtherapeutic levels of testosterone therapy, in which case the dosage could be increased (eg, for a gel) or the dose interval could be shortened (eg, for a long-acting injectable preparation). If symptoms persist despite attainment of testosterone levels above 250 ng/dL (>12 nmol/L), one should reassess whether other comorbidities may be contributing to symptoms. The patient should be asked whether the mode of testosterone administration "works for them." For instance, men with young children are often concerned about cross-contamination risks associated with gels. Conversely, men with pronounced peak and trough symptoms may respond better to either long-acting injections, implants, or daily preparations.

Prostate Safety

Testosterone deprivation causes prostatic atrophy. However, no statistical relationship exists between serum PSA levels and circulating testosterone levels in the eugonadal range (ie, the saturation hypothesis).[12] Furthermore, multiple studies have failed to show that testosterone therapy increases risks of de novo prostate cancer.[13,14] Therefore, patients can be reassured that testosterone therapy does not cause prostate cancer. However, an existing prostate cancer might be hidden by hypogonadism (causing gland and tumor shrinkage), and testosterone therapy might accelerate its growth. Prostate cancer is extremely rare in men younger than 40 years, and no monitoring is recommended for this age group. Endocrine Society guidelines recommend prostate surveillance prior to and during testosterone treatment for men older than 40 years.[1] This includes serum PSA measurement and digital rectal examination. Any abnormality on digital rectal examination, a PSA increase of 1.4 ng/mL (1.4 µg/L) within 12 months, or a serum PSA

Table. Available Testosterone Formulations Used to Treat Male Hypogonadism

Formulation and dosage	Administration and monitoring	Advantages	Disadvantages
Transdermal topical testosterone gels and axillary solution 20 to 80 mg testosterone in transdermal gel once daily 60 to 120 mg of testosterone solution applied in the axillae once daily (not available in the United Kingdom)	Clear alcohol gel available in sachets, tubes, and pumps; applied to dry, clean skin on shoulders, abdomen, upper arms, or thighs (avoid genital area) Monitor total testosterone 2 to 6 hours after gel application and 2 to 3 weeks after treatment initiation or dosage adjustment, aiming for midnormal value	Physiological levels of serum testosterone with no "peak and troughs" between applications; dosage easily adjustable to individual needs; no pain of injections	Skin irritation for some patients; takes time to apply; potential transfer to female partner or child
Long-acting testosterone undecanoate intramuscular injections 750 to 1000 mg in ampoule of oily preparation every 8 to 14 weeks	Injected slowly into the gluteal muscle Second injection (loading dose) may be given at 6 weeks and subsequent doses are typically every 8 to 14 weeks Injection interval is adjusted based on trough total testosterone level, aiming for lower end of normal reference range; monitor trough total testosterone and hematocrit at least annually	Less noticeable "peak and trough" symptoms Convenient due to infrequent administration	Requires large muscle bulk for injection Slow withdrawal of effect if reversal is required Rare pulmonary microembolism presenting with severe coughing during injection Cannot be self-administered
Short-acting testosterone injections 1. Combined testosterone esters, eg, 250 mg/mL intramuscularly every 3 to 4 weeks containing propionate, 30 mg; phenylpropionate, 60 mg; isocaproate, 60 mg; decanoate, 100 mg 2. Testosterone enanthate or cypionate, 150 to 200 mg intramuscularly every 2 weeks or 50 to 100 mg intramuscularly or subcutanenously once weekly	Can be self-administered Injection interval is adjusted based on trough total testosterone level, aiming for lower end of normal reference range; monitor trough total testosterone and hematocrit at least annually	Dose flexibility and convenient administration, relatively inexpensive	Sometimes marked "peak and trough" symptoms due to supraphysiological testosterone levels after injection Erythrocytosis due to higher overall testosterone exposure vs other preparations
Bioadhesive buccal testosterone tablet 30-mg controlled-release tablets applied to the upper gum twice daily	Testosterone is absorbed from the buccal mucosa over 12 hours; monitor testosterone levels 2 to 6 hours after tablet application, aiming for midnormal reference range	Easy and fast to apply Serum testosterone levels remain within physiological range without significant peaks and troughs	Risk of gum-related adverse events May detach when eating shortly after application
Subcutaneous testosterone implants Testosterone pellets, 100 or 200 mg (to a total of 600 to 1200 mg testosterone per dose)	3 to 6 pellets every 4 to 6 months Pellets implanted under local anaesthetic	Convenient—twice or thrice a year application	Painful procedure with risk of infection Risk of spontaneous extrusion of pellets
Oral testosterone undecanoate capsules, 40 mg 1 to 3 capsules (40 to 120 mg) twice or thrice daily with meals	Absorption improved when taken with fatty meal Swallow without chewing	Easy and convenient administration Suitable for patients who cannot tolerate other forms of treatment	Low bioavailability and very high interindividual and intraindividual variability in absorption Testosterone levels are often subtherapeutic

Not all preparations are available within individual countries. The suggested dosing may require an individualized regimen.[2,10,11]

Adapted from Jayasena CN et al. *Clin Endocrinol (Oxf)*, 2022;96(2) © John Wiley & Sons Ltd.

concentration above 4 ng/mL (>4 µg/L) should trigger urological referral. It is therefore important to ask men about new or worsening lower urinary tract symptoms within the first few months of initiating testosterone treatment, particularly if they have other risk factors such as Black ethnicity, strong family history of prostate cancer, or are older than 65 years.

Hematocrit

A recent observational study suggested that testosterone treatment was associated with increased risk of venous thromboembolism.[15] Men should be told that testosterone treatment can increase the risk of thrombosis, but that the absolute risk is low. Annual hematocrit measurement is mandatory to ensure that erythrocytosis is avoided.[1] If hematocrit is elevated above 50% (>0.50), the testosterone dosage could be reduced, the dose interval could be lengthened, or the patient's regimen could be switched to transdermal testosterone treatment, which has a lower risk of erythrocytosis than injectable testosterone.[16] If hematocrit reaches 54% (0.54), testosterone therapy should be stopped until levels drop again, and hematological referral should be considered. One should evaluate for secondary causes of elevated hematocrit.

Cardiovascular Safety

There is controversy about the effects of testosterone treatment on cardiovascular risk. Interventional and observational studies have reported contradictory results regarding cardiovascular event risk, but no interventional studies have been published that have been powered to assess cardiovascular safety.[17,18] The National Institutes of Health testosterone trials reported increases in noncalcified plaque volume and total plaque volume following testosterone treatment vs placebo.[19] The US FDA recommends that men on testosterone treatment be advised of the potential cardiovascular risks,[20] but other regulatory agencies have concluded that there is insufficient evidence to link testosterone treatment to increased cardiovascular risk.[21]

In summary, testosterone treatment has uncertain effects on cardiovascular and cerebrovascular risk. In men with low cardiovascular risk, concerns about cardiovascular safety should not be a factor discouraging the initiation of testosterone treatment. However, men with high cardiovascular risk should be counseled that the cardiovascular safety of testosterone therapy is uncertain. The US FDA–mandated TRAVERSE study will provide robust evidence on this topic.[22]

Bone Mineral Density

Testosterone increases bone mineral density[23] and would be predicted to reduce fracture risk in hypogonadal men (although fracture reduction has not been proven). There is currently insufficient evidence to justify routine bone densitometry. However, assessment should be considered in individuals at high risk, such as those with known fractures, with hypogonadism onset during early adulthood, or who are on glucocorticoid treatment.

Clinical Case Vignettes

Case 1

A 38-year-old man has been experiencing low mood, reduced libido, inability to maintain erections during intercourse, and loss of early-morning erections over the last 6 months. His symptoms have been progressively worsening. He underwent orchidectomy following testicular torsion 11 years ago. He has never been treated for cancer and has no comorbidities. He takes no medications and has a BMI of 24.7 kg/m².

Laboratory test results:

> Serum LH = 12.5 mIU/mL (2.0-10.0 mIU/mL) (SI: 12.5 IU/L [2.0-10.0 IU/L])
> Serum FSH = 14.2 mIU/mL (2.0-10.0 mIU/mL) (SI: 14.2 IU/L [2.0-10.0 IU/L])
> Total testosterone (9 AM, fasting) = 282 ng/dL and 303 ng/dL (SI: 9.8 nmol/L and 10.5 nmol/L)
> SHBG = 41 µg/mL (20-60 µg/mL) (SI: 365 nmol/L [178-534 nmol/L])
> Hematocrit = 38% (40%-54%) (SI: 0.38 [0.40-0.54])

Is testosterone treatment indicated?

A. Yes

B. No

Answer: A) Yes

This case illustrates the importance of corroborative evidence when serum testosterone levels are borderline. One of the testosterone measurements is above a common "threshold" for diagnosis (300 ng/dL [10.4 nmol/L]), but assays are subject to variation. He has specific (sexual) symptoms of hypogonadism. Orchidectomy confers a higher risk of hypogonadism, and his elevated gonadotropins show that he has testicular failure. Furthermore, he has borderline anemia, which supports the diagnosis of hypogonadism. Testosterone treatment is indicated (Answer A).

Case 2

A 61-year-old man has been experiencing tiredness, low mood, low libido, and inability to put on muscle bulk when exercising for the last 2 years. He does not experience early-morning erections but can maintain erections during intercourse. He has high cholesterol treated with a stain, hypertension treated with a calcium channel blocker, and type 2 diabetes treated with metformin. His BMI is 33.7 kg/m^2.

Laboratory test results:

> Serum LH = 2.5 mIU/mL (2.0-10.0 mIU/mL)
>   (SI: 2.5 IU/L [2.0-10.0 IU/L])
> Serum FSH = 3.3 mIU/mL (2.0-10.0 mIU/mL)
>   (SI: 3.3 IU/L [2.0-10.0 IU/L])
> Total testosterone (9 AM, fasting) = 256 ng/dL
>   (SI: 8.9 nmol/L) and 265 ng/dL (SI: 9.2 nmol/L)
> SHBG = 1.35 µg/mL (2.25-6.74 µg/mL)
>   (SI: 12 nmol/L [20-60 nmol/L])
> Calculated free testosterone = 8.07 ng/dL
>   (SI: 0.28 nmol/L)
> Hematocrit = 42% (40%-54%) (SI: 0.42 [0.40 to 0.54])

Is testosterone treatment indicated?

A. Yes

B. No

Answer: B) No

Low serum testosterone is common. However, only 2% of men aged 40 to 90 years fulfilled the criteria for late-onset hypogonadism defined by European Male Ageing Study as: (1) low libido, loss of morning erections and loss of spontaneous erections; (2) low testosterone defined as total testosterone less than 230 ng/dL (<8 nmol/L) or a combination of testosterone less than 317 ng/dL (<11 nmol/L) and calculated free testosterone less than 6.3 ng/dL (220 pmol/L). This man has a low SHBG level, so his calculated free testosterone is normal. His comorbidity may be contributing to his symptoms, and weight loss should be offered as an alternative to testosterone therapy. Thus, testosterone therapy should not be offered (Answer B).

Case 3

A 71-year-old man has been experiencing low libido, inability to maintain erections during intercourse, and loss of early-morning erections. His symptoms have been worsening over the last year. He had a myocardial infarction 3 years ago with left anterior descending coronary stenting. He takes nitrates, aspirin, a statin, and an ACE inhibitor. His BMI is 27.3 kg/m^2.

Laboratory test results:

> Serum LH = 15.5 mIU/mL (2.0-10.0 mIU/mL)
>   (SI: 15.5 IU/L [2.0-10.0 IU/L])
> Serum FSH = 27.1 mIU/mL (2.0-10.0 mIU/mL)
>   (SI: 27.1 IU/L [2.0-10.0 IU/L])
> Total testosterone (9 AM, fasting) = 176 ng/dL
>   (SI: 6.1 nmol/L) and 170 ng/dL (SI: 5.9 nmol/L)
> SHBG = 2.9 µg/mL (2.2-6.7 µg/mL)
>   (SI: 26 nmol/L [20-60 nmol/L])
> Calculated free testosterone = 8.1 ng/dL
>   (SI: 0.28 nmol/L)
> Hematocrit = 37% (40%-54%) (SI: 0.37 [0.40-0.54])

DXA documents a lumbar T-score of –2.7 and femoral neck T-score of –1.6.

Is testosterone treatment indicated?

A. Yes

B. No

Answer: A) Yes

This patient has anemia, osteoporosis, elevated gonadotropins, and unequivocally low serum testosterone. Under normal circumstances, testosterone treatment would be a straightforward decision. However, he has a strong history of cardiac disease. The patient and his cardiologist should discuss the uncertain cardiac effects of testosterone. However, the benefits of treatment for sexual health, bone health, and anemia are substantial. Therefore, testosterone treatment should be considered if possible (Answer A).

References

1. Bhasin S, Brito JP, Cunningham GR, et al. Testosterone therapy in men with hypogonadism: an Endocrine Society clinical practice guideline. *J Clin Endocrinol Metab.* 2018;103(5):1715-1744. PMID: 29562364

2. Jayasena CN, Anderson RA, Llahana S, et al. Society for Endocrinology guidelines for testosterone replacement therapy in male hypogonadism. *Clin Endocrinol (Oxf).* 2022;96(2):200-219. PMID: 34811785

3. Ponce OJ, Spencer-Bonilla G, Alvarez-Villalobos N, et al. The efficacy and adverse events of testosterone replacement therapy in hypogonadal men: a systematic review and meta-analysis of randomized, placebo-controlled trials. *J Clin Endocrinol Metab.* 2018 [online ahead of print] PMID: 29562341

4. Travison TG, Vesper HW, Orwoll E, et al. Harmonized reference ranges for circulating testosterone levels in men of four cohort studies in the United States and Europe. *J Clin Endocrinol Metab.* 2017;102(4):1161-1173. PMID: 28324103

5. Brambilla DJ, Matsumoto AM, Araujo AB, McKinlay JB. The effect of diurnal variation on clinical measurement of serum testosterone and other sex hormone levels in men. *J Clin Endocrinol Metab.* 2009;94(3):907-913. PMID: 19088162

6. Wu FCW, Tajar A, Beynon JM, et al; EMAS Group. Identification of late-onset hypogonadism in middle-aged and elderly men. *N Engl J Med.* 2010;363(2):123-135. PMID: 20554979

7. Goldman AL, Bhasin S, Wu FCW, Krishna M, Matsumoto AM, Jasuja R. A reappraisal of testosterone's binding in circulation: physiological and clinical implications. *Endocr Rev.* 2017;38(4):302-324. PMID: 28673039

8. Fiers T, Wu F, Moghetti P, Vanderschueren D, Lapauw B, Kaufman JM. Reassessing free-testosterone calculation by liquid chromatography-tandem mass spectrometry direct equilibrium dialysis. *J Clin Endocrinol Metab.* 2018;103(6):2167-2174. PMID: 29618085

9. Handelsman DJ. Free testosterone: pumping up the tires or ending the free ride? *Endocr Rev.* 2017;38(4):297-301. PMID: 28898980

10. Llahana S. Testosterone therapy in adult men with hypogonadism. In: Llahana S, Follin C, Yedinak C, Grossman A, eds. *Advanced Practice in Endocrinology Nursing.* Springer International Publishing; 2019:885-902.

11. Bhasin S, Jameson JL. Disorders of the testes and male reproductive system In: Jameson JL, ed. *Harrison's Endocrinology.* 4th ed. McGraw Hill Education; 2017:159-185.

12. Morgentaler A, Traish AM. Shifting the paradigm of testosterone and prostate cancer: the saturation model and the limits of androgen-dependent growth. *Eur Urol.* 2009;55(2):310-320. PMID: 18838208

13. Lenfant L, Leon P, Cancel-Tassin G, et al. Testosterone replacement therapy (TRT) and prostate cancer: an updated systematic review with a focus on previous or active localized prostate cancer. *Urol Oncol.* 2020;38(8):661-670. PMID: 32409202

14. Santella C, Renoux C, Yin H, Yu OHY, Azoulay L. Testosterone replacement therapy and the risk of prostate cancer in men with late-onset hypogonadism. *Am J Epidemiol.* 2019;188(9):1666-1673. PMID: 31145457

15. Walker RF, Zakai NA, MacLehose RF, et al. Association of testosterone therapy with risk of venous thromboembolism among men with and without hypogonadism. *JAMA Intern Med.* 2020;180(2):190-197. PMID: 31710339

16. Jick SS, Hagberg KW. The risk of adverse outcomes in association with use of testosterone products: a cohort study using the UK-based general practice research database. *Br J Clin Pharmacol.* 2013;75(1):260-270. PMID: 22574772

17. Xu L, Freeman G, Cowling BJ, Schooling CM. Testosterone therapy and cardiovascular events among men: a systematic review and meta-analysis of placebo-controlled randomized trials. *BMC Med.* 2013;11:108. PMID: 23597181

18. Corona G, Maseroli E, Rastrelli G, et al. Cardiovascular risk associated with testosterone-boosting medications: a systematic review and meta-analysis. *Expert Opin Drug Saf.* 2014;13(10):1327-1351. PMID: 25139126

19. Budoff MJ, Ellenberg SS, Lewis CE, et al. Testosterone treatment and coronary artery plaque volume in older men with low testosterone. *JAMA.* 2017;317(7):708-716. PMID: 28241355

20. US Food and Drug Administration. Drug safety communication: FDA cautions about using testosterone products for low testosterone due to aging; requires labeling change to inform of possible increased risk of heart attack and stroke with use. January 2014. Available at: https://www.fda.gov/media/91048/download

21. European Medicines Agency EMA/706140/2014: No consistent evidence of an increased risk of heart problems with testosterone medicines. November 21, 2014. Available at: https://www.ema.europa.eu/en/documents/referral/testosterone-article-31-referral-no-consistent-evidence-increased-risk-heart-problems-testosterone_en.pdf

22. A study to evaluate the effect of testosterone replacement therapy (TRT) on the incidence of major adverse cardiovascular events (MACE) and efficacy measures in hypogonadal men (TRAVERSE). Available at: https://www.clinicaltrials.gov/ct2/show/NCT03518034

23. Snyder PJ, Kopperdahl DL, Stephens-Shields AJ, et al. Effect of testosterone treatment on volumetric bone density and strength in older men with low testosterone: a controlled clinical trial. *JAMA Intern Med.* 2017;177(4):471-479. PMID: 28241231

Management Strategies for Primary Ovarian Insufficiency in Adolescence: Protecting Long-Term Health

Lawrence C. Layman, MD. Reproductive Endocrinology, Infertility, and Genetics, Department of Obstetrics and Gynecology, Medical College of Georgia at Augusta University, Augusta, GA; E-mail: lalayman@augusta.edu

Learning Objectives

As a result of participating in this session, learners should be able to:

- Discuss the clinical presentation of primary ovarian insufficiency (POI) in adolescence.

- Describe a rational diagnostic approach to the adolescent with POI.

- Explain how POI affects long-term health.

- Guide the management of POI.

Main Conclusions

- Diagnosis of POI in adolescent patients rests upon amenorrhea and elevated gonadotropins with estrogen deficiency.

- Chromosomal abnormalities, particularly a 45,X cell line, must be excluded in all adolescents with primary amenorrhea who have POI and should be considered in adolescents with secondary amenorrhea and POI depending upon stature.

- The absence of somatic anomalies should not be a reason to dismiss Turner syndrome.

- Autoimmune disorders, pathogenic variants in genes associated with POI, and history of chemotherapy/radiation should be considered.

- Hormone treatment with estrogen may alleviate vasomotor and urogenital symptoms and lower the risk for future osteoporosis and cardiovascular disease.

- Practically speaking, fertility is extremely unlikely in women with POI without an egg donor.

Significance of the Clinical Problem

POI, formerly known as premature ovarian failure, is usually defined as hypoestrogenic amenorrhea for 3 to 6 months and elevated gonadotropins on at least 2 occasions 4 weeks apart. POI has been typically stated to occur in approximately 1% of women younger than age 40 years in the United States (globally 2%-3%).[1] Ovarian function may cease prior to, during, or after puberty has been completed. Affected patients present with amenorrhea and hypoestrogenism with elevated gonadotropins. Particular attention should be given to pubertal development and stature. Potential etiologies include chromosomal, genetic, autoimmune, and history of chemotherapy and/or radiation.[1,2]

It is important to recognize and exclude a 45,X cell line (Turner syndrome), as this has important consequences for long-term health, particularly cardiovascular complications consisting of cardiac valve abnormalities and aortic dilatation predisposing to dissection.[3] If a patient has a 46,XX karyotype, fragile X syndrome and associated autoimmune disorders should be excluded.[1,2,4]

Hormone treatment with estrogen and progesterone is important to treat vasomotor and urogenital symptoms and to prevent osteoporosis and cardiovascular disease.[1,2] Fertility, in most cases, requires egg donation and in vitro fertilization.

Barriers to Optimal Practice

- It is not normal to have absent breast development by age 13 years, no period by age 15 years, or be amenorrheic for more than 4 to 6 months. In any of these circumstances, an evaluation is necessary.

- POI can be diagnosed in adolescence prior to the onset of puberty, during puberty, or once puberty is completed.

- There is fear/misunderstanding that hormone therapy conveys risks similar to those of treatment in natural menopause.

Strategies for Diagnosis, Therapy, and/or Management
Diagnosis of POI

Girls without breast development by age 13 to 14 years and/or without menarche by age 15 to 16 years, as well as adolescents with suspected hypogonadism, should be examined and evaluated. Pubertal milestones should be ascertained, including thelarche, pubarche, growth velocity, peak height velocity, and menarche. A thorough history of these timepoints is important, as well as the presence of any other associated disorders, including thyroid disease, adrenal disease, or other autoimmune phenomena. A history of malignancy with exposure to chemotherapy and/or radiation

should be determined. A family history, preferably a pedigree, should be obtained, documenting relatives with other associated disorders, anomalies, and/or POI.

A complete physical examination should be performed with particular attention to height, weight, thyroid gland, and Tanner staging of breast development and pubic hair. A full pelvic examination is challenging to perform in these hypogonadal girls and is best avoided (particularly, a speculum exam).[5] If the patient allows, a Q-tip can be placed into the vagina to document a patent outflow tract, which is expected if the patient has POI. If no vagina is identified, etiologies other than POI must be considered.

Female adolescents without breast development (Tanner stage 1) or impaired breast development (Tanner stage 2 to 3) by age 13 to 14 years are nearly always hypoestrogenic. Similarly, female adolescents with breast development without menarche are also likely to be hypoestrogenic. If the adolescent has had normal breast development with menarche and then ceases to menstruate, it must be determined whether she is hypoestrogenic. Typically, amenorrhea of 3 to 6 months' duration should be investigated.[2,5] This may be accomplished in several different ways, including serum estradiol measurement, progestin withdrawal test, or vaginal maturation index. It is important to know whether the estradiol assay used is able to discriminate low from low-normal values (normal follicular-phase levels 30-300 pg/mL [110.1-1101.3 pmol/L]; hypogonadism <30 pg/mL [<110.1 pmol/L]). Administering 7 to 10 days of medroxyprogesterone acetate may be helpful if the estradiol value is inconclusive. A normal eugonadal response is a full period; spotting and absence of bleeding within a week of the last pill suggests hypoestrogenism. A vaginal maturation index with a preponderance of parabasal cells (small cells with large nucleus, which indicate hypoestrogenism) rather than estrogenic superficial cells (large cells with a small pyknotic nucleus) when collected with a Q-tip inserted into the vagina also suggests hypogonadism.[5]

Laboratory studies include the measurement of serum estradiol, FSH, LH, TSH (with or without free T$_4$), and prolactin. In the United States, patients with POI typically have FSH levels greater than 40.0 mIU/mL (>40.0 IU/L) (in Europe >25.0 mIU/mL [>25.0 IU/L]) on 2 occasions 4 weeks apart, elevated LH levels, and normal thyroid function and prolactin levels.[1,2] Once hypergonadotropic hypogonadism is diagnosed, karyotype analysis is indicated for all patients with primary amenorrhea and for those with short stature (<63 in [<160 cm]) with secondary amenorrhea. This is true regardless of whether the individual has Turner syndrome stigmata. A 45,X cell line requires lifetime medical surveillance for cardiac and kidney dysfunction. If the patient has a 46,XX karyotype, fragile X syndrome testing should be offered to assess for the presence of an *FMR1* premutation CGG expansion. If fragile X testing is negative, a targeted POI gene panel can be considered, as 20% to 25% of affected patients possess pathogenic variants in 1 of approximately 30 genes. Because of the common (30%) association of autoimmune disease, including autoimmune thyroiditis, Addison disease, and type 1 diabetes, ordering fasting glucose measurement, as well as TPO antibodies and 21-hydroxylase antibodies should be considered. Alternatively, 8-AM cortisol measurement is also reasonable.[1,2]

Therapy

A discussion with the patient and involved family members is important to address the psychologic stress that comes from knowing that there is impaired ovarian function and that pregnancy chances are extremely low. Patients with primary amenorrhea, particularly those without breast development, will benefit from estradiol administration by either oral or transdermal routes. Once breast development is adequate (which may take 6 to 12 months depending on development) or the patient has a menstrual bleed, adding progestin for 7 to 10 days per month helps protect the endometrium from long periods of unopposed estrogen and subsequent hyperplasia and malignancy. If the adolescent already has breast development, estradiol with cyclic progestin is indicated.[1,2] For convenience, oral contraceptives are an acceptable convenient alternative in most patients. This therapy can be administered until the patient has reached the age of menopause (~early 50s) and should not be perceived to have the same risks as menopausal hormone replacement. Estradiol is important for protecting against bone loss that could lead to osteoporosis, preventing urogenital atrophy and dyspareunia, and preventing cardiovascular disease.[1,2]

Management

Discussion regarding the management of the adolescent with POI involves multiple facets. Estrogen treatment is important for prevention of osteoporosis and cardiovascular disease. Fertility is very unlikely without an egg donor because expectant management, oral medications such as clomiphene citrate, injectable gonadotropins, or in vitro fertilization all result in very low—but not zero—pregnancy rates (~5%). This is particularly true for patients with Turner syndrome.[1,2] If the patient has Turner syndrome, cardiac echocardiography is indicated to exclude a dilated aorta, bicuspid aortic valve, or other cardiac anomaly.[3] Regular follow-up is suggested to reduce the likelihood of aortic dissection, which may complicate 2% of pregnancies. For this reason, egg donation in a patient with Turner syndrome is usually discouraged. Baseline kidney ultrasonography is also indicated to exclude congenital anomalies such as horseshoe kidney or unilateral kidney agenesis.

In patients with a normal karyotype, pregnancy with egg donation appears to be safe. It is important to determine whether the patient has an *FMR1* premutation, which increases the risk of having affected male offspring (50% of males will be affected; 50% of females will be carriers). Even if the patient's chance of pregnancy is low, her diagnosis could be beneficial to share with other family members. Gene panels can help to determine the etiology of POI in patients with a 46,XX karyotype, but most cases are due to autosomal recessive inheritance, so do not present significant risks for offspring should the patient conceive.

Yearly assessments for thyroid function, diabetes mellitus, and cortisol should be considered, and studies should be performed, especially if symptoms develop.[1,2] If 2 or more autoimmune disorders are present, then autoimmune polyglandular syndrome is diagnosed.[6] Autoimmune polyglandular syndrome type I is a rare monogenic disorder due to pathogenic variants in the *AIRE* gene and is characterized by mucocutaneous candidiasis, hypoparathyroidism, Addison disease, type 1 diabetes, and hypothyroidism. More than 50% of affected females develop POI. Types II though IV are adult diseases: autoimmune polyglandular syndrome type II (Addison disease + another endocrine disorder), type III (type 1 diabetes + autoimmune thyroid disease), and type IV (2 or more other endocrinopathies). These adult types are more common than type I and are multifactorial vs autosomal dominant in some cases.[6]

Clinical Case Vignettes

Case 1

An 18-year-old woman seeks evaluation because she has never had a period. She has Tanner stage 3 breast development. Her referring physician gave her 7 days of medroxyprogesterone, and she did not bleed.

On physical examination, a Q-tip was able to be inserted into her vagina.

Her estradiol concentration is 10 pg/mL (30-50 pg/mL [follicular phase]) (SI: 36.7 pmol/L [110.1-183.6 pmol/L]).

Which of the following is the best next step?

A. Expectant management

B. Karyotype analysis

C. Serum FSH measurement

D. Transabdominal ultrasonography

Answer: C) Serum FSH measurement

Although it looks like she had some breast development (ie, estrogen exposure), delayed puberty is usually defined as no breast development by age 13 to 14 years and/or no period by age 15 to 16 years. She is clearly beyond this and needs evaluation. Thus, expectant management (Answer A) is incorrect.

She did not bleed in response to progestin and has a low estradiol level, so she has hypogonadism. Serum FSH measurement (Answer C) (usually along with LH) will help delineate whether the defect is hypothalamic/pituitary or gonadal.

Outflow obstruction is unlikely since a vagina is present. Thus, transabdominal ultrasonography (Answer D) will not add much at this point. The uterus and ovaries are small, which could be observed in a patient with hypogonadism from any cause (or even be missed by ultrasonography).

Karyotype analysis (Answer B) is not needed since it is not yet known whether she has hypergonadotropic hypogonadism or hypogonadotropic hypogonadism.

Case 1 (Continued)

Laboratory test results:

FSH = 57.0 mIU/mL (3.0-10.0 mIU/mL) (SI: 57.0 IU/L [3.0-10.0 IU/L])
LH = 33.0 mIU/mL (3.0-10.0 mIU/mL) (SI: 33.0 IU/L [3.0-10.0 IU/L])

Repeated measurement 4 weeks later shows an FSH concentration of 25.0 mIU/mL (25.0 IU/L) and LH concentration of 22.0 mIU/mL (22.0 IU/L). Her vital signs are normal. Her height is 61 in (155 cm) and BMI is 22 kg/m².

Which of the following is the best next step?

A. Brain MRI

B. DXA

C. Gene panel

D. Karyotype analysis

Answer: D) Karyotype analysis

Karyotype analysis (Answer D) is necessary to rule out a chromosomal abnormality, namely Turner syndrome. In this case, it is prudent to ask the laboratory to count chromosomes in 50 cells rather than the standard 20 to exclude 45,X cell-line mosaicism. Most patients with Turner syndrome are shorter than 60 in (<152 cm), and this patient is 61 in (155 cm). Counting approximately 30 cells excludes 10% mosaicism, and counting 50 to 60 cells excludes 5% mosaicism.[3] She could have a 45,X cell line with or without mosaicism (46,XX or 47,XXX; 46,XY is unlikely, as she has had some breast development). Alternatively, she could have a karyotype demonstrating 46,XX with an Xp deletion, an Xq deletion, an isochromosome X in which she has an X chromosome with 2 long (q) arms (and missing the p arm), or a translocation involving an autosome or a Y chromosome with X. If she has Turner syndrome, there is a high risk of cardiovascular anomalies and an increased risk of kidney anomalies, which would be important to know to guide her management.[3]

Brain MRI (Answer A) is important if gonadotropins are low or normal (hypogonadotropic hypogonadism), but not in this case.

Although DXA (Answer B) will be important for long-term management, it is not important in the diagnosis.

A gene panel (Answer C) is not appropriate yet, as it would not be necessary if she has Turner syndrome.

Case 1 (Continued)

Her karyotype is reported as 46,XX with 50 cells counted. A more detailed family history is obtained, and she states that her mother had menopause at age 33 years and a maternal aunt never had children but had some type of tremor. She also has a first cousin with autism.

Which of the following genes should be considered for testing?

A. *FMR1*

B. *FOXL2*

C. *FSHR*

D. *SHOX*

Answer: A) FMR1

Fragile X syndrome is an X-linked dominant disorder due to full expansion of the triplet repeat in the *FMR1* gene (Answer A). Affected male patients typically have varying degrees of intellectual disability or autism, facial abnormalities, and macroorchidism. Female patients with the full expansion can have intellectual disability, which is usually less severe, but they do not have POI. Females in a family with known fragile X syndrome and who have the premutation have an increased risk of POI (15% to 20%). If the proband is ascertained because of POI, the risk for a premutation is about 3% to 4% if no other family members are affected, but the risk is 10% to 15% if 2 or more family members are affected. In this patient's family history, the first-degree cousin with autism and the family history of POI are suggestive of fragile X syndrome. Male and female patients with a premutation have increased risk of tremors/ataxia when they get older.

FSHR (Answer C) pathogenic variants are associated with resistant ovary syndrome, in which patients have multiple follicles and POI.

SHOX (Answer D) pathogenic variants may cause short stature, Leri-Weill dyschondrosteosis, and Langer mesomelic dysplasia, both of which have skeletal anomalies among others.

FOXL2 (Answer B) pathogenic variants have blepharophimosis-ptosis epicanthus syndrome, in which eyelid abnormalities are accompanied by POI.

None of these disorders is associated with the intellectual disability or tremor/ataxia that can be associated with *FMR1* pathogenic variants.

Case 1 (Continued)

This 18-year-old patient with POI asks about treatment, including questions about fertility.

She should be counseled that her chances of fertility are:

A. 5%

B. 25%

C. 50%

D. 75%

Answer: A) 5%

Treatment consisting of expectant management, ovulation induction, or in vitro fertilization using the patient's own eggs offers very low pregnancy rates. POI, particularly in patients with a normal karyotype, may wax and wane, so they should not be counseled that they will never conceive—however, the chances are low (Answer A). Only egg donation has the potential to result in pregnancy rates of approximately 50%, depending on sperm and uterine factors.

References

1. Stuenkel CA, Gompel A, Davis SR, Pinkerton JAV, Lumsden MA, Santen RJ. Approach to the patient with new onset secondary amenorrhea: is this primary ovarian insufficiency? *J Clin Endocrinol Metab.* 2022;107(3):825-835. PMID: 34693971

2. McGlacken-Byrne SM, Conway GS. Premature ovarian insufficiency. *Best Pract Res Clin Obstet Gynaecol.* 2021 [Online ahead of print] PMID: 34924261

3. Zhong Q, Layman LC. Genetic considerations in the patient with Turner syndrome--45,X with or without mosaicism. *Fertil Steril.* 2012;98(4):775-779. PMID: 23020909

4. Layman LC. Would combined glucocorticoid and gonadotropin therapy improve pregnancy rates in women with primary ovarian insufficiency? *F S Rep.* 2020;1(3):171-172. PMID: 34223237

5. Layman LC, Reindollar RH. The diagnosis and treatment of pubertal disorders. *Adolesc Med.* 1994;5(1):37-56. PMID: 10358259

6. Kahaly GJ, Frommer L. Polyglandular autoimmune syndromes. *J Endocrinol Invest.* 2018;41(1):91-98. PMID: 28819917

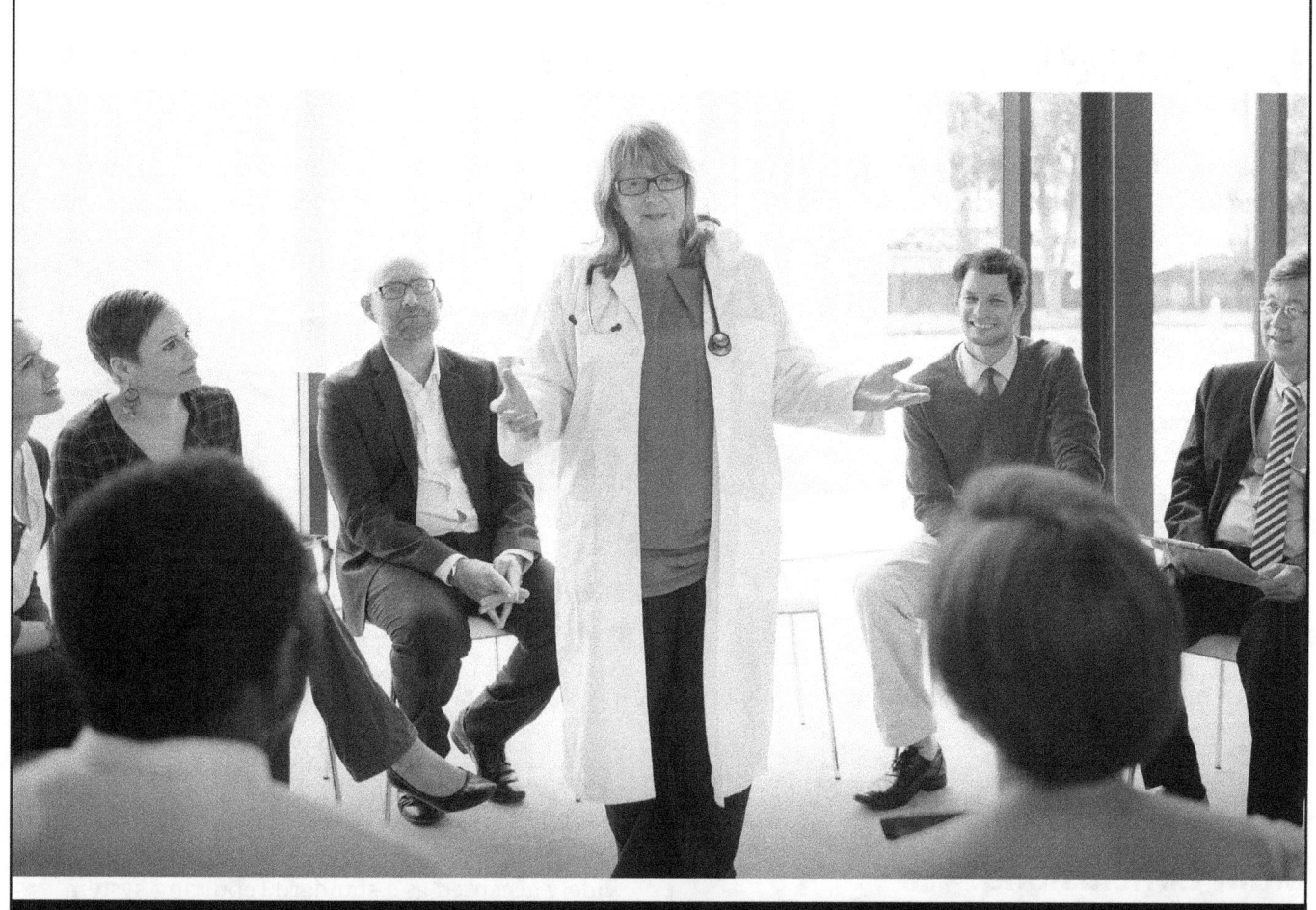

THYROID

Molecular Diagnosis of Indeterminate Thyroid Nodules

Bryan R. Haugen, MD. Division of Endocrinology, Metabolism and Diabetes, University of Colorado School of Medicine, Aurora, CO 80045. E-mail: bryan.haugen@cuanschutz.edu

Sarah E. Mayson, MD. Division of Endocrinology, Metabolism and Diabetes, University of Colorado School of Medicine, Aurora, CO 80045. E-mail: sarah.mayson@cuanschutz.edu

Learning Objectives

- Appropriately assess the strengths and limitations of molecular testing in patients with indeterminate thyroid nodule cytology.

- Summarize what is known about the long-term outcomes of nonoperatively managed thyroid nodules with indeterminate cytopathology and negative molecular testing.

Main Conclusions

- Currently available molecular tests have high sensitivity to rule out malignancy and reasonable specificity to rule in malignancy for patients with indeterminate thyroid nodule cytology.

- Sonographic features of the thyroid nodule must be considered when interpreting molecular test results for patients with indeterminate cytology.

- Certain pathogenic variants can be associated with familial syndromes. Providers should be aware of these variants and consider referral to genetic counseling when appropriate.

- The presence of higher-risk pathogenic variants (*TERT* promoter, *TP53*, *PIK3CA*, etc) may help guide more or less aggressive management/monitoring, but more studies are needed.

Significance of the Clinical Problem

FNA is recommended to evaluate for malignancy in thyroid nodules meeting criteria for biopsy according to validated ultrasound risk stratification systems, including the 2015 American Thyroid Association (ATA) Guidelines for Patients with Thyroid Nodules and Differentiated Thyroid Cancer and the American College of Radiology (ACR) Thyroid Imaging Reporting and Data System (TI-RADS). The Bethesda System for Reporting Thyroid Cytopathology (TBSRTC) is widely accepted as a standard reporting system for thyroid cytopathology. This system includes 3 indeterminate reporting categories (Bethesda III-V), each of which is associated with a different predicted risk for malignancy. The 2017 TBSRTC proposes that the risk for malignancy for atypia of undetermined significance/follicular lesion of undetermined significance (AUS/FLUS) (Bethesda III) cytology is 6% to 18% when noninvasive follicular thyroid neoplasm with papillary-like nuclear features (NIFTP) is considered benign and 10% to 30% when NIFTP is considered malignant.[1] Furthermore, the predicted risk for malignancy for follicular neoplasm/suspicious for follicular neoplasm (FN/SFN) (Bethesda IV) is 10% to 40% when NIFTP is considered benign and 25% to 40% when NIFTP is considered malignant. The risk for malignancy associated with both categories remains low enough to not justify surgical resection for all patients, yet high enough to not justify monitoring for all.

The historical management of patients with indeterminate cytopathology, especially prior to TBSRTC, was diagnostic thyroid surgery (ie, lobectomy) to definitively rule in or rule out cancer. This approach has many disadvantages, including financial costs and operative risks, and leads to overtreatment or undertreatment in up to 60% of patients. Postoperative hypothyroidism necessitating lifelong thyroid hormone replacement occurs in approximately 20% of patients after lobectomy and is even more prevalent in patients with underlying chronic autoimmune thyroiditis who have normal thyroid function before surgery.

Since 2011, a number of molecular platforms have been developed to assist in the diagnostic evaluation of thyroid nodules with indeterminate cytopathology. Molecular testing can help identify nodules that are unlikely to be malignant (posttest probability of malignancy ≤5%), allowing these nodules to be triaged to clinical rather than operative management. In addition, some molecular tests can identify specific genetic alterations in the nodule, which may help to inform patient management.

Barriers to Optimal Practice

- Regional or institutional variation in the prevalence of malignancy/NIFTP of Bethesda III-IV thyroid nodules influences the performance of molecular tests used in clinical practice.

- There are limited studies evaluating the longer-term outcomes of thyroid nodules with indeterminate cytopathology and negative results for the molecular tests that are currently available.

- More research is needed to clearly define the prognostic and therapeutic implications of the many genetic alterations that can be identified through molecular testing.

Strategies for Diagnosis, Therapy, and/or Management

Before being adopted into clinical practice, molecular tests should be evaluated to confirm their analytical validity, clinical validity, and clinical utility. Analytical validation refers to the accuracy of the test to measure what it is intended to measure in the context of limited input material or in the presence of contamination (eg, blood), as well as the reproducibility of the test to produce the same results over repeated runs. Clinical validation evaluates the ability of a diagnostic test to rule out disease (sensitivity, negative predictive value [NPV]) and rule in disease (specificity, positive predictive value [PPV]). Both sensitivity and specificity are inherent properties of the diagnostic test and thus can be compared among different studies in different populations. However, PPV and NPV are influenced by disease prevalence. NPV increases and PPV decreases as prevalence falls, while the opposite is observed when prevalence rises. Clinical utility refers to the psychological, social, and economic consequences of testing and impact on health outcomes in the context of the individual, family, and society.

Molecular platforms for the evaluation of indeterminate thyroid nodules use different testing approaches. These include assessment for single nucleotide variants (point mutations), insertions/deletions, gene fusions, chromosomal copy number alterations, and/or abnormal gene expression using DNA, mRNA, miRNA, or a combination thereof. The Afirma Genomic Sequencing Classifier (GSC) and Xpression Atlas (XA), ThyroSeq v3 Genomic Classifier (GC), and ThyGeNEXT/ThyraMIR are currently the best studied, most widely available molecular diagnostic tests in the United States. All are based on earlier versions of the same/similar tests.

Afirma GSC requires a fresh FNA specimen that is immediately placed into a proprietary collection vial. The test primarily uses mRNA expression and machine-learned algorithms to risk stratify indeterminate thyroid nodules as benign or suspicious. An upstream mutation/fusion panel allows for specific gene variants highly correlated with thyroid cancer (*BRAF* V600E, *RET/PTC1*, or *RET/PTC3* fusions) to be identified, thus bypassing the core classifier. There are additional upstream components to identify parathyroid tissue and medullary thyroid carcinoma. The Afirma GSC clinical validation study was a blinded multicenter study of 191 Bethesda III/IV thyroid nodules, which used retained samples from the prospective Afirma Gene Expression Classifier (GEC) validation trial. The overall sensitivity was 91%, specificity was 68%, NPV was 96%, and PPV was 47%. The prevalence of thyroid cancer was 24% (NIFTP prevalence not known). One of the key improvements of Afirma GSC over the earlier version (GEC) is its improved specificity, mostly owed to its superior performance in Hurthle-cell nodules (specificity of 58.8% for GSC vs 11.8% for GEC in Hurthle-cell nodules).[2] Afirma XA is a separate test that can be ordered reflexively when GSC is positive. XA uses whole-transcriptome RNA sequencing to identify gene variants and fusions. The original version of XA included 511 thyroid-related genes, while the current expanded panel includes 593 genes (905 variants and 235 fusion pairs). A recent study of more than 16,000 GSC suspicious Bethesda III/IV nodules detected 1 or more mutation/fusion in 42% of nodules using the original panel and 44% using the expanded panel.[3] Because XA is an RNA-based test, it cannot detect mutations/fusions that are present in noncoding regions of DNA (eg, *TERT* promoter).

ThyroSeq v3 GC has been analytically validated for use with fresh FNA specimens and FNA smears. Better preservation of nucleic acid material is observed with ethanol-fixed vs air-dried smears.[4] ThyroSeq GC uses next-generation sequencing of DNA and mRNA to evaluate for 5 classes of genetic alterations in 112 thyroid cancer-related genes. These include point mutations, insertions/deletions, gene fusions, chromosomal copy number alterations, and gene expression alterations. Each genetic alteration that is identified is assigned a score between 0 and 2, and the total score is calculated for the sample. A score of 2 or more is considered positive. In addition to a binary positive/negative result, all ThyroSeq GC test results include a detailed report of the genetic alterations that were identified and the estimated risk of malignancy associated with the identified variants. The ThyroSeq GC clinical validation study was a prospective blinded multicenter study of 286 Bethesda III-V thyroid nodules, including 154 Bethesda III and 93 Bethesda IV nodules. The overall sensitivity was 94%, specificity was 82%, NPV was 97%, and PPV was 66%. The prevalence of cancer/NIFTP was 28%. The study included 11 nodules (4%) that were NIFTP on histopathology, all of which were classified as positive.[5]

The performance of Afirma GSC and ThyroSeq GC was recently compared in a single-center randomized pragmatic clinical trial that included 372 indeterminate thyroid nodules.[6] The majority of nodules with negative molecular results were managed nonoperatively. The prevalence of cancer/NIFTP was 19.6%. Overall, 49% of patients were able to avoid diagnostic surgery. Importantly, there was no significant difference in the observed sensitivity, specificity, NPV, or PPV of Afirma GSC and ThyroSeq GC. This trial provides real-world data that the 2 tests perform similarly well in clinical practice.

ThyGeNEXT/ThyraMIR can be performed using fresh FNA specimens, formalin-fixed histopathologic specimens, or ethanol-fixed FNA smears. This multiplatform test combines next-generation sequencing of DNA and mRNA to evaluate for 42 gene variants and 38 gene fusions with qRT-PCR to measure expression levels of 10 miRNAs. The test uses a proprietary algorithm to ultimately yield a positive, negative, or "moderate" result. The ThyGeNEXT/ThyraMIR clinical validation study was a multicenter retrospective cross-sectional cohort study with pathologist blinding. The initial study set included 309 archived samples, while the final study set included 197 Bethesda III/IV nodules after 59 were excluded due to insufficient material and 53 samples were excluded because of lack of histopathology consensus. The prevalence of cancer/NIFTP was 30%. The observed sensitivity was 93%, specificity was 90%, NPV was 95%, and PPV was 74%. The risk of disease with a moderate result was 30%. When calculating test sensitivity, the authors counted the 15 moderates with malignant histopathology as true positives. When calculating test specificity, they counted the 35 moderates with benign histology as true negatives. Finally, the authors separately reported prevalence-adjusted statistical parameters. Following adjustment of disease prevalence to 14%, the test sensitivity was 95%, specificity was 90%, NPV was 97%, and PPV was 75%. The risk of disease with a moderate result was 39%.[7] The performance of ThyGeNEXT/ThyraMIR should ideally be confirmed in a prospective multicenter clinical validation study.

Molecular diagnostic testing has become a commonly used tool to help triage indeterminate thyroid nodules into 2 groups: (1) those that are likely to be benign and can be managed nonoperatively, similar to benign (Bethesda II) nodules, and (2) those that are likely to represent thyroid cancer or NIFTP and should be treated surgically. In addition, some molecular tests can identify specific genetic alterations that are associated with indolent, or conversely, aggressive forms of thyroid cancer. In this context, molecular test results also have the potential to inform clinical management decisions, as we will discuss in some of the cases that follow.

Clinical Case Vignettes

Case 1

A 70-year-old man with no risk factors for thyroid cancer underwent initial evaluation of a left thyroid nodule 2.5 years ago. Ultrasound examination demonstrated a 3.2-cm isoechoic solid nodule with well-defined regular borders and no suspicious lymph nodes. Ultrasound-guided FNA demonstrated AUS (Bethesda III) cytopathology with architectural atypia. Molecular testing with Afirma GSC was negative. The patient has pursued clinical and ultrasonography follow-up for his nodule. Today his neck examination and ultrasonography demonstrate stable size and appearance of the nodule and normal-appearing cervical lymph nodes. The patient has no compressive symptoms.

What is the most appropriate management to recommend for this patient? What proportion of thyroid nodules deemed benign on molecular testing are eventually resected, and what is the frequency of malignancy? Are there are any clinical or radiographic risk factors that predict missed thyroid cancer?

Published studies of thyroid nodules with indeterminate cytology and negative molecular testing that are followed nonoperatively are generally reassuring. A recent study from the University of California Los Angeles group found that patients with nodules classified as benign on molecular testing who were followed longitudinally with ultrasound surveillance did not experience a decline in health-related quality of life or worsening anxiety or depression over time.[8]

Reported rates of surgical resection of thyroid nodules classified as benign on molecular testing range from 5% to 25%, but missed malignancies are uncommon.[9-12] Studies assessing the longer-term outcomes of molecularly benign thyroid nodules evaluated with currently available tests are presently limited, but would be expected to yield similarly low false-negative rates. A prospective cohort of 95 indeterminate thyroid nodules with negative molecular testing (Afirma GEC or ThyroSeq v2) were followed for a median of 26.7 months to determine the frequency of delayed resection and the false-negative rate of molecular testing. Immediate surgery was performed for 12 nodules (11 benign, 1 NIFTP) and delayed surgery for 10 (6 benign, 4 malignant). The overall false-negative rate was 5.8%. Change in nodule appearance on ultrasonography (increase in size and/or development of suspicious features) was correlated with malignancy.[12] A larger retrospective study of 289 molecular benign nodules (Afirma GEC or GSC) found that the false-negative rate was significantly higher for thyroid nodules that were considered to have high risk for malignancy based on ultrasound risk stratification.[11]

In conclusion, molecularly benign thyroid nodules that have high-risk sonographic findings at baseline or develop suspicious features during follow-up are most likely to represent missed thyroid cancers. The interval development of suspicious sonographic findings should prompt further evaluation of the nodule (eg, repeat FNA) and possible resection. In contrast, the thyroid nodule described in this case demonstrated low-risk sonographic findings at baseline, which have been stable on subsequent imaging follow-up. Continued clinical and ultrasonography follow-up would be the most appropriate management to recommend for this patient.

Case 2

A 33-year-old man undergoes neck ultrasonography for "fluctuating neck adenopathy" after COVID vaccination. Imaging demonstrates a left 1.4-cm isoechoic nodule with coarse internal hyperechoic echoes. He has no neck symptoms. Serum TSH concentration is 1.8 mIU/L. Ultrasound-guided FNA cytology is categorized as AUS (Bethesda III) with a microscopic description of "many nuclear grooves and rare nuclear pseudoinclusions." Results of Afirma GSC testing are suspicious and identify the *BRAF* V600E pathogenic variant.

What is the best way to sonographically evaluate for extrathyroidal extension? What are the best next steps for this patient? Does cancer location in the thyroid influence the approach (monitoring vs surgery)?

Isoechoic nodules are generally classified as having a low sonographic risk pattern.[13] This nodule would be classified as TI-RADS TR4 (4 points, moderately suspicious).[14] Still images may be useful to identify potential extrathyroidal extension, which is most easily identified in the anterior thyroid. If there is question of extrathyroidal extension on still images, video clips, when available, can be helpful.

In general, a suspicious Afirma GSC result confers approximately 50% risk of malignancy,[15]

but the *BRAF* V600E variant confers nearly 100% risk of thyroid cancer.[16] There is increasing evidence that many patients with small papillary thyroid carcinoma (PTC) (<1 cm) may safely undergo active surveillance or deferred therapy instead of immediate surgery.[17-19] Of note, younger patients (<40 years) tend to have a higher rate of disease progression than older patients.[17] Studies are ongoing to determine whether properly selected patients with PTC up to 1.5 to 2 cm could be candidates for active surveillance.

There are multiple components to "properly selected patients," but one important component is tumor location. Tumors with clear normal tissue surrounding them on ultrasonography are at lowest risk for extrathyroidal extension and are good candidates for surveillance. Surgical resection is generally recommended when there is a question of extrathyroidal extension on ultrasonography and for those tumors located posteriorly, with potential for posterior or tracheal extension. This patient underwent a planned left lobectomy that was converted to thyroidectomy when the surgeon noted tumor adherence to the trachea. Final pathology noted extrathyroidal extension.

Case 3

A 28-year-old woman with a history of a uterine fibroid tumor and stage I breast cancer presents for evaluation of a left thyroid nodule detected on PET/CT imaging done in the context of her recent breast cancer diagnosis. The thyroid nodule was not noted to be fluorodeoxyglucose-avid. The patient's mother died of breast cancer. The patient's father and older sister are healthy. Her younger brother has a nonsevere form of autism spectrum disorder.

Subsequent neck ultrasonography confirms the presence of a 1.6-cm isoechoic solid nodule in the left mid pole of the thyroid gland with well-defined regular borders and no contralateral nodules or abnormal lymph nodes. Her serum TSH concentration is 2.0 mIU/L. The patient undergoes ultrasound-guided FNA of the thyroid nodule, which reveals AUS cytology (Bethesda III), and molecular testing with ThyroSeq v3 is positive for a *PTEN* variant (c.388C>T [p.R130]). This is identified in the sample at 50% allele frequency. No additional genetic alterations are detected.

What is the significance of the identified PTEN gene variant? Does the reported allelic frequency have potential significance? How should this patient be managed?

Pathogenic variants in the phosphatase and tensin homolog gene (*PTEN*) are observed in both benign and malignant thyroid tumors and can occur as either germline or sporadic events. PTEN is a phosphatase that negatively regulates AKT, leading to the induction of apoptosis. Loss of this tumor suppressor leads to increased cell survival. A study of 95 sporadic thyroid neoplasms documented *PTEN* alterations in 11 tumors: in 26% of benign or atypical adenomas and in 6% of thyroid carcinomas.[20] *PTEN* alterations have been associated with thyroid cancer tumor progression. A study of 779 advanced differentiated and anaplastic thyroid cancers documented *PTEN* pathogenic variants in 11% of anaplastic cancers. In the group of advanced differentiated cancers, *PTEN* alterations were identified in 17% of Hurthle-cell carcinomas, in 14% of follicular thyroid carcinomas (FTCs), and in only 2% of PTCs.[21] Another study screened 259 unselected patients with differentiated thyroid cancer for germline *PTEN* pathogenic variants. The frequency of *PTEN* alterations was only 0.8% across all thyroid cancers, but it was 4.8% when only follicular cancers were considered.[22]

Germline pathogenic variants in *PTEN* may lead to the *PTEN* hamartoma tumor syndrome, one of the most common known causes of syndromic nonmedullary thyroid cancer. *PTEN* hamartoma tumor syndrome encompasses several distinct phenotypes, including Cowden syndrome, Bannayan-Riley-Ruvalcaba syndrome, and Proteus and Proteus-like syndromes.[23] Cowden syndrome is an autosomal dominant disorder resulting from inherited or de novo *PTEN* pathogenic variants. It is associated with a high risk of benign and malignant tumors (breast, thyroid, kidney, and endometrium), trichilemmomas, papillomatous papules, gastrointestinal polyposis, and macrocephaly. Cowden syndrome has been estimated to affect 1 in 200,000 to 250,000 persons, but it is most likely underrecognized.

Thyroid involvement in Cowden syndrome is usually multinodular and bilateral. Benign thyroid nodules and thyroid cancer occur in approximately 75% and 35% of affected individuals, respectively.[24] Thyroid cancer is most often diagnosed in women and young adults, but it can be present at any age, even in early childhood. Although both PTC and FTC are observed in Cowden syndrome, FTC in particular is overrepresented compared with its incidence in the general population. The National Comprehensive Cancer Network recommends age-based screening for breast, uterine, and thyroid cancers, as well as renal ultrasonography and colonoscopy for patients with Cowden syndrome. Initiation of annual screening thyroid ultrasonography begins at the time of diagnosis in adults and at age 7 years in children.[25]

The thyroid nodule in this case was documented to have the *PTEN* c.388C> T (p.R130) variant through molecular testing; this specific pathogenic variant has been recurrently associated with *PTEN* hamartoma tumor syndrome.[24] The variant was detected in the sample at an allele frequency of 50%, where the allele frequency is the proportion of sequencing reads containing the gene variant divided by the total number of reads through the locus. Documentation of an allele frequency near 50% should raise concern for a germline pathogenic variant. However, evaluation for the same variant in nonneoplastic tissue is required to prove that the alteration is not somatic. Referral to a genetic counselor should be offered to the patient in the context of the molecular test results and her personal and family history of Cowden syndrome features. A genetic counselor can discuss genetic testing with the patient and her family and provide information on the mode of inheritance and clinical implications of a germline *PTEN* pathogenic variant.

The patient met with a genetic counselor, and testing confirmed the presence of a germline *PTEN* pathogenic variant. Because the documented

PTEN variant is germline, it can be concluded that the thyroid nodule in question has no genetic alterations that are somatic and is very likely benign. The nodule can thus be managed conservatively without surgery at this time; however, the patient will require routine screening for thyroid cancer on an ongoing basis with annual clinical neck examination and thyroid ultrasonography.[25]

Case 4

A 63-year-old woman is noted to have an isoechoic 3.5-cm left thyroid nodule during evaluation for amiodarone-induced thyrotoxicosis (AIT) type 2. AIT resolves. Results from FNA of the thyroid nodule are benign. The nodule slowly grows over 6 years. Results from repeated FNA are follicular neoplasm (Bethesda IV). Based on growth and cytology, the patient undergoes left lobectomy, which demonstrates a 6.4-cm minimally invasive FTC (no angioinvasion seen). Based on the size, the patient has completion thyroidectomy (no additional cancer) and rhTSH-stimulated radioiodine remnant ablation with 30 mCi [131]I (uptake in thyroid bed region only, thyroglobulin = 409 ng/mL [409 µg/L]). Three months after treatment, findings on neck ultrasonography are normal, her TSH concentration is 0.17 mIU/L, and thyroglobulin concentration is 1.7 ng/mL (1.7 µg/L) with negative thyroglobulin antibodies. At 12 months, her serum thyroglobulin and TSH concentrations are 20.0 ng/mL (20.0 µg/L) and 0.5 mIU/L, respectively.

How accurate are assessments of angioinvasion and capsular invasion in FTC >4 cm? Is the postoperative stimulated thyroglobulin concentration concerning? Is there a role for molecular testing in large, minimally invasive FTC? If she has persistent cancer, what are the most likely sites of persistent disease? What is the most appropriate next management step for this patient?

Minimally invasive FTC generally has an indolent course and can often be treated with lobectomy alone.[26] Risk factors for distant metastases in patients with minimally invasive FTC are age and tumor size.[27] Multivariate analyses from 292 patients with minimally invasive FTC showed that tumor size larger than 4 cm was an independent predictor of worse disease-free survival and disease-specific survival.[28] Therefore, patients with minimally invasive FTC larger than 4 cm should be approached differently than patients with smaller tumors. Furthermore, this patient had an rhTSH-stimulated thyroglobulin concentration of 409 ng/mL (409 µg/L) after thyroidectomy, which is also a very concerning feature. The 2 most common sites for distant metastases in patients with FTC are the lungs and bone. Imaging of the lungs (generally with noncontrast chest CT) and/or bones (nuclear medicine scan, skeletal MRI) would be reasonable next steps for this patient.

When the thyroglobulin concentration of 20.0 ng/mL (20.0 µg/L) on levothyroxine therapy was noted, the patient underwent a diagnostic ^{123}I whole-body scan and was noted to have an iliac crest lesion on SPECT imaging. After treatment with 146 mCi ^{131}I, the patient was noted to have multiple bone metastases (bilateral iliac crests, left femur, left fifth rib, inferior pubic ramus) and a left lower lung nodule.

Tissue was sent for ThyroSeq GC testing, which revealed an *HRAS* Q61R variant and a *TERT* 124C>T promoter variant. *RAS* variants are common in FTC. *TERT* promoter variants are rare in minimally invasive FTC but are associated with poor prognosis in differentiated thyroid cancer.[29,30] There are no studies exploring the utility of genetic testing in minimally invasive FTC, but this could be considered in older patients and in patients with larger tumors to determine whether higher-risk variants are present (*TERT* promoter, *TP53*, *PIK3CA*, etc) if monitoring with or without radioiodine is being considered.

Acknowledgment

The authors would like to thank Dr. Yuri Nikiforov, MD, PhD, from the Division of Molecular and Genomic Pathology at the University of Pittsburgh Medical Center, for providing the ThyroSeq report that served as the basis for Case 3.

References

1. Cibas ES, Ali SZ. The 2017 Bethesda system for reporting thyroid cytopathology. *Thyroid.* 2017;27(11):1341-1346. PMID: 29091573

2. Patel KN, Angell TE, Babiarz J, et al. Performance of a genomic sequencing classifier for the preoperative diagnosis of cytologically indeterminate thyroid nodules. *JAMA Surg.* 2018;153(9):817-824. PMID: 29799911

3. Hu MI, Waguespack SG, Dosiou C, et al. Afirma genomic sequencing classifier and Xpression Atlas molecular findings in consecutive Bethesda III-VI thyroid nodules. *J Clin Endocrinol Metab.* 2021;106(8):2198-2207. PMID: 34009369

4. Nikiforova MN, Lepe M, Tolino LA, et al. Thyroid cytology smear slides: an untapped resource for ThyroSeq testing. *Cancer Cytopathol.* 2021;129(1):33-42. PMID: 32697051

5. Steward DL, Carty SE, Sippel RS, et al. Performance of multigene genomic classifier in thyroid nodules with indeterminate cytology: a prospective blinded multicenter study. *JAMA Oncol.* 2019;5(2):204-212. PMID: 30419129

6. Livhits MJ, Zhu CY, Kuo EJ, et al. Effectiveness of molecular testing techniques for diagnosis of indeterminate thyroid nodules: a randomized clinical trial. *JAMA Oncol.* 2021;7(1):70-77. PMID: 33300952

7. Lupo MA, Walts AE, Sistrunk JW, et al. Multiplatform molecular test performance in indeterminate thyroid nodules. *Diagn Cytopathol.* 2020;48(12):1254-1264. PMID: 32767735

8. Schumm MA, Nguyen DT, Kim J, et al. Longitudinal assessment of quality of life following molecular testing for indeterminate thyroid nodules. *Ann Surg Oncol.* 2021;28(13):8872-8881. PMID: 34292427

9. Deaver KE, Haugen BR, Pozdeyev N, Marshall CB. Outcomes of Bethesda categories III and IV thyroid nodules over 5 years and performance of the Afirma gene expression classifier: a single-institution study. *Clin Endocrinol (Oxf).* 2018;89(2):226-232. PMID: 29791966

10. Angell TE, Frates MC, Medici M, et al. Afirma benign thyroid nodules show similar growth to cytologically benign nodules during follow-up. *J Clin Endocrinol Metab.* 2015;100(11):E1477-E1483. PMID: 26353010

11. Endo M, Porter K, Long C, et al. Features of cytologically indeterminate molecularly benign nodules treated with surgery. *J Clin Endocrinol Metab.* 2020;105(11):e3971-e3980. PMID: 32772084

12. Zhu CY, Donangelo I, Gupta D, et al. Outcomes of indeterminate thyroid nodules managed nonoperatively after molecular testing. *J Clin Endocrinol Metab.* 2021;106(3):e1240-e1247. PMID: 33394039

13. Haugen BR, Alexander EK, Bible KC, et al. 2015 American Thyroid Association management guidelines for adult patients with thyroid nodules and differentiated thyroid cancer: the American Thyroid Association Guidelines Task Force on Thyroid Nodules and Differentiated Thyroid Cancer. *Thyroid.* 2016;26(1):1-133. PMID: 26462967

14. Tessler FN, Middleton WD, Grant EG, et al. ACR Thyroid Imaging, Reporting and Data System (TI-RADS): white paper of the ACR TI-RADS Committee. *J Am Coll Radiol.* 2017;14(5):587-595. PMID: 28372962

15. Patel KN, Angell TE, Babiarz J, et al. Performance of a genomic sequencing classifier for the preoperative diagnosis of cytologically indeterminate thyroid nodules. *JAMA Surg.* 2018;153(9):817-824. PMID: 29799911

16. Rossi M, Buratto M, Bruni S, et al. Role of ultrasonographic/clinical profile, cytology, and BRAF V600E mutation evaluation in thyroid nodule screening for malignancy: a prospective study. *J Clin Endocrinol Metab.* 2012;97(7):2354-2361. PMID: 22535974

17. Miyauchi A, Kudo T, Ito Y, et al. Estimation of the lifetime probability of disease progression of papillary microcarcinoma of the thyroid during active surveillance. *Surgery.* 2018;163(1):48-52. PMID: 29103582

18. Ho AS, Luu M, Zalt C, et al. Mortality risk of nonoperative papillary thyroid carcinoma: a corollary for active surveillance. *Thyroid.* 2019;29(10):1409-1417. PMID: 31407637

19. Molinaro E, Campopiano MC, Pieruzzi L, et al. Active surveillance in papillary thyroid microcarcinomas is feasible and safe: experience at a single Italian center. *J Clin Endocrinol Metab.* 2020;105(3):e172-e180. PMID: 31652318

20. Dahia PL, Marsh DJ, Zheng Z, et al. Somatic deletions and mutations in the Cowden disease gene, PTEN, in sporadic thyroid tumors. *Cancer Res.* 1997;57(21):4710-4713. PMID: 9354427

21. Pozdeyev N, Gay LM, Sokol ES, et al. Genetic analysis of 779 advanced differentiated and anaplastic thyroid cancers. *Clin Cancer Res.* 2018;24(13):3059-3068. PMID: 29615459

22. Nagy R, Ganapathi S, Comeras I, et al. Frequency of germline PTEN mutations in differentiated thyroid cancer. *Thyroid.* 2011;21(5):505-510. PMID: 21417916

23. Yehia L, Eng C. 65 years of the double helix: one gene, many endocrine and metabolic syndromes: PTEN-opathies and precision medicine. *Endocr Relat Cancer.* 2018;25(8):T121-T140. PMID: 29792313

24. Yehia L, Eng C. *PTEN* Hamartoma Tumor Syndrome. In: Adam MP, Ardinger HH, Pagon RA, et al, eds. GeneReviews. PMID: 20301661

25. NCCN clinical practice guidelines in oncology.: National Comprehensive Cancer Network (NCCN). 2021.

26. Goffredo P, Cheung K, Roman SA, Sosa JA. Can minimally invasive follicular thyroid cancer be approached as a benign lesion?: a population-level analysis of survival among 1,200 patients. *Ann Surg Oncol.* 2013;20(3):767-772. PMID: 23111705

27. Sugino K, Ito K, Nagahama M, et al. Prognosis and prognostic factors for distant metastases and tumor mortality in follicular thyroid carcinoma. *Thyroid.* 2011;21(7):751-757. PMID: 21615311

28. Ito Y, Hirokawa M, Masuoka H, et al. Prognostic factors of minimally invasive follicular thyroid carcinoma: extensive vascular invasion significantly affects patient prognosis. *Endocr J.* 2013;60(5):637-642. PMID: 23327839

29. Moon S, Song YS, Kim YA, et al. Effects of coexistent BRAFV600E and TERT promoter mutations on poor clinical outcomes in papillary thyroid cancer: a meta-analysis. *Thyroid.* 2017;27(5):651-660. PMID: 28181854

30. Liu R, Bishop J, Zhu G, Zhang T, Ladenson PW, Xing M. Mortality risk stratification by combining BRAF V600E and TERT promoter mutations in papillary thyroid cancer: genetic duet of BRAF and TERT promoter mutations in thyroid cancer mortality. *JAMA Oncol.* 2017;3(2):202-208. PMID: 27581851

What's Wrong With This Picture? Challenging Cases in Thyroid Ultrasonography

Jennifer A. Sipos, MD. Division of Endocrinology, The Ohio State University, Columbus, OH; E-mail: Jennifer.Sipos@osumc.edu

Learning Objectives

As a result of participating in this session, learners should be able to:

- Define suspicious sonographic findings on ultrasonography of thyroid nodules and categorize thyroid nodules using the American Thyroid Association (ATA) and the American College of Radiology (ACR) Thyroid Imaging Reporting and Data System (TI-RADS) sonographic risk stratification systems (SRSSs).

- Discuss the strengths and limitations of the ATA and ACR TI-RADS SRSSs.

Main Conclusions

Sonographic characterization is an effective means to triage thyroid nodules and provide insight into the malignancy risk. Several sonographic features are highly predictive of identifying papillary thyroid carcinoma, including invasive margins, taller-than-wide shape, and punctate echogenic foci in a solid nodule. All of the SRSSs identify these lesions similarly well. Nodules that have less specific and/or low-risk findings still harbor a nonnegligible risk of malignancy and may warrant further investigation based on their size and the patient's clinical scenario.

Significance of the Clinical Problem

Thyroid nodules are a common clinical entity, and the sheer volume in the general population precludes aspiration of all identified lesions. Furthermore, most thyroid nodules are benign. It is incumbent on the clinician to risk stratify nodules and thereby enrich the pool of clinically concerning nodules that harbor a higher likelihood of malignancy. Several SRSSs[1,2] have been created to aid in the decision of which nodules warrant additional evaluation. Uncertainty exists, however, regarding which SRSS is optimal for nodule classification. Ideally an SRSS should provide both high sensitivity and high specificity. The ATA system[2] provides high sensitivity but lower specificity, while ACR TI-RADS[1] provides improved specificity at the expense of lower sensitivity for detection of malignancy.[3] Nonetheless, both systems perform similarly well for the identification of intermediate- and high-risk nodules. The main difference between these SRSSs lies in the size thresholds for FNA.[4]

This session will help the clinician understand the pitfalls of each SRSS while also providing real-time feedback regarding nodule classification. Furthermore, this session will examine the physics behind ultrasonography and its associated artifacts to aid the clinician in diagnosing the underlying pathophysiology seen on bedside ultrasonography.

Barriers to Optimal Practice

- Clinician confidence and reference standards to accurately classify nodules.

- Adequate time allotment in a busy clinic for carefully performing ultrasonography to characterize the nodule and optimize image captures.

- Each SRSS has specific limitations in its usage and classification of thyroid nodules.

Strategies for Diagnosis, Therapy, and/or Management

Ultrasonography is an invaluable tool for the evaluation of thyroid nodules; it helps stratify a large proportion of nodules into higher- or lower-risk categories. It is also important, however, for clinicians using ultrasonography for nodule triage to familiarize themselves with the strengths and limitations of this technology.

Suspicious sonographic features such as irregular/infiltrative margins, taller-than-wide shape, and punctate echogenic foci have a high specificity for predicting malignancy. These features are typically associated with papillary thyroid carcinoma. Indeed, SRSSs generally perform very well in identifying papillary thyroid carcinomas. Follicular-patterned tumors, however, are more likely to have a less specific appearance; they are often isoechoic, have well-defined margins, and typically lack suspicious sonographic features.[5] Thus, many histologically follicular-patterned tumors, such as follicular carcinoma, noninvasive follicular tumor with papillary like nuclear features (NIFTP), and follicular variant of papillary thyroid cancer fall into lower sonographic risk categories (low/intermediate risk with ATA and TR2 or TR3). A major limitation of the current literature evaluating the efficacy of SRSSs for malignancy risk prediction is that many studies eliminate nodules with indeterminate cytology, which disproportionately excludes follicular-patterned tumors. Consequently, very few studies have a sufficient number of nodules to carefully examine the performance of a given SRSS in diagnosing follicular tumors.

An additional limitation of sonographic evaluation of thyroid nodules is interobserver variability of reporting individual sonographic features. The features associated with the highest interobserver variability are the presence of capsular invasion, microcalcifications, and nodule margins.[6] ACR TI-RADS is thus subject to the potential for overscoring or underscoring a nodule using a summation of nodule features. The ATA SRSS uses pattern-based recognition in an attempt to lessen the impact of this potential bias.[2] Unfortunately, with this pattern-based system, not all types of nodules are currently characterized and some nodules are unable to be risk stratified.

An additional concern with sonographic evaluation of thyroid nodules is the relative weight assigned to individual features for malignancy risk prediction. A recent study[7] using artificial intelligence to stratify biopsy-proven thyroid nodules validated ACR TI-RADS but found that the assignment of new scores to individual features improved the specificity while still maintaining the sensitivity. The findings suggested that hyperechogenicity or isoechogenicity should not be assigned any points and that microcalcifications or coarse calcifications should be the only types of calcifications for which points are given.

Finally, it is important for clinicians to approach a thyroid nodule from within the framework of the clinical scenario, considering patient age, family history, radiation exposure, and comorbidities. None of the current SRSSs consider the patient's clinical context when assigning malignancy risk. These patient-related factors can significantly influence the decision to perform FNA and/or guide the optimal evaluation strategy. Because most thyroid cancers are indolent tumors, patients with certain comorbid conditions may be more suitable for observation alone rather than undergo FNA, even in the setting of a sonographically suspicious nodule. However, a young, healthy patient with a strong family history of thyroid cancer may be an appropriate candidate for a lower threshold for FNA if an indeterminate or high-risk nodule is identified.

Clinical Case Vignettes

Case 1

A 24-year-old nonbinary patient presents to the endocrine clinic for evaluation of a thyroid nodule incidentally detected during the evaluation of neck injury after a motor vehicle accident. There are no compressive symptoms, history of radiation exposure, or family history of thyroid cancer. The radiologist who performed ultrasonography described a 1.4 × 1.2 × 1.6-cm ACR TI-RADS 4 nodule (5 points) (*see Figure*). The report indicated a spongiform nodule (0 points) with infiltrative margins (2 points) (*asterisk*) and linear calcifications (2 points) (*arrows*).

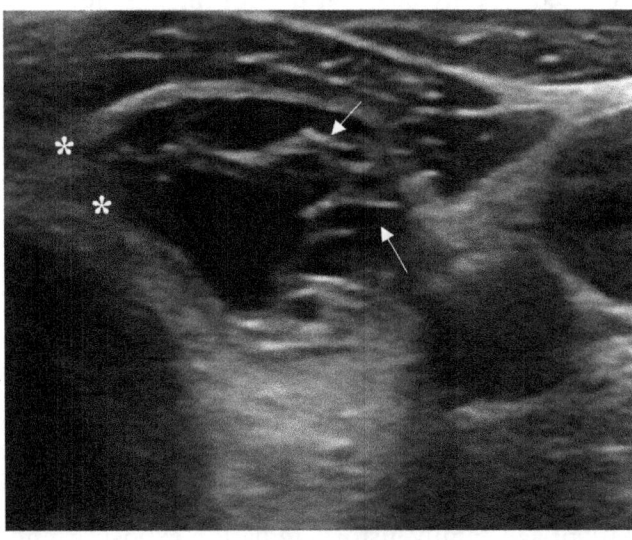

The patient is referred for consideration of FNA of the intermediate-risk nodule.

Which of the following is the best next step in this patient's management?

A. Evaluate with elastography

B. Order ^{123}I or technetium scan

C. Perform FNA

D. Reassure the patient

E. Refer for ethanol ablation

Answer: D) Reassure the patient

This is a spongiform nodule. These lesions have a very low risk of malignancy (<3%). The ATA guidelines recommend *either* FNA *or* observation of these lesions if they are larger than 2.0 cm. The nodule does not meet the size threshold for FNA (Answer C), so reassuring the patient (Answer D) is correct.

Scintigraphy with ^{123}I or technetium (Answer B) is not needed in this case unless the TSH concentration is low. It would be reasonable, however, to measure the patient's serum TSH since it has not yet been done.

Ethanol ablation (Answer E) is incorrect because nodules should be aspirated twice to definitively rule out malignancy before referral for the procedure.

Elastography (Answer A) can be helpful in the assessment of thyroid nodules for further refining malignancy risk, but it is not necessary in this setting, as the nodule is already clearly a very low-risk lesion. Furthermore, elastography cannot be used for nodules that are predominantly cystic.

A very important question in this case is how are the 2 SRSSs so divergent in the malignancy risk of this nodule? According to the radiology report that used ACR TI-RADS, this nodule has an intermediate risk of malignancy. In contrast, using the ATA SRSS, it is a very low-suspicion lesion. One of the limitations of ACR TI-RADS is the potential for overassigning risk in a given nodule due to the use of individual features. The one situation where pattern recognition is recommended for use with ACR TI-RADS is in the setting of a spongiform nodule. The first step in evaluating a nodule with ACR TI-RADS involves determination of the nodule composition. If a nodule is composed of more than 50% small cystic spaces, it is classified as spongiform and further points should not be added for the other categories (echogenicity, shape, margins, or echogenic foci). In this case, the radiologist continued to assign points for the individual nodule features and the malignancy risk was falsely elevated. If used appropriately, both systems would accurately categorize this nodule as low risk. But in this scenario, the radiologist inappropriately continued to assign the ACR TI-RADS point in the assessment of this spongiform nodule.

One final note: the areas of "linear calcifications" seen in this nodule are not actually calcifications. Rather, these represent linear areas of posterior acoustic enhancement that are visible in the septations located posterior to a cystic area. These are commonly seen in spongiform nodules. It is an artifact due to the change in acoustic impedance between a cystic area and a solid septation. A strong reflection of waves back to the ultrasound occurs when the wave moves from the cystic medium to the solid, resulting in a brighter-than-expected appearance of the septations.

Case 2

A 75-year-old man is referred for a nodule that was incidentally noted on ^{18}F-fluorodeoxyglucose PET done for prostate cancer staging. The nodule is metabolically active, with a standard uptake value of 15. On ultrasonography, the nodule measures 1.6 × 1.5 × 2.2 cm (*see Figures*).

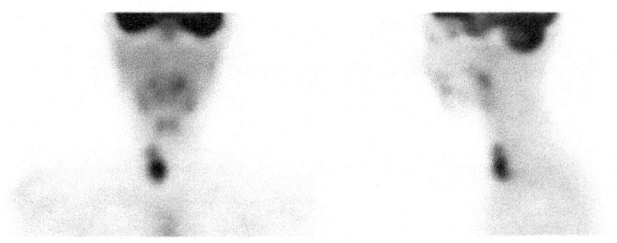

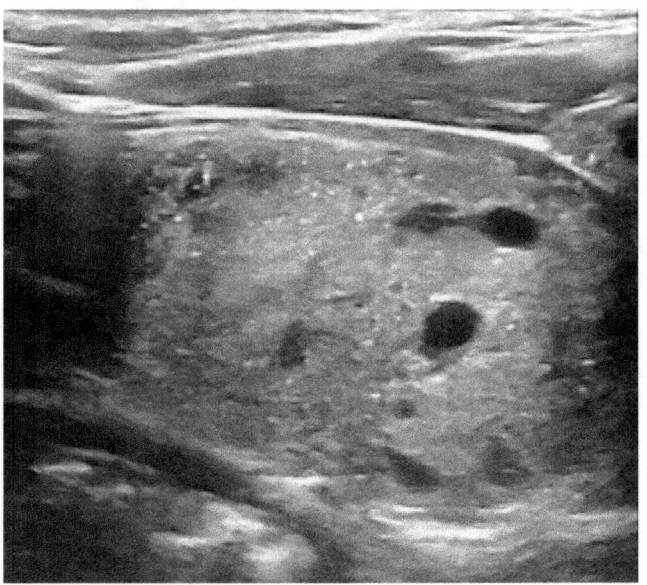

Which of the following is the ATA risk classification of this nodule?

A. Very low suspicion

B. Low suspicion

C. Intermediate suspicion

D. High suspicion

E. Nonclassifiable

Answer: E) Nonclassifiable

This nodule is isoechoic, partially cystic, and has punctate echogenic foci. It is not spongiform because it is less than 50% cystic. This nodule is nonclassifiable (Answer E) with the ATA SRSS. It is ACR TI-RADS TR4 (solid [2], isoechoic [1], regular margins [0], wider than tall [0], microcalcifications [3] = 6 points).

Several types of nodules are currently not captured with the ATA SRSS. These include isoechoic or cystic nodules with 1 or more suspicious sonographic feature(s), including taller-than-wide shape, infiltrative margins, or punctate echogenic foci. Additionally, coarse calcifications are not captured with the ATA system. In these scenarios, ACR TI-RADS may be used to classify the nodule.

The frequency of ATA nonclassifiable lesions is variably reported in the literature, between 2.7% and 17.9%.[8,9] The malignancy risk associated with ATA nonclassifiable lesions is also variably reported, between 9.4% and 18.8%,[10,11] which overlaps with risk associated with the intermediate suspicion category of nodules in the ATA SRSS (10%-20%).[2]

References

1. Tessler FN, et al. ACR thyroid imaging, reporting and data system (TI-RADS): white paper of the ACR TI-RADS committee. *J Am Coll Radiol.* 2017;14(5):587-595.

2. Haugen BR, et al. 2015 American Thyroid Association management guidelines for adult patients with thyroid nodules and differentiated thyroid cancer: the American Thyroid Association Guidelines Task Force on Thyroid Nodules and Differentiated Thyroid Cancer. *Thyroid.* 2016;26(1):1-133.

3. Kim PH, et al. Unnecessary thyroid nodule biopsy rates under four ultrasound risk stratification systems: a systematic review and meta-analysis. *Eur Radiol.* 2021;31(5):2877-2885.

4. Yim Y, et al. Concordance of three international guidelines for thyroid nodules classified by ultrasonography and diagnostic performance of biopsy criteria. *Korean J Radiol.* 2020;21(1):108-116.

5. Jeh SK, Jung SL, Kim BS, Lee YS. Evaluating the degree of conformity of papillary carcinoma and follicular carcinoma to the reported ultrasonographic findings of malignant thyroid tumor. *Korean J Radiol.* 2007;8(3):192-197. PMID: 17554185

6. Grani G, Lamartina L, Cantisani V, Maranghi M, Lucia P, Durante C. Interobserver agreement of various thyroid imaging reporting and data systems. *Endocr Connect.* 2018;7(1):1-7. PMID: 29196301

7. Wildman-Tobriner B, Buda M, Hoang JK, et al. Using artificial intelligence to revise ACR TI-RADS risk stratification of thyroid nodules: diagnostic accuracy and utility. *Radiology.* 2019;292(1):112-119. PMID: 31112088

8. Grani G, Lamartina L, Ascoli V, et al. Reducing the number of unnecessary thyroid biopsies while improving diagnostic accuracy: toward the "right" TIRADS. *J Clin Endocrinol Metab.* 2019;104(1):95-102. PMID: 30299457

9. Gao L, Xi X, Wang J, et al. Ultrasound risk evaluation of thyroid nodules that are "unspecified" in the 2015 American Thyroid Association management guidelines: a retrospective study. *Medicine (Baltimore).* 2018;97(52):e13914. PMID: 30593211

10. Ruan J-L, Yang H-Y, Liu R-B, et al. Fine needle aspiration biopsy indications for thyroid nodules: compare a point-based risk stratification system with a pattern-based risk stratification system. *Eur Radiol.* 2019;29(9):4871-4878. PMID: 30715590

11. Ha EJ, Na DG, Baek JH, Sung JY, Kim J-H, Kang SY. US fine-needle aspiration biopsy for thyroid malignancy: diagnostic performance of seven society guidelines applied to 2000 thyroid nodules. *Radiology.* 2018;287(3):893-900. PMID: 29465333

Unmet Needs in Hypothyroidism

Elizabeth A. McAninch, MD. Division of Endocrinology, Gerontology and Metabolism, Stanford University School of Medicine, Stanford, CA; E-mail: lizzymac@stanford.edu

Learning Objectives

As a result of participating in this session, learners should be able to:

- Identify patients with hypothyroidism who may benefit from a trial of combination therapy and counsel them on the potential risks and benefits of combination therapy.

- Perform a trial of combination therapy for eligible patients with hypothyroidism.

Main Conclusions

The standard of care for treatment of hypothyroidism remains levothyroxine at dosages to achieve a normal serum TSH concentration. Most patients do well with this approach with restoration of clinical and biochemical euthyroidism. However, a minority of patients experience residual hypothyroid symptoms despite normalization of serum TSH. Evaluation for other potential etiologies should be performed in these patients. In more than a dozen clinical trials, superiority of combination therapy has not been consistently demonstrated. A roadmap for designing new, better clinical trials has been outlined, but in the meantime, clinicians can consider a trial of combination therapy (levothyroxine plus liothyronine) in nonpregnant adults with residual symptomatology due to hypothyroidism.

Currently available liothyronine formulations exhibit pharmacokinetic properties that do not well mimic physiologic, stable serum T_3 levels (supraphysiologic serum peaks and short half-life). There are potential safety concerns due to insufficient long-term outcome data, but many recent clinical trials have shown no increased morbidity or mortality. Further longitudinal safety studies are needed. The safety of liothyronine is unknown in patients with comorbid osteoporosis, psychiatric disease, cardiovascular disease, or atrial fibrillation.

For individuals on levothyroxine with a normal serum TSH level, combination therapy can be initiated by decreasing the levothyroxine dosage by 12 to 25 mcg daily and adding liothyronine, 2.5 to 5 mcg once or twice daily. For monitoring peak levels, serum T_3 should be assessed 2 to 4 hours after liothyronine consumption. Normalization of serum TSH and optimization of symptoms remain the treatment goals. If no symptomatic improvement is noted, levothyroxine monotherapy can be resumed.

Significance of the Clinical Problem

In endogenous euthyroidism, the thyroid gland secretes about 5 to 6.5 µg of T_3 daily.[1,2] Most T_3 (~20 µg) is produced in the periphery by deiodination pathways. The sum of these contributors results in remarkably stable serum T_3 levels in euthyroid individuals.[3] Hypothyroidism is highly prevalent, affecting about 5% of the population in iodine-sufficient regions.[4] Treatment standard of care is levothyroxine,[1] which is consistently one of the most prescribed pharmaceuticals in the United States.[5] It is increasingly well-recognized that a minority (about 14% in one study[6]) of hypothyroid patients on levothyroxine experience symptoms that could be consistent with residual symptoms of hypothyroidism. In voluntary patient surveys (subject to sampling bias), dissatisfaction is even more prominent.[7,8] Given the high prevalence of hypothyroidism, the proportion of those struggling with residual symptomatology represents a significant number of individuals. It is well-established that hypothyroid patients treated with levothyroxine exhibit higher serum T_4-to-T_3 ratios.[9-12] The acknowledgment of residual symptomatology and altered T_4-to-T_3 ratios exhibited by levothyroxine-treated hypothyroid patients has fueled the hypothesis that these symptoms may be due to relative T_3 deficiency within the peripheral tissues.

In an effort to ameliorate residual symptomatology and better approximate physiologic serum T_4-to-T_3 ratios, combination therapy with levothyroxine plus liothyronine has been explored with mixed results, failing to demonstrate consistent superiority in clinical trials.[13] However these trials were heterogenous in design and recruitment.[14] One of the potential barriers in such trials is the lack of FDA-approved sustained-release T_3 preparations. The American, British, and European Thyroid Associations have outlined proposals for the design of new trials,[14] but until those can be accomplished, clinicians ultimately must balance the biochemical parameters, symptomatology, and any comorbidities within individual patients. Several recent studies have shown no morbidity or mortality with combination therapy.[15-17] Combination therapy is more complex to prescribe (multiple doses daily), more costly, and more complex to monitor than monotherapy. Despite these complexities, many clinicians are prescribing combination therapy.[18] Some helpful prescribing parameters have been proposed by experts in the field.[19,20] Most agree that the treatment goal in hypothyroidism is to restore euthyroidism, but exactly how to best achieve this remains controversial.

Barriers to Optimal Practice

- Residual symptoms are often subjective and nonspecific.

- Liothyronine pharmacokinetics are challenging (short half-life, supratherapeutic peak).

- Clinical trial results of combination therapy inconsistently demonstrate "superiority."

- More long-term safety data of liothyronine are needed. The safety in individuals with preexisting comorbidities such as psychiatric disease, cardiovascular disease, atrial fibrillation, and osteoporosis is unknown.

- Should achieving a physiologic T_4-to-T_3 ratio be a therapeutic goal? If so, when should T_3 be measured?

Strategies for Diagnosis, Therapy, and/or Management

Since the 1970s, the standard of care for hypothyroidism has been levothyroxine monotherapy at dosages to achieve a normal serum TSH level.[21] That the deiodinases convert T_4-to-T_3 in the periphery[22] provided justification for this approach. In more recent years, however, this dogma has been the subject of intense study, with many groups of investigators finding that levothyroxine-treated hypothyroid patients with normal serum TSH levels may not be systemically euthyroid.[9,14,23,24] Even when only considering levothyroxine, there is strong evidence if its pervasive overuse[25,26] and inadequate/inefficient dosing,[27,28] perhaps suggesting that even its use is not entirely straightforward.

Objectively, despite normal serum TSH, LDL cholesterol and total cholesterol can remain elevated[24,29,30] and the metabolic rate is slower[23,31,32] in population studies. Compared with individuals with endogenous euthyroidism, hypothyroid patients report lower metabolic equivalents, weigh more, and report more antidepressant and statin use.[9] Subjectively, patients can experience residual fatigue, "brain fog,"[33] and have mood complaints.

These findings are all supported by rodent models where animals with hypothyroidism have a lower metabolic rate and higher serum lipid profiles despite treatment with levothyroxine monotherapy.[34,35] All thyroid professional societies now acknowledge that some patients with hypothyroidism can experience residual symptoms despite treatment with levothyroxine at dosages that normalize serum TSH.[36]

Patients may be dissatisfied with therapy and feel that their symptoms are dismissed by providers.[7] The finding that levothyroxine + liothyronine combination therapy could improve symptoms was heralded,[6] but interestingly, this has not been consistently demonstrated in clinical trials,[13] creating major controversy in the field. There are important limitations due to liothyronine pharmacokinetics: it has a short half-life and supratherapeutic peak, necessitating multiple daily doses to even approach mimicking physiologic replacement. It is not known whether, if physiologically dosed, the combination therapy trial results would offer more clarity. Although exciting new liothyronine formulations and thyroid transplant technologies are on the horizon,[37-39] clinicians are left dealing with this highly prevalent clinical dilemma in the present. The field currently lacks substantial knowledge of exactly what liothyronine's risks are, ineligibility criteria for combination therapy, treatment goals (Serum TSH only? Serum T_4-to-T_3 ratios? Subjective symptoms/preference?), treatment monitoring, and the specific dosing ratios and timing of levothyroxine + liothyronine.[14] Thus, how to best restore thyroid hormone homeostasis in patients with hypothyroidism is a rapidly evolving topic.

Risk-to-Benefit Ratio

The American, British, and European Thyroid Association guidelines have recently evolved in their recognition of the potential limitations of levothyroxine.[36] This shift is reflected in prescribing patterns: physician use of combination therapy is prevalent and possibly increasing.[18]

The guidelines suggest that patients who feel "unwell," "not benefited," or who have "persistent complaints" could be considered for an n-of-1 trial of combination therapy.[1,19] Clinical trial results have been inconsistent, but some trials have shown benefits, including improved weight management and preference for combination therapy.[13,15,16,40]

The clinical syndrome of T_3 thyrotoxicosis due to Graves disease has well-defined consequences that include increased risks of psychosis, fracture, osteoporosis, atrial fibrillation, and cardiovascular events. Before the development of the TSH radioimmunoassay,[41] much higher dosages of thyroid hormone replacement in hypothyroidism were used and such adverse effects were not uncommon.[21] In the modern era, despite a reliable serum TSH assay, concern for these potentially devastating risks persists. These concerns are perhaps amplified by the pharmacokinetic profile of liothyronine, which results in fluctuating serum levels, often with transient hypertriiodothyroninemia at its peak.[42] That being said, there has not been a modern study showing serum T_3 fluctuations within the reference range (while preserving normal serum TSH) to be associated with adverse events[19]; the longest of these studies followed patients for 1 year. In a large population study conducted over 17 years (more than 250,000 person-years total follow-up), individuals on liothyronine therapy were found to have double the risk of receiving an incident antipsychotic prescription, but no increased risk of fracture, atrial fibrillation, or cardiovascular events.[17] Further, rigorous exploration of the safety of levothyroxine + liothyronine combination therapy is needed before the risks can be fully described to patients and likely before the routine use of combination therapy can be recommended by professional society guidelines. There have been no safety studies performed in elderly participants or in those with preexisting cardiovascular disease, atrial fibrillation, or osteoporosis, so clinicians are unable to adequately describe the risks to patients and obtain informed consent.

Prescribing Levothyroxine + Liothyronine

The physiologic T_4-to-T_3 ratio secreted by the human thyroid is approximately 14:1, of which about 5 to 6.5 mcg of T_3 is secreted daily.[1,2] There are several combination pills with various fixed T_4-to-T_3 ratios in Europe (10:1, 5:1, 4:1).[43] In the United States, the only such combination formulation is in desiccated porcine thyroid, where the T_4-to-T_3 ratio is approximately 4:1; this is not FDA-approved. In the United States, liothyronine is available in 5-, 25-, and 50-mcg tablets, so multiples of 2.5 mcg (half tablet) or 5 mcg are usually used. Liothyronine to levothyroxine dose equivalency is considered to be about 3:1.[44] As the guidelines currently state, all patients should be prescribed levothyroxine at initial diagnosis, with the dosage titrated to achieve a normal serum TSH level. Once the clinician has identified an appropriate candidate for an n-of-1 therapeutic trial, in theory, one has the advantage of knowing the levothyroxine dosage that normalized the patient's serum TSH. Levothyroxine + liothyronine combination therapy can then be estimated in the context of these known variables.

For example, if patient A has a normal serum TSH concentration on levothyroxine, 88 mcg daily, a reasonable first option would be to decrease the levothyroxine dosage to 75 mcg and add liothyronine, 2.5 mcg twice daily or 5 mcg once daily (T_4-to-T_3 ratio = 15:1). If patient B has a normal serum TSH concentration on levothyroxine, 150 mcg daily, a reasonable option would be to decrease the levothyroxine dosage to 125 mcg daily and add liothyronine, 5 mcg twice daily (T_4-to-T_3 ratio = 12.5:1). Measuring serum TSH about 6 weeks after the dosage change is the minimum requirement, and if one wishes to evaluate for hypertriiodothyroninemia, total T_3 can be measured within 2 to 4 hours of the morning liothyronine dose. As with levothyroxine dosing, there is no simple formula that predicts the "correct" dose in every patient and dosage adjustments may be needed depending on serum thyroid function tests and symptoms.

Anecdotal Experience

Since 2014, I have been offering to prescribe levothyroxine + liothyronine to select, dissatisfied patients struggling with residual hypothyroid symptoms. In my clinical practice, I have patients whose symptoms do not improve on combination therapy after a few dosage adjustments, so they agree to resume levothyroxine monotherapy. I also have had patients experience palpitations, exacerbation of menopausal hot flashes, insomnia, and anxiety while on combination therapy, which leads to them to ask to have their regimen converted back to levothyroxine monotherapy. Interestingly, even in these patients, I have observed that the serum T_3 measured at its peak to be within the normal range when using doses of 2.5 to 5 mcg liothyronine. There are patients who feel the extra cost and dosing schedules do not justify any benefit, whose regimens are thus converted back to levothyroxine monotherapy. Most of my patients (who had residual symptoms on levothyroxine and thus opted to embark on a therapeutic trial— selection bias!) prefer levothyroxine + liothyronine combination therapy over levothyroxine monotherapy. Most of my patients on combination therapy are prescribed dosages of 2.5 mcg liothyronine twice daily or 5 mcg liothyronine once or twice daily. Anecdotally, among my long-time patients, the dosages of liothyronine that maximize clinical benefit/preference vary from 2.5 mcg liothyronine every morning (postmenopausal patient with Hashimoto thyroiditis) to 7.5 mcg liothyronine twice daily (athyreotic athlete). Thrice-daily liothyronine is too burdensome for most of my patients. I take great care to listen to them and provide the most therapeutic environment that I can, as I believe that the patient-physician relationship must be optimized to embark on this exploratory journey together to evaluate these often subjective, *je ne sais quoi*, symptoms.

Clinical Case Vignettes

Case 1

A 57-year-old postmenopausal woman presents with large, symptomatic, nontoxic multinodular goiter. She is otherwise healthy. After several FNA biopsies of dominant nodules over the years demonstrating benign characteristics, she opts to proceed with thyroidectomy for worsening compressive symptoms. She has total thyroidectomy with a high-volume thyroid surgeon and starts levothyroxine replacement at 1.6 mcg/kg per day (150 mcg daily).

She has a follow-up appointment 4 weeks postoperatively. She feels wonderful! She is very pleased that she had surgery, after years of bothersome, progressing, compressive symptoms.

Laboratory test results:

> Serum TSH = 2.01 mIU/L (0.45-4.50 mIU/L)
> Serum PTH, normal
> Serum calcium, normal

One month later (8 weeks postoperatively), the patient sends a message through the electronic health record: "My energy has been pretty low. I'm tired almost all the time. I cannot function at work. I know my blood work was in the "normal" range, but is there anything that can be done? Our next appointment isn't until the end of next month, which seems too long to wait." Blood counts and metabolic panel are normal.

Laboratory test results:

> Serum TSH = 1.8 mIU/L (0.45-4.50 mIU/L)
> Free T_4 = 1.5 ng/dL (0.82-1.77 ng/dL)
>   (SI: 19.3 pmol/L [10.6-22.8 pmol/L])
> Total T_3 = 87 ng/dL (71-180 ng/dL)
>   (SI: 1.34 nmol/L [1.09-2.8 pmol/L])

Which of the following is the most appropriate next step in this patient's management?

A. Continue levothyroxine at same dosage

B. Increase the levothyroxine dosage to 175 mcg daily, aiming to achieve low-normal serum TSH

C. Offer a therapeutic trial with desiccated thyroid

D. Offer a therapeutic trial with levothyroxine, 125 mcg daily, plus liothyronine, 5 mcg twice daily

E. Offer a therapeutic trial with levothyroxine, 137 mcg daily, plus liothyronine, 2.5 mcg twice daily

Answer: D or E) Offer a therapeutic trial with levothyroxine, 125 mcg daily, plus liothyronine, 5 mcg twice daily or offer a therapeutic trial with levothyroxine, 137 mcg daily, plus liothyronine, 2.5 mcg twice daily

This healthy, previously hormonally asymptomatic patient presents with acute-onset symptoms after thyroidectomy that could be associated with hypothyroidism. She has no known cardiac or bone disease. Reassurance that her thyroid function test results are normal does not address her symptoms, so continuing levothyroxine at the same dosage (Answer A) is incorrect.

Increasing the levothyroxine dosage while serum TSH remains within reference range has not been shown to improve symptoms in randomized controlled clinical trials (Answer B).[23]

Desiccated thyroid (Answer C) is not FDA-approved and contains supraphysiologic T_3 doses for humans.

A therapeutic trial with levothyroxine and liothyronine could be offered, and both dosing regimens listed (Answers D and E) are reasonable; they represent more physiologic serum T_4-to-T_3 ratios.[19,20]

Case 2

A 50-year-old woman is a night-shift worker who has been on long-term thyroid hormone treatment (about 20 years), after initially presenting with weight gain, fatigue, and increased hair shedding. She seeks a third opinion. She recalls that her initial diagnostic evaluation yielded thyroid function test results that were within the reference range but that her reverse T_3 was "off." One year ago, she sought a second opinion from an endocrinologist because of continued symptoms, and that physician recommended changing to a brand-name, gluten-free levothyroxine formulation and adding liothyronine.

She is a single parent to 2 school-aged children whom she transports and cares for during the day. During the 2 to 4 hours of sleep she gets per day, she snores. She feels fatigued, reports difficultly losing weight, and has noticed that her hair is shedding excessively. Her symptoms have not improved since thyroid hormone initiation 20 years ago, or since the initiation of combination therapy last year. She has no history of depression, hopelessness, or suicidal ideation. Twenty-four–hour urinary free cortisol excretion is within the reference range. Four hours after her levothyroxine (63 mcg daily) and liothyronine (5 mcg every morning) are administered, blood is collected for analysis.

Laboratory test results:

> Serum TSH = 0.246 mIU/L (0.45-4.50 mIU/L)
> Free T_4 = 1.54 ng/dL (0.82-1.77 ng/dL)
>   (SI: 19.8 pmol/L [10.6-22.8 pmol/L])
> Total T_3 = 130 ng/dL (71-180 ng/dL)
>   (SI: 2.0 nmol/L [1.09-2.77 pmol/L])
> Free T_3 = 4.0 pg/mL (2.0-4.4 pg/mL)
>   (SI: 6.1 pmol/L [3.1-6.8 pmol/L])

Which of the following should be advised?

A. Continue current regimen and evaluate for other causes of fatigue

B. Decrease liothyronine, repeat thyroid function tests in 4 to 6 weeks

C. Discontinue liothyronine, repeat thyroid function tests in 4 to 6 weeks

D. Discontinue levothyroxine, repeat thyroid function tests in 4 to 6 weeks

E. Discontinue levothyroxine and liothyronine, repeat thyroid function tests in 4 to 6 weeks

Answer: E) Discontinue levothyroxine and liothyronine, repeat thyroid function tests in 4 to 6 weeks

The symptoms of hypothyroidism are nonspecific; therefore, a biochemical diagnosis must be consistent with hypothyroidism before treatment can be appropriately initiated. However, many individuals with endogenous euthyroidism are inappropriately treated with thyroid hormone supplementation,[26] perhaps due to nonspecific symptomatology.[1] This patient has a history suggestive of endogenous euthyroidism. Thyroid hormone supplementation should not be continued (Answers A, B, C, and D) until a concrete biochemical diagnosis of hypothyroidism can be established. After discontinuation of thyroid hormone (Answer E), the following laboratory values were documented:

> Serum TSH = 1.67 mIU/L
> Free T_4 = 1.21 ng/dL (SI: 15.6 pmol/L)
> Total T_3 = 97 ng/dL (SI: 1.5 nmol/L)
> Free T_3 = 2.6 pg/mL (SI: 4.0 pmol/L)

She was diagnosed with moderate obstructive sleep apnea and shift-work disorder.

Case 3

A 27-year-old G0P0 woman with history of postsurgical hypothyroidism (benign goiter at age 20 years) presents to establish care. She is otherwise healthy. Her menses are regular, and she has a copper intrauterine device. She plans to remove the intrauterine device in about 5 years to conceive. Immediately after thyroidectomy, her previous physician had prescribed desiccated porcine thyroid extract, 120 mg every morning. She has never tried another thyroid hormone replacement regimen. She has no palpitations, fluctuating energy levels, heat intolerance, anxiety, or weight change. She exercises a few times per week and has no dyspnea on exertion, muscle aches, or weakness. She feels normal and has no concerns. She is satisfied with her current regimen. Her physician retired recently, so she is seeking to establish care.

On physical examination, her weight is 125.6 lb (57 kg) (BMI = 21 kg/m^2). Her pulse rate is 76 beats/min, and blood pressure is 108/68 mm Hg. Cardiac auscultation reveals no murmurs, and remaining examination findings are normal.

Laboratory test results:

Serum TSH = 2.0 mIU/L (0.45-4.50 mIU/L)
Free T$_4$ = 0.9 ng/dL (0.82-1.77 ng/dL)
  (SI: 11.6 pmol/L [10.6-22.8 pmol/L])
Total T$_3$ (sample collected 3 hours after
  ingestion of desiccated thyroid
  extract) = 160 ng/dL (71-180 ng/dL)
  (SI: 0.01 nmol/L [1.09-2.77 nmol/L])

You counsel her on the goals of therapy in hypothyroidism for nonpregnant adults, treatment options, and pregnancy and hypothyroidism.

After a thorough discussion of the risks and benefits, which of the following options would be appropriate to offer?

A. Continue desiccated thyroid extract, 120 mg daily

B. Discontinue desiccated thyroid extract and initiate levothyroxine, 1.6 mcg/kg daily

C. Discontinue desiccated thyroid extract and initiate levothyroxine, 200 to 250 mcg daily

D. Split desiccated thyroid extract dose into 60 mg twice daily

E. Transition to levothyroxine + liothyronine combination therapy at dosages to achieve normal serum TSH

Answer: B or E) Discontinue desiccated thyroid extract and initiate levothyroxine, 1.6 mcg/kg daily, or transition to levothyroxine + liothyronine combination therapy at dosages to achieve normal serum TSH

Levothyroxine is the standard of care due to its efficacy and safety (Answer B). Two grains (120 mg) of desiccated thyroid contain about 76 mcg T$_4$ and 18 mcg T$_3$. If the pharmacodynamic equivalence of T$_4$ to T$_3$ is around 3:1,[44] then one could translate her current dosage as equivalent to about 260 mcg levothyroxine (Answer C). However, this would be about 4.5 mcg/kg and would be highly likely to suppress her serum TSH.

Desiccated thyroid extract is not FDA-approved or regulated (Answer A), but she is asymptomatic, has no contraindications, and has normal serum T$_3$ level measured near its peak. If the patient were experiencing fluctuating symptoms (thyrotoxic at peak and hypothyroid in trough), consideration could be made to splitting the dose to twice daily (Answer D), but this could interfere with her meal schedule.

Levothyroxine and liothyronine are FDA-approved and regulated (Answer E) and would also provide combination therapy, with established efficacy and safety standards.

However, she opted for Answer A because she felt well. Continued surveillance over years is notable for stable biochemical parameters and treatment satisfaction.

References

1. Jonklaas J, Bianco AC, Bauer AJ, et al; American Thyroid Association Task Force on Thyroid Hormone Replacement. Guidelines for the treatment of hypothyroidism: prepared by the American Thyroid Association task force on thyroid hormone replacement. *Thyroid*. 2014;24(12):1670-1751. PMID: 25266247

2. Pilo A, Iervasi G, Vitek F, Ferdeghini M, Cazzuola F, Bianchi R. Thyroidal and peripheral production of 3,5,3'-triiodothyronine in humans by multicompartmental analysis. *Am J Physiol*. 1990;258(4 Pt 1):E715-E726. PMID: 2333963

3. Abdalla SM, Bianco AC. Defending plasma T3 is a biological priority. *Clin Endocrinol (Oxf)*. 2014;81(5):633-641. PMID: 25040645

4. Taylor PN, Albrecht D, Scholz A, et al. Global epidemiology of hyperthyroidism and hypothyroidism. *Nat Rev Endocrinol*. 2018;14(5):301-316. PMID: 29569622

5. The IQVIA Institute. Medicine Use and Spending in the U.S. A Review of 2018 and Outlook to 2023 Institute Report. May 2019. Available at: https://www.iqvia.com/insights/the-iqvia-institute/reports/medicine-use-and-spending-in-the-us-a-review-of-2018-and-outlook-to-2023. Accessed for verification April 14, 2022.

6. Saravanan P, Chau W-F, Roberts N, Vedhara K, Greenwood R, Dayan CM. Psychological well-being in patients on 'adequate' doses of l-thyroxine: results of a large, controlled community-based questionnaire study. *Clinical Endocrinol (Oxf)*. 2002;57(5):577-585. PMID: 12390330

7. Peterson SJ, Cappola AR, Castro MR, et al. An online survey of hypothyroid patients demonstrates prominent dissatisfaction. *Thyroid*. 2018;28(6):707-721. PMID: 29620972

8. Mitchell AL, Hegedus L, Zarkovic M, Hickey JL, Perros P. Patient satisfaction and quality of life in hypothyroidism: An online survey by the british thyroid foundation. *Clin Endocrinol (Oxf)*. 2021;94(3):513-520. PMID: 32978985

9. Peterson SJ, McAninch EA, Bianco AC. Is a normal TSH synonymous with "euthyroidism" in levothyroxine monotherapy? *J Clin Endocrinol Metab*. 2016;101(12):4964-4973. PMID: 27700539

10. Gullo D, Latina A, Frasca F, Le Moli R, Pellegriti G, Vigneri R. Levothyroxine monotherapy cannot guarantee euthyroidism in all athyreotic patients. *PloS One*. 2011;6(8):e22552. PMID: 21829633

11. Stock JM, Surks MI, Oppenheimer JH. Replacement dosage of L-thyroxine in hypothyroidism. A re-evaluation. *N Engl J Med*. 1974;290(10):529-533. PMID: 4811096

12. Ingbar SH, Woeber KA. Thyroid hormone deficiency. In: Williams RH, ed. *Williams Textbook of Endocrinology*. 5th ed. WB Saunders Company; 1974:191-212.

13. Akirov A, Fazelzad R, Ezzat S, Thabane L, Sawka AM. A systematic review and meta-analysis of patient preferences for combination thyroid hormone treatment for hypothyroidism. *Front Endocrinol (Lausanne)*. 2019;10:477. PMID: 31396154

14. Jonklaas J, Bianco AC, Cappola AR, et al. Evidence-based use of levothyroxine/liothyronine combinations in treating hypothyroidism: a consensus document. *Thyroid*. 2021;31(2):156-182. PMID: 33276704

15. Shakir MKM, Brooks DI, McAninch EA, et al. Comparative effectiveness of levothyroxine, desiccated thyroid extract, and levothyroxine+liothyronine in hypothyroidism. *J Clin Endocrinol Metab*. 2021;106(11):e4400-e4413. PMID: 34185829

16. Millan-Alanis JM, Gonzalez-Gonzalez JG, Flores-Rodriguez A, et al. Benefits and harms of levothyroxine/L-triiodothyronine versus levothyroxine monotherapy for adult patients with hypothyroidism: systematic review and meta-analysis. *Thyroid*. 2021;31(11):1613-1625. PMID: 34340589

17. Leese GP, Soto-Pedre E, Donnelly LA. Liothyronine use in a 17 year observational population-based study - the tears study. *Clin Endocrinol (Oxf)*. 2016;85(6):918-925. PMID: 26940864

18. Jonklaas J, Tefera E, Shara N. Short-term time trends in prescribing therapy for hypothyroidism: results of a survey of American Thyroid Association members. *Front Endocrinol (Lausanne)*. 2019;10:31. PMID: 30761091

19. Idrees T, Palmer S, Maciel RMB, Bianco AC. Liothyronine and desiccated thyroid extract in the treatment of hypothyroidism. *Thyroid*. 2020;30(10):1399-1413. PMID: 32279609

20. Wiersinga WM, Duntas L, Fadeyev V, Nygaard B, Vanderpump MPJ. 2012 ETA guidelines: the use of L-T4 + L-T3 in the treatment of hypothyroidism. *Eur Thyroid J*. 2012;1(2):55-71. PMID: 24782999

21. McAninch EA, Bianco AC. The history and future of treatment of hypothyroidism. *Ann Intern Med*. 2016;164(1):50-56. PMID: 26747302

22. Braverman LE, Ingbar SH, Sterling K. Conversion of thyroxine (T4) to triiodothyronine (T3) in athyreotic subjects. *J Clin Invest*. 1970;49(5):855-864. PMID: 4986007

23. Samuels MH, Kolobova I, Antosik M, Niederhausen M, Purnell JQ, Schuff KG. Thyroid function variation in the normal range, energy expenditure, and body composition in L-T4-treated subjects. *J Clin Endocrinol Metab*. 2017;102(7):2533-2542. PMID: 28460140

24. McAninch EA, Rajan KB, Miller CH, Bianco AC. Systemic thyroid hormone status during levothyroxine therapy in hypothyroidism: a systematic review and meta-analysis. *J Clin Endocrinol Metab*. 2018;103(12):4533-4542. PMID: 30124904

25. Burgos N, Toloza FJK, Singh Ospina NM, et al. Clinical outcomes after discontinuation of thyroid hormone replacement: a systematic review and meta-analysis. *Thyroid*. 2021;31(5):740-751. PMID: 33161885

26. Brito JP, Ross JS, El Kawkgi OM, Maraka S, Deng Y, Shah ND, Lipska KJ. Levothyroxine use in the United States, 2008-2018. *JAMA Internal Med*. 2021;181(10):1402-1405. PMID: 34152370

27. Miccoli P, Materazzi G, Rossi L. Levothyroxine therapy in thyrodectomized patients. *Front Endocrinol (Lausanne)*. 2020;11:626268. PMID: 33584551

28. Brun VH, Eriksen AH, Selseth R, et al. Patient-tailored levothyroxine dosage with pharmacokinetic/pharmacodynamic modeling: a novel approach after total thyroidectomy. *Thyroid*. 2021;31(9):1297-1304. PMID: 33980057

29. Lee YK, Lee H, Han S, et al. Association between thyroid-stimulating hormone level after total thyroidectomy and hypercholesterolemia in female patients with differentiated thyroid cancer: a retrospective study. *J Clin Med*. 2019;8(8):1106. PMID: 31349714

30. Ito M, Miyauchi A, Hisakado M, et al. Biochemical markers reflecting thyroid function in athyreotic patients on levothyroxine monotherapy. *Thyroid*. 2017;27(4):484-490. PMID: 28056660

31. Samuels MH, Kolobova I, Smeraglio A, Peters D, Purnell JQ, Schuff KG. Effects of levothyroxine replacement or suppressive therapy on energy expenditure and body composition. *Thyroid*. 2016;26(3):347-355. PMID: 26700485

32. Gorman CA, Jiang NS, Ellefson RD, Elveback LR. Comparative effectiveness of dextrothyroxine and levothyroxine in correcting hypothyroidism and lowering blood lipid levels in hypothyroid patients. *J Clin Endocrinol Metab*. 1979;49(1):1-7. PMID: 447807

33. Ettleson MD, Raine A, Batistuzzo A, et al. Brain fog in hypothyroidism: understanding the patient's perspective. *Endocr Pract*. 2022;28(3):257-264. PMID: 34890786

34. Werneck de Castro JP, Fonseca TL, Ueta CB, et al. Differences in hypothalamic type 2 deiodinase ubiquitination explain localized sensitivity to thyroxine. *J Clin Invest*. 2015;125(2):769-781. PMID: 25555216

35. Escobar-Morreale HF, del Rey FE, Obregon MJ, de Escobar GM. Only the combined treatment with thyroxine and triiodothyronine ensures euthyroidism in all tissues of the thyroidectomized rat. *Endocrinology*. 1996;137(6):2490-2502. PMID: 8641203

36. McAninch EA, Bianco AC. The swinging pendulum in treatment for hypothyroidism: from (and toward?) combination therapy. *Front Endocrinol (Lausanne)*. 2019;10:446. PMID: 31354624

37. Idrees T, Price JD, Piccariello T, Bianco AC. Sustained release T3 therapy: animal models and translational applications. *Front Endocrinol (Lausanne)*. 2019;10:544. PMID: 31456749

38. Dumitrescu AM, Hanlon EC, Arosemena M, et al. Extended absorption of liothyronine from poly-zinc-liothyronine: results from a phase 1, double-blind, randomized, and controlled study in humans. *Thyroid*. 2022;32(2):196-205. PMID: 34641706

39. Posabella A, Alber AB, Undeutsch HJ, et al. Derivation of thyroid follicular cells from pluripotent stem cells: insights from development and implications for regenerative medicine. *Front Endocrinol (Lausanne)*. 2021;12:666565. PMID: 33959101

40. Hoang TD, Olsen CH, Mai VQ, Clyde PW, Shakir MK. Desiccated thyroid extract compared with levothyroxine in the treatment of hypothyroidism: a randomized, double-blind, crossover study. *J Clin Endocrinol Metab*. 2013;98(5):1982-1990. PMID: 23539727

41. Utiger RD. Thyrotrophin radioimmunoassay: another test of thyroid function. *Ann Intern Med*. 1971;74(4):627-629. PMID: 5551168

42. Jonklaas J, Burman KD, Wang H, Latham KR. Single-dose T3 administration: kinetics and effects on biochemical and physiological parameters. *Ther Drug Monit*. 2015;37(1):110-118. PMID: 24977379

43. Dayan C, Panicker V. Management of hypothyroidism with combination thyroxine (T4) and triiodothyronine (T3) hormone replacement in clinical practice: a review of suggested guidance. *Thyroid Res*. 2018;11:1. PMID: 29375671

44. Celi FS, Zemskova M, Linderman JD, et al. The pharmacodynamic equivalence of levothyroxine and liothyronine: a randomized, double blind, cross-over study in thyroidectomized patients. *Clin Endocrinol (Oxf)*. 2010;72(5):709-715. PMID: 20447070

Management of Hereditary Medullary Thyroid Cancer

Uriel Clemente-Gutierrez, MD. Department of Surgical Oncology, Section of Surgical Endocrinology, University of Texas MD Anderson Cancer Center, Houston, TX; E-mail: ueclemente@mdanderson.org

Bernice L. Huang, MD. Department of Surgical Oncology, Section of Surgical Endocrinology, University of Texas MD Anderson Cancer Center, Houston, TX; E-mail: bhuang2@mdanderson.org

Danica M. Vodopivec, MD. Department of Endocrine Neoplasia and Hormonal Disorders, University of Texas MD Anderson Cancer Center, Houston, TX; E-mail: dmvodopivec@mdanderson.org

Nancy D. Perrier, MD. Department of surgical Oncology, Section of Surgical Endocrinology, University of Texas MD Anderson Cancer Center, Houston, TX; E-mail: nperrier@mdanderson.org

Learning Objectives

As a result of participating in this session, learners should be able to:

- Identify the clinical manifestations and define the appropriate workup for hereditary medullary thyroid carcinoma (MTC).

- Explain the role of specific *RET* pathogenic variants and their prognostic implications regarding the timing of prophylactic thyroidectomy based on the American Thyroid Association risk categories.

- Summarize recommended follow-up for patients with MTC.

- Describe the surgical management of hereditary MTC, including the indications for therapeutic and prophylactic cervical lymph node dissection.

- Determine the indications of targeted therapies in advanced and recurrent MTC.

Main Conclusions

MTC is an infrequent cancer arising from the parafollicular cells. This thyroid neoplasia is hereditary in 25% of affected adults and in 75% of affected children, and it is part of multiple endocrine neoplasia (MEN) type 2 syndrome.

Clinical evaluation must include neck inspection and imaging with ultrasonography, assessment for signs and symptoms of calcitonin excess, and investigation for nonendocrine manifestations, including cutaneous lichen amyloidosis, Hirschsprung disease, and oral/eyelid ganglioneuromas. The clinical presentation is based on the *RET* proto-oncogene codon alteration. As part of the initial workup, basal levels of secretory products of the C cells, calcitonin and carcinoembryonic antigen (CEA), should be measured. Genetic counseling and testing are necessary for patients with a new diagnosis of MTC. If a *RET* gene variant is identified, patients should undergo prophylactic or therapeutic thyroidectomy, depending on the clinical context.

The timing and indications of prophylactic thyroidectomy are based on the aggressiveness of their MTC, which depends on the patient's genotype. In the case of therapeutic thyroidectomy (ie, the patient has preoperative evidence of MTC), prophylactic unilateral central lymphadenectomy is indicated. The management of cervical lateral compartment lymph nodes is based on the calcitonin level and documented lymphadenopathy, among other factors.

Follow-up after thyroidectomy consists of clinical, radiologic, and laboratory evaluation every 6 months for the first year and thereafter on a yearly basis, adjusted based on the calcitonin and CEA levels and trends. In case of recurrent disease, targeted therapies have specific indications.

Significance of the Clinical Problem

MTC is a neuroendocrine tumor derived from the C cells in the thyroid gland, and it accounts for up to 3% to 4% of all thyroid cancers. MTC has a wide range of clinical behaviors, varying from indolent to invasive tumors, with a reported 10-year survival of 69% to 89%. Hereditary MTC has the potential to be treated early with prophylactic thyroidectomy, contributing to high cure rates and low morbidity when appropriately managed by a high-volume, multidisciplinary thyroid treatment team. Lymph node metastases in MTC depend on the size of the primary lesion in the thyroid, as well as the preoperative calcitonin and CEA levels. Timely prophylactic intervention can prevent extrathyroidal spread of the disease and is associated with surgical remission.

Barriers to Optimal Practice

- Difficulty in diagnosing MTC due to heterogeneity of clinical presentation.
- Establishing a correlation between genotype and phenotype in hereditary MTC.

- Defining the optimal timing and extension of prophylactic surgery for pediatric patients.
- Treatment and follow-up are required in referral centers due to the complexity of the disease.
- Targeted therapies have specific indications.

Strategies for Diagnosis, Therapy, and/or Management

Clinical Presentation and Diagnostic Workup

Hereditary MTC is one of the main features of MEN type 2A and MEN type 2B. When this thyroid neoplasia is diagnosed, it may present in the index patient as a palpable thyroid nodule with or without symptoms of calcitonin excess such as diarrhea. In contrast, when MTC is diagnosed as a result of screening in a kindred with known hereditary MTC, it often presents as an asymptomatic or nonpalpable thyroid nodule. Surveillance and timing are critical, and knowledge of the recommendations to proceed with prophylactic thyroidectomy is key.

MEN type 2 can present with different phenotypes and thus has different clinical manifestations. MEN type 2A represents 95% of MEN type 2 cases, and it is characterized by the development of MTC, hyperparathyroidism, and pheochromocytoma. Nonendocrine manifestations such as cutaneous lichen amyloidosis and Hirschsprung disease are rare and are associated with pathogenic variants in *RET* codons 634/804 and 609/611/618/620, respectively. MEN type 2B accounts for 5% of all MEN type 2 cases. Its clinical manifestations are early-onset MTC (within the first year of life); pheochromocytoma; and nonendocrine physical features, including alacrima (newborn period), hypotonia, constipation, failure to thrive, tongue/lip neuromas (first year of life), elongated/marfanoid facies and body habitus, and ganglioneuromas (affecting the aerodigestive tract, lacrimal duct, and eyelids by age 5 years). These clinical manifestations are highly suggestive of MEN type 2B and should prompt workup in the pediatric population (*Figure*). Failure to clinically recognize MEN type 2B leads to delayed diagnosis with a coincident high rate of patients who have metastatic disease at the time of surgical intervention and failure to achieve surgical remission.

Initial workup should be the same as with any thyroid nodule and include thyroid function tests, cervical ultrasonography, and FNA. Signs and symptoms indicating excess calcitonin secretion or metastatic disease should be addressed, especially flushing, diarrhea, and bone pain. A biochemical evaluation for hyperparathyroidism and pheochromocytoma should be performed in all patients, without exception. The biochemical workup includes measurement of serum levels of secretory products of parafollicular C cells, which are used as tumor markers, particularly calcitonin and CEA. Some pathologic conditions may lead to falsely elevated calcitonin, including chronic kidney disease, hypercalcemia, some neuroendocrine tumors (ie, gastrinomas), the presence of heterophilic antibodies to calcitonin, and the use of certain medications (eg, glucocorticoids, β-adrenergic blockers, and proton-pump inhibitors). Basal serum calcitonin concentrations in MTC often correlate with tumor burden; nonetheless, normal calcitonin levels with high CEA levels could reflect tumor differentiation.

In adults, 25% of MTC cases are hereditary. In addition, up to 7% of patients with apparently sporadic MTC are found to have a *RET* pathogenic variant. Hence, genetic counseling and testing should be offered to all new patients. In children, 75% of MTC cases are hereditary with the exception of MEN type 2B, which has a higher rate (50% or more) of de novo mutation. The American Thyroid Association guidelines on

Figure. Genotype-Phenotype Correlations in MEN Type 2

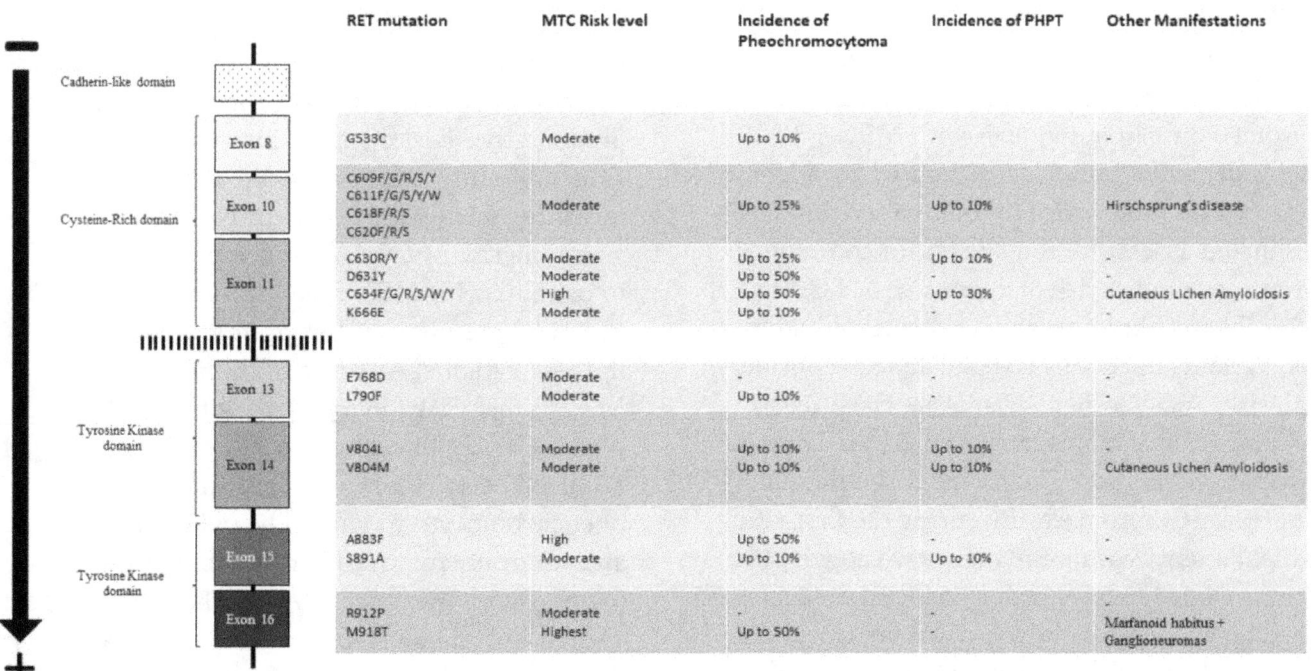

RET mutation	MTC Risk level	Incidence of Pheochromocytoma	Incidence of PHPT	Other Manifestations
G533C	Moderate	Up to 10%	-	-
C609F/G/R/S/Y C611F/G/S/Y/W C618F/R/S C620F/R/S	Moderate	Up to 25%	Up to 10%	Hirschsprung's disease
C630R/Y	Moderate	Up to 25%	Up to 10%	-
D631Y	Moderate	Up to 50%	-	-
C634F/G/R/S/W/Y	High	Up to 50%	Up to 30%	Cutaneous Lichen Amyloidosis
K666E	Moderate	Up to 10%	-	-
E768D	Moderate	-	-	-
L790F	Moderate	Up to 10%	-	-
V804L	Moderate	Up to 10%	Up to 10%	-
V804M	Moderate	Up to 10%	Up to 10%	Cutaneous Lichen Amyloidosis
A883F	High	Up to 50%	-	-
S891A	Moderate	Up to 10%	Up to 10%	-
R912P	Moderate	-	-	Marfanoid habitus + Ganglioneuromas
M918T	Highest	Up to 50%	-	

The diagram shows the RET receptor (left) with the reported codons affected in different exons (encoding different domains in the receptor). The table summarizes the associated endocrine and nonendocrine characteristics and their incidence. The closer the activating pathogenic variant is to the kinase domain in the RET receptor, the more aggressive MTC could be. Adapted with permission from Kouvaraki MA et al. *Thyroid*, 2005; 15(6) © Mary Ann Liebert, Inc.

MTC management suggest that patients with suspected hereditary MTC should undergo genetic testing via a tiered approach, beginning with the most commonly mutated "hotspots" and then proceeding to analysis of other exons if needed. However, more recently, there has been availability and decreasing cost of next-generation sequencing technology, allowing some commercial genetic testing laboratories to offer sequencing of the entire coding region (and certain intronic and noncoding) of the gene.[1] More than 100 pathogenic variants in the *RET* gene have been identified in patients with hereditary MTC; the most commonly described pathogenic variants in MEN type 2A are those affecting the cysteine codons in exons 10 and 11. Ninety-five percent of patients with MEN type 2B have a pathogenic variant in exon 16 (M918T); in the remaining 5% of cases, there is a variant in exon 15 (A883F). If a *RET* variant is identified, genetic counseling should be offered for at risk-risk family members.

Prophylactic Thyroidectomy: Timing, Indications, and Follow-Up

The aggressiveness of MTC and, hence, the recommended timing of prophylactic thyroidectomy in individuals with MEN type 2 is largely dependent on the specific *RET* pathogenic variant. The American Thyroid Association has designated a classification system for common *RET* variants to predict risk of aggressive MTC.[2] The M918T pathogenic variant is considered highest risk, variants in codons 634 and 883 are considered high risk, and all other variants are classified as moderate risk. Patients in the American Thyroid Association's highest-risk category should undergo prophylactic thyroidectomy during the first year of life. Patients within the high-risk category are recommended to have prophylactic thyroidectomy based on age, *RET* pathogenic variant, calcitonin levels, and family preference. Thyroidectomy should be offered around age 5 or 6 years, and factors such as school and family dynamics are important for psychologic welfare. Therefore, surgical procedures are usually scheduled during summer or school breaks. If calcitonin levels are found to be elevated or there is evidence of a rising trend before age 5, thyroidectomy should be performed earlier. Patients in the moderate-risk category must be screened on a 6-month to annual basis, starting at age 5 years. Physical examination, neck ultrasonography, and calcitonin levels are the screening tools. Thyroidectomy is indicated based on a proven trend of rising calcitonin levels or identification of any thyroid abnormalities on ultrasonography. Long-term screening can be a concerning topic for some parents. If this is the case, prophylactic thyroidectomy could be considered based on timing that is appropriate given input from the family, endocrinologist, and endocrine surgeon.

Studies in patients with MEN type 2A have demonstrated that lymph node metastases are rare in patients younger than age 11 years and in patients with a preoperative calcitonin concentration less than 40 pg/mL (<11.7 pmol/L). Therefore, for all American Thyroid Association risk categories, prophylactic central neck dissection, which would place the recurrent laryngeal nerve and parathyroid glands at significantly increased risk, is not indicated unless worrisome lymph nodes are encountered during preoperative assessment or intraoperatively. Concomitantly, calcium should always be measured during the preoperative workup given the risk of primary hyperparathyroidism in patients with MEN type 2A. However, MTC generally presents before parathyroid disease in these patients. As a rule of thumb, when MTC is diagnosed in a patient with MEN type 2A or 2B, pheochromocytoma must be excluded before thyroidectomy and, if detected, pheochromocytoma should be medically blocked and surgically removed before the thyroid. In patients with MEN type 2A who have a pathogenic variant in codon 634, pheochromocytoma can develop as early as 8 years of age.[3] In general, screening for pheochromocytoma in these patients is recommended to start at age 11 years.

After prophylactic thyroidectomy has been performed in patients with hereditary MTC, the suggested follow-up strategy is to evaluate with physical examination, neck ultrasonography, and biochemical tests (calcitonin and CEA measurement) every 6 months for the first postoperative year and annually thereafter. If serum calcitonin is elevated but less than 150 pg/mL (<43.8 pmol/L), doubling times are evaluated with measurement of calcitonin and CEA every 3 to 6 months. If it is found that doubling occurs in less than 6 months or the calcitonin concentration is greater than 150 pg/mL (>43.8 pmol/L), imaging studies should be used to evaluate for recurrent and metastatic disease.

What Should Be the Extension of Thyroidectomy and Lymph Node Dissection?

When index family members with hereditary MTC presents for medical evaluation, they usually present with a palpable thyroid nodule. Lymph node involvement is found in more than 70% of affected individuals (this presentation is much more similar to that seen in patients with sporadic MTC). In this case, the standard therapeutic treatment of MTC is total thyroidectomy and, depending on preoperative serum calcitonin levels, neck ultrasound findings, and intraoperative evaluation, compartmental cervical lymph node dissection may proceed as well. More than 70% of patients with MTC have central compartment involvement,[4] and involvement of the compartment ipsilateral to the thyroid lesion is frequently observed. Contralateral lymphadenopathy has been documented when preoperative calcitonin levels are greater than 200 pg/mL (>58.4 pmol/L). For this reason, prophylactic ipsilateral central compartment lymphadenectomy (level VI) is recommended in all cases, lateral compartment dissection (levels II, III, IV, and V) is indicated when abnormal lymphadenopathy is documented in preoperative ultrasonography, and contralateral prophylactic lymphadenectomy can be considered if calcitonin levels are above 200 pg/mL (>58.4 pmol/L).[2,5]

Factors other than the presence or absence of cervical lymphadenopathy or calcitonin levels have been studied to potentially omit or recommend prophylactic lymphadenectomy in specific population subgroups. The absence of desmoplastic stromal reaction is a favorable prognostic factor, and prophylactic lymphadenectomy might be of poor utility in this group of patients.[6] Interestingly, specific RET pathogenic variants such as those occurring in exons 11 and 13 have been associated with elevated risk of cervical lymph node metastases.

Recurrent Disease: Indications for When to Start Systemic Therapy

Many patients with distant metastases have indolent disease—with stable to slow-growing lesions and tumor markers increasing at a slow pace—that requires active surveillance without the need for systemic therapy for years. Systemic therapy is reserved for metastatic disease with at least 1 of the following characteristics: (1) progressive (by RECIST) within 12 to 14 months, (2) symptomatic and not treatable with local or symptom-specific therapies, (3) compromises nearby structures and not treatable with localized therapies, (4) calcitonin or CEA doubling time less than 6 months with structural evidence of clinically significant disease, and (5) severe, intractable MTC-related diarrhea or Cushing syndrome with lack of an alternative effective treatment.

FDA-approved tyrosine kinase inhibitors for the treatment of MTC are divided into 2 different categories: (1) multikinase inhibitors[7]: vandetanib[8] and cabozantinib[9,10] and (2) selective RET inhibitors: selpercatinib and pralsetinib. Selpercatinib[11] and pralsetinib[12] are considered first choice because they are receptor specific and hence better tolerated (fewer adverse effects).

In general, if small-volume oligometastatic disease is stable in all but one area, systemic therapy should be deferred and localized treatment (to the single area of growth) would be preferred. Localized treatments include external-beam radiation, surgical resection, embolization, or cryoablation. Starting systemic therapy should not be taken lightly, as it confers toxicities, is not curative, requires long-term use for disease control, and loses efficacy over time due to acquired resistance. In conclusion, the take-home message is that the use of systemic treatment for advanced MTC is reserved for patients with progressive, unresectable, locally advanced, or metastatic disease not amenable to other treatments.

Clinical Case Vignettes

Case 1

A 6-year-old boy with no family history of endocrinopathies and who is otherwise healthy presents to clinic for evaluation. His mother states that since early in the patient's life, she has noted lesions on his lips and tongue. She points out that, peculiarly, similar lesions have appeared on his eyelids, causing corneal irritation.

Physical examination confirms what the mother has described and reveals a 2-cm anterior cervical mass. After appropriate workup with cervical ultrasonography, FNA, and biochemical laboratory tests, MTC is diagnosed.

Which of the following statements about genetic testing in this patient's case is correct?

A. Genetic testing is not indicated in this patient because he does not have family history indicating a hereditary condition

B. Genetic testing with a tiered approach will probably identify pathogenic variants in exons 10 and 11

C. The most common *RET* pathogenic variant causing MEN type 2B is located in exon 15

D. The *RET* M918T pathogenic variant is the most probable cause of this patient's condition

Answer: D) The RET M918T pathogenic variant is the most probable cause of this patient's condition

All patients with newly diagnosed MTC should undergo genetic counseling and testing, especially when syndromic characteristics are identified, such

as ganglioneuromas described in this case (thus, Answer A is incorrect).

This patient has a phenotype consistent with MEN type 2B, including ganglioneuromas of the oral cavity and eyelids. These nonendocrine manifestations are not seen in patients with MEN type 2A, who predominantly have pathogenic variants in exons 10 and 11 (thus, Answer B is incorrect).

The *RET* M918T pathogenic variant (Answer D) is identified in 95% of patients with MEN type 2B, and this is the most probable cause of this patient's condition. The A883F pathogenic variant in exon 15 (Answer C) is found in the remaining 5% of patients with MEN type 2B.

Case 2

A 10-year-old girl who is otherwise healthy presents to clinic for evaluation. Her mother was recently diagnosed with MEN type 2A, and the patient has tested positive for the same pathogenic variant in codon 634 of the *RET* gene that her mother has. Cervical ultrasonography does not reveal abnormalities of the thyroid gland or concerning lymph nodes.

Laboratory test results:

> TSH, normal
> Free T$_4$, normal
> Basal calcitonin = 17 pg/mL (<8 pg/mL)
>   (SI: 4.96 pmol/L [<2.34 pmol/L])
> Calcium = 9.3 mg/dL (8.2-10.2 mg/dL)
>   (SI: 2.3 mmol/L [2.1-2.6 mmol/L])

Which of the following is the most appropriate next step in this patient's management?

A. Surveillance

B. Total thyroidectomy

C. Total thyroidectomy with bilateral central neck dissection

D. Total thyroidectomy with bilateral central neck dissection and bilateral lateral neck dissection

E. Total thyroidectomy with subtotal parathyroidectomy

Answer: B) Total thyroidectomy

For patients with a high-risk pathogenic variant (eg, C634 or A883F), MTC often develops early in life, and annual screening with physical examination, cervical ultrasonography, and biochemical evaluation is recommended to start at age 3 years, with the timing of prophylactic thyroidectomy generally considered at age 5 to 6 years. For these reasons, total thyroidectomy (Answer B) is the correct answer in this case. If calcitonin levels are noted to be elevated or rising prior to this age, thyroidectomy should be performed earlier.

Surveillance (Answer A) is incorrect because in the setting of hereditary MTC, after age 5 or 6 years, this strategy would be indicated only in patients with a moderate-risk pathogenic variant.

Prophylactic lymph node dissection (Answers C and D) in pediatric patients with hereditary MTC is not routinely performed, and lymphadenectomy is only indicated when there are clearly affected lymph nodes.

Subtotal parathyroidectomy (Answer E) would only be indicated in case of confirmed hyperparathyroidism.

Case 2 (continued)

The patient's surgical pathology demonstrates a medullary microcarcinoma, 0.15 cm in largest dimension, with 2 lymph nodes that are negative for carcinoma. Her calcitonin level 3 months after surgery is undetectable.

What further treatment and surveillance for persistent or recurrent disease are recommended for this patient?

A. Biochemical studies (thyroid function tests, calcitonin and CEA measurement) every 3 months

B. Cervical ultrasonography and biochemical studies every 6 months indefinitely

C. Physical examination, cervical ultrasonography, and biochemical studies every 6 months for the first year and annually thereafter

D. TSH suppression with levothyroxine

E. No further treatment or surveillance indicated

Answer: C) Physical examination, cervical ultrasonography, and biochemical studies every 6 months for the first year and annually thereafter

The suggested follow-up dictated by the American Thyroid Association for patients with a high-risk pathogenic variant, which is the case of the patient presented in the clinical vignette, is to continue postoperative surveillance with physical examination, ultrasonography of the cervical region, and measurement of serum levels of calcitonin and CEA every 6 months for the first year and annually thereafter (Answer C).

Answers A, B, and E do not satisfy these recommendations.

TSH suppression with levothyroxine (Answer D) is incorrect because MTC is not a follicular neoplasm; postoperative replacement therapy with levothyroxine should be administered with the objective of maintaining serum TSH levels in the normal range.

Case 3

A 34-year-old woman with a personal and family history of a germline exon 10 *RET* C620R pathogenic variant leading to MEN type 2A (American Thyroid Association level: moderate risk) presents to clinic for active surveillance.

Her relevant medical history dates to approximately 1.5 years ago when metastatic MTC and a pheochromocytoma in the right adrenal gland were diagnosed. Preoperative calcitonin and CEA measurements are shown in the table. Preoperative staging scans showed metastatic disease in lateral cervical lymph nodes, bilateral subcentimeter lung nodules, and a single small liver metastasis (biopsy-proven MTC). Surgical resection of the pheochromocytoma was addressed first through a posterior retroperitoneoscopic

Measurement	Preoperative (time of initial diagnosis)	Preoperative (3 months after pheochromocytoma resection)	Postoperative (6 months after neck surgery)	Postoperative (12 months after neck surgery; today's clinic visit)
Calcitonin	4968 pg/mL (SI: 1451 pmol/L)	4972 pg/mL (SI: 1452 pmol/L)	1145 pg/mL (SI: 334 pmol/L)	1202 pg/mL (SI: 351 pmol/L)
CEA	47.6 ng/mL (SI: 47.6 µg/L)	50.9 ng/mL (SI: 50.9 µg/L)	25.5 ng/mL (SI: 25.5 µg/L)	30.2 ng/mL (SI: 30.2 µg/L)

Reference ranges: calcitonin, ≤7.6 pg/mL (SI: ≤2.2 pmol/L); CEA, ≤3.8 ng/mL (SI: ≤3.8 µg/L).

approach. Three months after adrenalectomy, in the absence of biochemical and structural evidence of pheochromocytoma, as well as restaging scans showing stable distant metastatic disease, the patient underwent total thyroidectomy with bilateral central and lateral neck dissection.

At today's clinic visit (12 months after neck surgery), the patient has no concerns, including no flushing or diarrhea. Her calcitonin and CEA levels are both rising. Imaging shows stable metastatic lesions in the lungs and a 3-mm increase in the size of the liver lesion over a 12-month interval (1.1 to 1.4 cm). Liver enzymes are within normal limits, the liver lesion is not causing any bile duct obstruction, and it is not located close to the Glisson capsule.

Which of the following is the best next step in this patient's management?

A. Continue to observe

B. Give external radiotherapy targeting the liver metastasis

C. Start immune check-point inhibitor therapy

D. Start intravenous chemotherapy

E. Start a tyrosine kinase inhibitor

Answer: A) Continue to observe

In patients with MEN type 2 who have pheochromocytoma, this tumor must be resected first to avoid cardiovascular complications in future operative interventions. In this case, with known distant metastatic disease at the time of initial diagnosis, the intent of neck surgery was not to cure but to control disease burden in the neck to prevent tumor invasion into the trachea, esophagus, or wrapping around major neck vessels in the future. If the 3-month restaging scans after adrenalectomy had shown rapid metastatic disease progression, a selective RET inhibitor would have been started and the neck surgery deferred. Even though this patient has metastatic disease, the lesions are not rapidly growing and she is asymptomatic. Thus, continuing to observe (Answer A) is the most appropriate recommendation.

Starting intravenous chemotherapy (Answer D) is incorrect not only because the patient does not meet indications to start systemic treatment, but also because with the advent of precision oncology, tyrosine kinase inhibitors have completely replaced cytotoxic chemotherapy. However, starting tyrosine kinase inhibitor therapy (Answer E) is incorrect because over a 12-month period, the lung metastases have not grown and remain subcentimeter in size, the single liver lesion has slightly increased in size (3 mm), and there are no new lesions. These findings translate to indolent metastatic disease—not rapidly progressing—and the patient is asymptomatic.

Immunotherapy (Answer C) has not been approved for the treatment of MTC and is being studied in clinical trials.

External radiotherapy targeting the liver metastasis (Answer B) would have been appropriate if in the presence of stable metastatic disease in all other areas, the single liver lesion was continuing to rapidly grow, cause biliary obstruction, or cause pain due to its proximity to the Glisson capsule.

References

1. Hyde SM, Cote GJ, Grubbs EG. Genetics of multiple endocrine neoplasia type 1/multiple endocrine neoplasia type 2 syndromes. *Endocrinol Metab Clin North Am.* 2017;46(2):491-502. PMID: 28476233

2. Wells SA Jr, Asa SL, Dralle H, et al; American Thyroid Association Guidelines Task Force on Medullary Thyroid Carcinoma. Revised American Thyroid Association guidelines for the management of medullary thyroid carcinoma. *Thyroid.* 2015;25(6):567-610. PMID: 25810047

3. Rowland KJ, Chernock RD, Moley JF. Pheochromocytoma in an 8-year-old patient with multiple endocrine neoplasia type 2A: implications for screening. *J Surg Oncol.* 2013;108(4):203-206. PMID: 23868299

4. Moley JF, DeBenedetti MK. Patterns of nodal metastases in palpable medullary thyroid carcinoma: recommendations for extent of node dissection. *Ann Surg.* 1999;229(6):880-887; discussion 887-888. PMID: 10363903

5. Machens A, Dralle H. Biomarker-based risk stratification for previously untreated medullary thyroid cancer. *J Clin Endocrinol Metab.* 2010;95(6):2655-2663. PMID: 20339026

6. Niederle MB, Riss P, Selberherr A, et al. Omission of lateral lymph node dissection in medullary thyroid cancer without a desmoplastic stromal reaction. *Br J Surg.* 2021;108(2):174-181. PMID: 33704404

7. Cabanillas ME, Hu MI, Jimenez C. Medullary thyroid cancer in the era of tyrosine kinase inhibitors: to treat or not to treat--and with which drug--those are the questions. *J Clin Endocrinol Metab.* 2014;99(12):4390-4396. PMID: 25238206

8. Wells SA Jr, Robinson BG, Gagel RF, et al. Vandetanib in patients with locally advanced or metastatic medullary thyroid cancer: a randomized, double-blind phase III trial. *J Clin Oncol.* 2012;30(2):134-141. PMID: 22025146

9. Elisei R, Schlumberger MJ, Müller SP, et al. Cabozantinib in progressive medullary thyroid cancer. *J Clin Oncol.* 2013;31(29):3639-3646. PMID: 24002501

10. Schlumberger M, Elisei R, Müller S, et al. Overall survival analysis of EXAM, a phase III trial of cabozantinib in patients with radiographically progressive medullary thyroid carcinoma. *Ann Oncol.* 2017;28(11):2813-2819. PMID: 29045520

11. Wirth LJ, Sherman E, Robinson B, et al. Efficacy of selpercatinib in RET-altered thyroid cancers. *N Engl J Med.* 2020;383(9):825-835. PMID: 32846061

12. Subbiah V, Hu MI, Wirth LJ, et al. Pralsetinib for patients with advanced or metastatic RET-altered thyroid cancer (ARROW): a multi-cohort, open-label, registrational, phase 1/2 study. *Lancet Diabetes Endocrinol.* 2021;9(8):491-501. PMID: 34118198

What's New in the Treatment of Differentiated Thyroid Cancer?

Benjamin J. Gigliotti, MD. Department of Medicine, Division of Endocrinology, University of Rochester, Rochester, NY; E-mail: Benjamin_Gigliotti@urmc.rochester.edu

Learning Objectives

As a result of participating in this session, learners should be able to:

- Identify appropriate candidates for conservative treatment of low-risk differentiated thyroid cancer (DTC) and summarize the pros and cons of active surveillance, hemithyroidectomy, and emerging focally ablative methods.

- Develop a personalized approach to treating patients with advanced and metastatic thyroid cancers, including identification of aggressive and/or radioiodine-refractory disease, and determine when to consider and refer for "targeted" therapies.

Main Conclusions

- Management of thyroid cancer has been a moving target in recent years and has become increasingly personalized and risk-adapted. Treatment of low-risk thyroid carcinoma is becoming increasingly conservative, and the molecular era has provided new insights and treatment options for patients with advanced disease.

- Hemithyroidectomy is an attractive initial surgical approach for patients with indeterminate cytopathology or low-risk intrathyroidal DTC smaller than 4 cm, especially if the contralateral lobe and central/ lateral nodal stations are radiographically normal and there is no history of neck radiation or family history of thyroid cancer.

- Active surveillance is a reasonable management option for adults, especially if certain patient factors (accepting of surveillance philosophy, good adherence, high surgical risk) and tumor factors (smaller than 1.5 cm with normal surrounding parenchyma, no extrathyroidal extension, no nodal or distant metastases, no high-risk cytopathologic features) are present, along with access to high-quality ultrasonography and willingness of the health care team to facilitate surveillance.

- Focal ablative technologies such as percutaneous radiofrequency, microwave, laser, and ethanol ablation are being actively studied in the treatment of papillary thyroid microcarcinomas and locoregional nodal disease, although they are not yet widely available.

- Advanced thyroid cancers are uncommon and exhibit a wide range of behavior. Defining their size, location, and growth trajectory is helpful in management, as is working in or referring to experienced multidisciplinary teams. For clinically significant disease that is refractory to surgery, radioactive iodine (RAI), TSH suppression, and, when appropriate, external-beam radiation, local ablative therapies, and molecular targeted therapies are invaluable and rapidly evolving treatment modalities.

Significance of the Clinical Problem

The incidence of thyroid cancer has been steadily increasing over the last 3 decades. Small indolent papillary thyroid carcinomas (PTCs) account for much of the rise, which suggests overdiagnosis, most likely due to increasing sensitivity and availability of thyroid ultrasonography and FNA. While recent data suggest there may be a small rise in the incidence of more aggressive thyroid cancers (to which obesity may be contributory), along with a modest increase in mortality, nearly all of these additional cases are not lethal.[1,2]

Given widespread recognition that most DTCs are indolent and carry an excellent prognosis, coupled with epidemiologic data that overtreatment increases morbidity, management of thyroid cancer has become increasingly conservative. Active surveillance, hemithyroidectomy rather than total thyroidectomy, more judicious use of RAI, and local ablative technologies have all garnered significant attention and have expanding evidence to support their use. However, thoughtful application of conservative strategies requires proper identification of appropriate "low-risk" patients who are unlikely to be harmed from receiving less up-front therapy.[3] Most clinicians have cared for relatively uncommon but memorable patients with "low-risk" disease who experienced poor outcomes. Refining the definition of "low risk" is an important ongoing effort, including active research to more explicitly quantify tumor size, volume, and multifocality, define the extent of margin positivity, and handle increasingly ubiquitous molecular data.

On the opposite end of the disease spectrum, a small but clinically significant subset of patients with thyroid cancer experience locoregional recurrence and distant metastasis. Improved understanding of the molecular pathogenesis of thyroid cancer has shed new light on the pathogenetic drivers behind more aggressive behavior (including refractoriness to RAI) and the development of poorly differentiated and undifferentiated (anaplastic) histologies. The nearly dizzying expansion of available molecular targeted therapies has made many of these oncologic alterations "actionable," dramatically increasing treatment options for patients with aggressive disease. However, the optimal agent and/or sequence of agents, patient/tumor characteristics, and timing of initiation are not always clear. In other words, we are left with the same fundamental questions as for patients with low-risk disease: who and when?

The changing landscape of thyroid cancer management has made this an equally exciting and bewildering time to care for patients. The purpose of this chapter is to briefly review several of these new and evolving management strategies, focusing on low-risk thyroid cancer, which is significantly more common and relevant to clinicians in endocrinology, as well as the rarer but more vexing scenario of advanced disease, through the lens of practical clinical application.

Barriers to Optimal Practice

- Active surveillance is most successful in the setting of specific patient and tumor characteristics and requires local expertise as well as high-quality neck ultrasonography.

- Long-term surveillance after hemithyroidectomy is more challenging than surveillance after total thyroidectomy followed by RAI.

- Local ablative therapies continue to benefit from innovation in technology and expanding indications, but they require specialized equipment and expertise and are not yet widely available.

- Advanced and metastatic thyroid carcinomas are uncommon and follow a variable course. Most systemic therapies are effective, although they remain palliative and carry the risk of significant adverse effects. Tumors eventually develop resistance. Optimal use scenarios and timing of initiation are not always clear.

Strategies for Diagnosis, Therapy, and/or Management

Low-Risk DTC

DTC collectively includes PTC and follicular thyroid carcinoma (FTC); Hürthle-cell carcinoma and poorly differentiated carcinoma are also included in the 2017 World Health Organization classification. While distinct in biology and behavior, PTC and FTC are often grouped together because their prognosis is generally very good, and clinical management strategies, including thyroidectomy and RAI, are similar.[4] Contemporary thyroid cancer management relies on a risk-adapted approach; the American Thyroid Association Management Guidelines for Adult Patients with Thyroid Nodules and Differentiated Thyroid Cancer have articulated a shared lexicon to stratify "risk of structural disease recurrence" using evidence-based clinicopathologic variables, supplemented by molecular diagnostics and dynamic risk restratification over time.[3] According to the most recent guidelines, low-risk DTC is defined as follows.

- Intrathyroidal PTC with:

  - No locoregional tissue invasion, local metastases, or distant metastases on axial or ^{131}I scanning

  - Conventional or follicular variant histology and absence of aggressive histology (eg, tall-cell variant, hobnail variant, columnar variant) or vascular invasion

  - All macroscopic tumor resected (R0) and no macroscopic or microscopic invasion of perithyroidal soft tissues

  - No suspicious lymph nodes on ultrasonography, ≤5 lymph node micrometastases <2 mm in largest dimension

- Intrathyroidal FTC with capsular invasion, but <4 foci of vascular invasion

It is worth noting that encapsulated follicular variant PTC were included in the low-risk category at the time the 2015 American Thyroid Association guidelines were published because they have long been recognized to be unusually indolent. Since that time, they have been reclassified as noninvasive follicular thyroid neoplasms with papillary-like nuclear features (NIFTP), rather than carcinoma, although "carcinoma in situ" may be a more precise description. While NIFTP has relatively strict diagnostic criteria (eg, no evidence of capsular invasion after complete examination of the tumor capsule), these lesions are definitively treated with hemithyroidectomy and unequivocally do not require additional therapy.[5]

Hemithyroidectomy

Hemithyroidectomy, or thyroid lobectomy, involves removal of the ipsilateral thyroid lobe and isthmus.[5] Despite fairly widespread use of hemithyroidectomy for the treatment of thyroid cancer in the past, total thyroidectomy followed by RAI became increasingly common practice since the 1970s because of several studies showing a reduction in tumor recurrence and mortality. Since that time, various risk-stratification tools have been designed and validated, enabling better prediction of the risk of disease recurrence/mortality, and defining who may benefit most (and least) from RAI. While the debate about the ideal clinical use of RAI has, and continues to be, a vibrant one, it is clear that more judicious use of RAI in a risk-tailored approach is successful.[6] The 2009 American Thyroid Association thyroid cancer management guidelines pioneered the first recurrence-focused risk system and recommended against routine use of RAI in patients at low risk, given convincing data of little-to-no benefit.[1] The 2015 American Thyroid Association guidelines went a step further to refine the definitions of risk categories and added that hemithyroidectomy rather than total thyroidectomy may be a reasonable initial surgical option for low-risk disease, especially since one of the arguments for total thyroidectomy is to remove iodine-avid healthy thyroid tissue to facilitate RAI.

Table. Pros and Cons of Hemithyroidectomy

Pros	Cons
Reduced likelihood of needing postoperative thyroid hormone (risk factors for replacement include baseline TSH >2-2.5 mIU/L, positive antithyroid antibodies or ultrasonographic evidence of autoimmunity, smaller thyroid volume, female sex)	Therapeutic RAI and diagnostic RAI whole-body scanning cannot be performed without completion lobectomy or residual lobe RAI ablation
Lower surgical risk of recurrent laryngeal nerve injury, hypoparathyroidism, hematoma/seroma, especially when done by a lower-volume surgeon	Potential need for a second surgery if pathology reveals higher-risk features
No increased risk of mortality	Decreased sensitivity of thyroglobulin in detecting tumor persistence/recurrence due to "noise" from the residual lobe
Potential savings in cost and increased quality-of-life scores	At most a small increased recurrence risk

Ideal Candidates

- Absence of contralateral nodules/goiter
- Absence of abnormal lymph nodes in the central/lateral compartments
- Nodules <4 cm (especially <1 cm) without extrathyroidal extension
- Absence of risk factors, including prior head/neck radiation and a strong family history of thyroid cancer
- Bethesda 3 or 4 indeterminate cytopathology
- Strong preference for hemithyroidectomy
- Low operative risk, even if 1 or more surgery is needed

Reasonable Candidates

- Low-risk contralateral nodules (with benign FNA, if indicated by ultrasonographic features and size)
- Bethesda 5 or 6 cytopathology

Indications for Completion Thyroidectomy (With or Without Compartment-Oriented Lymph Node Dissection)

- American Thyroid Association intermediate- or high-risk histopathologic features
- Development of new abnormal central or lateral compartment lymph nodes (ideally after confirming malignancy with FNA and, if acellular, thyroglobulin washout)
- A markedly elevated postoperative thyroglobulin value, especially if locoregional or distance disease is suspected or found
- A positive margin is controversial; a wide rather than focal extent of the margin, and posterior more than anterior margin involvement appears to carry higher risk
- Tumor multifocality is controversial; if contralateral nodules are present, or there are additional risk factors (family history, history of neck radiation), completion thyroidectomy is attractive

Active Surveillance

Serial ultrasonographic surveillance of biopsy-confirmed or suspected thyroid cancer. Active surveillance was first proposed and implemented for patients with papillary thyroid microcarcinoma (<1 cm) in Japan in the early 1990s, based on observations that small occult PTCs were common and indolent.[8] In their landmark study, only 8% of patients experienced tumor growth of 3 mm or more over 10 years, and the 3.8% of patients who required a salvage definitive surgery for new lymph node metastases had similar outcomes to those who underwent up-front surgery. These findings have been corroborated in Korea and now in the United States, confirming the overall safety of the active surveillance strategy and identifying predictors and patterns of tumor progression that continue to undergo active study. Active surveillance was added to the 2015 American Thyroid Association guidelines as an acceptable management strategy for appropriately selected patients, and a clinical framework was subsequently published to guide adoption for when the right confluence of patient, tumor, and medical team characteristics are present.[3,9]

Ideal Circumstances

- Patient factors

    ○ Age >60 years

    ○ Accepting of the active surveillance philosophy and potential need for future surgery

    ○ Reliable and adherent to clinical and ultrasonography follow-up

    ○ High risk of surgery, significant comorbidities, and/or limited life expectancy

- Nodule/tumor factors

    ○ Size <1 cm

    ○ Solitary well-defined thyroid nodule with >2 mm of surrounding normal gland parenchyma

    ○ No evidence of extrathyroidal extension on ultrasonography

    ○ Size stability over time

    ○ No clinical evidence of nodal or distant metastases

    ○ No high-risk cytopathologic or molecular features (as of this writing, there are no clear molecular features that preclude active surveillance)

- Medical team factors

    ○ Multidisciplinary team with endocrinologists, high-volume thyroid surgeons, and sonographers/radiologists

    ○ Physician comfort

    ○ Availability of high-quality neck ultrasonography

    ○ Robust ancillary support to ensure follow-up and adherence to surveillance protocols

Less Ideal, But Appropriate Characteristics

- Age 18 to 59 years

- Size <1.5 cm (most studies use a 1.5-cm cutoff, but up to 2 cm may be appropriate; all numerical thresholds in medicine are informed by available data, rather than a sacrosanct biological cutoff)

- Multifocal papillary thyroid microcarcinoma

- Indistinct tumor margins or a heterogeneous or multinodular thyroid parenchyma

- Nodule ^{18}F-fluorodeoxyglucose avidity on positron emission tomography (if <1 cm)

- Subcapsular nodule location, as long as it is away from regions harboring critical anatomy (eg, the recurrent laryngeal nerve, trachea, esophagus)

Suggested Surveillance Protocols

- Baseline thyroid ultrasonography with axial dimension measurement and tumor volume calculation

- Serial thyroid ultrasonography every 6 months for 2 to 3 years, then annually (if stable)

Indications to Abort Active Surveillance

- ≥3 mm or more increase in the axial dimension

- >50% increase in tumor volume, especially if there is a short doubling time or the tumor is adjacent to the thyroid capsule

- Radiographic evidence of invasion through the thyroid capsule

- Development of cervical lymph node metastasis (or more rarely, distant metastasis)

Locally Ablative Technologies

A cadre of focally delivered ablative therapies have been used in the treatment of benign and malignant thyroid disease, including percutaneous ethanol ablation, radiofrequency, or microwave ablation, cryoablation, laser ablation, chemoembolization, and high-intensity focused ultrasonography. While varying widely in technique, they are often grouped together because of an image-guided minimally invasive approach, compared with conventional surgical excision. As with any specialized medical technology, their study and clinical application have been a moving target, including use in the treatment of benign cystic and solid thyroid nodules, oligometastatic disease in neck lymph nodes or distant sites, and salient to the topic of low-risk DTC in the nonsurgical management of papillary thyroid microcarcinoma. Percutaneous radiofrequency, microwave, laser, and ethanol ablation have data to support their use in this setting.[10,11] Potential pros of percutaneous ablation include similar outcomes in select patients, lower cost, an attractive safety profile, and potentially higher quality-of-life scores. Use of these methods is actively being codified into management guidelines position statements.[12,13] Patients who are interested may be directed to centers within the United States and abroad that have developed expertise and have active clinical programs and/or trials.

Advanced DTC

Up to 30% of patients with DTC experience locoregional recurrence (or more precisely, persistence). While most of these patients do well, a subset experience repetitive recurrence with related morbidity, and 1% to 5% of patients develop distant metastases.[14] Poorly differentiated and undifferentiated tumors exhibit more consistently aggressive behavior, and may arise de novo or due to dedifferentiation of an existing DTC.[15] While uncommon, these patients are often a source of worry and uncertainty for practicing clinicians, especially in the context of rapidly evolving understanding of the molecular pathogenesis underlying aggressive behavior, and an overwhelming cadre of systemic therapies. My mentor, Dr. Gilbert Daniels from the Massachusetts General Hospital Thyroid Unit, provides us with a guiding axiom in his primer on clinical endocrinology in the *Williams Textbook of Endocrinology, 12th edition:* "With most innocent or nonaggressive thyroid cancers, the rule is to think and act like an endocrinologist. With more aggressive thyroid and other endocrine cancers, a good rule is to think like an oncologist, and to refer the patient to one of them if necessary."[16]

An important first step in the management of patients with advanced or dedifferentiated DTC is to recognize the presence of aggressive features and clinical behavior. Potential characteristics of more aggressive disease include the following:

- High-risk of recurrence and/or tumor/node/metastasis stage
- Rapid tumor growth trajectory
- Large, locally invasive tumors, especially involving or encasing critical structures such as the trachea, esophagus, prevertebral fascia, and carotid artery or mediastinal vessels
- Presence of distant metastasis
- Multiple recurrent or progressive tumors in the central or lateral neck, especially if unresectable
- Failure to respond to surgical resection, RAI, and TSH suppression

The recognition of failure to respond to our most widely used and usually successful tools (surgery, RAI, and TSH suppression), is particularly important. Given the importance of surgery as first-line management, relying on the expertise of a skilled and high-volume thyroid surgeon, and obtaining a second opinion, if necessary, is important before deciding that surgery is no longer a good option. Defining the clinical utility of radioactive iodine, however, often falls to us. Unfortunately, no international consensus has been reached on a precise and encompassing definition of RAI-refractory disease. A recent joint statement from international experts in the field nicely captures areas of consensus and controversy and articulated the following common clinical scenarios as being suggestive of reduced likelihood of response to RAI:

- No ^{131}I uptake in tumor foci on a diagnostic (pretreatment) scan or a posttreatment ^{131}I scan

- [131]I uptake is present in some but not other tumor foci, or is lost over time

- Presence of metastasis(es) that progress despite ^{131}I uptake or a cumulative ^{131}I activity of >600 mCi (>22.2 GBq)

However, it is important to note that response to RAI exists in a spectrum, and no single criterion definitively excludes benefit in every clinical scenario. Therefore, multidisciplinary collaboration with nuclear medicine (and referring for a second opinion at a high-volume center, if necessary) is critical, especially in light of changes on the horizon due to new treatment strategies and emerging "redifferentiation" protocols aimed at restoration of iodine uptake in recalcitrant tumors through the use of small molecule inhibitors.

Advances in understanding the genetic alterations that drive thyroid cancer have shed new light on the mechanisms underlying more aggressive disease. For instance, most thyroid cancers harbor alterations (mostly mutations and fusions) in the mitogen-activated protein kinase (MAPK) pathway, with *BRAF* V600E representing the most common alteration in PTC. Certain gain-of-function pathogenic variants within the MAPK pathway, including *BRAF* V600E, can decrease downstream sodium-iodine symporter expression, conveying refractoriness to RAI. The development of tyrosine kinase inhibitors that target multiple pathways in angiogenesis and cell growth, along with inhibitors specific for altered and wild-type proteins in the MAPK pathway, among others, have become the mainstay for patients with progressive disease.[17] A total of 9 systemic therapies (sorafenib, lenvatinib, dabrafenib/trametinib, selpercatinib, pralsetinib, larotrectinib, entrectinib, cabozantinib) are currently approved by the US FDA for the treatment of thyroid cancers of follicular cell origin. However, these therapies have important limitations:

- Response rates are variable

- Treatment is mostly tumoristatic and palliative; most have shown an improvement in progression-free survival, but not mortality

- Adverse effects can be significant, although newer/more specific therapies such as RET inhibitors selpercatinib and pralsetinib appear to have a gentler adverse effect profile

- Development of resistance is nearly inevitable, although mechanisms of resistance and strategies to circumvent them are being actively investigated

To address these limitations, several therapies and strategies are in the research pipeline. There is ongoing identification of driver alterations with expanding drug options to target them, application of immunotherapy and peptide receptor therapy, leveraging of targeted therapies to increase iodine uptake and retention through restoration of sodium-iodine symporter function, exploration of sequential or combinatorial treatment protocols to attempt to maximize response and minimize development of resistance.

While some endocrinologists have developed particular expertise in the use of targeted therapies, most notably the Endocrine Neoplasia and Hormonal Disorders Department at MD Anderson, most of us rely on oncology colleagues who have more experience with systemic therapies along with a more robust clinical infrastructure to procure, prescribe, and monitor them. However, as the longitudinal providers for most patients with thyroid cancer, clinicians in endocrinology are best suited to identify potential candidates for systemic therapy and to refer to oncology when needed. Since even recalcitrant or metastatic thyroid cancer can still be relatively indolent, our main task is to differentiate clinically significant and progressive disease from cancers that are simply detectable (eg. indolent metastases) and warrant active surveillance. Tumor size, growth trajectory, location, and symptoms from organ involvement are critical variables to consider, as is whether a disease site is amenable to local-directed therapies. Consideration of systemic therapy is most appropriate for patients who exhibit the following:

- Tumor foci ≥1 to 1.5 cm or in immediate adjacency to critical structures

- Rapid growth trajectory over 6 to 12 months or less (the role of an isolated rise during biochemical surveillance, eg, thyroglobulin doubling without radiographic correlate, is less clear)

- Presence of symptoms related to disease burden (eg, shortness of breath or hemoptysis associated with lung metastases)

- Failure to respond to TSH suppression, radioactive iodine, and if disease foci are oligometastatic and accessible, failure to respond to external-beam radiation and/or focal therapies such as resection and percutaneous ablation

If unsure whether to refer, most oncologists are happy discuss or see the patient in consultation; I have found comanagement to be an effective, team-building, and educational strategy.

Conclusion

Management of DTC is increasingly moving towards a personalized and risk-adapted approach, and active research continues to refine risk categories and the most appropriate therapeutic options for each group. While treatment of low-risk DTC has become progressively more conservative, and treatment of advanced disease has become more team-based, our options are only increasing in number, and staying abreast of new changing practice patterns has never been more challenging. The importance of collaborating with each other, as well as with colleagues in other specialties cannot be overstated. Working in a multidisciplinary team with experienced thyroid surgeons, nuclear medicine specialists, radiologists, pathologist, oncologists, and radiation oncologists is an effective way to care for patients across the disease spectrum. However, thanks to our longitudinal relationships with our patients,

clinicians in endocrinology remain at the heart of the treatment team, and our role has remained the same: to lead, coordinate (and occasionally, herd), support, and innovate.

Clinical Case Vignettes

Case 1

A 78-year-old man presents for evaluation of multinodular goiter incidentally identified on chest CT during workup for new-onset hemoptysis, which is eventually attributed to chronic bronchitis. His medical history is notable for chronic obstructive pulmonary disease on maximal medical therapy and 2 L of oxygen via nasal cannula (40 pack-year smoking history, quit after starting oxygen), heart failure with preserved ejection fraction, hypertension, hyperlipidemia, diet-controlled type 2 diabetes mellitus, obesity, low back pain, and benign prostatic hypertrophy. TSH and free T_4 concentrations are normal. Thyroid ultrasonography at an outside imaging center reveals a well-demarcated, 1.4-cm, right-sided, hypoechoic, taller-than-wide nodule with microcalcifications in the anterior/mid aspect of the lobe with at least 4 mm of normal surrounding parenchyma. There is no sonographic evidence of extrathyroidal extension. Additional nodules include a nearby right 1.2-cm complex nodule and a left 2.5-cm complex nodule, both of which lack suspicious features. Lateral neck lymph nodes were not examined. He has no history of radiation exposure or family history of thyroid cancer. Ultrasound-guided FNA of the right 1.4-cm nodule reveals Bethesda V "suspicious for PTC," while the left 2.5-cm nodule is interpreted to be a benign colloid nodule. He lives roughly 10 miles from your clinic and always attends medical appointments. He has a minimalist philosophy to medical care and wants to pursue the least invasive management option, "as long as it's not going to hurt me." He has no compressive neck symptoms.

Which of the following is the most appropriate initial management strategy for this patient?

A. Measurement of thyroid nodule size and volume and locoregional node examination in anticipation of active surveillance

B. Referral to interventional radiology for radiofrequency ablation of the right 1.4-cm nodule

C. Referral to thyroid surgery for consideration of right hemithyroidectomy

D. Referral to thyroid surgery for consideration of total thyroidectomy

Answer: A) Measurement of thyroid nodule size and volume and locoregional node examination in anticipation of active surveillance

This elderly man has a Bethesda V 1.4-cm thyroid nodule without extrathyroidal extension. The nodule is in a favorable location for active surveillance. He is high risk for perioperative complications and has a limited life expectancy, no significant risk factors for thyroid cancer, and a minimalist philosophy. He engages in reliable follow-up. The only less ideal (but still reasonable) variable is the presence of multinodular goiter, although his suspicious nodule has a distinct border and the other nodules are low risk and the largest has benign findings on FNA. Provided that his physician is comfortable following him and that high-quality ultrasonography is available (with accurate measurements and normal regional lymph node morphology), active surveillance (Answer A) is most consistent with the patient's request.

Right hemithyroidectomy (Answer C) is not unreasonable, although his high operative risk, his desire for minimal invasiveness, and the presence of a contralateral, albeit asymptomatic, nodule make hemithyroidectomy less attractive.

Total thyroidectomy (Answer D) is reasonable but invasive; the patient should be counseled that it may yet be necessary if significant growth of the suspicious nodule is noted.

Radiofrequency ablation (Answer B) is inappropriate given limited data to support efficacy and safety for suspicious nodules larger than 10 mm, along limited availability.

Case 2

A 59-year-old woman presents for evaluation of a neck mass after total thyroidectomy 7 years ago. Medical records document that she had a 4-cm "minimally invasive" FTC with fewer than 4 foci of angioinvasion. She did not receive radioactive iodine and does not recall any recent bloodwork or ultrasound surveillance. Her medical history is otherwise insignificant. Ultrasonography reveals a 3-cm hypoechoic and hypervascular nodule in the right thyroid bed, and findings on ultrasound-guided FNA are interpreted to be follicular neoplasm.

Her TSH concentration is 2.2 mIU/L on levothyroxine, 125 mcg of daily, and her thyroglobulin concentration is 0.24 ng/mL (0.24 ug/L) with negative antithyroglobulin antibodies.

She undergoes revision thyroid surgery by a high-volume thyroid surgeon, and pathology reveals a 3-cm angioinvasive FTC; no nodes were submitted. Postoperative ^{131}I diagnostic (using a 3 mCi, 0.111 GBq dose) whole-body scanning reveals scant central neck uptake but no other sites of iodine avidity. A 100 mCi (3.7 GBq) adjuvant dose of ^{131}I is given, and the posttreatment scan is unchanged. A postoperative and post RAI thyroglobulin concentration is less than 0.1 ng/mL.

One year after revision surgery, she develops calf swelling and shortness of breath after a long car ride. CT chest reveals a small pulmonary embolism, as well as innumerable small pulmonary nodules, the largest of which is 1 cm. Bronchoscopy is performed and FNA is positive for the presence of follicular epithelial cells. A repeated diagnostic whole-body ^{131}I scan is negative, and no treatment is given. Her shortness of breath resolves with anticoagulation, and her TSH is suppressed and maintained at a concentration less than 0.10 mIU/L. Over the next 7 years, her pulmonary nodules slowly grow by approximately 1 mm/year until sudden growth is noted, coinciding with the development of hemoptysis and shortness of breath.

Which of the following is the most appropriate next step in this patient's management?

A. Referral to oncology for consideration of systemic therapy

B. Referral to radiation oncology for consideration of external-beam radiation therapy

C. Referral to thoracic surgery

D. Repeated ^{131}I whole-body scanning

Answer: A) Referral to oncology for consideration of systemic therapy

This patient has developed rapidly progressive, symptomatic, metastatic (lung) angioinvasive FTC after 7 years of indolent growth during active surveillance. Thus, she is a good candidate for systemic therapy (Answer A). Her relatively low thyroglobulin level despite high tumor burden and lack of iodine avidity at diagnosis is consistent with dedifferentiated RAI-refractory FTC. Given the large size of her original tumor, it is possible that more significant angioinvasion was missed due to incomplete sectioning.

Thoracic surgery (Answer C) is incorrect. Oligometastatectomy may improve survival in select patients with localized pulmonary metastases.

Repeated ^{131}I whole-body scanning (Answer D) is low yield given lack of uptake on 2 diagnostic ^{131}I whole-body scans, including a post-100 mCi treatment scan.

Referral for radiation (Answer B) is also not likely to be fruitful given the widespread pattern of pulmonary metastasis; it would be more reasonable if there were regional oligometastases that were not amenable to resection.

References

1. Kitahara CM, Sosa JA. The changing incidence of thyroid cancer. *Nat Rev Endocrinol.* 2016;12(11):646-653. PMID: 27418023

2. Lim H, Devesa SS, Sosa JA, Check D, Kitahara CM. Trends in thyroid cancer incidence and mortality in the United States, 1974-2013. *JAMA.* 2017;317(13):1338-1348. PMID: 28362912

3. Haugen BR, Alexander EK, Bible KC, et al. 2015 American Thyroid Association management guidelines for adult patients with thyroid nodules and differentiated thyroid cancer: the American Thyroid Association Guidelines Task Force on Thyroid Nodules and Differentiated Thyroid Cancer. *Thyroid.* 2016;26(1):1-133. PMID: 26462967

4. Schlumberger M, Leboulleux S. Current practice in patients with differentiated thyroid cancer. *Nature Rev Endocrinol.* 2021;17(3):176-188. PMID: 33339988

5. Addasi N, Fingeret A, Goldner W. Hemithyroidectomy for thyroid cancer: a review. *Medicina (Kaunas).* 2020;56(11):586. PMID: 33153139

6. Hay ID, Kaggal S, Iniguez-Ariza NM, Reinalda MS, Wiseman GA, Thompson GB 2021 Inability of radioiodine remnant ablation to improve postoperative outcome in adult patients with low-risk papillary thyroid carcinoma. *Mayo Clin Proc.* 2021;96(7):1727-1745. PMID: 33743997

7. American Thyroid Association (ATA) Guidelines Taskforce on Thyroid Nodules and Differentiated Thyroid Cancer, Cooper DS, Doherty GM, et al. Revised American Thyroid Association management guidelines for patients with thyroid nodules and differentiated thyroid cancer. *Thyroid.* 2009;19(11):1167-1214. PMID: 19860577

8. Lohia S, Hanson M, Tuttle RM, Morris LGT. Active surveillance for patients with very low-risk thyroid cancer. *Laryngoscope Investig Otolaryngol.* 2020;5(1):175-182. PMID: 32128446

9. Brito JP, Ito Y, Miyauchi A, Tuttle RM. A clinical framework to facilitate risk stratification when considering an active surveillance alternative to immediate biopsy and surgery in papillary microcarcinoma. *Thyroid.* 2016;26(1):144-149. PMID: 26414743

10. van Dijk SPJ, Coerts HI, Gunput STG, et al. Assessment of radiofrequency ablation for papillary microcarcinoma of the thyroid: a systematic review and meta-analysis. *JAMA Otolaryngol Head Neck Surg.* 2022;148(4):317-325. PMID: 35142816

11. Hay ID, Lee RA, Kaggal S, et al. Long-term results of treating with ethanol ablation 15 adult patients with cT1aN0 papillary thyroid microcarcinoma. *J Endocr Soc.* 2020;4(11):bvaa135. PMID: 33073159

12. Orloff LA, Noel JE, Stack BC Jr, et al. Radiofrequency ablation and related ultrasound-guided ablation technologies for treatment of benign and malignant thyroid disease: an international multidisciplinary consensus statement of the American Head and Neck Society Endocrine Surgery Section with the Asia Pacific Society of Thyroid Surgery, Associazione Medici Endocrinologi, British Association of Endocrine and Thyroid Surgeons, European Thyroid Association, Italian Society of Endocrine Surgery Units, Korean Society of Thyroid Radiology, Latin American Thyroid Society, and Thyroid Nodules Therapies Association. *Head Neck.* 2022;44(3):633-660. PMID: 34939714

13. Mauri G, Hegedus L, Bandula S, et al. European Thyroid Association and Cardiovascular and Interventional Radiological Society of Europe 2021 clinical practice guideline for the use of minimally invasive treatments in malignant thyroid lesions. *Eur Thyroid J.* 2021;10(3):185-197. PMID: 34178704

14. Kim WW, Lee J, Jung JH, et al. Predictive risk factors for recurrence or metastasis in papillary thyroid cancer. *Int J Thyroidology.* 2020;13(2):111-117.

15. Fagin JA, Wells SA, Jr. Biologic and clinical perspectives on thyroid cancer. *N Engl J Med.* 2016;375(11):1054-1067. PMID: 27626519

16. Melmed S, Polonsky K, Larsen PR, Kronenberg HM eds. *Williams Textbook of Endocrinology.* 12th ed. Elsevier Saunders; 2011.

17. Fullmer T, Cabanillas ME, Zafereo M. Novel therapeutics in radioactive iodine-resistant thyroid cancer. *Front Endocrinol (Lausanne).* 2021;12:720723. PMID: 34335481

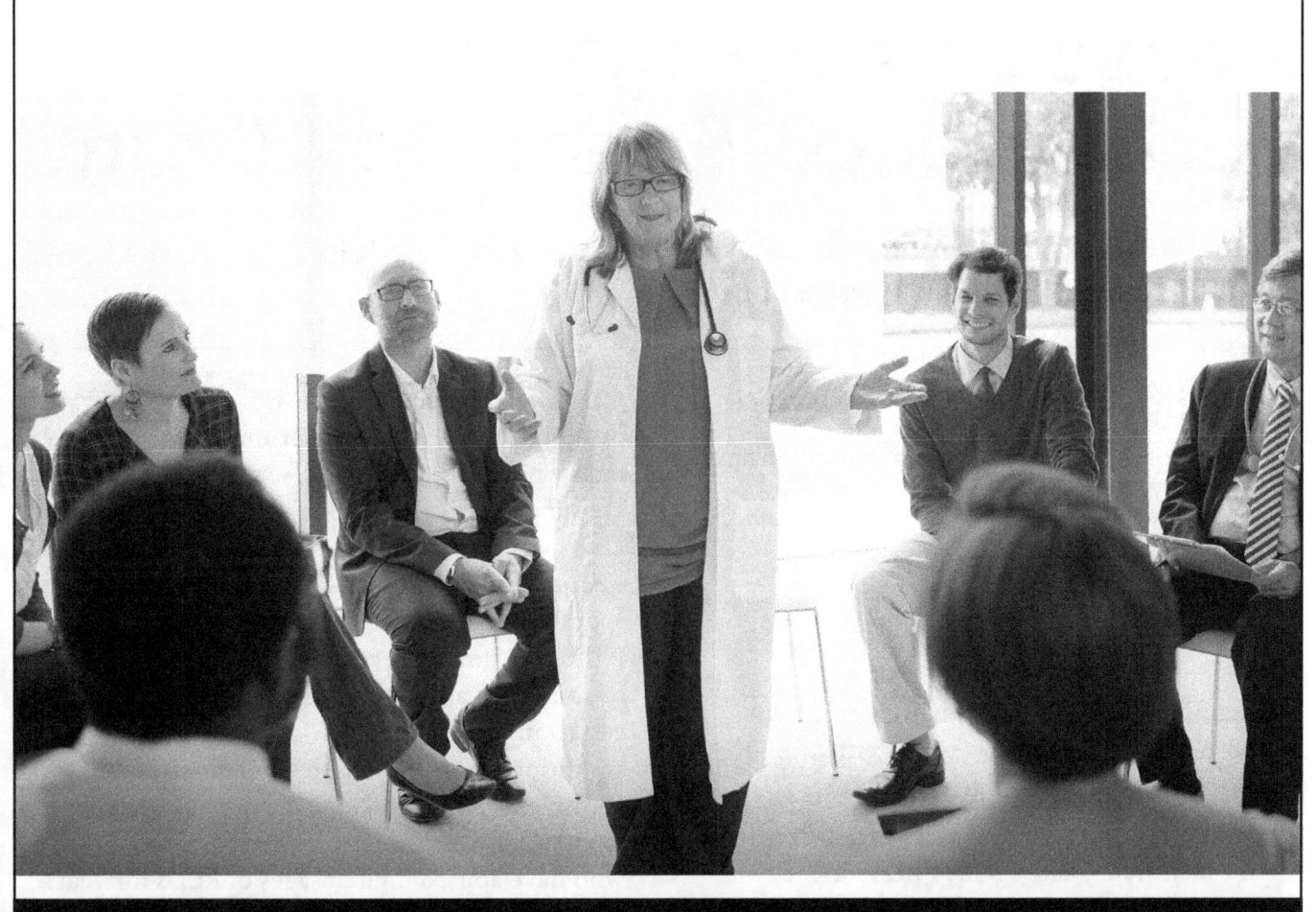

MISCELLANEOUS

Doping With Androgens: Abuse of Androgenic Performance-Enhancing Drugs

Bradley D. Anawalt, MD. University of Washington School of Medicine, Seattle, WA;
E-mail: banawalt@medicine.washington.edu

Learning Objectives

As a result of participating in this session, learners should be able to:

- Recognize the clinical presentation of androgenic performance-enhancing drug (PED) abuse (including infertility).

- Recognize the history and physical examination findings and pattern of serum hormone results that are consistent with specific forms of androgenic PED abuse.

- Identify the laboratory studies that are useful for identifying androgenic PED abuse.

- Develop a rational approach to the use of psychotherapy and hormone therapy in the management of patients who wish to discontinue androgenic PED abuse.

Main Conclusions

Androgens and drugs that raise endogenous androgen production are the most commonly abused PEDs. In clinical practice, androgenic PEDs are used almost exclusively by men. The proven health consequences include infertility, acne, and erythrocytosis in men. Other potential adverse effects include increased cardiovascular disease, hepatopathy (with oral alkylated androgens), neuropsychopathology, and ruptured upper-extremity tendons. The common clinical presentations of androgenic PED abuse are male infertility and requests for testosterone prescriptions to treat low serum testosterone. In men who abuse androgens, serum gonadotropins are suppressed, and seminal fluid analyses show azoospermia or very low sperm concentrations. Recovery of gonadal axis function occurs spontaneously after discontinuation of androgenic PEDs; the time to recovery is related to duration of abuse. Treatment consists of encouraging cessation by respectful and nonjudgmental education about the health consequences of androgenic PEDs and management of underlying anxiety and depressive disorders. For some men who have abused high dosages of PEDs for years, there might be a role for adjunctive hormone therapy with a short course of testosterone or clomiphene to treat anabolic androgenic steroid withdrawal syndrome or a short course of gonadotropin or clomiphene therapy to hasten spermatogenic recovery and improve fertility.

Significance of the Clinical Problem

Many drugs are used to enhance athletic performance and appearance, including androgens and drugs that increase serum androgen concentrations, insulin, and growth hormone. Androgens administered at pharmacological dosages are the most commonly used PEDs, and they are the only class of drugs with definitive evidence that they enhance strength and athletic performance. Members of the general public are much less likely to use growth hormone, insulin, and other nonandrogens as potential PEDs. For the purposes of this review and session, the focus will be on androgenic PED abuse, and the use of pharmacological dosages of androgens or drugs that increase endogenous androgens will be defined as androgenic PED use. Individuals who are eugonadal and take androgenic PEDs are abusing them; prescription of androgen and gonadotropin replacement to hypogonadal patients is not PED abuse.

It has been difficult to assess the prevalence of androgenic PED abuse, but the lifetime prevalence of ever using these PEDs is probably 1% to 5% in men worldwide.[1] There is a trend toward decreased incidence in teenagers and young adults, but there might be a small increasing incidence in middle-aged and older men. The prevalence of androgenic PED abuse is much higher in men than in women (>50:1), and long-term abusers are almost exclusively male. Most chronic androgenic PED abusers begin in their twenties and are former elite or near-elite athletes or weightlifters with a fixation on being more muscular (often referred to as muscle dysmorphia or bigorexia).

Assessing the short-term and long-term adverse effects of androgenic PEDs has also been difficult. There are well-described adverse effects of androgen therapy, including acne (more common in younger patients), erythrocytosis (more common in older patients), and infertility.[1,2] Chronic androgenic PED use accelerates male-pattern alopecia and causes hirsutism, alopecia, and defeminization and virilization in women. Hepatopathy occurs with use of oral alkylated androgens only, and there appears to be increased risk of tendinous ruptures, particularly in muscles of the arms and chest.[3,4] There is increasing evidence that there is an androgenic PED withdrawal syndrome of depressed mood, anxiety, and low self-esteem after acute cessation.[5,6]

High dosages of androgenic PEDs might increase the incidence of cardiovascular disease, hypertension, and psychiatric disorders.[3,7] The causal relationship is unclear because chronic androgenic PED abusers are also more likely to have baseline depression and anxiety and are more likely to use tobacco and marijuana products, alcohol, illicit drugs, and high dosages of dietary supplements and nutraceuticals that have not been studied rigorously for safety. In addition, androgenic PEDs are often purchased on the open market or through the internet, and these drugs might contain or be contaminated with unsafe substances.

Barriers to Optimal Practice

- Social stigma and laws against androgenic PED abuse are barriers to disclosure of abuse.

- Many clinicians do not recognize the clues of possible androgenic PED abuse.

- Except for disclosure of androgenic abuse by the patient, there are no methods of making a definitive diagnosis of androgenic PED abuse in members of the general public.

- There are very limited data on the best therapeutic approach for individuals who abuse androgenic PEDs and want to discontinue.

- The data about the short-term and long-term effects of androgenic PED abuse are based on case reports, case series, and cross-sectional studies with numerous confounders.

Strategies for Diagnosis, Therapy, and/or Management
Clinical Presentation of Androgenic PED Abuse

Men who chronically abuse androgenic PEDs typically present with infertility or with requests for evaluation for testosterone therapy. These men may present with androgenic PED withdrawal syndrome, with symptoms and signs of hypogonadism, or with infertility. The use of aromatizable androgenic PEDs can cause gynecomastia, and the use of nonaromatizable androgenic PEDs may be associated with sexual dysfunction.

Women who chronically abuse androgenic PEDs are almost exclusively elite athletes and are rarely seen by most endocrinologists; they may present with amenorrhea, infertility, and variable degrees of defeminization and virilization. This session will not address this rare endocrine disorder.

Diagnosis of Androgenic PED Abuse

The diagnosis of androgenic PED abuse should be suspected in muscular men who present with infertility or request an evaluation for testosterone therapy. Most men who abuse androgenic PEDs exercise frequently and many lift weights regularly. These men usually have bigorexia or muscular dysmorphia, a distorted body image that they are not muscular enough.[1] They often spontaneously report that their strength and muscle bulk benefit have plateaued in the weight room. Another clue that may suggest chronic androgenic PED abuse is a history of use of nutraceuticals and supplements to build muscles (eg, creatine powder).

In addition to increased musculature, the physical examination may demonstrate gynecomastia and small testes, but these findings are not sensitive or specific. The history and the physical examination may also offer clues to the type of androgenic drug being used (*Table*). Androgenic drugs that increase aromatization of testosterone to estradiol are more likely to cause breast growth, breast pain, and tenderness and gynecomastia. Androgen precursor abuse increases the serum estradiol concentration disproportionately to the serum testosterone concentration and is also more likely to cause

symptomatic or new-onset gynecomastia. Chronic androgenic PED abuse that causes gonadotropin suppression is associated with variably decreased testicular volumes (typically ~25%-35%), but men with baseline testicular volumes of 25 mL or more may not have small testes after chronic androgenic PED abuse. Testicular texture (eg, softness or firmness) is not a specific or sensitive physical examination finding of androgenic PED abuse.

The biochemical evaluation for suspected androgenic PED abuse begins with measurement of serum testosterone and gonadotropins in a blood sample obtained between 7 and 10 AM. Serum testosterone and gonadotropin concentrations differ depending on the type of androgenic PED use (*Table*). The use of nontestosterone androgenic anabolic steroids (eg, nandrolone, oxandrolone, danazol, stanozolol, or tetrahydrogestrinone) is associated with low testosterone and gonadotropin concentrations. The standard evaluation for secondary hypogonadism, including sellar imaging and measurement of serum prolactin, should be done in patients with this biochemical profile who do not report the use of androgenic PEDs. If androgenic PED use is suspected in a patient with laboratory evidence of secondary hypogonadism, it is worthwhile to repeat a respectful and nonjudgmental enquiry about androgenic PED use. Sometimes, patients will report androgenic PED use if they understand that further evaluation for other secondary causes of hypogonadism will cost them time and money.

Table. Serum Hormone Concentrations During Androgenic PED Use

Androgenic PED	New-onset or tender gynecomastia	Testes <15 cc	Serum testosterone	Serum FSH	Serum LH
Testosterone	Uncommon	More common	↑	↓	↓
Testosterone precursors*	More common	More common	↑	↓	↓
Nontestosterone androgenic steroids	More common**	More common	↓	↓	↓
hCG	Common	No	↑	↓	↓
Aromatase inhibitor alone	Uncommon	No	↑	↑	↑
Clomiphene	?	No	↑	↑	↑

* Very high dosages are required.

** If an aromatizable androgen.

Androgens increase serum hematocrit and decrease serum HDL cholesterol, SHBG, and thyroxine-binding globulin. In patients with suspected androgenic PED use, it is useful to measure hematocrit and often helpful to measure HDL cholesterol, SHBG, and/or thyroxine-binding globulin. Seminal fluid analyses generally show azoospermia or very low sperm concentrations.

There are methods for detecting androgenic PEDs and their metabolites in urine samples of elite athletes, but these methods are not available in most commercial laboratories.[8] In addition, there are many ways to create spurious results, including dilution, substitution of someone else's sample, and submitting a sample at a time when the patient is not using androgenic PEDs. For elite athletes, urine samples are obtained under very strict circumstances, including random times and observed micturition into a sample container. Thus, methods to accurately measure androgenic PEDs and their metabolites in urine are not relevant diagnostic studies in clinical practice.

Treatment of Androgenic PED Abuse and Withdrawal Syndrome

There are no clinical trials or guidelines on the management of patients who abuse androgenic PEDs or the management of cessation of androgenic PEDs and androgenic PED withdrawal syndrome. Therefore, care of patients who abuse androgenic PEDs is based on the following: (1) readiness to cease androgenic PEDs; (2) duration and intensity of androgenic PED abuse; (3) near-team goals for fertility; and (4) a risk-benefit analysis of the treatment options compared with continuation or resumption of androgenic PED use.[1]

A key principle for the care of androgenic PED users is the establishment a relationship of trust based on respectful and nonjudgmental behavior. While this principle guides all patient-clinician relationships, it is particularly important for this group of patients. They are often distrustful of traditional health care providers and scientists.

After all, scientists disputed the benefits of androgenic PEDs decades after athletes empirically proved the performance-enhancing effects; why should androgenic PED abusers believe scientists and clinicians about potential adverse effects? All androgenic PED users must be queried about anxiety and depression and abuse of alcohol or illicit drugs and offered a referral for treatment if appropriate.

Some men are not prepared to stop using androgenic PEDs. The endocrinologist should counsel patients about the known adverse effects (including reduced fertility that might take 1 to 2 years to normalize after discontinuation of androgenic PEDs, erythrocytosis, and dyslipidemia) and potential adverse effects with a focus on the cardiovascular system. Some men who are not willing to discontinue androgenic PEDs are willing to "convert" to prescription testosterone. Conversion to intramuscular testosterone formulations at up to 2 to 3 times the usual replacement dosage with a tapering of the dosage over several months is likely to be safer than very high dosages of androgenic PEDs of unknown safety and purity purchased from unregulated sources. High dosages of testosterone are initially required because androgenic PED users generally use high dosages of various androgens simultaneously ("stacking"), and they will experience symptoms of withdrawal if immediately converted directly to typical testosterone replacement dosages used for treatment of male hypogonadism. This approach permits the establishment of a relationship between the patient and clinician over time; this might facilitate eventual discontinuation of androgenic PED use.

For men who are ready to quit androgenic PED use, there are the following options: (1) immediate discontinuation without medical therapy; (2) conversion to testosterone therapy with a tapering dosage over many months (see above); (3) discontinuation with initiation of a limited course of subcutaneous hCG therapy, or (4) discontinuation with initiation of a limited course of oral clomiphene therapy.

Immediate discontinuation of androgenic PEDs without additional medical therapy is the best choice for men who have used these drugs for 1 year or less. Based on limited, low-quality data, it appears that after androgenic PED discontinuation, serum gonadotropin concentrations spontaneously normalize within 3 to 6 months, followed by recovery of serum testosterone to normal serum concentrations within 6 months in most men who report a year or less of androgenic PED use. Spermatogenesis typically returns to normal 3 to 6 months after serum testosterone normalizes.[1,9]

For men who report chronic androgenic PED use longer than 1 year, there is a higher risk of withdrawal syndrome, and the gonadal axis may take years to recover.[1,10-12] Intramuscular testosterone that is tapered over many months might be a good option for many of these men, but this approach is not an option for men who are interested in conceiving. Exogenous testosterone therapy will continue to suppress spermatogenesis and fertility. For men who are infertile because of androgenic PED use for more than 1 year and who want to have a child within the next 2 years, the best options may be hCG therapy or clomiphene therapy. Clinical experience and safety data are much more robust for hCG therapy than for clomiphene, but there are scanty data on the effectiveness for improving spermatogenesis and fertility in this setting for either drug.

Clinical Case Vignettes

Case 1

A 32-year-old man requests evaluation for testosterone or clomiphene therapy. He confides that he has been taking anabolic androgenic steroids for the past year. He reports taking a combination of several at once ("stacking") and rotating the combination ("cycling"). His wife has been urging him to stop taking them because she is concerned about his health. He is under the care of a mental health professional for treatment of anxiety and depression.

On physical examination, his blood pressure is 135/85 mm Hg, pulse rate is 80 beats/min, respiratory rate is 12 breaths/min, and BMI is 21 kg/m². He is muscular. There is no gynecomastia, and testes are 12 mL bilaterally. No acne is observed.

Laboratory test results:

> Hematocrit = 46% (38%-48%)
> Serum total testosterone = 110 ng/dL (264-870 ng/dL)
>   (SI: 3.8 nmol/L [9.2-30.2 nmol/L])
> Serum FSH = 0.2 mIU/mL (1.0-7.0 mIU/mL)
>   (SI: 0.2 IU/L [1.0-7.0 IU/L])
> Serum LH = 0.1 mIU/mL (1.0-9.0 mIU/mL)
>   (SI: 0.1 IU/L [1.0-9.0 IU/L]

You advise him to abstain from using androgenic steroids. You also inform him that he might feel sluggish and tired for several weeks while his hypothalamic-pituitary-testicular axis recovers within 3 to 6 months.

The patient returns 6 months later with his wife. He reports that he has felt tired and despondent since stopping androgenic PEDs. He has low libido and low sexual satisfaction. He now reports that he has been taking androgenic PEDs for many years. His wife confirms these symptoms and reports that they have been trying to conceive for the past 6 months. She confirms that he took testosterone for "about a year" and that he had a marked increase in libido during that year.

Laboratory test results at this clinic visit:

> Hematocrit = 37% (38%-48%)
> Serum total testosterone = 80 ng/dL (264-870 ng/dL)
>   (SI: 2.8 nmol/L [9.2-30.2 nmol/L])
> Serum FSH = 0.3 mIU/mL (1.0-7.0 mIU/mL)
>   (SI: 0.3 IU/L [1.0-7.0 IU/L])
> Serum LH = 0.2 mIU/mL (1.0-9.0 mIU/mL)
>   (SI: 0.2 IU/L [1.0-9.0 IU/L])
> Seminal fluid analysis, no sperm

Which of the following would you recommend?

A. Anastrozole therapy

B. Evaluation for hypothalmic or pituitary causes of hypogonadism

C. hCG therapy

D. Intramuscular testosterone taper

E. Reassurance

Answer: B) Evaluation for hypothalmic or pituitary causes of hypogonadism

This man continues to be significantly hypogonadal 6 months after cessation of androgenic PED abuse. His decline in hematocrit supports that he has discontinued PEDs. It is unusual to have no sign of recovery the hypothalamic-pituitary-testicular axis after 6 months of abstinence from androgen use. Most men younger than 50 years regain normal serum gonadotropin and testosterone concentrations within 1 to 3 months of discontinuing androgen use of 1 year or less.[1] With the use of longer-acting formulations, recovery might take a little longer, but there should be significant recovery or normalization of serum testosterone 6 months after discontinuing androgen use of 1 year or less.

His wife's comments suggest that the patient might have had underlying hypogonadism prior to using illicit androgenic steroids; his sustained increase of libido after initiating androgenic steroids is unusual in normal eugonadal men because there is a ceiling effect for testosterone on sexual function. There might be a transient placebo effect to increase libido with the initiation of androgens in eugonadal men, but that effect does not generally persist except in men with hypogonadism.

This man should be evaluated for causes of pituitary dysfunction (Answer B), including hyperprolactinemia, iron overload, and pituitary macroadenoma. Gonadotropin replacement therapy should be considered for this couple that is trying to conceive.

Case 2

A 21-year-old man seeks evaluation of breast growth and tenderness for the past 3 months. He reports that he does not get the same "cut" look (increased muscles) that his friends at the gym do. He reports no change in libido. He has no weight loss. He went through puberty at age 13 years. He reports no history of medical illness and no surgeries. He states that he does not take any medications or anabolic androgenic steroids ("steroids"), opioids, or other illicit drugs. He does not drink alcohol.

On physical examination, his blood pressure is 110/70 mm Hg, pulse rate is 72 beats/min, respiratory rate is 12 breaths/min, and BMI is 21 kg/m². He has a beard and normal musculature. There is 2.5 cm of slightly tender gynecomastia, and testes are 15 mL bilaterally. There are no scrotal masses. Findings on skin examination are normal with no striae or ecchymoses. He has mild acne on his back.

Laboratory test results (ordered by the referring clinician):

> Hematocrit = 48% (38%-48%)
> Serum total testosterone = 880 ng/dL (264-916 ng/dL) (SI: 30.6 nmol/L [9.2-30.2 nmol/L])
> Serum DHEA-S = 556 μg/dL (211-494 μg/dL) (SI: 15.1 μmol/L [5.72-13.39 μmol/L])
> Serum FSH = 0.2 mIU/mL (1.0-7.0 mIU/mL) (SI: 0.2 IU/L [1.0-7.0 IU/L])
> Serum LH = 0.1 mIU/mL (1.0-9.0 mIU/mL) (SI: 0.1 IU/L [1.0-9.0 IU/L])

Which of the following is the most likely diagnosis?

A. Adrenal cortical carcinoma

B. hCG use

C. Leydig-cell tumor

D. Nandrolone use

E. Testosterone use

Answer: B) hCG use

This man is in the demographic that is most likely to abuse androgens (male, age ~16-25 years, weightlifter or body builder). Testosterone (Answer E) and hCG (Answer B) abuse are both consistent with the presentation of a high serum testosterone concentration and low serum gonadotropin concentrations, but hCG abuse is much more likely to cause acute breast growth and tenderness. Because hCG has LH activity that increases aromatase activity and conversion of testosterone to estradiol, hCG is more likely to cause gynecomastia.

The high serum testosterone concentration excludes abuse with a nontestosterone androgenic PED such as nandrolone (Answer D); nontestosterone androgens suppress serum testosterone and gonadotropins.

A Leydig-cell tumor (Answer C) can produce testosterone or estradiol and could explain this patient's presentation, but these tumors are uncommon and occur mostly in prepubertal boys.

This patient's presentation is inconsistent with adrenal cortical carcinoma (Answer A), which generally does not present with evidence of excess production of androgens or estrogens until the tumor is large (might be palpable) and symptomatic with weight loss, abdominal pain, anorexia, and/or nausea. Although his serum DHEA-S is elevated, modest elevations are usually idiopathic and not due to adrenal pathology (eg, adrenal carcinoma).

References

1. Anawalt BD. Diagnosis and management of anabolic androgenic steroid use. *J Clin Endocrinol Metab.* 2019;104(7):2490-2500. PMID: 30753550

2. Christou MA, Christou PA, Markozannes G, Tsatsoulis A, Mastorakos G, Tigas S. Effects of anabolic androgenic steroids on the reproductive system of athletes and recreational users: a systematic review and meta-analysis. *Sports Med.* 2017;47(9):1869-1883. PMID: 28258581

3. Pope HG Jr, Wood RI, Rogol A, Nyberg F, Bowers L, Bhasin S. Adverse health consequences of performance-enhancing drugs: an Endocrine Society scientific statement. *Endocr Rev.* 2014;35(3):341-375. PMID: 24423981

4. Kanayama G, DeLuca J, Meehan WP 3rd, et al. Ruptured tendons in anabolic-androgenic steroid users: a cross-sectional cohort study. *Am J Sports Med.* 2015;43(11):2638-2644. PMID: 26362436

5. Onakomaiya MM, Henderson LP. Mad men, women and steroid cocktails: a review of the impact of sex and other factors on anabolic androgenic steroids effects on affective behaviors. *Psychopharmacology (Berl).* 2016;233(4):549-569. PMID: 26758282

6. Piacentino D, Kotzalidis GD, Del Casale A, et al. Anabolic-androgenic steroid use and psychopathology in athletes. A systematic review. *Curr Neuropharmacol.* 2015;13(1):101-121. PMID: 26074746

7. Baggish AL, Weiner RB, Kanayama G, et al. Cardiovascular toxicity of illicit anabolic-androgenic steroid use. *Circulation.* 2017;135(21):1991-2002. PMID: 28533317

8. Anawalt BD. Detection of anabolic androgenic steroid use by elite athletes and by members of the general public. *Mol Cell Endocrinol.* 2018;464:21-27. PMID: 28943276

9. Liu PY, Swerdloff RS, Christenson PD, Handelsman DJ, Wang C; Hormonal Male Contraception Summit Group. Rate, extent, and modifiers of spermatogenic recovery after hormonal male contraception: an integrated analysis. *Lancet.* 2006;367(9520):1412-1420. PMID: 16650651

10. Kanayama G, Hudson JI, DeLuca J, et al. Prolonged hypogonadism in males following withdrawal from anabolic-androgenic steroids: an under-recognized problem. *Addiction.* 2015;110(5):823-831. PMID: 25598171

11. Rasmussen JJ, Selmer C, Østergren PB, et al. Former abusers of anabolic androgenic steroids exhibit decreased testosterone levels and hypogonadal symptoms years after cessation: a case-control study. *PLoS One.* 2016;11:e0161208. PMID: 275532478

12. Anawalt BD. Male fertility after androgenic steroid use: how little we know. *J Clin Endocrinol Metab.* 2021;106(7):e2813-e2815. PMID: 33861859

E-Consults: An Evolving Area of Endocrine Care

David Saxon, MD. Division of Endocrinology, Metabolism, and Diabetes, University of Colorado School of Medicine and Rocky Mountain Regional VA Medical Center, Aurora, Colorado; E-mail: david.saxon@cuanschutz.edu

Varsha Vimalananda, MD. Center for Healthcare Organization and Implementation Research (CHOIR), Bedford VA Medical Center, Bedford, Massachusetts; Section of Endocrinology, Diabetes, and Nutrition, Boston University School of Medicine, Boston, Massachusetts; E-mail: varsha.vimalananda@va.gov

Learning Objectives

As a result of participating in this session, learners should be able to:

- Explain the use and benefits of electronic consultations (e-consults), as well as barriers to their use, in the field of endocrinology.

- Recognize various e-consult models that have been used for endocrine care and describe how these models might be used to a greater extent to improve endocrine care in the future.

- Describe considerations related to reimbursement for e-consults.

- Identify the elements of a high-quality e-consult response.

Main Conclusions

E-consult use is growing within the United States and internationally. As a lab-based specialty with expertise in many common diseases, endocrinology is one of the most popular subspecialties for e-consults. Various models of e-consult care have been used. E-consults across specialties increase access to care (ie, more appropriate use of specialist visits) and improve management of some conditions (at the individual patient and population levels). Endocrine disease-specific scenarios where e-consults have shown benefit are also reported in the literature. Reimbursement for e-consults is improving but remains a concern for those who practice in fee-for-service systems. "High-quality" e-consult responses are specific, practical, educational, and often give anticipatory guidance, so that the patient can remain under the care of their primary care clinician.

Significance of the Clinical Problem

Timely access to specialty care is a longstanding and worsening challenge. Endocrinology as a field faces a clinical workforce shortage, exacerbating access challenges for our specialty. E-consults offer an approach to overcoming problems of access while improving use of health care resources and maintaining high patient and provider satisfaction.

E-consults are asynchronous, consultative, provider-to-provider communications within a shared electronic medical record (or web-based platform). Patients are not directly involved in this mode of care delivery. Many diabetes and endocrine questions can be answered in a useful and succinct way by endocrinologists without the need for a face-to-face patient visit. This session will review the growing use and utility of e-consults with a specific focus on use in the endocrine space.

Barriers to Optimal Practice

- Lack of or unpredictable reimbursement for this type of care.

- Concern about the legal ramifications of providing e-consult care without physically seeing the patient whose issue is being addressed.

- Insufficient technological support to create and maintain a robust e-consult platform.

- Lack of clarity and agreement across services about elements of a good e-consult request and response.

- Added work for the primary care provider and specialist.

Use and Benefits of E-Consults

E-Consult Systems Are Increasingly Common

Historically, "curbside consults" have been commonplace in medicine. However, face-to-face and phone communication among clinicians has decreased as the electronic medical record has taken over as the primary channel by which colleagues in large hospital systems interact. Furthermore, in many health care settings, limited access to timely specialty care has necessitated the development of clinical workflows that address this issue. It is within this changing nature of medical practice that e-consults have arisen as a model for clinical care.

E-consults are now used in many health care systems in the United States and internationally. Additionally, since 2014 the American Association of Medical Colleges has partnered with more than 40 academic medical centers, children's hospitals, and health care organizations to implement e-consults as a part of Project CORE (Coordinating Optimal Referral Experiences). There are also national network, third-party contractors who provide e-consult services. Studies of e-consult use have consistently shown that endocrinology is one of the most highly used

medical subspecialties.[1-3] Endocrinologists can reasonably anticipate that e-consults will become a routine aspect of their clinical practice at some point during their career.

Endocrinology Is Well-Suited to E-Consults

Studies at both single institutions and large health care systems have consistently shown that endocrinology is one of the more commonly e-consulted specialties. Certainly, the lab-based nature of our specialty is one of the main drivers of this popularity. In the Veterans Health Administration from 2012 to 2018, more than 3 million e-consults were completed across 41 specialties. Endocrinology ranked as the third most used specialty overall.[1]

Benefits of E-Consults

E-consults allow primary care clinicians to access specialty expertise through chart review and often result in avoiding a face-to-face patient visit. Even if the consultant decides a face-to-face visit is ultimately needed, an e-consult beforehand can guide the primary care clinician in a previsit workup (eg, laboratory tests and imaging) that could be completed in time for review at the initial endocrinology visit. This preparatory work results in a more efficient face-to-face consultation and potentially avoids at least 1 visit.

Compared with face-to-face visits, e-consults result in faster access to specialty input, allow specialists to triage and prioritize patients for face-to-face care, and reduce wait times for face-to-face visits. E-consults have been shown to reduce the total cost of care by 36% to 83%, including for endocrinology.[4] Patient, primary care clinician, and specialist satisfaction with e-consults is high across studies. There are limited data on safety and clinical outcomes, but the existing literature suggests that e-consults are safe and not associated with worse clinical quality of care.[5]

Benefits of E-Consults for Endocrine Care

Benefits of e-consults that are applicable to endocrine practice include their feasibility and flexibility across a variety of settings, as well their ability to facilitate timely specialty advice (while reducing unnecessary or inappropriate consultations).[6] Also, e-consults present an opportunity for the endocrinologist to provide succinct (often templated) education to their primary care colleagues on commonly encountered endocrine problems, an experience that many find to be enjoyable.

Several experiences in endocrine-related e-consult care have been published. In one series, the most common reasons for endocrinology e-consults were thyroid diseases, osteoporosis, and adrenal insufficiency.[7] The majority of answered e-consults suggested the need for further testing, and nearly 95% of the consults were answered within 3 or fewer business days. When thyroid fine-needle aspirations were preceded by an endocrinology e-consult, there were timelier workups and similar guideline concordance as compared with fine-needle aspirations preceded by endocrinology face-to-face visits.[8] In the inpatient setting, use of targeted automatic e-consults (referred to as a "virtual glucose management service") to manage diabetes at 3 University of California San Francisco hospitals over a 12-month period was shown to decrease the proportion of patients with hyperglycemia or hypoglycemia by 39% and 36%, respectively.[9]

E-Consult Models

E-consults are flexible in their application. Common models include:

1. **E-consult option—optional pathway model:**

   In this model (see *Figure*), primary care clinicians request an e-consult up front. In many systems, specialists retain the option to convert e-consults to face-to-face referrals or request additional information.

Especially if the goal of the e-consult is to avoid a face-to-face visit, the primary care clinician should discuss the e-consult with the patient prior to requesting it. Patient consent is a required component for Medicare reimbursement.

Figure. Optional Pathway Model

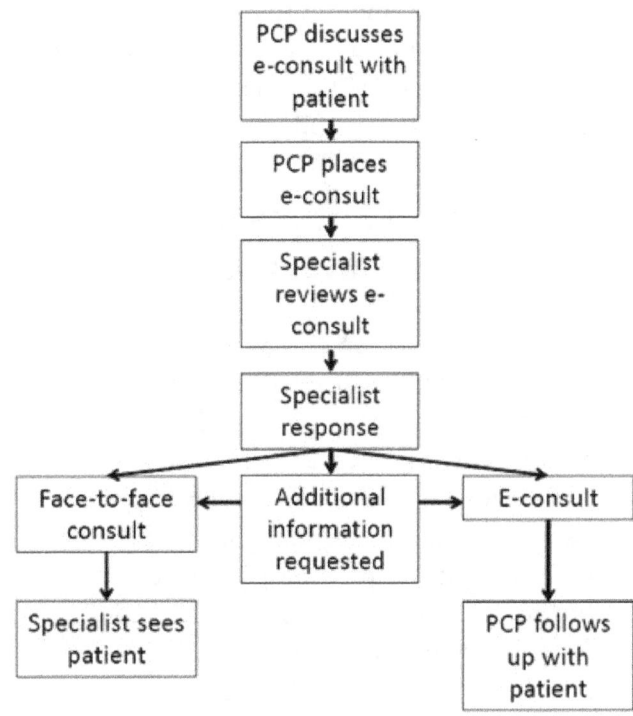

Reprinted from Vimalananda VG et al. *Journal of Telemedicine and Telecare*, 2015;21(6) © SAGE Publications.

2. **E-consult first—single pathway model:**

   In this model, specialists make the judgment about an e-consult vs face-to-face care. The e-consult is reviewed by a specialty clinician who then either recommends that the patient be seen in person or resolves the e-consult request without a visit by providing needed information regarding management of the condition. When this model was deployed in the Los Angeles County Department of Health Services, the average e-consult response time was 1 day and 25% of all e-consults were resolved without a specialist visit.[10]

3. **Targeted automatic e-consults:**

Patients are prospectively identified using electronic medical record data. Relevant clinical information is then presented on a dashboard to consultants who provide written recommendations as a "virtual consult" without the request being initiated by the primary care clinician. This model has been used to identify and improve care for patients with hip fractures who may be candidates for medical therapy and to optimize treatment for patients with uncontrolled diabetes.[9,11]

The Potential Future of Endocrine E-Consult Care

- There are many scenarios where targeted e-consults could be used in the outpatient setting to triage care, improve the appropriateness of care rendered at a population level, and address some clinical issues that may have gone ignored. Some examples include providing guidance on hormonal workup of radiological endocrine incidentalomas, suggesting appropriate next laboratory tests and imaging for newly identified thyroid disorders, improving the clinical diagnosis of familial hypercholesterolemia, or providing advice on next steps for optimizing diabetes medication prior to a primary care visit.

- Greater use of specialty-to-specialty e-consults could be deployed, such as direct e-consultation between endocrinology and urology regarding use of testosterone in a man with a history of prostate cancer.

- Systematic incorporation of e-consults as part of an "expanding spectrum of modalities of care" that includes both patient-involved (eg, synchronous video, remote patient monitoring) and clinician-clinician (eg, teleconsultation by email or phone, Project ECHO).

- With wider reimbursement, e-consults are likely to spread even more broadly.

Guidance on Reimbursement

In many integrated health care systems, clinicians are not reimbursed directly for responding to e-consults. Other arrangements include reimbursement per e-consult completed or time spent completing an e-consult. Another option is to reimburse e-consults as a mode of care delivery. In 2019, the Centers for Medicare and Medicaid adopted 2 new codes for interprofessional internet consultation, and these are used for e-consults.

Consulting Clinician

99451: "Interprofessional telephone/internet/ electronic health record assessment and management service provided by a consultative physician including a written report to the patient's treating/requesting physician or other qualified health care professional, 5 or more minutes of medical consultative time"

- Can be reported for new or established patients

- Can be reported for a new or exacerbated problem

- Are reported only by a consultant when requested by another physician/qualified health professional

- Cannot be reported more than once per 7 days for the same patient

- Are reported based on cumulative time spent, even if that time occurs on subsequent days

- Are not reported if a transfer of care or request for a face-to-face consultation occurs because of the consultation within the next 14 days

- Are not reported if the patient was seen by the consultant within the past 14 days

- Require that the request and the reason for the request for the consult be documented in the record

- Require verbal consent for the interprofessional consultation from the patient/family documented in the patient's medical record

Code	Reported by:	Concluded with:	Time required	How time is spent	2021 wRVU
99451	Consultant	Written report required to treating/requesting physician/qualified health professional	≥5 min	Review pertinent medical records, laboratory tests/imaging studies, medication profile, etc, and medical consultative verbal or internet discussion	0.7
99452	Requestor	NA	≥16 min	Preparing for the consult and/or the actual time spent communicating with the consultant	0.7

Features of High-Quality E-Consult Responses

In endocrinology, e-consults are perhaps best used for clinical scenarios where there are either minor laboratory abnormalities or where the primary care clinician is already managing the endocrine condition but needs advice about the best next step in the patient's management.

Excellent e-consult responses reduce the likelihood that patients will ultimately need a face-to-face visit. Rigorous consensus methods identify the features of a "high-quality" e-consult correspondence: specific, up-to-date, patient-individualized, and practical advice (with anticipatory guidance) that a primary care provider can effectively implement.[12] Anticipatory guidance is critical given that management of the condition is intended to remain with the primary care clinician. Thus, it is helpful to list any indications for face-to-face referral. Responses are enhanced when they are educational for the consulting clinician; this may include pertinent professional society guidelines and other relevant literature. Endocrinologists might consider developing templates for common questions that can be tailored for the individual patient. Templates can ease the burden of responding to the same question repeatedly while ensuring all relevant components of a response are covered.

Clinical Case Vignettes

Case 1

Question from primary care provider
"Does this patient with subclinical hyperthyroidism need further evaluation or can these labs just be monitored?"

Response

Endocrinologist's chart review:
A 70-year-old woman with a history of hypertension and osteopenia was found to have a TSH value of 0.33 mIU/L (reference range, 0.45-5.30 mIU/L) on routine laboratory tests in March 2021. No previous TSH values are documented in the electronic medical record. Follow-up testing performed in April 2021 included normal free T_4 and free T_3 levels (TSH and total T_3 were not measured). Current medications include amlodipine, 5 mg daily; lisinopril, 5 mg daily; and vitamin D_3, 2000 units daily. There is no prior neck imaging in her record. A recent primary care clinical note states that the patient has been in good health and does not mention any symptoms concerning for hyperthyroidism or neck discomfort. There is no mention of herbal or over-the-counter medications or supplements.

Endocrinologist's recommendation(s):
This patient has a mildly low TSH value documented on one occasion. The clinical significance of this finding is unknown, and many patients with such an abnormality have normalization of TSH on repeated testing. TSH values that are fully suppressed (ie, TSH <0.1 mIU/L) merit a more extensive workup. In the case of an only slightly low TSH value, the best next step is to ensure this is not a spurious result. When subclinical hyperthyroidism is present (ie, fully suppressed TSH, but normal free T_4 and total T_3 values), treatment is recommended for older patients because this situation poses an increased risk of bone loss and atrial fibrillation. Please perform a thorough

physical examination to assess for palpable thyroid nodules or signs of Graves disease. Also, FYI, we generally avoid measuring free T_3 levels because the assay is thought to be unreliable. Please send a follow-up e-consult or refer the patient for a clinic visit if repeated thyroid testing or physical exam warrants further assessment and management.

Evidence supporting e-consult response:

- Ross DS, Burch HB, Cooper DS, et al. 2016 American Thyroid Association Guidelines for diagnosis and management of hyperthyroidism and other causes of thyrotoxicosis. *Thyroid.* 2016;26(10):1343-1421.

E-consult outcome:
Following this e-consult, the primary care physician measured TSH again 5 and 8 months later. Both TSH values fell within the normal range and no further workup was performed.

Case 2
Question from primary care provider
A 53-year-old man presents with asymptomatic hypercalcemia. He reports that his calcium has been high in the past, but we do not have copies of previous lab results. Current laboratory test results:

> Calcium = 11.6 mg/dL (SI: 2.9 mmol/L)
> Calcium (ionized) = 6.1 mg/dL (SI: 1.5 mmol/L)
> PTH = 193 pg/mL (SI: 193 ng/L)
> 25-Hydroxyvitamin D = 32 ng/mL (SI: 79.9 nmol/L)
> Creatinine = 1.35 mg/dL (SI: 119.3 μmol/L)
> Estimated glomerular filtration rate =
>   58 mL/min per 1.73 m²

DXA shows the lowest T-score is –1.2 at the left femoral neck. No history of kidney stones. Do you recommend that I observe patient, send to endocrine, or send to surgery?

Response

Endocrinologist's chart review:
Laboratory test results from 3/22/2021:

> Calcium = 11.6 mg/dL (SI: 2.9 mmol/L)
> PTH = 193 pg/mL (SI: 193 ng/L)
> 25-Hydroxyvitamin D = 13 ng/mL (SI: 32.4 nmol/L)
> Creatinine = 1.35 mg/dL (SI: 119.3 μmol/L)
> Estimated glomerular filtration rate =
>   58 mL/min per 1.73 m²
> Hemoglobin A_{1c} = 5.7% (39 mmol/mol)

On 4/9/2021, DXA documents lowest T-score is –1.2 at left femoral neck, and findings are otherwise normal.

Endocrinologist's recommendation(s):
This patient very likely has primary hyperparathyroidism. The only other test to order is a 24-hour urinary calcium with creatinine just to make sure that he does not have FHH (familial hypocalciuric hypercalcemia), which is a genetic disorder that runs in families and can mimic primary hyperparathyroidism. In patients with FHH, the urinary calcium is very low, whereas in primary hyperparathyroidism the urinary calcium is generally normal or high. FHH is very rare but needs to be ruled out because missing that diagnosis can result in a patient going to surgery who does not need it. If the urine test result is not concerning for FHH, then the best and most appropriate treatment option for primary hyperparathyroidism is parathyroidectomy because it is definitive. He meets guideline criteria for parathyroidectomy given that his calcium level is a full point above the upper limit of normal. Please write back with questions or concerns.

Evidence supporting e-consult response:
Primary hyperparathyroidism is diagnosed by finding an elevated serum calcium level associated with a serum PTH level that is elevated or in the mid- to high-normal range >20 pg/mL [>20 ng/L]). Serum PTH levels are less than 10 pg/mL (<10 ng/L) or undetectable in all other causes of hypercalcemia except one rare genetic syndrome. For asymptomatic patients, indications for surgery include the following: serum calcium

greater than 1 mg/dL above the upper limit of normal, bone mineral density T-score less than −2.5 or a fragility fracture, creatinine clearance less than 60 mL/min, 24-hour urinary calcium greater than 400 mg/24 h, kidney stones, or age younger than 50 years. Surgery should be offered to symptomatic patients and to asymptomatic patients who meet 1 or more of these criteria. For asymptomatic patients who don't meet any of these criteria, surgery is still an option, but it is also reasonable to monitor such patients without surgery with measurement of serum calcium and creatinine every 6 to 12 months and DXA every 1 to 2 years. When low bone mineral density is the only criterion met, an alternative is to treat with a bisphosphonate or other osteoporosis medication.

- Zhu CY, Sturgeon C, Yeh MW. Diagnosis and management of primary hyperparathyroidism. *JAMA.* 2020;323(12):1186-1187.
- Bilezikian J. Guidelines for the management of asymptomatic primary hyperparathyroidism: summary statement from the Fourth International Workshop. *J Clin Endocrinol Metab.* 2014;99(10):3561-3569.

E-consult outcome:
The patient was referred directly to endocrine surgery without need for a face-to-face endocrinology consultation and underwent successful single-gland parathyroidectomy for a parathyroid adenoma.

References

1. Saxon DR, Kaboli PJ, Haraldsson B, Wilson C, Ohl M, Augustine MR. Growth of electronic consultations in the Veterans Health Administration. *Am J Manag Care.* 2021;27(1):12-19. PMID: 33471457

2. Leyton C, Zhang C, Rikin S. Evaluation of the effects of the COVID-19 pandemic on electronic consultation use in primary care. *Telemed J E Health.* 2022;28(1):66-72. PMID: 33794114

3. Kirsh S, Carey E, Aron DC, et al. Impact of a national specialty e-consultation implementation project on access. *Am J Manag Care.* 2015;21(12):e648-e654. PMID: 26760427

4. Thielke A, King V. Electronic consultations (eConsults): a triple win for patients, clinicians, and payers. *Milbank Memorial Fund.* 2020. Available at: http://resource.nlm.nih.gov/101775057

5. Vimalananda VG, Orlander JD, Afable MK, et al. Electronic consultations (E-consults) and their outcomes: a systematic review. *J Am Med Inform Assoc.* 2020;27(3):471-479. PMID: 31621847

6. Vimalananda VG, Gupte G, Seraj SM, et al. Electronic consultations (e-consults) to improve access to specialty care: a systematic review and narrative synthesis. *J Telemed Telecare.* 2015;21(6):323-330. PMID: 25995331

7. Wasfy JH, Rao SK, Essien UR, et al. Initial experience with endocrinology e-consults. *Endocrine.* 2017;55(2):640-642. PMID: 27507674

8. Yoon SS, Wong DH, Wormwood JB, Reisman JI, Vimalananda VG. Impact of electronic consultation on timeliness and guideline concordance of workups leading to thyroid nodule fine-needle aspiration biopsy. *Endocr Pract.* 2021;27(10):1011–1016. PMID: 33766654

9. Rushakoff RJ, Sullivan MM, MacMaster HW, et al. Association between a virtual glucose management service and glycemic control in hospitalized adult patients: an observational study. *Ann Intern Med.* 2017;166(9):621-627. PMID: 28346946

10. Barnett ML, Yee HF Jr, Mehrotra A, Giboney P. Los Angeles safety-net program eConsult system was rapidly adopted and decreased wait times to see specialists. *Health Aff (Millwood).* 2017;36(3):492-499. PMID: 28264951

11. Lee RH, Pearson M, Lyles KW, Jenkins PW, Colon-Emeric C. Geographic scope and accessibility of a centralized, electronic consult program for patients with recent fracture. *Rural Remote Health.* 2016;16(1):3440. PMID: 26745338

12. Tran C, Liddy C, Pinto N, Keely E. Impact of question content on e-consultation outcomes. *Telemed J E Health.* 2016;22(3):216-222. PMID: 26281010